Health Social Science

Health Social Science

A Transdisciplinary and Complexity Perspective

Nick Higginbotham
Glenn Albrecht
Linda Connor

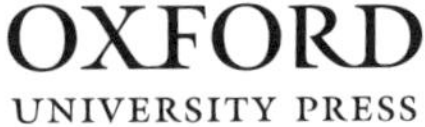

UNIVERSITY PRESS

OXFORD
UNIVERSITY PRESS

253 Normanby Road, South Melbourne, Australia

Oxford University Press is a department of the University of Oxford.
It furthers the University's objective of excellence in research, scholarship, and education by publishing worldwide in

Oxford New York

Athens Auckland Bangkok Bogotá Buenos Aires Calcutta
Cape Town Chennai Dar es Salaam Delhi Florence Hong Kong Istanbul
Karachi Kuala Lumpur Madrid Melbourne Mexico City Mumbai Nairobi
Paris Port Moresby São Paulo Shanghai Singapore Taipei Tokyo Toronto Warsaw

with associated companies in Berlin Ibadan

OXFORD is a registered trade mark of Oxford University Press in the UK and in certain other countries

First published 2001

National Library of Australia
Catalogue-in-publication data:

Higginbotham, Nick.
Health social science: a transdisciplinary and complexity perspective.

Bibliography.
Includes index.
ISBN 0 19 550787 8.

1. Public health personnel—Australia. 2. Health education—Australia.
3. Public health—Research—Australia. 4. Social medicine—Research—Australia.
I. Connor, Linda, 1950– . II. Albrecht, Glenn. III Title.

362.10420994

Edited by Sandra Goldbloom Zurbo
Cover designed by Polar Design Pty Ltd
Typeset by Solo Typesetting, Adelaide
Printed in Malaysia through Bookpac P/L

To our mentors

Robert Preston Price II
Anthony J. Marsella
Julius Kovesi
Jero Tapakan Tibubolong
Douglas Miles

Contents

List of Figures

List of Tables

Contributors

Glenn Albrecht, PhD

Dr Glenn Albrecht is a senior lecturer in Environmental Studies in the School of Geosciences at the University of Newcastle, Australia, and has research interests in environmental philosophies, environmental ethics, environmental politics, ecologically sustainable development, bioregionalism, animal care and ethics, Australian environmental history, and transdisciplinary theories of human health.

Julie Byles, BMed, PhD

Julie Byles is the acting director of and senior lecturer in Clinical Epidemiology and Biostatistics at the Centre for Clinical Epidemiology and Biostatistics, University of Newcastle, Australia, and director of the Hunter Institute of Aging Research. Julie's current research interests are cancer screening, women's health, and preventative health for older Australians. She is currently a member of the management committee of Women's Health Australia and the Veterans' Home Care Reference Group, and directs the Veterans' Affairs Preventive Care Trial as well as the Hunter Cervical Screening Network for the Hunter Area Health Service. Julie has recently been instrumental in the development of a new centre, the Hunter Institute of Ageing Research.

Linda Connor, PhD

Linda Connor teaches anthropology and research methods at the University of Newcastle, Australia. Awarded a PhD from the University of Sydney in 1982, she has carried out field research in Indonesia, North India, and Australia over the last two decades. Linda has written on Indigenous healing in the context of global transformation and modernity, and has used ethnographic approaches to the study of medical pluralism in Australia. With Timothy and Patsy Asch she is the author of *Jero Tapakan: Balinese Healer* (Ethnographics Press 1996, 2nd edn), as well as being the author of a number of ethnographic films on Balinese healing and articles on healing and culture. Linda's recent publications include *Staying Local in the Global Village: Bali in the Twentieth Century* (co-edited with Raechelle Rubinstein, University of Hawai'i Press, 1999), and *Healing Powers and Modernity: Shamanism, Science and Traditional Medicine in Asian Societies* (co-edited with Geoffrey Samuel, Bergin and Garvey, 2000).

Kate D'Este, PhD

Kate D'Este is a senior lecturer in Biostatistics at the Centre for Clinical Epidemiology and Biostatistics, University of Newcastle, Australia, and supervises a wide range of post-graduate and research higher degree students. Kate has contributed to numerous cardio-vascular disease and cancer screening research projects. Her methodological interests are analysis of correlated data, sampling methods, and missing data. Kate has helped to establish and maintain the Hunter Area Heart and Stroke Register, and is a member of the Hunter Area Heart and Stroke Health Outcomes Council. For several years she has served as a Committee Member of the NH&MRC Regional Grant Interview Committees and Discipline Panels.

Sonia Freeman, BA

Sonia Freeman is a social science researcher at the Centre for Clinical Epidemiology and Biostatistics and the Clinical Unit in Ethics and Health Law at the University of Newcastle, Australia. Over the past 8 years she has worked on a number of transdisciplinary research projects including the Oceanpoint Community Health Study and the Coalfields Heart Disease study. Sonia is the co-author of 'Complexity and Human Health: The Case for a Transdisciplinary Paradigm', published in 1998 in *Culture Medicine and Psychiatry*, and 'Cultural Constructions of Risk: The Case of Heart Disease in the New South Wales Coalfields, Australia', published in *Applying Health Social Science: Best Practice from the Developing World*.

Richard F. Heller, MB BS, MD, FRCP, FRACP, FFPHM

Richard Heller is currently the Chair of Public Health at the University of Manchester, Britain. Between 1984 and 2000 he held the positions of professor of Community Medicine and Clinical Epidemiology at the Faculty of Medicine, and of director of the Centre for Clinical Epidemiology and Biostatistics at the University of Newcastle, Australia. Dick has been a member of the International Clinical Epidemiology Network since 1984. He has made a major contribution to the development of clinical epidemiology in Australia and internationally.

Nick Higginbotham, PhD

Associate professor Nick Higginbotham directs graduate studies and is the head of Community Medicine at the Centre for Clinical Epidemiology and Biostatistics, University of Newcastle, Australia. Since receiving his doctorate in clinical psychology from the University of Hawai'i in 1979, he has helped to establish community psychology training in New Zealand (University of Waikato) and promoted the development of health social science internationally through the International Clinical Epidemiology Network (INCLEN) and the International Forum for Social Sciences and Health (IFSSH). Nick has authored a monograph on cross-cultural mental health (*Third World Challenge to Psychiatry: Culture Accommodation and Metal Health Care*, University of Hawai'i Press, 1984) and a clinical psychology text, *Psychotherapy and Behaviour Change: Social, Cultural and Methodological Perspectives* (Pergamon Press 1988). With Roberto Briceno-Leon and Nancy Johnson, Nick has completed another text in this field: *Applying Health Social Science: Best Practice from the Developing World*.

Jenny Porteous, PhD, MBBS, DipClinEpi, FAFPHM
Jenny Porteous has a medical degree from the University of New South Wales, Sydney, a postgraduate degree in clinical epidemiology from the University of Newcastle, Australia, and a PhD in nutritional and behavioural epidemiology from the Australian National University, Canberra. Jenny has a strong interest in combining qualitative and quantitative research techniques and in the methodology and philosophy of transdisciplinary research. She has been involved in the teaching of quantitative, qualitative, and transdisciplinary research methods in both the developed and developing worlds.

Ann Saul, BA Hons
Ann Saul studied at Girton College in Cambridge, Britain, where she completed her Social Science degree in 1974. She has been involved in research and consumer activism related to maternity issues in Britain and Australia for many years. Since 1992 Ann has taught social science to health science students and professionals at the University of Newcastle, Australia. Her PhD research is a qualitative study of midwifery and childbirth options in New South Wales.

Nelson K. Sewankambo, MD, MSc
Dr Nelson Sewankambo is the dean of Makerere University Medical School, Kampala, Uganda, and a Trustee of the International Clinical Epidemiology Network (INCLEN). He teaches and conducts research in internal medicine, clinical epidemiology, and medical anthropology. An HIV/AIDS clinical specialist, he is engaged in several HIV intervention studies in southwestern Uganda, as well as in behavioural research. Nelson is deeply committed to reshaping medical education in Uganda by incorporating transdisciplinary research using the Rakai community as an educational and research field station.

Carla Treloar, PhD
Carla Treloar is currently a lecturer in social interventions for public health in the Department of Social Science and Medicine at Imperial College School of Medicine, London. She has an interest in health inequalities, particularly the health of minority ethnic communities, and in examining 'joined up' interventions for complex health problems. Prior to joining Imperial College, Carla was a lecturer in health social science with the Centre for Clinical Epidemiology and Biostatistics at the University of Newcastle, Australia. In this capacity, she worked in a number of areas developing the Centre's focus on qualitative research methods.

Dennis Willms, PhD
Dennis Willms, a medical anthropologist, is associate professor in the Department of Anthropology at McMaster University, Ontario, Founding Director of the Salama SHIELD Foundation (*salama* is Swahili for health and SHIELD is the acronym for Sustaining Health Initiatives, Enabling Local Development), and a co-principal investigator of the CIDA/NGO-funded project, The Health NGO of the 21st Century: Redefining research capacities and needs for translating evidence into compelling health interventions. Dennis is keenly interested in participatory action research and in the development of a health intervention science that incorporates translational research methodologies. His recent publications include *Nurtured by Knowledge: Learning to Do Participatory-Action Research* (Apex Press and IDRC, New York and Ottawa). Current research activities include HIV/AIDS interventions among traditional healers in Zimbabwe and among adolescents in Uganda.

Acknowledgments

The authors appreciate the assistance of the many people who helped us bring this book to fruition. Comments on drafts were graciously offered by Jillian Albrecht and colleagues at the Centre for Clinical Epidemiology & Biostatistics: John Attia, Natalie Johnson, Rhonda Walker, Patrick Fitzgerald, Michael Dibley, Karla Karinen, and John Page. We acknowledge the contribution of the many researchers who worked with us in the TD teams whose work forms the basis of the examples and case studies in this book. In particular, we thank those who took part in the Coalfields Healthy Heartbeat project, the Oceanpoïnt project, the Care Aware study, the Rakai District study in Uganda, and the traditional healer investigation in Zimbabwe.

We are grateful to international health colleagues who encouraged development of this book, including health social scientists in INCLEN, IFSSH, APNET, SOMA-Net, COHRED, the Carnegie Corporation of New York, and the Ford Foundation. Patricia Rosenfield provided early visions for TD thinking among our group. Scott Halstead, then Director of the Rockefeller Foundation Health Sciences Division, made it possible for health social science to become part of the INCLEN family, while Richard Heller ensured that it survived and thrived in Australia and internationally. Annette Dobson was a vital ally and guide. We also thank our graduate students whose intellectual and career experiences inspired much of what is contained in this text.

Glenn Albrecht would especially like to acknowledge Roger Woods, sociologist at Curtin University, who was the first mentor to encourage him to think beyond the existing boundaries, and to some of the lecturers in philosophy at the University of Western Australia (UWA) who drove him away from British empiricism into Hegelian dialectics. Glenn's search for an organically unified understanding of no less than the whole world was greatly assisted by the late Julius Kovesi at UWA and Bill Doniela at the University of Newcastle, who were willing to feel the rhythm of the dialectic. Glenn also expresses appreciation to Jillian Albrecht, his partner in transdisciplinary adventures and fellow explorer of the beauty and perils of complexity.

Technical assistance was kindly provided by graphic designer Carly Briscoe and IT wizards Bill Plaizier and Jane Gibson. Alan Freeman played an important logistical role. Jill Henry at OUP provided wise counsel at various stages, and Sandra Goldbloom Zurbo contributed valuable copy editing suggestions. We acknowledge our children, Nicolas, Damien, Anthony, and Claire, who endured our many hours of parental preoccupation as we worked on this text over the years.

We also gratefully acknowledge the copyright permission granted by the following publishers.

Chapter 1

Cambridge University Press for an extract from McMichael, A. J. 1993, *Planetary Overload: Global Environmental Change and the Health of the Human Species*, Cambridge University Press, Cambridge, p. 154. Copyright © Cambridge University Press 1993. Reproduced with the permission of Cambridge University Press; Omni Publications International, Ltd for an extract from McAuliffe, K. 1990, 'The Killing Fields: Latter-day Plagues', *Omni*, May, pp. 52–3, p. 96. Copyright © Omni Publications International, Ltd., reprinted by permission; Norman Swan for an extract from 'Return of the Deadly Diseases', reproduced in the *Sunday Telegraph*, 9 May 1993, p. 122 from the SBS Film Australia Series, *Invisible Enemies*, written and narrated by Norman Swan. Copyright © Film Australia 1992; Farrar, Straus and Giroux, for an extract from Garrett, L. 1994, *The Coming Plague: Newly Emerging Diseases in a World Out of Order*, pp. 171–2, 189–90, London, Virago Press. Copyright © Laurie Garrett. Reprinted by permission of Farrar, Straus, and Giroux, LLC. Copyright © USA and its dependencies, the Philippines, Canada and the open market; Little, Brown and Company (UK) for an extract from Garrett, L. 1994, *The Coming Plague: Newly Emerging Diseases in a World Out of Order*, pp. 171–2, 189–90, London, Virago Press. Copyright © UK and Commonwealth, excluding Canada; Westview Press, a member of Perseus Books, LLC, for an extract on pp. 38–41, in A. McElroy, and P.K. Townsend, 1999, *Medical Anthropology in Ecological Perspective* (3rd edn), Macmillan Education Australia. Copyright © 1996 Westview Press, Inc. Reprinted by permission of Westview Press, a member of

Perseus Books, LLC; The Text Publishing Company for an extract by Watkin Tench, 'Transactions of the Colony in April and May 1789', in T. Flannery (ed.), *Watkin Tench 1788*, 1996, The Text Publishing Company, Melbourne, pp. 102–10; Kluwer Academic Publishers and Marilyn Nations for an extract from Nations, M. 1986, 'Epidemiological Research on Infectious Disease: Quantitative Rigor or Rigormortis?', in C. Janes, R. Stall and S.M. Gifford (eds), *Anthropology and Epidemiology*, Reidel Publishing, Boston, pp. 97–9. Copyright © 1986 by D. Reidel Publishing Co. Reprinted with kind permission from Kluwer Academic Publishers; *The Cessnock Advertiser* and Jennifer Pont for an extract from Pont, J. 1990, 'Heart Attack . . . We Believe it Will Never Happen To Us', *Cessnock Advertiser*, 24 October 1990, p. 44.

Chapter 2

The American Psychiatric Association and Peter A. Engel (on behalf of George L. Engel), for figure 2.4, 'Hierarchy of Natural Systems' in George L. Engel 1980, 'The Clinical Application of the Biopsychosocial Model', *American Journal of Psychiatry*, vol. 137, pp. 535–44. Copyright © 1980 American Psychiatric Association; Elsevier Science for figure 2.5, 'Three Tiers of Causes of High Rates of Child Mortality', p. 255, in A.V. Millard 1994, 'A Causal Model of High Rates of Child Mortality', *Social Science and Medicine*, vol. 38, no. 2, pp. 253–68. Copyright © 1994 Elsevier Science. Reprinted with permission from Elsevier Science.

Chapter 3

Heart Foundation (Qld Division) for figure entitled 'Atherosclerosis and the heart' on p. 5 of *Promoting Heart Health: An Educational Resource Manual for Rural and Remote Health Workers*, n.d., Heart Foundation, Queensland; Kresh, J.Y. et al. 2000, for the 'Phase-plane portrait (Poincaré plots) of heart-beat interval time-series from a healthy individual', in *Journal of Thoracic and Cardiovascular Surgery*, in press.

Chapter 4

Kluwer Academic Publishers for sections of text; table 1, 'The Character of Transdisciplinary Research', p. 59; figure 4.1, 'The Transdisciplinary Dynamic',

p. 64, and figure 4.3, 'The Dynamic Process of Transdisciplinary Thinking', p. 65, in G. Albrecht, S. Freeman and N. Higginbotham 1998, 'Complexity and Human Health: The Case for a Transdisciplinary Paradigm', *Culture, Medicine and Psychiatry*, vol. 22, no. 1, pp. 55–92. Copyright © 1998 Kluwer Academic Publishers.

Chapter 5

Australian and New Zealand Journal of Public Health for table 4, 'Comparison of Coalfields and Newcastle Respondents' (%) Intensity of Worry About Health Problems', p. 317, in N. Higginbotham et al. 1993, 'Community Worry About Heart Disease: A Needs Survey in the Coalfields and Newcastle Area of the Hunter Region', *Australian Journal of Public Health*, vol. 17, pp. 314–21. Copyright © *Australian and New Zealand Journal of Public Health* 1993; Elsevier Science for table 1, 'Coalfields Healthy Heartbeat Intervention Strategies: Levels of Participation and Years Initiated', in N. Higginbotham et al. 1999, 'Reducing Coronary Heart Disease in the Australian Coalfields: Evaluation of a Ten-Years Community Intervention', *Social Science & Medicine*, vol. 48, pp. 683–92. Copyright © 1999 Elsevier Science Ltd. Reproduced with permission from Elsevier Science; Kluwer Academic Publishers for figure 5.2, 'The Larrikin Heart as a Way of Transforming Order', p. 83, in G. Albrecht, S. Freeman and N. Higginbotham 1998, 'Complexity and Human Health: The Case for a Transdisciplinary Paradigm', *Culture, Medicine and Psychiatry*, vol. 22, no. 1, pp. 55–92. Copyright © 1998 Kluwer Academic Publishers.

Chapter 6

Zed Books, for the extract entitled 'Future Shock', pp. 1–2, in A. Chetley 1990, *A Healthy Business? World Health and the Pharmaceutical Industry*, Zed Books, London; *Green Left Weekly* for the extract entitled 'The Power Behind Your Doctor' by Ann Casey, in *Green Left*, 1993, April 7, pp. 14–15; Santi Rozario for a copy of a photograph labelled as figure 6.1: Over-the-Counter Medicine Shop in Dakkha.

Chapter 9

The Australasian Medical Publishing Company, for permission to reproduce the 'Critical Appraisal Worksheet', p. 390, in P.J. Darzins, B.J. Smith and R.F. Heller 1992, 'How to Read a Journal Article', *Medical Journal of Australia*, vol. 157, no. 6, 21 September, pp. 389–94. Copyright © 1992 *Medical Journal of Australia*—reproduced with permission.

Introduction

Rationale for health social science

As the twenty-first century unfolds, people the world over reflect on the many challenges facing the globe and wonder whether our present ways of dealing with these challenges are adequate for the future. One of our biggest challenges is to secure and sustain quality health for individuals, communities, whole nations, and, indeed, for the planet itself. Perhaps the most formidable barrier to achieving a healthier world is our inability to grasp the enormous complexity of the mixture of ingredients that determine human health.

At the close of the twentieth century leaders in health research and education acknowledged the complexity of the context for health. Bringing into active collaboration different disciplines and diverse knowledge bases, they began to seek entry points and pathways through the complexity that could lead to a deeper understanding of health in different contexts and to find more promising ways to improve it. In fact, a number of international programs have pursued work across many different fields of knowledge, a pursuit that has proven highly productive. Among these were efforts to reduce the spread and social impact of tropical diseases (World Bank/World Health Organization, Tropical Disease Research Program—WHO/TDR), prevent infant deaths from diarrhoeal diseases (Applied Diarrheal Disease Research Program—ADDRP), improve how medicines are prescribed and used (International Network for the Rational Use of Drugs—INRUD), address the neglect of women's reproductive health (the Ford Foundation), translate national research findings into effective health policies (Council on Health Research for Development—COHRED), change medical practices to follow the best evidence about effective, efficient, and community acceptable treatments (International Clinical Epidemiology Network—INCLEN), and ensure that the social and cultural dimensions of priority health problems are identified and included in the development of health services, policies, and research agendas (International Forum for Social Sciences in Health—IFSSH, the Carnegie Corporation of New York, the Ford Foundation).

Our experience from these programs and others shows clearly that social and behavioural science knowledge, along with understandings provided by the physical, biological, and health sciences, and by community members themselves are essential for unravelling the complexity of human health. In order to harness the spectrum of social science approaches and bring them into active engagement with the applied health sciences, a new perspective emerged in the 1980s—health social science. We see health social science not as a new discipline in competition with established fields. Rather, it is the transdisciplinary application of social and behavioural science theories and methods, in active partnership with complementary knowledge from biomedical and health sciences (including epidemiology and biostatistics) to gain a comprehensive understanding of a health problem. In addition, insights from fields as diverse as biology, ecology, physics, and climatology may be needed to complement the perspective of health social science. The totality of relevant perspectives can then be used to develop change strategies that are effective, sustainable, equitable, and acceptable.

Our definition of health social science has three emphases. First, it is inclusive of the spectrum of (sometimes competing) concepts and methods that make up the social and behavioural sciences. Each of these disciplines can play a role in mapping the reality of a health issue; leaving out perspectives weakens the potential of the overall social science contribution. Second, we see health social science as strenuously engaged in bridging the divide between the social and health/medical sciences. The core philosophy of this new perspective is collaboration and partnership of different but equally valid perspectives with the purpose of improving human health. Third, many different fields of knowledge are brought together by the mutual aim of solving a complex problem. This is done by synthesising complementary knowledge, and building up the best possible picture of the nature of the problem and its causes. It is then possible to implement the most likely means to bring about beneficial change within the limits of feasible action.

We use the term *transdisciplinary* (TD) to describe this process of synthesising diverse fields of knowledge in the quest for a creative understanding of the problem. In addition, the value position health social scientists adopt is that genuine health improvements are those that produce benefits in both clinical indicators and perceived quality of life, are sustainable in the context of the local environment, and are equitable across the society.

The purpose of *Health Social Science: A Transdisciplinary and Complexity Perspective* is to provide a practical learning resource for students and professionals who want to apply social science in order to better understand and improve human health in industrialised and postindustrial societies and/or in developing world regions. The book is written for people with social science backgrounds, such as psychology, anthropology, sociology, social work, geography, economics, or education, as well as for health scientists, whether their training is clinical medicine, nursing, nutrition, epidemiology, public health, occupational therapy, or another healing profession. This book is especially pertinent to practitioners of change and its management: those involved in health policy design, project management, organisational change, and community development who are already involved in interdisciplinary teams with problem-solving goals. The material presented respects the reader's current knowledge base—whether the reader is a social or health scientist, or health sector professional—and extends that knowledge into new ground. For example, by describing health research without disciplinary bias, those trained in quantitative methods will gain insight into qualitative methods, while practitioners of qualitative methods will learn about some basic tools of quantitative research.

Inspiration for this textbook in health social science came from our assignment to provide an education program that would prepare both social scientists and specialist physicians to work together within clinical epidemiology research groups. Such groups were being set up in Africa, Asia, and Latin America as part of the International Clinical Epidemiology Network (Halstead et al. 1991; Higginbotham 1994). No single textbook (or even a short list of textbooks) offered adequate coverage of the concepts and methods that we felt were essential for preparing social scientists to apply their background to the health field or assisting clinical epidemiologists to appreciate the relevance of such methods for their research needs. The present book is a result of 15 years teaching and research experience in an interdisciplinary environment and draws freely upon fields of knowledge such as psychology, epidemiology, medicine, nursing, sociology, anthropology, geography, ecology, philosophy, and history.

The unifying theme of this textbook is that health social science, by its very nature, requires transdisciplinary thought and action. Health problems are not owned by any single field of knowledge; they exist in their own reality (a kind of transdisciplinary space) that can best be illuminated and mapped by bringing together a full array of perspectives that have something to add to our understanding (Higginbotham and Albrecht 1988; Albrecht 1990). The special feature of a transdisciplinary health social science is to allow people with diverse backgrounds to understand each other and work in a team, incorporating each other's concepts and research tools. In this book we work through examples of transdisciplinary thinking and teamwork in areas such as coronary heart disease and AIDS prevention to illustrate the barriers to be overcome and the opportunities provided by this type of research practice.

The foundations of transdisciplinary thinking

Transdisciplinary thinking, as we elaborate in chapter 4, is thinking that goes beyond—transcends—the boundaries of existing fields of knowledge in order to more fully understand the interrelated complexity inherent in human existence in the natural world. Transdisciplinary thinking about health creates the richest possible description of the context within which health and disease are situated. The total health context (termed the *health hierarchy*; see chapter 2) encompasses a soft hierarchy of interdependent systems spanning physical, biological, and ecological foundations upon which the health of social, behavioural, and individual (body) components is built. Through the hierarchy, the reader is encouraged to conceptualise health status as dependent on the essential foundations of health. Such a concept involves the idea that there is a chain of dependency from the essentials of life delivered by physical systems (air, water, soil), to ecological systems (biota), and social systems (shelter, safety, socialisation). An individual human being, or indeed a whole population, sits on top of this foundation and optimal health is the ideal outcome of the consideration and use of all these factors. Put simply, if physical systems fail, there can be no ecological systems. If there are no ecosystems then social systems are impossible. Without social systems individual human beings cannot exist.

With such diversity and complexity comprising the health problem context, it is clear that we must pursue a mode of thinking that can span, integrate, and synthesise available knowledge and methods of attaining knowledge.

One way to understand transdisciplinary thinking is to contrast it with procedures of single, multiple, and interdisciplinary research activity. In this book, we use the term *disciplines* to refer to fields of study around which learning traditionally has been organised in educational institutions. Disciplines are formalised bodies of knowledge that are expressed through a great variety of communication technologies and patterns of social interaction between specialists or so-called experts, between specialists and laypeople, and between teachers and students. Disciplines not only delimit knowledge boundaries but also connect to social and political systems through access to funding, accreditation of professionals, and articulation with many other institutions of society. The organisation of disciplines changes over time, and particular disciplines may grow or decline in the amount of social and cultural resources they can attract. The growth of the discipline of computer science is an example of a rapidly growing and influential field. Several fields of study may merge to become new disciplines, such as clinical ecology (environmental health) or behavioural epidemiology. While disciplines are not fixed or immutable, at any one time they represent significant configurations of power and knowledge with considerable social force.

Many educational institutions have moved towards more interdisciplinary forms of organisation in recent decades. Institutionalised forms of collaboration in schools, research centres, and interdisciplinary programs of teaching are now common. Moreover, many professionalised fields of knowledge have a strong interdisciplinary foundation from which concepts and methods specific to the practice of the profession may emerge. While researchers and practitioners who were trained and already work in interdisciplinary fields of knowledge will approach health problems with a broader perspective, it is our observation that in many institutional contexts interdisciplinary fields of knowledge tend to operate in the same manner as disciplines, delimiting and restricting knowledge boundaries as part of the process of competing for funding and prestige.

In the field of health research, single disciplinary approaches use only the concepts and methods of their own domain to explain a health problem and elaborate specialist knowledge. Multidisciplinary research takes place with different disciplines working alongside each other on a common issue, but researchers stay within the boundaries of their own field. Interdisciplinary approaches move to synthesise discipline-specific insights and investigators are willing to see strict boundaries disappear for the purpose of resolving problems that are defined from within the interacting disciplines. However, other fields that are required to map the fullest understanding of the health context may not be considered in the collaboration. Transdisciplinary thinking takes the next significant step: it is committed to engaging all perspectives required to understand complex health problems as part of the evolution of complex, adaptive systems operating across multiple levels of the health hierarchy. When the collaboration is able to produce a common conceptual framework usable by all the disciplines involved, a transdisciplinary explanation emerges that can become a powerful tool for improving the health context.

While rigid knowledge boundaries are barriers to transdisciplinary thinking, disciplinary and interdisciplinary knowledge and methods themselves are essential compass points for mapping transdisciplinary space. TD thinking does not seek to do away with the perspectives of disciplines and interdisciplinary fields of study. Rather, it sets in motion processes and promotes new conceptual frameworks through which various perspectives can be joined to create an organically unified entity from what were formerly only partial views.

An increasing number of health planners, managers, funding agencies, researchers, academics, and consumer advocates alike now recognise that the fragmented approaches of the past—in which one field of knowledge is privileged over another—have limited use. While TD approaches are seen as new and innovative means for understanding health problems, exactly how they can be applied is less clear to many involved in research, community development, project management, and policy formulation. This textbook demonstrates the conceptual and methodological steps required to perform transdisciplinary research leading towards applications in a variety of health contexts. The volume is of practical use to students and professionals involved in health research. It will also inform medical and public health practitioners and health advocates at all levels who are grappling with major health problems in developed or developing world societies.

Health Social Science is organised in three main sections. It is possible for the reader to take two different approaches to the text. One approach is open to the reader who is already working in an interdisciplinary framework or predisposed to accept a transdisciplinary and complexity approach to health social science. This reader may wish to skip chapter 2, and briefly review our discussion of complexity theory in chapter 3 and transdisciplinarity in chapter 4. This reader can then move to our discussion of the application of such thinking from part II onwards.

The other approach is open to those readers who would like to discover for themselves the importance and relevance of complexity theory and TD thinking. For these readers, part I provides an extensive set of case studies and examples, with explanatory theory and discussion. In the chapters in this section we highlight the most important aspects of complexity and TD principles in relation to human health.

Nick Higginbotham
Glenn Albrecht
Linda Connor

Part I
Why a Transdisciplinary and Complexity Perspective

Preamble

Organisation of Part I

Part I sets out the nature and scope of the task facing health social science researchers.

Chapter 1 presents ten case studies of health problems that show how a broad sweep of forces work together to create the conditions necessary for the emergence of chronic diseases or the outbreak of epidemics.

Chapter 2 shows how these health problems can be arranged according to their main causes (for example, physical, biological, or social systems) to construct a hierarchy of health influences. We review prominent theories in health social science that strive to explain health problems by conceptualising their determinants at one or more of the levels in the health hierarchy.

In chapter 3, complexity theory is offered as an example of a unifying perspective for overcoming limitations of existing theories of health by conceptualising health problems as emergent properties of open, dynamic, social, and biological systems. Complexity theory is not the only possible TD perspective, but we find it particularly compelling and have thus given it some prominence in part I of the book.

Chapter 4, building on notions of complexity in health, introduces transdisciplinary thinking as a fundamental strategy for health research, and for policy makers and community practitioners seeking solutions to health problems.

1
Situating Health and Illness

GLENN ALBRECHT AND NICK HIGGINBOTHAM

1.1 Introduction

What is the best way to begin the journey towards understanding the complexity of human health and incorporating this knowledge into more effective health policy and practice? As a first step, we can look at several examples of well-documented health problems that show the broad sweep of forces operating at physical, biological, ecological, social, behavioural, and body levels. The new methodology that incorporates and goes beyond all these individual levels is what we term *transdisciplinary research*. Understanding the full impact of these forces on the health status of the human body and populations of humans is the ultimate goal of transdisciplinary research.

The need for a transdisciplinary (TD) approach grows more obvious as the disease profiles of all countries become increasingly complicated. The developing world continues to experience epidemics of the old diseases—cholera, measles, and malaria—but has the additional burden of new epidemics such as HIV/AIDS. Industrialised societies have a substantial burden of the so-called lifestyle diseases—heart disease, stroke, diabetes and lung cancer—but have also seen outbreaks of new epidemics of infectious diseases including antibiotic-resistant tuberculosis, legionnaires' disease and Lyme disease. As Levins argues:

> We are living in a period of extremely large-scale changes in society, the physical environment, populations, pathogens, knowledge, and also in the resources socially made available for coping with these problems. Therefore, we are living in a period in which increased encounters with both familiar and unfamiliar diseases are very likely to occur (Levins 1994, p. 405).

The case examples below show that no discipline alone has all the insights, explanations, or solutions to a particular health problem. Rather, each problem is sited in a unique context and can be approached by teasing out the many layers of causal influences that give rise to it. Different disciplinary tools are appropriate to use within each respective layer.

Assembling the disciplines and comparing the insights that arise from multiple perspectives are crucial elements of what we call transdisciplinary thinking. Transdisciplinary thinking requires that a health problem be reconceptualised within the full complexity of the systems in which it is embedded. This idea is the philosophical core of the book. While reading the case examples that follow, begin to identify for yourself the diverse and often diffuse connections among the elements influencing the health landscape.

1.2 Illness and complexity: case examples

1.2.1 Melanoma

In this example, the effect of naturally high levels of solar radiation on a person of fair skin is highlighted. The fear of serious skin cancers for such people is increased by the change in the ozone layer in the earth's atmosphere, leading to even higher levels of solar radiation for those who expose themselves to the sun.

> Dave was like any other young Australian in the 1950s. He loved the outdoors and spent many hours of each summer in the sun. A favourite place was the beach, where surfing, swimming, and sunbaking were his most popular activities. Sunburn and peeling of the skin were frequent results of such activity, but Dave thought nothing of these small pains: they were normal for the pale-skinned, fair-haired group of friends who he swam with. A good tan could not be achieved without a bit of burn and peeling and everybody wanted to have a good tan by the end of summer. Sunburn and evidence of peeling were seen as badges of honour by those who lived under the sun.
>
> In 1997 Dave became concerned about one of the many moles he had on his skin. It was spreading and looked different to others that he could see. The diagnosis from Dave's doctor confirmed his worst suspicions. Dave had a malignant melanoma that required urgent surgery and chemotherapy. Dave was one of the lucky ones, given that, in Australia, malignant melanoma kills about 850 people each year and, between 1980 and 1990, has doubled in prevalence. He now lives more carefully under

> the Australian sun and his own children are made to wear protective clothing and hats, and sunscreen lotion, which is now a vital part of the equipment needed to play in the sun.
>
> Dave is very concerned that the strength of the sun seems to have increased over the levels that he experienced as a child. He is worried about the hole in the earth's ozone layer that has become so large that his family is at risk of melanoma even with low levels of exposure to the sun.

1.2.2 Malaria

Anthony McMichael (1993) warns that there may be dramatic changes in the frequency and distribution of disease linked to climate change. Of particular concern is global warming due to the greenhouse effect, which itself is the result of industrial pollution. With the rate of drug-resistant malaria on the increase, any climate change that favours the mosquito could have devastating effects.

> In tropical countries . . . vector-borne diseases are a major cause of illness and death. For example, malaria and schistosomiasis pose health risks to 2100 million and 600 million people respectively, and the total numbers of infected persons are approximately 270 million and 200 million. Over 1 million deaths from malaria occur each year. In sub-Saharan Africa, which accounts for around 95 per cent of all malaria, half a million young children die from the infection each year. In eastern Africa, a relatively small increase in winter temperature would enable the malarial zone to extend 'upwards' to engulf the large urban highland populations that currently off-limits to the mosquito because of the cooler temperature at higher altitudes—for example, Nairobi (Kenya) and Harare (Zimbabwe). Indeed, such populations around the world, currently just outside the margins of endemic malaria, would provide early evidence of climate-related shifts in the distribution of this disease (Quoted from McMichael 1993, p. 154).

1.2.3 Ebola fever

As humans enter and change ecosystems where they have historically been absent, they come into contact with new pathogens that can cause epidemics of untreatable illness. When such pathogens are highly transmissible and create acute illness, they have the potential to create pandemics of a deadly new disease.

Near the fetid banks of the Ebola River in Northeastern Zaire, a horrible fever had seemingly sprung from nowhere. The year was 1976, and as Carl Johnson[1] arrived with an international team of investigators, fleeing villagers were being turned back at gunpoint by government authorities ordered to quarantine the entire province. None of the community would go near the bush hospital where the outbreak began. So the party of foreigners—with only surgical gowns, gloves, and face masks for protection—set off in jeeps to visit the sick in scattered villages. Johnson and his team saw very rapidly that the disease had an eighty to ninety percent fatality and had no idea how it was being transmitted. Compounding their fears, members of the team—all of whom had volunteered for the mission—kept getting splattered with blood while collecting medical samples. Meanwhile the villagers were unwittingly inviting death by participating in funerary rites that involved intimate contact with the deceased.

To Johnson's relief, the tribal chiefs awoke to the gravity of the threat, banned this ritual, and reinstituted stringent disease control practices used since antiquity in Africa to thwart the ravages of smallpox. The infected were isolated in a hut, where their only contact with the outside world was through food and water slipped under the door. 'If they walked out,' says Johnson, 'fine, if not, the hut was set on fire.'

Several hundred deaths later, the disease vanished as mysteriously as it had appeared. The researchers eventually determined that it was a blood-borne viral infection—unprecedented in medical history—precipitated at the hospital by the use of a few unsterilized syringes to administer hundreds of injections, and possibly spread by sex with infected individuals.

While Johnson struggled to stamp out the epidemic in Zaire, an identical disease broke out in another rural hospital in the Southern Sudan—600 miles away. Initially, it was assumed that the same virus had caused both epidemics. But to everyone's shock, laboratory analysis later revealed that two distinct—though related—strains of viruses were involved. 'It's a bizarre biological coincidence,' said Johnson. 'A disease never before encountered in recorded time strikes with the same vengeance, in the same season, 600 miles apart. It almost makes you think that some environmental factors were just right for this family of viruses to explode on the scene' (quoted from McAuliffe 1990, pp. 52–3).

1.2.4 Hantaan virus

Once again, in Norman Swan's example (1993), severe disturbance of a previously stable environment ushers in a new disease that has the potential to kill humans. In this case a war, which was the primary cause of disturbance to the environment, then exposed solders to wild-rodent faeces and urine carrying the Korean Hantaan virus.

> . . . on the docks of Baltimore, Maryland, a new infection is lying in wait and no one's sure why it hasn't already burst across the United States. It's a disease which emerged suddenly during the Korean War and attacked thousands of United Nations troops, killing many of them. The experts didn't know what it was but, since bleeding was a prominent feature, they called it Korean Haemorrhagic Fever.
>
> Nearly 20 years later, Korean scientists found the cause, a virus carried by mice in a tiny location near the Hantaan River in Korea. It had taken the environmental havoc of a war and the influx of thousands of vulnerable young men to create the circumstances for an infection which had probably been around for centuries to break out as an epidemic.
>
> Now relatives of this virus have been found in rats in the United States and Europe. No one knows if the infection has spread or been there for many years.
>
> Hantaan viruses may or may not be a real threat to developed nations but the message is that they're ready for the time when the infrastructure of our cities breaks down and the urban ghettoes become even more rat-infested than they already are (quoted from Swan 1993, p. 122).

1.2.5 Legionnaires' disease

The creation of artificial environments enables humans to live in ways that would be impossible if exposure to the elements were uncontrolled. Technologies such as airconditioners provide a comfort zone for humans in buildings. However, they can also harbour harmful organisms that are perfectly adapted to these new socially engineered environments. Laurie Garrett, in her timely book, *The Coming Plague,* highlights the emergence of new diseases from environments of our own creation.

> Few groups in the United States took patriotism as seriously as the American Legion, and in the country's bicentennial year [1976] it was more than appropriate that an organization dominated by World War II veterans should convene in Philadelphia, the cradle of the country's Declaration of Independence and constitution. For four days in July several hundred members of the Pennsylvania Legionnaires division held meetings, sat at banquets, danced and sipped cocktails in four Philadelphia hotels.
>
> Liquor flowed freely in the hospitality suites of thirteen candidates for Legionnaire offices. Scattered throughout the luxurious old Bellevue-Stratford Hotel, these suites were sites of energetic handshaking and free cocktails.
>
> On the second night of the meeting, two of the Legionnaires fell ill with symptoms that included fevers, muscle aches, and pneumonia. Because they were older men, these first cases raised no alarms.
>
> Within a week, however, the Pennsylvania Department of Health was flooded with reports of acute pneumonia illnesses and deaths among people who had been inside Philadelphia hotels during the latter half of July. The count would eventually reach 182 cases (78 percent males) and 29 deaths (quoted from Garrett 1994, pp. 171–2).

Garrett gave an account of the cause of the epidemic and the relationship discovered between new technology, our contemporary lifestyle, and exposure to pathogens.

> Further analysis revealed that the bacteria [*Legionella pneumophelia*, the cause of the disease] thrived in the Bellevue-Stratford Hotel's cooling tower. From that water supply, the hotel derived its air-conditioning. The Legionella organisms were hidden in biofilm 'scums' along the edges of the cooling tower, and were actively pumped into the hotel's hospitality suites during the hot month of July (quoted from Garrett 1994, pp. 189–90).

Garrett concludes her investigation of the history of the first outbreak with the following claim.

> In the case of Legionella, a new human disease had emerged in 1976, brought from ancient obscurity by the modern invention of air-conditioning (quoted from Garrett 1994, p. 190).

1.2.6 Kuru

Changes in cultural beliefs and associated rituals and practices can have important roles in the spread or termination of disease. In what was initially a very perplexing epidemic, McElroy and Townsend (1999) describe how knowledge of culture and ritual provided clues to the cause and to the end of the epidemic.

Kuru began with tremors. Despite her trembling and jerky motions, a South Fore woman in highland New Guinea could lean on her digging stick as she went about her work weeding her sweet potato garden and caring for her children. In several months, her coordination was worse; she could not walk unless someone supported her. Her eyes were crossed and her speech was slurred. Excitement made the symptoms of cerebellar dysfunction worse and she was easily provoked to foolish laughter. Within a year, she could no longer sit up and was left lying near the fireplace in her low grass-roofed house. Death was inevitable.

After her funeral was over, other women of the village prepared her body for cooking. The flesh, viscera, and brains were steamed with vegetables in bamboo tubes or in an earth oven with hot stones. Maternal relatives had a special right to their kinswoman's flesh, and specific kin had rights to certain body parts. A woman's brain was eaten by her son's wife or her brother's wife, for example. A woman's flesh was not eaten by her own parents, children or husband. South Fore warriors generally avoided eating human flesh, believing it made them vulnerable to the arrows of enemies. But in any case, they avoided women's flesh because women were believed to be polluting to men. It was mostly women who were cannibals and they shared the funeral meal with their children of both sexes. They would not eat a victim of certain diseases like dysentery and leprosy, but the flesh of kuru victims was acceptable.

Many different hypotheses were explored as possible explanations of kuru. In the early 1960s, the most widely accepted explanation was a genetic one, that a lethal mutation had arisen in this population. Analysis of genealogies showed that kuru did tend to run in families, though there were some odd, unexplained patterns. Most disturbing was the combination of high lethality and high incidence. How could the gene maintain itself in the population despite the high death rate from kuru, which would have been removing the gene from the population systematically? The gene must have conferred some powerful, but unknown, advantage to carriers of the gene who did not themselves develop kuru. Those who questioned the genetic hypothesis explored other possibilities, such as nutritional deficiencies, toxic substances, and psychosomatic causes.

At its peak, mortality from kuru was devastating. Between 1957 and 1968, over 1100 kuru deaths occurred in a South Fore population of 8000. Even as the kuru studies were continuing, the epidemiological patterns began to change: The incidence and mortality declined, first among the younger age groups and later in all age groups. It began to look as though kuru might eventually disappear although no treatment had yet been found. Although the Fore lacked written history or a system of dating events, cultural anthropologists Robert Glasse and Shirley Lindenbaum were able to probe the memories of older informants during field work in 1961–1962. They found that both cannibalism and kuru were relatively new to the Fore. The custom of cannibalism had been adopted about 1910, and the first cases of kuru had occurred some time later, with the disease becoming increasingly prevalent until the 1950s. They suggested that kuru was transmitted by cannibalism. As cannibalism declined, the disease was not being transmitted to children who had never tasted human flesh. Because of the long and variable incubation period, twenty years after cannibalism disappeared people were still coming down with the disease though they had been exposed many years earlier (quoted from McElroy and Townsend 1999, pp. 38–41).

1.2.7 Dengue

This case illustrates how changes in international trading in goods can promote the ecological expansion of species that are the vectors of disease. By unintentionally becoming part of the value-adding chain, even mosquitoes can successfully enter new environments and bring with them new diseases to a naïve population, as Kathleen McAuliffe describes (1990).

A viral infection transmitted by insects, dengue has been around in a mild form for centuries in Asia, causing flulike symptoms and aching joints in adults. In the fifties, however, the virus suddenly became much more virulent—especially in children. Young victims typically break out in a rash and begin bleeding from the nose and ears. Many of them then go into shock and die. More than 600 000 cases of this severe type of dengue were reported in Southeast Asia in 1987, compared with 2060 in 1967—a 300-fold increase in 20 years.[2]

> As if that were not bad enough, one type of mosquito that transmits the disease had been entering America since the early eighties aboard tyres for retreading. The insect's eggs, explains entomologist Bruce Eldridge of the University of California at Davis, hatch in water that collects inside the tyres when it rains. This highly successful invader is known as the Asian tiger mosquito and is now found in Texas, Missouri, and everywhere east of the Mississippi. So far it does not appear to be transmitting the deadly dengue virus—at least not within the continental USA. But there are plenty of mosquito carriers throughout the tropics—including Puerto Rico and Mexico, where haemorrhagic fever attacked more than 30 000 people in 1986. 'The disease is literally knocking at our back door,' warns Eldridge (quoted from McAuliffe 1990, p. 96).

1.2.8 Smallpox

Colonisation by the European powers in the sixteenth, seventeenth, and eighteenth centuries brought with it not only new technologies and culture, but also pathogens such as smallpox to new world populations that were completely naïve to such disease. In this 1789 eyewitness account by Watkin Tench, the horrifying impact of such a new disease on Australian Aborigines is graphically portrayed.

> An extraordinary calamity was now observed among the natives. Repeated accounts, brought by our boats, of finding bodies of the Indians [Australian Aborigines] in all the coves and inlets of the harbour, caused the gentlemen of our hospital to procure some of them for the purposes of examination and anatomy. On inspection, it appeared that all the parties had died a natural death. Pustules, similar to those occasioned by the smallpox, were thickly spread on the bodies; but how a disease to which our former observations had led us to suppose them strangers could at once have introduced itself, and have spread so widely, seemed inexplicable. Whatever might be the cause, the existence of the malady could no longer be doubted. Intelligence was brought that an Indian family lay sick in a neighbouring cove. The governor, attended by Arabanoo [Aborigine guide and translator] and a surgeon, went in a boat immediately to the spot. Here they found an old man stretched before a few lighted sticks and a boy of nine or ten years old pouring water on his head from a shell which he held in his hand. Near them lay a female child dead, and a little farther off, its unfortunate mother. The body of the woman showed that

famine, superadded to disease, had occasioned her death. Eruptions covered the poor boy from head to foot, and the old man was so reduced that he was with difficulty got into the boat. Their situation rendered them incapable of escape and they quietly submitted to be led away (Watkin Tench 1789, as quoted in Flannery 1996, pp. 102–10).

1.2.9 Enteric infections

Marilyn Nations (1986), an anthropologist researching child mortality in north-eastern Brazil, gives a dramatic explanation of how social, cultural, and behavioural factors lead to underreporting of early childhood deaths due to enteric infections in Brazil. Until insiders' perspectives to the child's life are taken into consideration, health authorities will not have a valid index of the burden of mortality in Brazil.

Quickly before death set in, the infant girl's tiny hands were tied around a matchbox in an attitude of prayer and her eyes pried open to see God. Then her body was placed on a crude wooden box in her home to remain, in the light of votive candles, until the next day when she would rest in a homemade coffin. Dona Fatima, the infant's mother, collapsed in her hammock, her only comfort the thought that her daughter no longer suffered: she was now an *angelhino*—a little angel innocent of sin—and, as such, she would fly directly to heaven avoiding purgatory where adults must languish to expiate their sins before reaching their destination. Still, Dona Fatima could not sleep. It was only three years since her son had died of the same *doenca de crianca*—'illness of the child'. Now Fatima stared at the body of her only daughter, questioning God's plan in taking the two children from her.

She had done everything she knew to protect her baby from the common childhood illnesses in Pacatuba: *quebranto* (evil eye), *susto* (fright disease), *sombra* (spirit intrusion) and *quintura* (intestinal heat). She had planted a *pihao* bush outside the house, strung a gold-leaf charm on a red ribbon and tied it to the child's wrists, been careful not to even expose her intentionally to loud noises or cross-roads, and never allowed her outside on the hot grounds without sandals. After such symptoms as vomiting or diarrhoea, Fatima collected medicinal leaves and roots and prepared the proper teas. When the baby had not improved, she went to Dona Mocina, an elderly *rezadeira* or 'praying woman', who began the appropriate healing ceremony. The old woman's incantations, herbal preparations and healing powers had always cured her four oldest children, but the baby was weak and plagued by an unusually powerful *quebranto* cast upon her by a menstruating woman, or so Dona Mocina had diagnosed. Every village mother knows this kind of curse can kill within a day, so Fatima spent her savings on an expensive antibiotic, but this too failed. The infant's fontanelle had already fallen, diarrhoea and vomiting increased, her lips became dry and cracked, and, worst of all, her glazed eyes sank deeply into their sockets, giving her 'angel eyes', the omen of death. When Fatima realised traditional remedies were unavailing, she borrowed money from her comadre to purchase a bus ticket to Fortaleza. Though she had travelled to the capital several times as a maid, she was still bewildered by its high-rise buildings, rushing crowds and noisy traffic. Carrying the dying baby in her arms, Fatima descended from the bus and walked past rows of offices and specialty medical clinics. She could not read the signs on the buildings, but knew from the past that these places did not treat 'illness of the child'. It was only after a ten-block walk that she came to her destination. After waiting nearly three hours, her infant, now nearly lifeless, was lifted from her arms by strangers in white. 'There is not much hope for this one', they scolded, 'you cannot wait until they are half dead and then expect us to perform a miracle!' Fatima lowered her head and nodded in silence; only God knew she had done everything to save her baby. The hospital attendants shaved smooth spots on her infant's head and repeatedly thrust a needle into her scalp. At last they tapped the small, blue vein and administered a balanced electrolyte solution in hopes of reversing the effects of severe dehydration.

Later, Fatima and her child returned home. The infant's fate was now in God's hands. Fatima would go to church at sunrise and make a vow to San Francisco to crawl on her knees to his shrine in Canede, to cut off her hair, to carve a wooden statue—anything if only her daughter would be allowed to live. But instead, Fatima felt only a heaviness in her arms; her baby was dead, now a 'little angel'. In all her twenty-seven years Fatima had never known such a weight as her dead child. She covered the child's bruised head with the old sheet she used as a blanket.

Morning came quickly. A crowd, mostly women and children, gathered around the wooden table. Prayers were recited, and Fatima said farewell to her baby. Four boys carried the open casket filled with flowers covering all but the child's face and hands, and led the procession of school children through the streets to the community cemetery. Fatima's husband lowered the sky-blue coffin into the ground then furiously shovelled dirt over his right shoulder. Exhausted, he walked away—never once looking back (quoted from Nations 1986, pp. 97–9).

1.2.10 Heart disease

In long-established industrial societies such as Australia, heart disease has become a major epidemic, accounting for close to 50 per cent of all fatalities. Lifestyle and behavioural factors are key elements in the understanding of this epidemic. In this case example, Jennifer Pont (1990) captures the experience of one man in the Coalfields region of New South Wales, revealing some of the common factors in the establishment of heart disease.

A major killer of Coalfields people is heart disease but many of us like to think that it won't happen to me.

Yet about 50 families in the Coalfields area each year lose a loved one from heart attack. Hundreds of other people have heart attacks but, fortunately, live to tell about it. In November 1989, John Knight was one of those people.

John Knight is a well known local identity. He has lived in the Coalfields all of his 60 years ('People here are better than anywhere else') and has been active in business, council and as Secretary/Manager of the local Rugby League Supporters Club. His life has been a busy one, a fact that Mr Knight considers put him at high risk of heart attack.

'My life was pretty hectic before the heart attack. I was working 12 hours a day, seven days a week, you would probably say I was a workaholic. I could probably have gotten away with less, but the club was growing and I accepted it as a challenge.'

Mr Knight's hectic life included diet and exercise habits that, in combination, put him in what is recognised as a 'high risk' group. 'I wasn't a big eater, I enjoyed baked dinners, traditional food, none of this fancy stuff, but if I was busy I would grab a [meat] pie or skip a meal. I would do things I shouldn't have, but I never had a weight problem, probably because I smoked so much. I used to smoke forty or fifty cigarettes a day. I think that certainly interferes with your appetite.

'Ironically enough, I had given up smoking six weeks before the heart attack. I had been threatening to do it for months and months. I had a touch of emphysema and I decided it was time to do something about it. My wife had given up a couple of years before, but I left it too late.

'Earlier in my life I had been a State swimming champion. I also played a bit of league (football). I had plenty of sport, but in later years I felt I didn't have time for exercise, or to sit around in doctors' waiting rooms for check ups. I was always getting in trouble with my family but I probably never thought I was putting myself at risk. I was enjoying myself and I had blinkers on just looking at the goal I set myself. I wasn't getting the priorities right.'

After his heart attack, Mr Knight made changes to his lifestyle to reduce the risk of it happening again. 'I used to come to work at seven o'clock, now I come in at nine o'clock. I get up and I have breakfast. I make sure I have time to eat it. I've cut down on dairy foods and eat low cholesterol everything. I go for regular walks. I used to work back at night. I don't now.'

Mr Knight's advice to other people is to make time for regular exercise, get regular check-ups and eat the right foods. 'Put yourself number one because you've got to.'

'I didn't think anything would happen to me. I think most people are like that. You think it will happen to somebody else, but never to me, you know' (quoted from Pont 1990, p. 44).

1.3 Comment

It is clear from the above case examples that various factors work together to create the conditions necessary for the outbreak of epidemics and occurrence of diseases. These factors range from global changes to the physical systems vital to life, to individual behaviours that expose humans to the damaging agents underlying lifestyle disease.

It is equally clear that knowledge of many disciplines is needed to understand these multiple influences and how they interact. In this book we show how health social scientists, using transdisciplinary thinking and working in partnership with other researchers, practitioners, and members of communities, can combine knowledge across disciplines to unlock the mysteries of modern epidemics and other puzzling health problems.

1.4 Questions to start TD thinking

Your own transdisciplinary thinking can begin by answering two types of questions about the case examples. First, what key factors have influenced the emergence and spread of each health problem? Second, how do the factors interrelate with each other as they play their part in disease causation? Specifically:

- How would changes in climate affect the frequency and distribution of disease?
- What part do cultural practices play in the spread of infectious diseases?
- In what ways can economic conditions alter the course of epidemics?
- What part do historical circumstances play in shaping the way people take action in response to epidemics?
- How may geographical and ecological factors impact on the emergence and spread of a virus?
- Why do some viruses suddenly become more virulent for a particular age group?
- What part do demographic changes play in the emergence and spread of viruses?
- How might health beliefs and economic circumstances affect the ability of people to gain timely health care?
- What is the impact of gender identity on people's willingness to change lifestyle to avoid chronic disease?

Notes

1 World-renowned expert on tropical infections then at the United States Center for Disease Control (CDC).

2 The case detection and reporting systems may have been different in the two time periods. Nevertheless, the increase in the incidence of dengue over the 20 years (1967–87) appears significant.

2
The Hierarchy of Health Influences

GLENN ALBRECHT, NICK HIGGINBOTHAM, AND SONIA FREEMAN

2.1 Introduction

In this chapter, we show that the case examples of health problems presented in chapter 1 can be loosely arranged according to their main causes. In doing so, we can construct a hierarchy of key elements that influence human health.

First, we define the health hierarchy as an ongoing process whereby optimal health status for an individual or population is only achieved when more basic conditions fundamental to health status are sustained.

Second, the main disciplines contributing to health and medicine are outlined. As a result of this exercise, we can begin the task of seeing health social science within the full spectrum of disciplinary knowledge dealing with health matters.

Third, we briefly review prominent fields of knowledge in the health social sciences that go beyond conventional discipline boundaries. These frameworks try to explain health problems by conceptualising health determinants at one or more of the levels in the health hierarchy. While some of the approaches focus on one level in the hierarchy (for example, behavioural), others move between levels. All of the fields of knowledge are interdisciplinary, with the aim of accounting for some of the complexity that surrounds health problems.

Fourth, we identify the main limitations of existing interdisciplinary theories of health. In the context of the health hierarchy, we see that these conceptual frameworks tend to favour a limited range of *elements of influence* along the full spectrum of potential influences.

2.2 The health hierarchy

Imagine the full spectrum of factors or elements influencing human health as arranged within a hierarchy. Like Abraham Maslow's (1968) hierarchy of needs, where full human psychological and social potential cannot be realised if basic foundational needs such as food, water, and shelter are not first met, optimum human health cannot be achieved unless several essential foundations are present. The health status of an individual or population is the outcome of complex

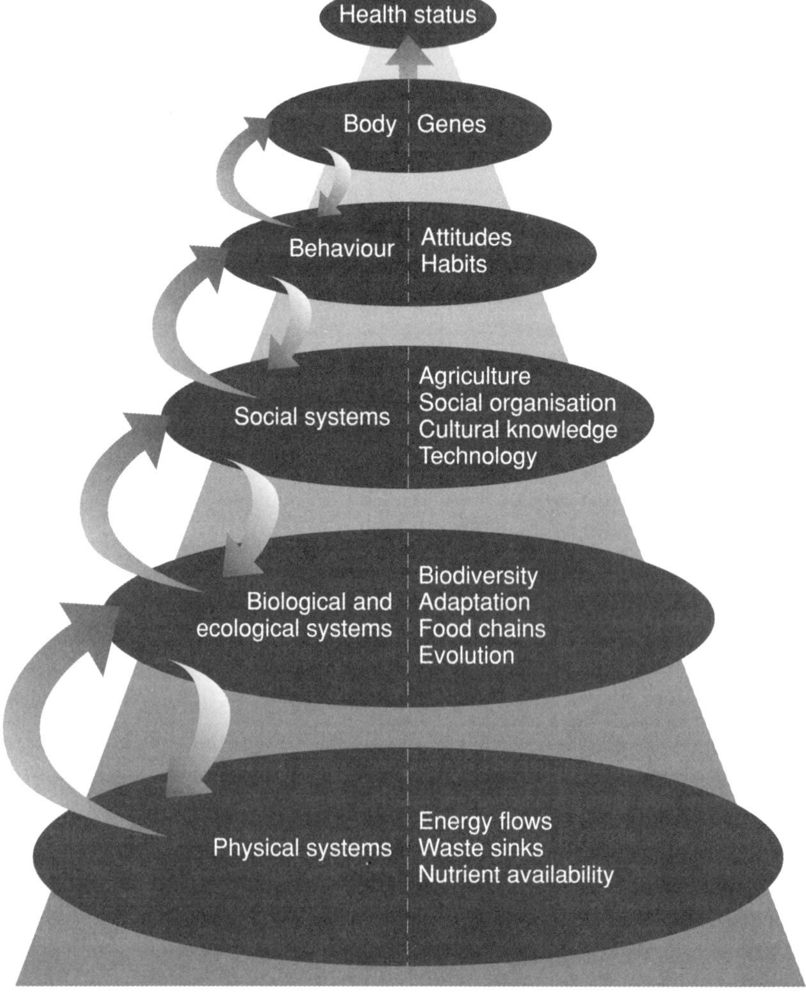

Figure 2.1 The health hierarchy

interactions between the elements that sustain human life. The hierarchy can be described as *soft* since there are no hard barriers between the levels present in what is in actual fact a complex interactive system. We argue, however, that there is some directionality present in the open system since complexity and diversity at the top of the hierarchy are built upon less complex and less diverse foundations. Human health can then be seen as the outcome of the elements shown in figure 2.1, which shows that the health status of a living system, be it an ecosystem or an individual organism, is the outcome of a series of interactions within and between the elements of the health hierarchy.

2.2.1 Physical systems

At the base of the hierarchy are the most basic physical necessities of life, such as solar energy, elements, nutrients, and waste sinks. These are the primary sources of the fundamentals of human social systems such as clean water, clean air, productive soil, and food.

2.2.2 Biological and ecological systems

Organisms use these physical necessities and when organisms coexist in complex interactive systems, ecosystems are the result. Biological and ecological systems convert the physical necessities of life into forms of energy that can be used by organisms, including humans, that are the secondary and tertiary consumers of such energy (see Miller 1995 for the details of the relationships between energy and ecosystems).

2.2.3 Social systems, culture, and behaviour

People, along with other secondary and tertiary consumers, can then interact with supporting environments to increase their supply of necessities. In human social systems this is done through technology, economies, and primary food production (for example, farming). Human social systems are critically dependent on physical, biological, and ecological systems for their existence and sustainability. Sustainability, in this context, means the ability of a given social system to continue indefinitely into the future and maintain its physical infrastructure and culture. Such a social system can continue to evolve and change, but it must do so within the physical limitations of the biological and ecological systems within which it must exist.

However, unlike the social systems of other animals, human social systems are influenced by much more than the physical and biological elements which support them. Culture, in the sense of knowledge that is learnt and transmitted from one generation to the next, is dynamic and evolving, and human behaviour can profoundly influence the structure and processes of human society. If human social systems, culture, and behaviour are adapted to exist harmoniously within the limits of the physical systems that support them, then health is likely to be maximised. On the contrary, if human social systems are maladapted to these basic systems, then human and social health is likely to be compromised and the hierarchy of interacting systems may become unsustainable. Thus, for example, if humans pollute their own environments to the point where, say, the capacity of the atmosphere to support life is compromised, then epidemics of respiratory disease will follow. London's killer fog of December 1952 is thought to have claimed up to 4000 lives and was the catalyst for the Clean Air Act of 1956 which put controls on the issue of smoke from domestic and industrial sources (Bellini 1986, p. 12).

2.2.4 The body

Finally, the human body and its genetic makeup are the products of perhaps millions of years of evolution within the limitations of the laws of physics and ecology. It is therefore likely that when social systems and behaviour are maladapted to our genetic legacy, outcomes that are harmful to health status will follow.

2.3 The health hierarchy and examples of human illness

Human health is the outcome of the interactions throughout the health hierarchy. As shown through the case examples in chapter 1 and figure 2.2. below, different diseases and conditions can be identified as operating predominantly at distinct levels in the health hierarchy. We have simplified the real complexity of some of the diseases and syndromes presented in order to clarify the theories of health and illness.

2.3.1 Physical systems

Humans have created a global network of industrial societies supported by complex technologies. In so doing, we have altered some of the fundamental conditions that form the physical basis of life. The most dramatic and measurable change to this domain is the depletion of the ozone layer in the upper atmosphere and the resultant increase in solar radiation hitting the earth. This increase in solar radiation is caused by gases such as chlorofluorocarbons (CFCs) literally eating the layer of ozone that has been the earth's protective sunscreen for approximately 450 million years.

The increase in solar radiation that hits the earth in turn causes an increase in the incidence of malignant melanoma and many other skin diseases in light-skinned people who are particularly susceptible to excessive sunlight. Other possible health problems associated with ozone depletion include cataracts of the eye and depressed immune systems (see McMichael 1993).

A distinct but related problem is global warming caused by the so-called enhanced greenhouse effect. Gases such as carbon dioxide, CFCs, methane, and

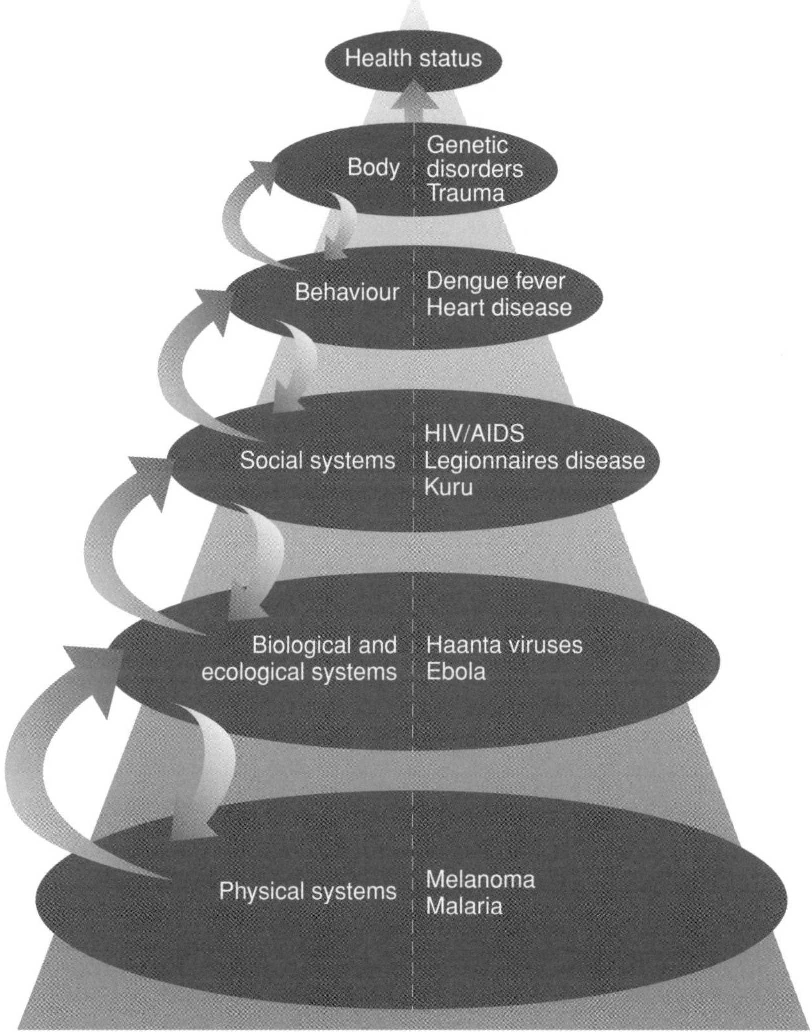

Figure 2.2 The health hierarchy and human illness

nitrous oxide all contribute to this warming of the planet. As output of these gases has increased over the past 200 years of industrial activity, there has been a steady increase in average surface temperature over the whole planet. Although scientists agree that human-induced (that is, *anthropogenic*) global warming is occurring, there is little agreement on the exact amount of warming. If the prediction of an increase of 2°C over a period of three or four decades were to prove correct, then the consequences for the distribution of ill health throughout the world would be profound. Such an increase in global temperature due to the greenhouse effect will, for example, shift malaria and other infectious diseases such as sleeping sickness further north and south from their present distribution in the tropics. This would be due to the fact that the insect species that are the carriers of disease will have a greater range of climate and habitat zones within which to complete their lifecycles (see Garrett 1994, pp. 566–9).

The combined effect of ozone depletion and depressed immunity together with increased exposure to pathogens due to global warming could see a wave of infectious disease epidemics that would severely challenge the health of human populations. These challenges would arise from changes induced in the physical foundations of life by humans themselves. This is the first time in the history of the planet that one species has been able to consciously change the basic conditions of life and, hence, the conditions for optimum health for all living things, including our fellow humans.

2.3.2 Biological and ecological systems

Anthropogenic change to environments can also be demonstrated in biological and ecological systems that are part of life-support systems. As humans move into previously uninhabited ecosystems and fundamentally disturb them by actions such as vegetation clearing, the conditions are created for exposure of humans to new pathogens. Ebola and Hantaan virus, as noted in chapter 1, have emerged from such previously undisturbed ecosystems.

2.3.3 Social systems

Changes in social systems and human culture can be directly linked to disease processes. Legionnaires' disease, for example, is the outcome of engineering artificial environments in the form of airconditioning units and cooling towers that produce perfect habitat and temperature for Legionella, the bacteria that cause the disease. This artificial environment is ideal for the reproduction of the organism in numbers large enough to cause epidemics of disease in those exposed to the organism.

The account of kuru in chapter 1 clearly indicates that cultural beliefs can exercise a powerful influence on disease outcomes. Eating the flesh of the deceased as a special mourning rite was the route by which the disease of the brain (a transmissible spongiform encephalopathie, or TSE) was passed through the population.

Culture impacts on the likelihood of so-called diseases of affluence with, for example, heart disease in advanced industrial countries influenced by attitudes to food, gender roles, social position, and conflict. Sexually transmitted diseases such as HIV/AIDS are powerfully influenced by the cultural context within which they occur. The large diversity of sexual norms in different cultures and subcultures can greatly enhance or minimise the likelihood of risk of exposure to this deadly virus.

2.3.4 Behaviour

Human behaviour significantly influences health, as we saw in the example of heart disease where a combination of cultural beliefs and behaviours hostile to the heart underlie the epidemic of this condition in Australia. Several mechanisms link behaviour to physical disease. Human action forms a common pathway linking wider social values, cultural roles, and economic constraints in the person's life with exposures (that is, environmental stimuli or biological processes) that harm or protect health. Indeed, people may deliberately or unintentionally act in ways that promote or undermine their own physical well-being. Cardiovascular disease and cancer are strongly linked to behaviours such as cigarette smoking, eating foods rich in saturated animal fats, physical inactivity, excessive consumption of alcohol, and obesity. Hepatitis C is reaching almost epidemic proportions in Australia; it is spread primarily through injecting drug users sharing and re-using unsterilised needles.

Another mechanism linking behaviour with disease is the person's reaction to becoming ill and the sick role. When someone overlooks the significance of symptoms, refuses to consider or delays seeking treatment, fails to adhere to the recommended treatment, or self-treats with pharmaceuticals that are not beneficial, then that person can prolong or exacerbate an illness condition. A large number of heart attack patients (perhaps as many as 50 per cent) delay seeking help, thereby diminishing their chances of survival. Similarly, the benefits of antibiotics are being lost because a growing number of people are not completing a full course of the medication, are taking too many of them, or are taking them when they are not indicated (for a viral infection, for example).

2.3.5 The body

The human body itself, quite independently of other immediate influences, can be a cause of disease. Genetic disorders such as Down syndrome and Parkinson's disease can emerge even though all other sectors of the health hierarchy may be present in optimal ways. However, if basic requirements such as nutritional levels fall, then a large number of opportunistic infections and diseases are more likely to invade the weakened body. A flawed social system can create the conditions for epidemics of injury and death due to motor vehicle and industrial accidents. Again, this is despite the fact that all other conditions in physical and ecological systems may be working towards optimum health for a given population.

Health in the human body—be it of an individual or whole populations—is critically dependent on all of the elements within the health hierarchy. These elements need to act synergistically, that is, they must work together to produce the best possible outcome for nutrition, growth, and resistance to disease. The health status of a human is the culmination of complex processes within the health hierarchy that all have an influence on mental and physical well-being.

2.4 The health hierarchy and health-related disciplines

At each level of the health hierarchy are various disciplines and fields of knowledge that address the occurrence of illness at that level.

2.4.1 Physical systems

The provision of the necessities of life such as clean air and water, productive soil, and nutritious food is the outcome of natural processes and cycles. When water becomes contaminated with excessive human waste, the chances are that infectious disease such as cholera will follow. The discovery that there is a direct link between human waste, water supply, and infectious disease led to the sanitation movement of the nineteenth century. Great gains in public health were made possible by cleaning the urban environment and constructing sewerage systems that separated sewage effluent from the water supply. The ecological public health movement continues the pioneering work of the sanitation movement.

Newer disciplines that cover the intersection of previously unrelated areas such as environmental epidemiology have been able to contribute further to our understanding of the links between such basic environmental factors as the levels of particulate matter (for example, dust) and the levels of modern epidemics such as asthma.

2.4.2 Biological and ecological systems

The traditional discipline areas of medicine that cover normal and diseased functioning of human biology are microbiology, virology, pathology, physiology, and immunology. These disciplines attempt to understand the basic structure and function of organisms that are implicated in human disease. Diseases are treated using agents that modify the pathological process: antibiotics kill bacteria that cause infections, steroids suppress inflammatory processes, chemotherapy retards the growth of tumours, antivirals reduce the ability of viruses to reproduce, and antihelminths rid the body of certain parasites.

New disciplines and interdisciplinary fields of study such as clinical ecology (environmental health) have focused on the links between ill health and exposure to chemicals in food and in the urban environment. It appears that hormone-disrupting chemicals such as polychlorinated biphenyls (PCBs) are now present throughout ecosystems (Colborn et al. 1996, pp. 12–28) and will have deleterious effects on the reproductive systems of all animals. The bio-accumulation of these toxins will particularly affect humans, as they are at the top of the food chain. Another emerging field, molecular epidemiology, uses techniques of molecular biology to detect genes that are linked with disease states, such as the BRCA1 and BRCA2 genes that place women at risk of breast cancer. The goals are:

- to identify an individual's (or population group's) risk of specific diseases, such as cancer, by looking at host cancer susceptibilities (for example, carcinogen metabolism, DNA repair and genetic alterations in tumour suppressor genes) and
- to understand biological evolution and maintenance of disease within and across populations (Hussain and Harris 1998).

2.4.3 Social systems

We shall examine social science approaches to human health in greater detail later in this chapter. However, we can briefly mention key social science disciplines and fields of study that deal specifically with culture and social processes in relation to health and illness.

The disciplines that have examined the relationship between human society and health have expanded from the work done by public health practitioners in the nineteenth century. Medical sociology examines the health implications of social institutions and processes, especially social class, gender roles, ethnicity, and power relations. The medico-industrial complex, including the pharmaceutical industry, is a key focus for understanding and evaluating preventative and curative medicine. Medical anthropology, while concerned with social processes, emphasises how culture shapes health patterns, including cultural perceptions of symptoms, local classification of illness, Indigenous healing knowledge and treatment preferences, and practices regarding nutrition, safety, hygiene, and communal living. Health economics addresses the question of how to maximise the benefits of the resources allocated to the formal health care sector in a society (that is, the *efficiency* of medical and public health services). Clinical economics applies economic methods to evaluate clinical strategies and inform clinical decision-making about the use of (often expensive) medical technology, such as computer-assisted diagnostic tests (CAT scans, ultrasound), and new generation pharmaceutical products (for example, anti-HIV drugs such as AZT and the protease inhibitors).

Occupational medicine deals with workplace-related diseases, especially how to prevent illness that may only become evident many years after the exposure (for example, mesothelioma from asbestos dust), or industrial injuries. The Healthy Cities movement is often described as part of the 'new public health' (see Ashton 1992, p. 5). It is an interdisciplinary field of study that has revived the idea that individual health is thoroughly embedded in healthy public policies that have city-wide relevance.

2.4.4 Behaviour

Health psychology is concerned with the role of psychological processes, including knowledge, attitudes, and practices, in maintaining health and the occurrence and course of illness (see below). Health promotion seeks to get groups of people in the population to increase control over their own health, through education and teaching new behaviours, as well as to take action against environmental determinants of ill health (for example, lack of healthy food choices).

Psychiatry is the medical discipline concerned with the diagnosis, treatment, and prevention of disorders of thinking, emotion, and behaviour. Psychiatric explanations of severe mental illness tend to favour genetic, biological, and neurochemical processes, although the role of learning and social context is also seen as important.

Behavioural epidemiology seeks to identify characteristics or behaviours of people who are associated with an increased probability of a health outcome, such as a chronic or communicable disease, injury, or death. Behavioural epidemiologists have been especially active in understanding the transmission of the HIV virus through unprotected sex, as well as the links between smoking, alcohol use, food habits, and physical exercise, and rates of non-communicable diseases in a population.

2.4.5 Body

Anatomy is the study of the normal structure of the human body. While it is also concerned with the mechanism of human movement, *pathology* addresses the changes in different anatomical structures (bones, organs, muscles, etc.) in various disease states.

Physiology is concerned with the functioning of the human body, at both the organ and cellular level, particularly in relation to the body's efforts to maintain a constant internal environment or homeostasis. *Pathophysiology* refers to the altered functioning of the human body in different disease states.

Clinical medicine deals with the investigation, diagnosis, and management of disease. More recently, the importance of the nature of the interaction between the doctor and patient and its impact upon the processes of investigation, diagnosis, and management is being increasingly recognised.

Surgery involves the practice of treating disease, injury, or deformity by manual operation. In many instances surgery aims to achieve a rapid cure or at least a partial return to normal function for different disease or disordered states. Historically, surgery has been viewed as dealing with more acute medical problems, and general medicine with more chronic illness, although in recent times this distinction has become blurred.

Alternative or *complementary medicine* are terms that encompass a variety of healing practices that are usually considered distinct from mainstream Western medicine practice. These general terms include, among others, the practice of acupuncture, chiropractic, osteopathy, homeopathy, naturopathy, and herbal medicine. A number of the alternative therapies have their basis in traditional medicine used in non-Western cultures and in earlier Western medical practices. In many cases these therapies are considered to be holistic, insofar as they take the whole person—an individual's mental, emotional, and environmental states, not just their physical symptoms and signs—into account in the diagnostic and therapeutic processes.

Clinical epidemiology extends the concepts used to study disease in populations to clinical decision-making, especially diagnosis and prognosis, decisions about treatment selection, and the use of resources. In particular, clinical epidemiology promotes 'evidence based medicine . . . the conscious, judicious and explicit use of current best evidence in making decisions about the care of the individual patient' (Sackett et al. 1996).

Biostatistics applies statistical principles to the analysis of information generated across many of the health-related disciplines, and thus is a core knowledge base operating at all levels of the health hierarchy.

2.5 Theories and frameworks that integrate health and social science

Over the past 20 years, a number of new approaches have been introduced in the health and social sciences in an attempt to integrate various disciplines or examine the totality of causes assumed to underlie health problems. These new interdisciplinary fields of study arise from the intersection of social and behavioural sciences such as psychology, sociology, and anthropology on the one hand, and clinical medicine, public health, and international health on the other. They have in common the aim of providing an account of the interrelationships and complexity that surround a health problem.

This section gives a brief overview of some of the well-established interdisciplinary fields of knowledge that we have found informative for our teaching and research. We classify them in terms of their emphasis on vertical reasoning (see below), ecology, political economy and globalisation, and health transition. By no means exhaustive, figure 2.3 shows how some of the major health-related disciplines and fields of study can be arranged within the hierarchy.

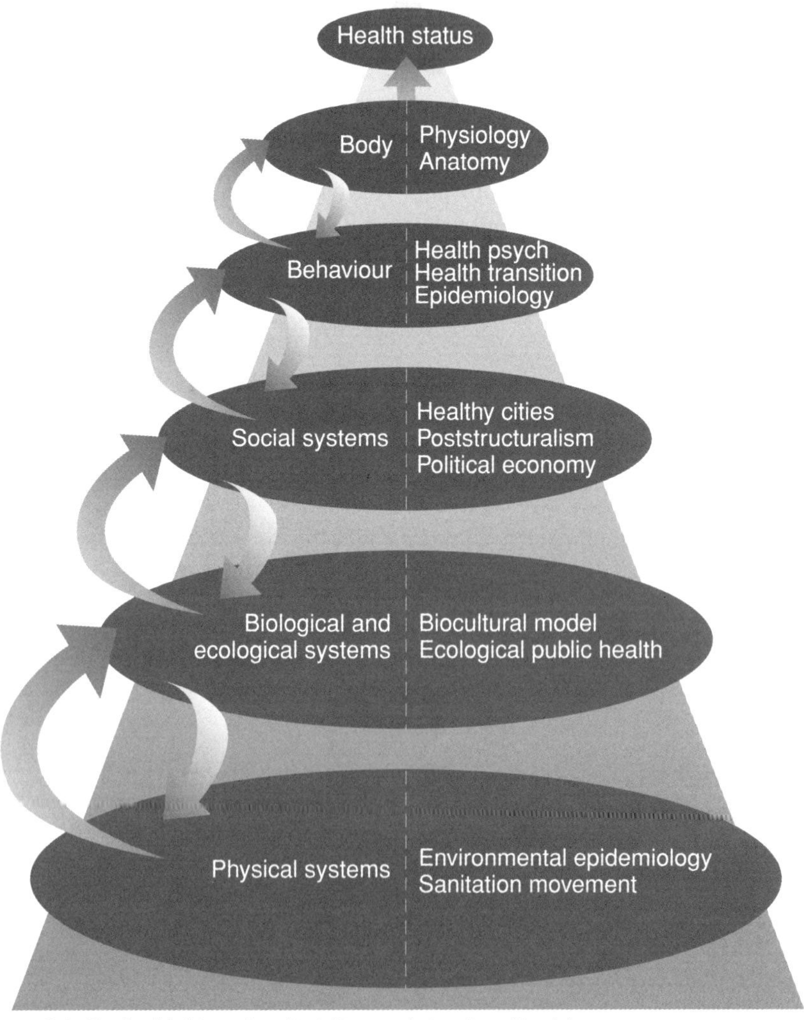

Figure 2.3 The health hierarchy: disciplines and theories of health

2.5.1 Vertical reasoning models

The first type of theoretical model emphasises the necessity of looking between different levels of analysis of a health problem in order to identify the key causal variables. The models all show that different levels of explanation, which are generally separated by discipline boundaries, can usefully be combined to take account of factors from the microbial to the global.

2.5.1.1 The biopsychosocial model

George Engel's (1977, 1980, 1982) biopsychosocial model was one of the first efforts to come to grips with the complexity of causal factors influencing health. His aim was to counter the reductionism of biomedicine that based diagnoses on physical signs and symptoms at the level of clinical anatomy and physiology and neglected the social and behavioural dimensions of causation (Anderson 1996). Figure 2.4 summarises Engel's idea that there is a 'hierarchy of natural systems' ranging from subatomic particles to global systems, including societies. This systems theory approach to health and illness maintains that all levels of organisation in any entity are linked to each other hierarchically; change in any one level will effect change in all the other levels. That is, health and illness are both caused by multiple factors and produce multiple effects (Taylor 1999).

Through Engel's hierarchy we see that, just as the array of factors influencing health are in dynamic relationship with each other, so too the disciplines describing these causal factors are in dynamic relationship with each other. In varying degrees of relevance, the physical, biological, and social sciences need to play an interactive part in explaining a particular health problem.

Marsden Blois (1988) extended Engel's model by arguing for the principle of vertical reasoning. He noted that each level in the hierarchy can be characterised by the nature of the disciplines (their paradigms and associated methods) that operate at that level. Vertical thinking requires one to range back and forth, consciously and effectively, from the mathematical descriptions of atoms to the statistical associations shown by complex biological systems, and to the natural-language description of human behaviour (Blois 1988, p. 81). Medical anthropologist Robert Anderson explains further the nature of vertical reasoning:

> It is the ability to integrate physics and chemistry with anatomy and physiology, with psychology and sociology, with political science and economics, and even with aesthetics and literature. It is a capacity for bringing basic and natural sciences to bear on a problem as well as the social sciences and the humanities. Vertical reasoning is based on an acknowledgment that human behavior is the most complex phenomenon in the universe (Anderson 1996, p. 36).

Anderson makes two additional points about vertical reasoning. First, effective reasoning will move across the levels in complex ways to identify multicausal

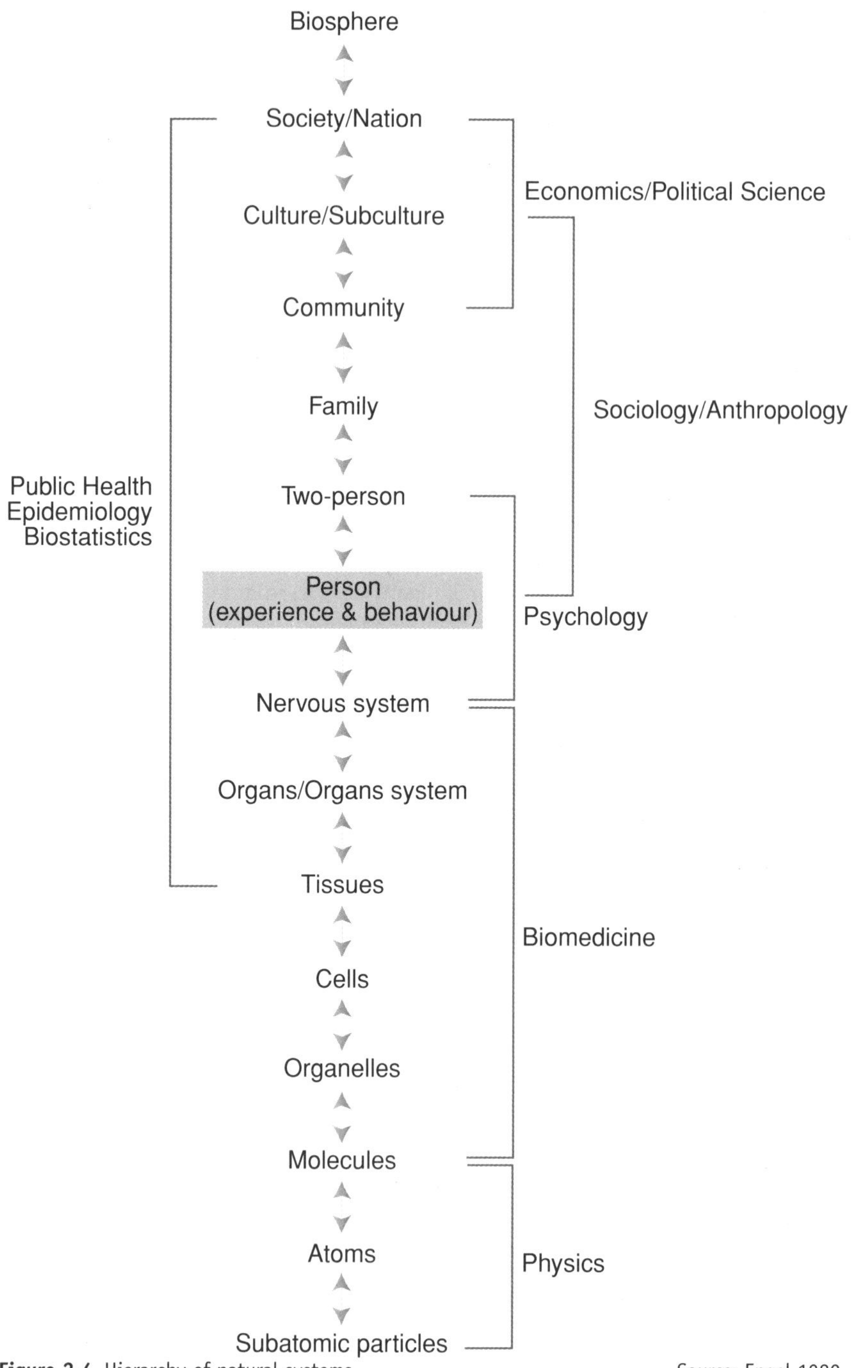

Figure 2.4 Hierarchy of natural systems *Source*: Engel 1980

chains, flowchart effects, and feedback loops. Second, analysis is necessarily multidisciplinary in nature, but the hierarchy does not operate in a reductionistic fashion nor privilege one level over another. Clearly, Anderson concludes, professionals working across disciplines need to practise 'intellectual stretching' in order to become more accomplished vertical thinkers (Anderson 1996).

2.5.1.2 The proximate determinants framework

An early example of vertical reasoning applied to a priority international health problem is Mosley and Chen's (1984) proximate determinants framework. Their framework was developed to improve research strategies directed towards child survival in developing countries. Mosley and Chen observed that social science approaches usually link wider socioeconomic factors with child mortality rates. In contrast, medical researchers look for disease causation factors, such as poor diet or environmental contamination, to explain morbidity and the prevalence of disease in the surviving population. Each approach has weaknesses. The way in which social structure causes disease is not explained in the first, while the second leaves out wider socioeconomic causes and does not include the burden of mortality as an effect. The proposed proximate determinants are intermediate variables or mechanisms, grouped into five areas, which explain how socioeconomic factors make an impact on the lives of individuals. The five determinants are:

- maternal factors (for example, age, parity)
- environmental contamination (for example, food, water, insect vectors)
- nutrient deficiency (for example, protein, vitamins)
- injury
- personal illness control (for example, personal prevention and medical care).

Subsequently, Ann Millard (1994) revised Mosley and Chen's framework to emphasise how the intermediate or proximate factors (such as mother's education or local dietary practices) depended on socioeconomic conditions in the 'ultimate tier' of causal influences. Millard found that some researchers place responsibility for proximate causes (for example, child spacing, poor diets, hygiene, childcare practices, failure to attend medical clinics) on the family or culture of the child. Millard's detailed local studies of child-rearing practices led her to query explanations blaming 'harmful' local customs or the supposed ignorance of mothers for high rates of child mortality. She argues that factors on the intermediate level in her framework arise from lack of resources, working outside the home for cash, or giving up subsistence farming to grow crops for sale. In turn, these may all be caused by wider economic trends, from local to global in scale, which affect the availability of food, types of childcare practices, and the exposure of children to pathogens. Consequently, these conditions determine how many and which

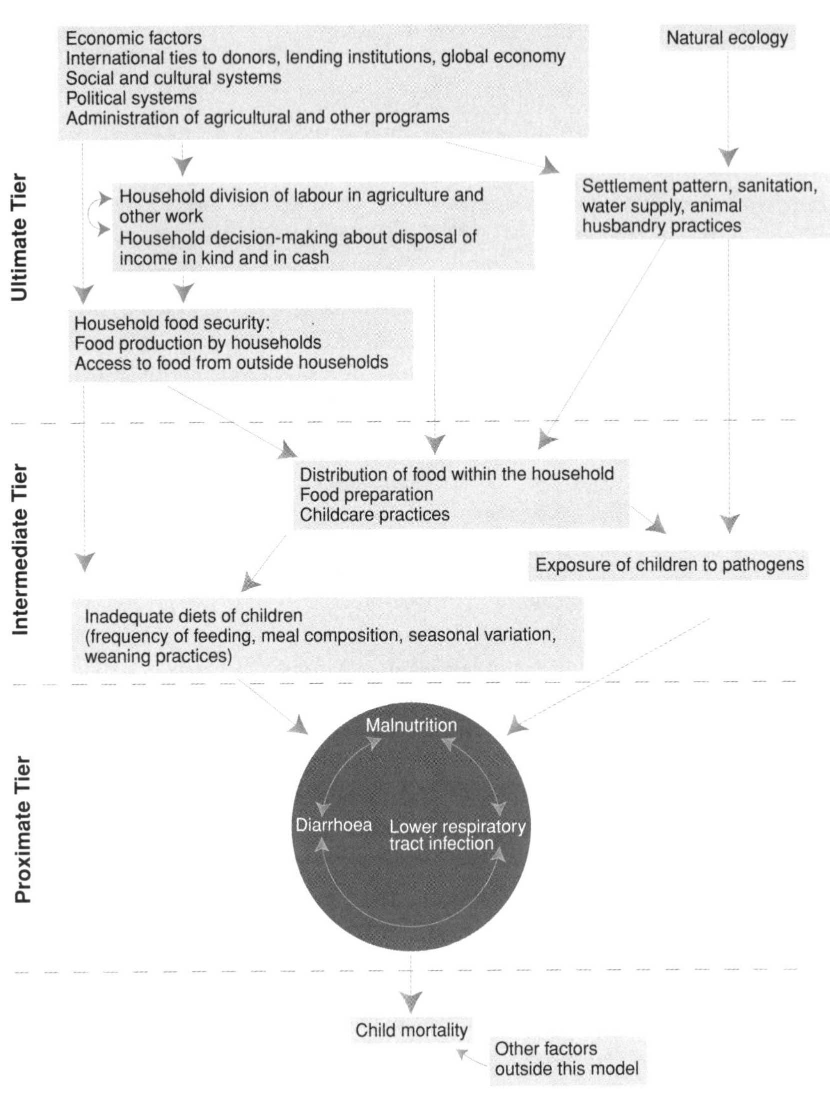

Source: Millard 1994

Figure 2.5 Three tiers of causes of high rates of child mortality

children will succumb to diseases such as the 'synergistic triad' of malnutrition, lower respiratory tract infection, and diarrhoea (Millard 1994) as shown in figure 2.5.

2.5.1.3 Health psychology frameworks

Health psychology, with its focus on the role of behaviour (thoughts, attitudes, beliefs, and actions) in the maintenance of health and in the development of illness, operates within a biopsychosocial model. It embraces vertical reasoning as a logical approach to studying health issues (Bloom 1988; Friedman and DiMatteo 1989; Kaplan et al. 1993; Taylor 1999). While there is a commitment in theory to study the natural interactions among the three domains—the biology, psychology, and sociology of health (Bloom 1988)—as yet little consensus has emerged on how best to conceptualise the connections between these different levels. Consequently, much of health psychology theorising and research still maintains a focus on the individual as the main level of analysis (see Spicer and Chamberlain 1996).

A notable exception to this is the pioneering work of Winette, King, and Altman (1989). These authors created a strategic framework for integrating health psychology and public health in order to more comprehensively understand health problems and design interventions for improving them. At the heart of their approach is the process of multilevel analysis (another name for vertical reasoning) in which a problem, such as smoking among teenagers, is systematically analysed from four perspectives: the personal, interpersonal, organisational, and institutional. Multilevel analysis will suggest interventions that combine individual change strategies (the forté of psychology) with system change strategies (tools of public health). Multilevel analysis will also specify how to evaluate a program's impact, involving multiple outcomes at multiple levels (Winette et al. 1989).

Limitations

While vertical reasoning encourages intellectual stretching to link disciplines and approaches that may be relevant to a problem, the means for systematically drawing together fields of knowledge have not been worked out among the theorists reviewed. Neither have criteria been developed for identifying relevant levels of analysis and choosing among knowledge bases. As a result, disciplines and whole fields of knowledge not considered in an exercise of vertical reasoning may be the most crucial for a full understanding of a problem.

2.5.2 Ecological frameworks

The term *ecology* refers broadly to 'the interrelationships between organisms and their environments' (Hawley, cited in Stokols 1992, p. 8). Three ecological approaches have evolved which use various assumptions and methods to address complex health problems:

1 *Biocultural* approaches integrate biological and cultural data on how humans adapt to various environments.
2 *Social ecology* analyses people–environment transactions in specific sociocultural and physical contexts.
3 *Ecological public health* emphasises the connection between humans and their physical and social environments and devises strategies for improving the health-enhancing ability of various settings, such as cities.

2.5.2.1 Biocultural approaches

The biocultural approach analyses the interactions between biological, cultural, and ecological factors that affect human well-being. It is found in several fields of study, including human biology, sociobiology, bioarchaeology, physical anthropology, and medical anthropology (mainly through theory and methods of medical ecology) (McElroy 1990a, p. 243).

The concept of *adaptation* is central to biocultural research. McElroy and Townsend have defined biocultural adaptation as 'changes and modifications that enable a person or group to survive in a given environment' (1999, pp. 11–12).

Theories of adaptation use the concept of an ecosystem defined as 'a set of relationships among organisms and their environment' (McElroy and Townsend 1999, p. 25). An ecosystem model of health is composed of the non-living physical (or abiotic) environment, the biotic environment, and the sociocultural environment. The three parts are interdependent and continually in interaction. Change in one variable often leads to change in another and may result in social, ecological, or physiological imbalances. Severe imbalances may result in stress or disease (McElroy and Townsend 1999, pp. 25–6).

Limitations

The biocultural approach has been criticised on a number of grounds. First, the central concept of adaptation lacks clarity and fails to recognise human agency in constructing environments (Leatherman 1996). Second, unstated assumptions and value judgments relating to consensus theory underpin analyses of ecosystems.[1] It presumes that any form of change threatens a part or the whole of the system and requires some form of adaptation to restore social equilibrium. The implication is that humans should not strive to change society but rather to maintain existing economic, political, and social arrangements—the status quo. It is difficult to reconcile this kind of thinking with political economy (see below) based on the notion that conflict between groups with differing social, economic, or political interests is the main mechanism for bringing about change in society. Third, biocultural researchers are criticised for not paying enough attention to macrosocial and political processes of ecological systems and in particular to political–economic factors.

Researchers using a political ecology approach have addressed this third criticism to some extent by incorporating analyses of interactions between various groups, classes, or nations that affect the ecology through changes in land use, shifts in population, or restrictions on access to resources (Leatherman 1996, p. 478; Brown 1998, p. 5). Political ecology also focuses on stratification caused by political systems and shows how it is related to patterns of disease (Brown et al. 1996, p. 200).

2.5.2.2 Social ecology

Social ecology provides a 'general framework for understanding the nature of people's transactions with their physical and sociocultural surroundings' (Stokols 1992, p. 7). Social ecology draws on insights from human ecology, ecological psychology, and social epidemiology. However, whereas these models are mainly concerned with biological processes and the geographical environment, social ecology places greater emphasis on 'social, institutional and cultural contexts of people–environment relations' (Stokols 1992, p. 7).

Multilevel analyses, which incorporate personal, organisational, and institutional features, are used to provide explanations of complex problems, including the dynamics of human health (Stokols 1992, p. 12). There is a commitment to interdisciplinary efforts that draw together knowledge from various fields. For example, in relation to a complex health issue, an environmental scientist might contribute information about air and water quality, a psychologist might contribute data about the impact of noise on stress levels, and an environmental designer might offer insight into the influence of physical space and lighting on well-being (University of California, Irvine, School of Social Ecology 1992, p. 2).

The concept of transactionalism is used to describe the interdependence between people and place. Occupants of various settings, rather than simply reacting to environmental stressors, actively participate in the creation and management of their surroundings (Stokols 1988, p. 233). Systems theory informs the idea that people–environment relations are dynamic rather than static, and are characterised as much by departures from equilibrium as by equilibrium maintenance (Stokols 1988, p. 235).

Social ecologists use a range of methods for assessing the healthfulness of settings and the well-being of individuals and groups (for example, medical examination, questionnaires, behavioural observations, environmental recordings, and epidemiologic analyses). They emphasis action research[2] and multilevel interventions combining complementary and synergistic behavioural and environmental strategies (Stokols 1992, p. 18).

While social ecologists focus on transactions in specific settings such as hospitals or neighbourhoods, analysis assumes that local behaviour and conditions exist as parts of broader regional or global contexts. Local and global settings are increasingly interdependent because of ease of travel, and technological and social changes. Hence, a real strength of the social ecology of public health is its attention to the dynamic interplay between local and global elements (for example, toxic waste, degraded natural resources, large-scale conflict) as they impact on health status (Stokols 1992, p. 7). Those working in the health promotion field have also been involved in the organisation and evaluation of the Healthy Cities movement (Greater Irvine Health Promotion Center 1993, pp. 4–5), discussed below.

Limitations

When social ecologists describe the people-environment relations in a particular cultural context, their analyses (following biopsychosocial traditions) fail to include ethnographic or phenomenological analyses of lived experiences. Furthermore, the social ecology model is extremely detailed, leading to problems in applying its concepts (for example, transactionalism). Even when appropriate research instruments are developed, social ecologists face a maze of interaction effects, making it difficult to translate research into action. What are the 'locations or levers for intervention' when, for example, complex interaction effects are discovered between family structure, race/ethnicity, neighbourhood poverty, parent perceptions of social disadvantage, and parental restrictiveness (Seidman 1994, p. 34)? Action researchers face the choice of either narrowing the scope of interventions or refining the nature of the ecological questions being asked (Seidman 1994).

2.5.2.3 Ecological public health and healthy cities

Ecological public health is an extension of the new public health, with its notion that 'health is intimately tied to overall living conditions'. The key to improving the health of populations lies outside the traditional domain of medicine and involves social reform (Chu 1994b, p. 3).

Health issues are assessed using the criteria of equity of access to resources (housing, education, social power), sustainability, defined as the capacity of social and economic developments to meet the needs of present and future generations, conviviality, expressed in terms of supportive social structures, harmonious interaction between community members, respect for non-human species, and preservation of the global environment through effective utilisation of resources (Chu 1994b, p. 4).

Strategies for promoting ecological public health are based on principles outlined in the 1986 *Ottawa Charter for Health Promotion* (Ashton 1986, p. 12). Projects are developed that promote health in various settings, including homes, schools, health service sectors, workplaces, communities, and cities

(Hancock 1992, p. 15). A key tool of ecological public health is the settings approach, a framework for coordinating a range of projects aimed at improving the environment and promoting health and quality of life for large populations (Chu 1994b, p. 2). WHO Healthy Cities movement is an example of a settings approach using the new public health principles to address links between sustainable development and health (Hancock 1992, p. 19). The Healthy Cities project started in European cities in 1986; by 1993 it had grown to an international movement with over 1200 projects, including about 100 in developing countries (Chu 1994a, p. 255).

In summary, ecological public health is 'multisectorial in scope', 'collaborative in strategy', and 'interdisciplinary in pursuit' (Kickbusch, cited in Chu 1994b, p. 1). It approaches a health problem holistically, examining the problem context as a whole system that has multiple causes and effects. Furthermore, democratic processes are encouraged, based on the view that research on communities needs to be participatory in nature (Hancock 1992, p. 8).

Limitations

Ecological public health is by no means a united framework. Differences arise because researchers use a variety of theoretical perspectives, including social exchange, ecology, functionalism, conflict theory, and general systems theory (Chu and Rickson 1994, p. 84). The role of natural science methods in analysing interrelationships between local and global social systems is one contested area, with some arguing that social theory and historical processes are more appropriate (Enzenberger, cited in Tesch 1988).

Another criticism is the universal application of the criterion of sustainable development and its underlying economic theory. Following the positivist[3] tradition, Labonte categorises economic theory as a natural science (1994, p. 21). This definition downplays the historical, social, and political forces and relations that influence the formation of economic theory and suggests a bias against dissent and change. Environmental impact statements derived from this perspective have been criticised as 'mostly a government means of controlling or reducing public dissent and participation in environmental affairs' (Chu and Rickson 1994, p. 83).

On the other hand, radical public health ecologists, defining the economy as a political process, address health issues relating to sustainable development in terms of the 'social, ecological and ethical implications of economic activity' (Hancock 1994, p. 42). These ecologists are committed to improving public health by 'replacing the fundamental ideology of economic thought', a stance that is 'subversive of the status quo' (Hancock 1994, p. 43). A practical limitation is that studies proposing radical structural solutions to health problems are ignored or underutilised by authorities; researchers adopting this perspective find it difficult to obtain funding (Singer 1995, pp. 81–2).

One premise of ecological public health is that it is relatively easy to achieve broad community agreement about the kind of improvements needed for a healthy city and that, generally speaking, the citizens are all pulling in a similar direction. However, such consensus may be an exceptional circumstance; ecological public health advocates may need to acknowledge that conflict and change are also part of a healthy city. Similarly, the settings strategy needs to more fully consider that there is no single urban way of life that can be identified and that ways of life do not necessarily correspond with geographic settings (see Higginbotham et al. 1999).

2.5.3 Political economy and globalisation theories

The political economy perspective is an example of a conflict model of society, as opposed to a consensus model.[4] Understood from the political economy perspective, diseases are only the 'proximate causes of suffering' which must be understood in terms of 'ultimate aetiologies' which derive from social, political, and economic inequality (Inhorn and Brown 1990, p. 109). Inequality is analysed in terms of power relations shaped primarily by social class, but also by race, ethnicity, and gender. *Dependency* or *world systems* theory, developed in the 1960s and 1970s, influenced many medical anthropologists concerned with health problems in developing countries (see Morgan 1987). Dependency theory, as espoused by writers such as Andre Gunder Frank and Emmanuel Wallerstein, holds that health problems in developing countries are 'inter-woven with the political–economic functioning of the capitalist world system' (Elling, cited in Morsy 1990, p. 34). Rather than dealing with health in reductionist terms which analyse biological or cultural properties in isolation from their association with lesser systems, political economy looks at health in terms of the imperative of capitalist investment (profit) and the role of the state (such as national governments) in supporting the capitalist economy. Thus, for political economists, economic systems, political power, and ideologies are dialectically related to biological, cultural, social, and experiential aspects of sickness and healing (Morsy 1996, p. 22).

Political economy analyses of the relationship between work and health are concerned with threats to individual workers from unsafe and exploitative work practices and dangerous environments, including harmful substances. Typically, these analyses examine how the social relations of capitalist production determine the conditions in the workplace that put the worker at risk of illness or injury. The emergence of increasingly globalised economic relationships has made it clear that arrangements between social groups that impact on health are not confined to local boundaries, such as a factory. Rather, they arise from power relationships operating at regional, national, or global levels (Morsy 1996, p. 24). Thus, an analysis of health problems linked to pollution from a factory in an industrialised country may look at the way power struggles between competing groups influence regulations governing protection of the environment and safety in the workplace. Power struggles on a global scale, such as competition between multinationals for world markets, or relationships between political élites, multinationals, and organisations governing world trade, may be relevant to health issues manifesting at a local level. In chapter 6 we use a political economy perspective to discuss the effect that globalisation has had on world trade as it relates to the production, sale, and distribution of pharmaceutical products.

Political economy also addresses social and power relations that affect the production and dissemination of knowledge. For example, Nash and Kirsch (1988) investigated corporate attempts in the United States of America to suppress epidemiological data supporting opposition to the production and use of health-threatening chemicals (PCBs) (cited in Morsy 1990, p. 38; Morsy 1996, p. 28). In other words, there is a focus on the power relations surrounding the discourse of medical science itself.

In brief, political economy of health, incorporating economic globalisation perspectives, develops the strong connection between the politics, economics, and history of a society or of an interdependent world system, the relative power and vulnerability of groups within it, and the consequent health status of populations and specific groups and categories of people. Specifically, in the political economy framework, the causes of disease among disadvantaged social groups are identified as powerlessness within an increasingly globalised economic order and lack of access to the basic resources that sustain health. For example, in capitalist society, alcoholism is redefined from a personal sickness to a feature of the economic system whereby the pursuit of profits (and taxes) promotes alcohol's use and abuse. Supporting this perspective is a large body of research that consistently shows a clear gradient linking social class position and health status; society's privileged enjoy the best health while those with increasingly less power and wealth have increasingly worse health (for example, Adler et al. 1994).

Limitations

The political economy approach attempts to overcome the limitations of other models that neglect macro social, political, and economic determinants of ill health. However, by analysing health largely in terms of capitalist social relations, political economy limits its universal application (not all social systems are capitalist to the same degree and in the same ways) and depersonalises health promotion and protection. To some extent, theories of economic globalisation address the shortcomings of political economy by shifting the focus from an ideal type of capitalist society to the situation of economic and political interconnectedness of all societies on a global scale. But theories such as political economy and economic globalisation imply that there is little that people can do to protect themselves from illness and that disease prevention is a macro process.

The world systems variant of political economy has been criticised on the basis that it depends on outdated ideal types (for example, 'core' and 'periphery') and that it focuses on the sphere of economic production to the neglect of distribution and consumption relations. Moreover, it has been suggested that it is unable to provide empirically satisfactory explanations for causes of ill health in precapitalist and socialist countries. To overcome these limitations, Donahue suggests that all health systems should be analysed in terms of the historically specific, concrete conditions of the particular political economy in which they are embedded. Research methods should address how specific health strategies are negotiated among several interest groups within the political economy and how the outcome compares to the stated goals of the political system (cited in Morsy 1990, p. 43).

A central argument of some political economists is that biomedicine maintains rather than alleviates inequality and that researchers who use biomedical categories have been 'co-opted by the intellectual hegemony of Western biomedicine' (Brown and Inhorn 1990, p. 109). This has led to criticism that political economy is a blaming or culprit-seeking perspective (Morsy 1990, p. 32). Such a stance represents a barrier to integrating material from the basic sciences or from frameworks that draw from the biomedical model.

2.5.4 Health transition

A final framework emerging from the intersection of demography, related social sciences, and epidemiology is termed *health transition* (Caldwell and Santow 1989). Previously, population scientists described changes across time for societies with reference to declines in childbirth rates (fertility transition), infant mortality or crude death rates (mortality transition), and infectious disease relative to chronic disease causes of morbidity and death (epidemiological transition). Health transition, as defined by Caldwell and his colleagues, is a broader concept, because it seeks to relate changes in a group's epidemiological profile to social change. Specifically, it is concerned with the cultural, social, and behavioural determinants of health, that is, nearly all the determinants except the material standards of living, medical interventions, and public health interventions (Caldwell 1994, p. 13). Health transition is a 'process through which high levels of mortality, morbidity and disability are reduced to low levels by influencing cultural, social and behavioural factors . . . such as educational levels among males and females, the age and sex composition of the population, and habits like alcohol consumption and smoking' (Reddy 1995, p. 250). In essence, change or transition is reflected in shifts in the ways that individuals and communities perceive and respond to their own health and ill health (Cleland and Hill 1991).

Early health transition research examined how individuals behave within households or local communities (Caldwell et al. 1990). As behaviour changes that more directly prevent disease or restore health occur, the historical course of a health transition is set in motion. Such a perspective attributes great importance to the history of literacy and education, especially among women, and makes men and women into agents of the health transition (Johansson 1995, p. 227). For example, the steep decline in infant mortality in some developing countries is seen as a symbiosis between educational and social change on the one hand, and increased access to curative and preventive medicine on the other. The specific role of maternal education in improving child survival is to fully and assertively make use of the health care system for their sick children without delay (Caldwell 1992, p. 213). More recently, the HIV/AIDS epidemic, particularly in sub-Saharan Africa, has commanded the attention of health transition researchers. Combining demographic surveys and ethnographic methods, this work seeks to understand how households and communities are functioning in the face of the epidemic and how social and cultural conditions affect vulnerability to HIV infection (for example, Ntozi et al. 1997; Caldwell et al. 1999).

Limitations

While health transition research is often policy oriented, there is the belief that its findings can have an enormous effect on health even if no specific interventions follow from them. This effect would be achieved directly through the public awareness of such findings, mainly through the media, as people achieve greater knowledge of themselves and institutions gain greater knowledge of the people (Caldwell 1995, p. 255). Unfortunately, a convincing demonstration of this trickle-down and through effect has yet to be performed. Meanwhile, there is growing evidence that intensely proactive methods are needed to translate research findings into institutional and behaviour change (for example, Lomas 1993).

2.6 Lessons from interdisciplinary frameworks for transdisciplinary health social science

What can we carry forward from our review of the interdisciplinary fields of study described above that can inform a transdisciplinary health social science that is responsive to the complexity inherent in human health and which brings diverse disciplines into productive relationships?

The value of the *vertical reasoning* frameworks is their demonstration that we must move across different levels of analysis, from micro to macro, to locate sets of health problem influences. In some way, we need to range back and forth between descriptions of molecules, bodies, ecologies, and so forth, to find connections and relationships. The researchers working across disciplinary traditions need to practise intellectual stretching to become vertical thinkers. A practical, visual tool for linking levels of influence is the flow diagram, as offered by Mosley and Chen (1984). A useful principle is presentation of pathways connecting immediate (proximate) influences with more remote determinants (intermediate and distal) of the health problem.

The *ecological* frameworks teach us to take a whole system approach, emphasising the often hidden interconnections between parts. A key principle of interrelation is the concept of 'energy flow'. For *biocultural* researchers, energy flow is a way of calculating ecological dynamics. If energy increases, the system is evolving to a new level of energy dynamics; depletion in energy indicates degradation of the environment and society (Anderson 1996, pp. 186–7). When analysed in terms of the principles of complexity theory (to be discussed in the next chapter), the concept of energy flow has the potential to be an integrating mechanism. It can free biocultural analyses from the limitations of reductionist consensus theories of equilibrium maintenance of a whole or a part of bounded systems.

One of the most useful aspects of *social ecology* is the emphasis on a diverse range of dynamic processes affecting human health. In the past, researchers from the health psychology and biopsychosocial fields have concentrated on links between psychological and behavioural factors in health. However, a more ecological version of health promotion examines the dynamic interplay between biological, psychological, and behavioural elements affecting health and well-being and multiple facets of both the physical and the social environments (Stokols 1992, p. 12). An important direction for future research, which has the potential to draw together many disciplines, is the identification of specific mechanisms by which these factors influence health and illness (Stokols 1992, pp. 12–13).

Ecological public health is inclusive and multisectorial, bringing together government representatives, professionals, community members, and other stakeholders from a variety of areas. This has resulted in a range of problems relating to integration of sometimes radically different points of view. While not all problems have been solved, ecological public health offers valuable insights into integrating researchers with other stakeholders in health problems. One persisting problem is confusion over who should have input into decision-making in various areas and what weight should be given to different knowledge bases. Will expert advice be sought in a variety of fields related to the project ('exhausted specialist mode') or will researchers interpret a little of every set of information ('superficial generalist mode') (Brown 1994, p. 58)? Furthermore, how are ecological public health researchers to forge connections between various knowledge bases and the 'relative emphases they give to various faces of the truth' (Brown 1994, p. 59)? These dilemmas suggest that as well as constructing conceptual frameworks for research, consideration needs to be given to the development of integrating guidelines for the practical application of multidisciplinary, multisectorial research.

Ecological public health researchers such as Hancock (1992) are open to new scientific developments, including chaos or complexity theory, which challenge old understandings of the world, particularly in relation to complex biological systems (Hancock 1992, p. 9). Finally, radical ecologists link public health with the quest for social justice, and argue that health promotion at the local level must address issues of peace, sustainability, and equity in terms of alternative economic models based on the concepts and values that underpin the Green political movement (Hancock 1994, pp. 42–5). These social justice connections are worth keeping in mind.

One of the most useful aspects of the *political economy* and *globalisation* approaches is the notion that micro and macro, local and global, or biological and social level analyses are not mutually exclusive. They are dialectically related. Dialectical explanations do not analyse parts in isolation from their relationship to wholes; they see the properties of parts as arising out of their associations. The bio-cultural view of health is 'a measure of how well a population has adapted to its environment' (Townsend and McElroy 1992, p. 11). The political economy perspective sees health as 'affected by an environment produced by the dialectical interaction of natural and sociocultural forces' (Baer 1996, p. 453).

2.7 The development of transdisciplinary thinking in health social science

Although scientists and philosophers offered insights into complex, dynamic systems for much of the twentieth century, it was not until the 1970s that systems thinking began to systematically challenge the linear and traditional disciplinary approach to human knowledge. Philosopher Erich Jantsch was one of the first scholars to argue that humans require a *transdisciplinary* way of thinking to interpret and understand dynamism and interaction (1972, pp. 215–41). Jantsch envisioned a transdisciplinary university to house the multilevel coordination of research, education, and innovation associated with the increasing complexity in all fields of human activity. He observed that 'the essential characteristic of a trans disciplinary approach is the coordination of activities at *all* levels of the education/innovation system' (1972, p. 234). While Jantsch's ideas have appealed to academics prepared to work beyond the constraints of a traditional university, transdisciplinary research and publications, until very recently, have been scarce.[5]

It was not until the 1990s that an international transdisciplinary movement began to take shape, including the 1994 First World Congress of Transdisciplinarity held in Portugal. This Congress issued a charter to guide like-minded researchers of all countries (Nicolescu 1998). The current textbook is the first monograph-length statement calling for recognition that, especially in the domains of environmental and human health, a new transdisciplinary paradigm[6] or way of knowing is a necessary next step in the understanding of complexity in all of its forms.

2.7.1 Teaching and promoting transdisciplinary thinking in health social science

In 1987 the International Clinical Epidemiology Network (INCLEN) sought to include social science perspectives in the Rockefeller-initiated program to build population health research capacity within key teaching hospitals in Asia, Latin America, and Africa (White 1991, chapter 8). In response to this opportunity, we created a new masters-level curriculum in 1988 aimed at teaching health social scientists how to apply a transdisciplinary perspective to conceptualise and study health problems (Higginbotham 1992). At that time we argued:

> The health social science perspective is part of a growing worldwide awareness of the importance of a *transdisciplinary* model that, together with biomedical level analysis, gives a comprehensive understanding of the aetiology of disease and restoration of human health (Higginbotham and Albrecht 1988, p. 3).

In essence, this textbook distils our transdisciplinary health social science curriculum as it has evolved since 1988, with contributions from our INCLEN colleagues globally as well as our own research experience. Subsequently, when the International Forum for Social Science in Health emerged as a global organisation for developing health social science as a scientific community and strengthening the social science contribution to improving human health, transdisciplinary thinking was adopted as a unifying philosophy among its members. Advancing a TD perspective became central to the organisation's mission (IFFSH 1993; Higginbotham 1994 and 1998; Higginbotham, Albrecht, and Freeman 1998).

Albrecht (1990) laid the philosophical foundation for a complexity-based approach to transdisciplinary thinking about human health that underpins our research and writing in this field. A core component of TD thinking, he argues, is the realisation that problems exist beyond the boundaries of all disciplines, in the realm of transdisciplinary space (Albrecht 1990, p. 5):

> Given that health problems arise from the interactions of multiple causative variables, each of which is the domain of a discipline, then the health problem itself can be said to exist in 'transdisciplinary space'. That is, the problem exists in a space that is beyond the explanatory power of any one discipline (Albrecht and Higginbotham 1992).

Patricia Rosenfield significantly advanced transdisciplinary research in the health social sciences by publishing the first definition of this new perspective and demonstrating its application to slowing the spread of malaria in the Brazilian Amazon (see below). Rosenfield showed how the transdisciplinary perspective works by encouraging discipline-based researchers to transcend their separate orientations in order to develop a shared approach to the investigation and to seek a 'common conceptual framework' (Rosenfield 1992, p. 1351). In chapter 4 we discuss common conceptual frameworks further, as an element of TD thinking.

2.8 Conclusion

A new transdisciplinary health social science, building on the insights above, would have several essential attributes. It would:

- engage vertical thinking (up and down the health hierarchy)
- adopt ecological principles (such as energy flows) that don't assume a closed system
- accept multiple sectors and stakeholders as essential actors
- use explicit guidelines for cross-disciplinary collaboration
- identify the mutual effects of local and global interactions
- acknowledge power relations and consensus in social organisation
- recognise that the totality of the health problem follows both historical (that is, dialectic) and evolutionary processes
- seek to create emergent conceptual frameworks.

Before completing this chapter, we need to raise a general problem to be avoided in building a transdisciplinary health social science. This is the temptation among researchers, imbued with the enthusiasm for holism, to incorporate aspects from other theories into their own perspective with little understanding of their theoretical bases. Mosley and Chen (1984) point out that biomedical researchers tend to treat social factors as 'explanatory black boxes—the internal mechanisms of which are unknown. Social scientists, on the other hand, may view physiological factors the same way' (cited in Kunstadter 1990, p. 353). For holistic research, drawing on several disciplinary fields and theories, we may require the 'non-discipline of cross-sectorial workers whose major task is to translate across existing disciplines' (see Nelson 1989, cited in Labonte 1992, p. 21).

The next chapter describes complexity theory as an important tool for health social scientists who have begun to understand that health and disease, like other phenomena, are expressions of complex adaptive systems. The role of disciplines and interdisciplinary fields of study in investigating the properties of evolving systems becomes clearer within this context. They all have a part to play in explicating the dynamics of such systems where factors that can influence evolution can range from the micro to the macro in scope and scale.

We have chosen to focus on complexity theory in the next chapter because it is a new transdisciplinary approach that displays the potential to unite previous disciplinary and interdisciplinary fields of study in the pursuit of common features and patterns of activity within all types of complex adaptive systems. Such an ambitious project seeks nothing less than the unification of the diverse approaches to health and disease—the social sciences with the physical, biological, and medical sciences. We are aware that many readers will already be operating within interdisciplinary fields of knowledge and that many will have already incorporated aspects of systems and complexity theory into their perspectives on health. In the next chapter, we attempt to systematically establish the relevance and importance of complexity theory to the transdisciplinary understanding of human health. However, readers who feel that they are already familiar with this approach may prefer to go directly to our discussion of transdisciplinary health social science in chapter 4.

Notes

1 Consensus theories are discussed in chapter 6 (see 6.2).

2 Action research is an empowering process in which the participants are 'partners in the research process' (Punch 1994, p. 89) and in which the goals are the solution to participant-identified problems.

3 Positivism is a theory of knowledge that emphasises the similarities between modes of research and explanation in the natural and the social sciences. In terms of positivism, scientific knowledge results from the observation of empirical phenomena and the formulation of laws about the relationships between phenomena. Ideally, the observer is a neutral and detached element in the research process and reality is independent of the observer's influence.

4 For an introductory discussion of these two types of social theory see chapter 6.

5 The word 'university' literally means 'towards unity'. The original function of a university was to educate people to enable them to obtain wisdom within the unity of knowledge.

6 Paradigm is a fairly loosely used word in the social sciences, and is often interchangeable with other terms such as 'framework', 'perspective', and 'approach'. In the more specific sense, stemming from the work of philosopher of science Thomas Kuhn, a paradigm is a way of understanding the world that implies certain theories that are linked to certain methods of conducting research. Trandisciplinary thinking can be viewed as a paradigm in this more specific sense.

3
Complexity and Human Health: Across the Health Hierarchy

GLENN ALBRECHT AND NICK HIGGINBOTHAM

3.1 Complexity theory: ideas that transcend disciplines

Human health is the outcome of complex processes that operate within and across physical, psychological, social, and ecological systems. Recognition of such processes pushes our way of thinking about health problems into frameworks that reflect this interrelatedness. Detailed knowledge of *complex, adaptive, dynamic systems* cannot come from within the narrow focus of specific traditional disciplines. We need to have the ability to situate health problems within networks of interrelated information and insight. To understand such interrelated phenomena, we need to understand complexity.

In the previous chapter we used the concept of the health hierarchy to explore how health problems can be seen as the result of interactions between humans, and between humans and their environment. We saw that these elements and their interactions range from individuals' subjective experiences and cultural influences to the impact of global climate change. In this chapter, we locate such interaction within the overarching theory of complexity. We summarise the new developments in complexity theory over the last decade that attempt to explain the full scope of these interactions. Complexity theory is now applied across a great variety of disciplines to more fully understand biophysical systems, human social systems, and expressions of human culture and creativity. We believe that complexity theory is capable of providing greater insight into both the nature of disorder and the emergence of new forms of order within systems, but especially within health-related systems.

We now describe the theoretical features of complexity theory in order to examine how it can be used to understand and inform problems of human health.[1] In order to understand the impact and novelty of complexity theory, we first examine earlier theories that attempted to describe complex systems and their characteristics.

3.2 The evolution of complexity theory

3.2.1 Newtonian reductionism and determinism

The image of the world that Newton (1642–1727) and his followers described was essentially machine-like (mechanistic) and deterministic (rule governed). In a Newtonian world, a finite number of rules or laws govern the motion of material bodies and these laws are universal. All other aspects of the 'world-machine' can similarly be determined; a complete account of the workings of parts of the machine is thought possible. In mechanistically unified structures, such as those Newton described, it is entirely valid to break down the structure of large things into smaller things in order to study them, because a complete account of the parts will constitute an account of the whole. An important outcome of this perspective, which is characterised as *reductionism* in the philosophy of science, is the idea that ultimately *all* things can be explained through mechanistic and deterministic laws. The use of the machine metaphor implies that regularity and order is the norm for complex systems and that instability or unpredictable change is the exception.

Newton's laws of motion worked well at one level of human experience. Newtonian laws have been successfully applied in producing technologies from sewing machines to jet aircraft. The relationships between the variables in mechanistically unified systems are described as *linear*. Within *linear systems* parts are related to each other in ways that do not change the nature of the whole. We can describe what will happen in linear systems and plot causally related variables on a graph. The relationship between cause and effect will be proportional, since under normal circumstances a large causal force will produce a large effect. With detailed knowledge of initial states and the environment within which they operate, linear systems are capable of precise mathematical description and offer high degrees of predictability. For example, a large input of energy into an engine will produce a proportionately large output of work or horsepower.

However, at more theoretical levels Newton's laws were counterintuitive. In a Newtonian universe, if we had absolute knowledge of all laws and rules governing matter, we could, with equal plausibility, reconstruct the past or predict the future since time sequences within linear systems are, in principle, reversible. As physicist and popular writer on complexity Paul Davies explains:

> Newtonian time derives from a very basic property of the laws of motion: they are reversible. That is, the laws do not distinguish 'time forwards' from 'time backwards'; the arrow of time can point either way. From the standpoint of these laws, a movie played in reverse would be a perfectly acceptable sequence of events (Davies 1989, p. 14).

Nineteenth-century physicists such as Clausius (1865) and Boltzmann (1872) challenged the idea of time's reversibility when they developed the idea that the universe is tending towards thermodynamic equilibrium. They were the first to develop what are called the first and second laws of thermodynamics. These laws state that:

1 The energy of the universe is constant.
2 Any closed system will tend spontaneously to a state of maximum possible disorder (entropy), that is the state of thermal equilibrium. Entropy is a measure of 'the degree of disorder' of a system (Pais 1991, p. 81).

The idea that entropy increases in a closed system (and, ultimately, in all open systems) suggests an 'inevitable element of irreversibility in mechanical systems in the course of time' (Pais 1991, p. 82). The implications of this view, however, were even more alarming than the theoretical Newtonian reversal of temporal order. The physicist von Helmholtz (1854) pointed out that if entropy always increases, then the universe is moving towards its own destruction. Paul Davies gives a graphic summary of this gradual running-down of the universe:

> The remorseless rise in entropy that accompanies any natural process could only lead in the end, said Helmholtz, to the cessation of all interesting activity throughout the universe, as the entire cosmos slides irreversibly into a state of thermodynamic equilibrium. Every day the universe depletes its stock of available potent energy, dissipating it into useless waste heat. This inexorable squandering of a finite resource implies that the universe is slowly but surely dying, choking in its own entropy (Davies 1989, p. 19).

The state of thermodynamic equilibrium can be understood with the help of an analogy. Consider what happens to a gas when it is put into a confined space, a see-through container. In the beginning, the gas is concentrated in a particular part of its container. If it were coloured, it would be seen to be swirling and moving in interesting ways. Different concentrations of the gas would appear as different shades or intensities of colour (that is, creative activity). However, once the supply is cut off and the container sealed, the gas is gradually dispersed or dissipated and takes up the entire volume of the container. At this point, we can describe the gas as evenly or homogeneously distributed within the container and its appearance as a uniform colour. *Equilibrium* has now been achieved and there is no longer any perceptible activity within the container. Hence, at the point of equilibrium, there is a cessation of all creative activity and process within the system. Conversely, the stage where creative activity takes place could be described as *far-from-equilibrium*.

According to the second law of thermodynamics (commonly known as the entropy law) the predicted fate of the heat death of the system within which we live (our planet) was not seriously challenged until the emergence of complexity theory in the 1970s. Complexity theory changed the nineteenth-century view of entropy as a force destructive of creative activity to one that might promote such activity.

The way physicists and others have come to this view is through the observation that systems that are open to an exchange of energy and matter (far-from-equilibrium) can display a creative tendency to self-organise in new and often unpredictable ways. Hence, in classical thermodynamics, there is order in the universe that is slowly dissipated or depleted into useless forms of energy. Such dissipation continues until all creative processes come to a halt at the point of equilibrium (movement from order to disorder). In what has come to be called *non-equilibrium thermodynamics* (NET), there is the suggestion that this process can be reversed in that there can be creative movement from disorder to order. It is important for readers who are unfamiliar with thermodynamics to appreciate this counterintuitive claim about the behaviour of complex systems and the terminology within complexity theory used to describe it. Disorder is ultimately connected to a state of equilibrium, while order is potentially connected to a state that is far-from-equilibrium.

3.2.2 Complex dynamic systems

A central claim of complexity theory is that spontaneous order and organisation can come from what appears to be flux and disorder in natural systems. The most recent form of complexity theory suggests that complex, open systems have distinctive properties that cannot be reduced to constituent parts. Paul Davies explains:

> In the traditional approach one regards complex systems as complicated collections of simple systems. That is, complex or irregular systems are in principle analysable into their simple constituents, and the behavior of the whole is believed to be reducible to the behavior of the constituent parts. The new approach treats complex or irregular systems as primary in their own right. They simply cannot be 'chopped up' into lots of simple bits and still retain their distinctive qualities (Davies 1989, p. 22).

Complexity theory advances perspectives on systems that run directly counter to all forms of reductionism and determinism. One strand of complexity theory, *chaos theory*, suggests that small, random changes to the parts of a system can give rise to large-scale or global changes to that system. Another strand of complexity theory emphasises the spontaneous generation of an emergent order in complex systems.[2] It is this *emergent order* that provides an alternative perspective on systems to the Newtonian paradigm. The production of greater complexity, new types of diversity, and novel spatial and temporal patterns and sequences in a variety of physical contexts suggests system behaviour more like that with which we are familiar in the biological realm. Hence, terms such as *adaptive*, *evolutionary*, and *self-organisation* can be applied to the understanding of matter and physical systems in general.

The new view of systems suggests that there is a class of systems that can be described as *complex adaptive systems* in that they actively change and evolve over time. *Adaptive* is the term used to describe the way complex systems change in response to changes in their environment. Complex systems are open to modify themselves in the face of pressure and perturbations from the wider environment within which they exist. They can co-evolve in interaction with other complex systems. Such systems display *non-linear* relationships between interacting variables whereby small changes to a small component of the system can produce a disproportionately large effect. Davies writes:

> In a non-linear system the whole is much more than the sum of its parts, and it cannot be reduced or analysed in terms of simple sub-units acting together. The resulting properties can often be unexpected, complicated and mathematically intractable (Davies 1989, p. 25).

3.2.3 Self-organisation and dissipative structures

A major claim within contemporary complexity theory is the idea that all the sciences, ranging from mathematics to biology and the social sciences, can now support the general hypothesis about the spontaneous evolution in life from the simple to the complex. The idea of increasing levels of complexity in an evolutionary view of the world is complemented by claims in complexity theory that all types of open systems have the potential to evolve *of their own accord* towards greater complexity. A constant theme that emerges in the literature is that new forms of complexity are achieved through spontaneous self-organisation. This means that there are no agents acting from outside the system that can account for the re-arrangement of the internal structure of a system to create greater order. The method by which this complexity evolves or self-organises is substantially explained through the idea of dissipative structures, or 'new dynamic states of matter' (Prigogine and Stengers 1984, p. 143).

Pioneering theorists of complexity, Prigogine and Stengers, describe this fundamental concept:

> We now know that far from equilibrium, new types of structures may originate spontaneously. In far-from-equilibrium conditions we may have transformation from disorder, from thermal chaos, into order. New dynamic states of matter may originate, states that reflect the interaction of a given system with its surroundings. We have called these new structures dissipative structures to emphasise the constructive role of dissipative processes in their formation (Prigogine and Stengers 1984, p. 12).

3.2.3.1 Dissipative structures

The most important discovery associated with complexity theory is that the second law of thermodynamics, the entropy law, while still having universal relevance, can be delayed or negated at local levels. By 'exporting entropy into its environment' (Davies 1989, p. 85), a dissipative structure can maintain its structural integrity and evade an increase in entropy. In order to maintain or increase coherence and complexity, a dissipative structure must exist in relationship with an *open system* where exchange of energy can take place. A dissipative structure creates an internal order that 'is far more efficient in utilising energy for organisation and maintenance than the background system within which the primary flux occurs' (Dyke, in Weber et al. 1988, p. 360).

The first law of thermodynamics states that the amount of energy in a closed system is constant. However, the second law also suggests that in a closed system (and open systems in a state far-from-equilibrium) the amount of usable energy (ranging from high to low) available for any process will always decrease. Within such systems there is an unequal distribution of energy available for use, ranging from high-level energy to useless waste heat. Left to its own devices, the system will inevitably move from a far-from-equilibrium situation to one that is termed *equilibrium*. There is movement from high-level energy to low-level energy, much like that involved in weather systems when the wind is caused by the movement of air from high- to low-pressure systems. We can term the difference between high and low pressure a *gradient*. This term is also applied to the differences between highly usable energy in a non-equilibrium system and energy that is highly degraded and in a system close-to-equilibrium.

At local levels, dissipative structures in non-living and living systems seem to defy the movement towards equilibrium and increasing disorder. Indeed, they increase complexity and diversity at local levels while entropy continues to increase at the global level. A reformulated second law of thermodynamics makes this apparent contradiction understandable. As Schneider and Kay explain, a restated second law states that 'the more a system is moved from equilibrium, the more sophisticated are its mechanisms for resisting being moved from equilibrium' (Schneider and Kay 1995, p. 165). As a result, any system self-organisation that assists in the process of eliminating the applied gradient will be an 'expected response of a system' (Schneider and Kay 1995, p. 165).

We can anticipate then that open, complex systems should adapt and self-organise to counteract the influence of an imposed energy gradient. The earth as a whole could be considered just such an open system, with the sun applying a large energy gradient upon it. Schneider and Kay argue that this energy challenge to the state of equilibrium is a major reason why the earth has its great diversity of life present in self-organising ecosystems. The diversity of life and ecosystem complexity is mainly a response to the imperative to dissipate energy in the gradient from high-quality (usable) to lower-quality (difficult to use) energy.

As evidence supporting such an hypothesis, Schneider and Kay point out that at the earth's equator, where five-sixths of the earth's solar radiation occurs, the greatest species diversity is present. They argue that:

> food chains are based on photosynthetic fixed material and further dissipate these gradients by making more highly ordered structures. Thus we would expect more species diversity to occur where there is more available energy (energy available to perform useful work) (Schneider and Kay 1995, p. 168).

Dissipative processes have been studied in many types of physical and biological systems and they are now being identified in human social systems. Examples of dissipative structures in physical systems include cyclones, twisters, autocatalytic chemical reactions, and convection cells. All types of biological systems can be considered to be dissipative structures.

In physical systems, a now well-known illustration of a dissipative process is the Belousov-Zhabatinski (BZ) autocatalytic chemical reaction. The experiment involves a number of chemicals that react with each other in a system kept open with pumps. When chemical throughput is slow there appears to be an even distribution of chemicals, as indicated by a lack of dominance of any one colour from dyes that are injected to indicate excess ions of a particular chemical. The system could be described as close-to-equilibrium. However, when the flow rate increases and the system moves far-from-equilibrium, the reaction changes such that it manifests a blue colour, indicating that a particular ion has increased its concentration. It stays blue for a short time then changes to red, indicating that another ion has come to predominate. The system then oscillates from blue to red with regularity so precise that Prigogine calls the reaction a 'chemical clock'. Barton explains that this regularity

> occurs because the chemical processes that result in the red state coming into existence become linked to the processes resulting in the blue state. When this happens, the two states codetermine one another in a cyclical, nonlinear fashion (Barton 1994, p. 7).

The BZ reaction and other similar observations of emergent self-organisation such as the Bénard convection cell (Sandar and Abrams 1999, pp. 75–6) reveal in experimental contexts forms of self-organising behaviour in matter. These sorts of self-organisation discovered in chemical and other non-living processes were previously thought only to operate at more complex levels in living systems. Complexity theory has developed to the point where theorists have speculated on the possibility that there might be common properties and dynamic processes operating across all types of complex natural systems. Complexity theorist Stuart Kauffman argues for the concept of a background natural order with which all other ordering processes interact. Kauffman suggests that:

> contrary to our deepest intuitions, massively disordered systems can spontaneously 'crystallize' a very high degree of order. Much of the order we see in organisms may be the direct result not of natural selection but of the natural order selection was privileged to act on (Kauffman 1993, p. 173).

The problem for students of complexity, despite the idea that all complex systems may be subject to common physical laws, is that such systems can change in ways that are unpredictable when in a state far-from-equilibrium. There is potential for either greater complexity or greater disorder; unless one has complete knowledge of all initial and boundary conditions, uncertainty will dominate. In simple systems, where boundary conditions can be accurately specified (such as controlled chemical reactions), we know that dissipative structures will become more complex as they adapt and change over time. This insight offers some hope that complexity can be clearly understood. Davies also suggests that we can develop 'idealised complex or irregular systems' (Davies 1989, p. 23) that will assist in approximating the features of real systems. The concept of an *attractor* within complex systems provides further opportunity to offer detailed explanation of the order that arises out of dynamically changing systems.

3.2.4 Factors that influence the evolution of complex adaptive systems

This section examines two factors that can influence the evolution of complex adaptive systems. First, regularities are discoverable within systems that display apparently chaotic behaviour in the face of disturbances. Second, *attractors* are features within a system that determine or influence the course of its evolution.

3.2.4.1 Disturbance or perturbation

When complex systems are disturbed we might expect that such disturbances could contribute to system breakdown or failure. Indeed, this is often the case if the magnitude or speed of disturbance (for example, a volcanic eruption such as that of Krakatau in 1883) is so great that adaptive responses to the change induced is impossible. In addition, systems that are already unstable will experience great changes even if small disturbances affect them. Small changes to the initial conditions of a chaotic system can lead to cascades of unpredictable change in that system.

However, complexity theorists have suggested that certain levels of disturbance can generate creative system reconfiguration. They have developed the concept of a state called 'the edge of chaos', where the forces of order and disorder come into competition. Such competition produces order within the system but it is order which is in constant tension as possibilities for interactive relationships become exhausted. When a system reaches a state where it appears to have maximum order, it also has the potential to self-organise into a new form of order because it verges on the edge of chaos. Such creative self-organisation is possible because of the richness of the interactions that occur within the chaotic state, generating potential for the novel exchange and processing of information. Kauffman provides us with a biological example of how such concepts might be applied:

> With high connectedness (within an ecosystem), any single change is likely to propagate hectically throughout the system, with many large avalanches. This is the chaotic state. At the intermediate state, the edge of chaos—with internal and between species interactions carefully tuned—some perturbations provoke small cascades of change, others trigger complete avalanches, equivalent to mass extinctions (Kauffman, in Lewin 1993, p. 62).

The physicist Per Bak has expanded on the idea of the edge of chaos to describe what he calls 'self-organised criticality' (Bak and Chen 1991). Bak suggests that complex adaptive systems have the ability to evolve towards a 'critical state' where the system 'shows waves of change and upheaval on all scales as if the size of the changes follows a power law' (in Waldrop 1994, p. 308). A mathematical *power law* can be described as the likelihood of a major change in a dynamic system such as a pile of sand that has new grains being constantly added to it. As summarised by Waldrop, such a system can exhibit all kinds of behaviours:

> But the steadily drizzling sand triggers cascades of all sizes—a fact that manifests itself mathematically as the avalanches' 'power-law' behavior: the average frequency of a given size of avalanche is inversely proportional to some power of its size (Waldrop 1994, p. 305).

Thus the concept of self-organised criticality assists in the understanding of systems that exhibit patterned behaviour. Cascades of change in all types of dynamic systems might follow power laws and such laws are, in principle, discoverable.

In the last decade the potentially constructive role of disorder and perturbation in the creation of complexity and diversity has also emerged within conventional ecological theory. Some ecological biologists now argue that *non-equilibrium* determinants of ecological order may be far more significant in the production of the biological diversity currently present on the planet than are the processes tied to the maintenance of equilibrium (Reice 1994). The role of natural disturbance in the form of flood, storm, and fire, for example, is such that it creates new energy gradients and hence new opportunities for evolution, and subsequently, biological diversity as the system in question recovers from the impact of the last perturbation or change. Such a view of the control of community structure transforms the way we see the origins of ecological complexity. High levels of complexity are caused and maintained by regular disturbance that is continually prompting dynamic readjustment from within the ecosystem in question (see Reice 1994, pp. 424–35).

3.2.4.2 Attractors

As complex systems evolve they are subject to forces that influence the course of such evolution. The term *attractor* has been used to describe the tendency of an evolving system to move towards a particular end state. We can think of attractors in two equally important and related ways:

- as specific points or features within a system that exert an influence on its future evolution
- as states towards which a system evolves (Prigogine and Stengers 1984, p. 140).

Kauffman encourages the student of complexity to understand the role of attractors within the spatial metaphor of a landscape such as a water catchment system or basin. Attractors are features within that basin which limit the number of possible configurations or states that it can achieve. Kauffman distinguishes between 'point attractors' and the 'basin of attraction' which he explains in the following topographical terms:

> The idea of basins of attraction and steady-state point attractors is essentially the same idea of a mountainous region with hills, ridges, valleys, lakes, and a water drainage system. Lakes correspond to point attractors; drainage basins, to the basin of attraction. Just as a mountainous region may have many lakes and drainage basins, so may a dynamical system have many attractors, each draining to its own basin. Therefore, it is natural to conceive of the state space as being partitioned into disjoint basins of attraction (Kauffman 1993, p. 176).

Goodwin (1995, pp. 169–73) has applied the idea of attractors within complexity theory to explain the evolution of the eye, a structure that has evolved independently in about forty different evolutionary lines. Following patterns laid out in embryonic development and other forms of cellular growth, the recognisable form of an eye is the result of pattern emergence within a sea of possibilities. As Goodwin explains it, 'there's a large attractor in morphogenic space that results in a functional visual system' (in Lewin 1993, p. 40). Rather than a situation of infinite flexibility and possibilities, certain 'laws of form' might operate in all kinds of contexts where complexity exists and emergence is possible.

Some attractors may exert very powerful forces on a system and maintain a pattern of order over very long periods of time. This is clearly the case for the attractor for the eye and other anatomical features that are found everywhere in nature. Others may have only short-term influence and a perturbation will shift the system towards some new attractor or leave the system in a state of chaos for some time. The rapid evolution of micro-organisms will come under the influence of a dynamic field or 'landscape' containing attractors that rise and ebb in importance. The fitness, or evolutionary success, of such micro-organisms will be determined by the total interaction of all attractors within the field of attraction (fitness landscape).

3.2.4.3 Characteristics of complex systems

From this brief summary of the features of complexity, we can distil a number of interrelated characteristics of complex systems:

- Local interaction can produce global order and global order can affect local behaviour.
- The role of disturbance (perturbation) can be both creative and destructive.
- Small changes to initial conditions can generate massive changes to system behaviour.
- The dynamic interaction of local and global levels of complex systems determines their properties. Such interaction might be subject to ordering influences that are internal to the system or may be universal features of all types of complex adaptive systems.
- Interactive causal relationships exist within and between entities and are at their richest at the edge of chaos, the point between order and disorder.
- Complex systems can self-organise and evolve towards states of increased complexity.
- Complex adaptive systems can form patterns and follow predictable paths of development. The identification of attractors or states, to which a system finally settles, is one clue as to why certain patterns (order) and not others are created.
- The properties of complex adaptive systems cannot be reduced to their constituent parts.
- There is order in what appears to be chaotic; order can spontaneously arise from fluctuations or perturbations within a system.

3.2.4.4 Attractors and social systems

Human social systems have evolved within the context of self-organised ecological and physical systems. So it should come as no surprise that we can apply the idea of attractors influencing order to the complex dynamic systems that are human societies. *Social attractors* act as catalysts in the production of regularities or patterns that can be discovered and studied in society. Such attractors of social order can range from charismatic individuals to ideological systems (that is, influential ideas and symbols). Lewin suggests that attractors for cultural evolution might include 'bands, tribes, chiefdoms, and states' (Lewin 1993, p. 21). Rather than a situation of anything goes, it is possible that the number of states to which any dynamic system settles will be determined by a finite number of attractors.

At different scales of human social systems, different attractors define the range of possible configurations of order. Some cities, for example, under the influence of a wide range of pressures, may be conceived of as attractors in the context of the global economic order, pulling in enormous amounts of energy, information, and technology and growing as a consequence while others degenerate and lose resources. Within cities, different attractors, such as working and sleeping hours, can produce very different patterns of order, for example, the congestion of traffic during peak hours producing a uniform distribution of vehicles and the random distribution of traffic late at night and very early morning (see Sandar and Abrams 1999, pp. 132–3).

At smaller scales of human interaction, quite different sets of attractors may be found that limit the number of possible patterns of interaction. Something as simple as the quality of coffee at a particular coffee shop may explain the popularity of a particular establishment in a sea of competing businesses. The promise of complexity theory is that it invites those who are attempting to understand the dynamics of complex systems to look not only for obvious attractors but also broad ordering principles that animate system dynamics.

3.3 Complexity and human health

The long-standing World Health Organization definition declares that health is 'a state of complete physical, mental and social well-being and not merely the absence of disease or infirmity' (WHO 1947). This perspective, while innovative for its era, gave a static image of what we view as a complex process. By the early 1990s, an emerging understanding of the importance of ecosystems saw the elevation of environmental concerns that have generated ecologically minded public health policy within some sections of WHO (see Chu and Simpson 1994). The clearly complex nature of major environmental problems highlights the need for new conceptions that locate health and disease within complex adaptive systems existing at all geographical scales, from local and national to continental and planetary.

Informed by complexity theory, we can outline a general view of optimal health. *Optimal health* implies the self-regulation and maintenance of all relevant systems promoting ongoing physical, ecological, psychological, and social well-being. This latter definition gives us a sharper understanding of what ill health is. Namely, *ill health* is the loss, for an individual or a community, of the ability to self-regulate, and the disintegration of support systems. Failure to self-regulate for health leads to the necessity for some form of intervention. Within the perspective of complex adaptive systems, intervention is directed towards restoration of all relevant support systems in order for health again to be self-generated and self-regulated.

In order to achieve optimal health, we need to discover all key causal influences for health and disease and map their interconnections. Stated in the language of complexity theory, research is required to find new attractors that may be exerting their influence on the system, pulling or pushing it into new health/disease configurations. Interventions sensitive to the need for the system to find new ways of self-regulating towards health will attempt to promote the value of existing causal influences (that is, attractors) to regain system health. Maintenance of health requires self-organisation in the support systems and maintenance of health attractors; intervention to restore health requires detailed knowledge of the dynamics leading to loss of self-regulation (disease attractors) so as to intervene or perturbate the system in a way that fosters a return to balance.

A useful point of entry into the study of complexity in human health is the identification of health-related attractors that influence health outcomes at the various scales of relevance from the microbiological to the transnational and global. Health attractors are health or disease states towards which health-related systems eventually settle and they can range from specific genetic and somatic pulls to broad social and political pushes that shape the health landscape. These pulls and pushes can create either order or disorder in the complex systems within which health is embedded. One way of looking at these opposing forces is to conceptualise health as existing in dialectical tension between the most basic attractors of life (dissipative structures) and death (entropy).

At microbiological levels the major factors that influence the organisms that affect human health are evolutionary and ecological. The HIV retrovirus evolves under the selection pressure exerted by the human host's immune system. Many strains of enteric bacteria are now evolving under the influence of the routine use of antibiotics in animal livestock management. This practice means that selection pressures in bacteria now include the expanded environments of medical (humans) and veterinary (animals) use of antibiotics. In such expanded environments, it should come as no surprise that resistant strains of bacteria are now emerging and are major threats to public health (Saradamma et al. 2000).

Attractors at this level include normal environmental selection pressures that determine the likely success of adaptive responses between host and organism, and new attractors such as the industrialisation of animal husbandry and the use of antibiotic drugs to maximise animal health, productivity, and hence, profitability. A beef cattle feedlot might be conceptualised as a new basin of attraction containing new types of interactions between attractors such as farmers, cattle, antibiotics, protein supplements, and consumers that were formerly related in different ways. The feedlot defines a new space of possibilities, also called a *fitness landscape* (see Kauffman, in Lewin 1993, p. 57), for the interaction of all these variables, one quite different from the space of possibilities for free-range beef.

Other new attractors in the fitness landscape for pathogenic micro-organisms are created by new environments produced by human technologies that are designed to maximise human comfort. These new artificial fitness landscapes include airconditioning cooling towers, and mass population water supply systems.

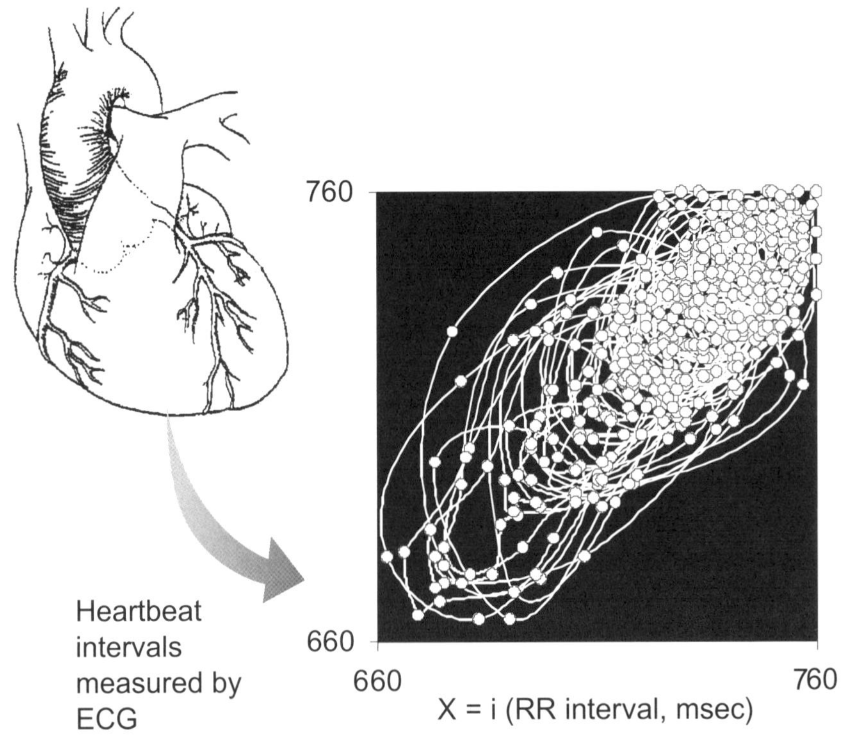

Source: Heart Foundation (Qld division), n.d., and J.Y. Kresh et al. 2000 (in press), *Journal of Thoracic Cardiovascular Surgery*

Figure 3.1 The heart's attractor

At the level of the human body, one attractor that has been the object of considerable study is the attractor for effective beating of the heart (see Figure 3.1).

It seems that when the heart experiences a heart attack or cardiac arrest, this is not caused simply by the heart ceasing to beat in rhythm. As Firth explains:

> In the physiological sphere, one would suppose the human heart to have an oscillatory attractor. In fact there are indications that the healthy heartbeat is actually slightly irregular, indeed chaotic. Be that as it may, it must have a fixed point attractor (cardiac arrest) into which it can be 'kicked' from the normal state by an electrical or other shock. With luck or skill, or both, it can sometimes be kicked back again: resuscitation (Firth 1991, p. 1567).

Goodwin (1995, p. 60) notes that ventricular fibrillation (uncoordinated and ineffective contractions) in the heart muscle can be caused by the presence of infarcts, or small patches of damaged tissue. These infarcts act as an attractor for the waves of heart contraction, breaking the normal rhythm and creating a new pattern (ventricular fibrillation) that is unable to sustain pumping functions compatible with the maintenance of life. The action of defibrillation machines is to shock or perturbate the muscle of the heart to leave the infarct attractor and to resume normal rhythm (around its chaotic attractor) with normal pumping activity.[3]

At the level of human social systems we can identify attractors that exert their influence on health status. Such attractors range from social and cultural pressures on diet and lifestyle to the influence that multinational corporations in the medico-industrial complex exert on the availability of drugs worldwide. Byrne (1998, pp. 108–21) argues that inequalities in health within the populations of cities can be understood in relation to attractor forms based on socioeconomic criteria such as inequality and the life chances (for example, poverty) that are structurally connected to them. Byrne argues for this position with respect to tuberculosis (TB) that 'We can say here that an unequal world city will have a TB problem, but that it is possible for us to recast the city as more equal and in that attractor state there will not be a TB problem' (Byrne 1998, p. 119).

At the level of small-scale human interaction, factors such as human values and their expression in policy and management will act as endpoint determinants or attractors. Miller et al. (1998) have used attractors in this sense to understand the dynamics of a social example of a complex adaptive system, a group of doctors operating a primary care clinical practice. They suggest that:

> Practice attractors can include a particular income goal, a specific understanding of patient care success, meeting patient and community expectations, or a particular practice vision. Attractors can also be understood as the motivators and values of the practice (Miller et al. 1998, p. 371).

Dean (1997) argues that 'human nature' itself might be subject to deep underlying structures that can be understood by complexity theory. Social and health problems such as drug and alcohol dependence (intoxication) might be explained by factors such as 'security' and 'status' that are 'forms of *primary selective categories*' or attractors for the evolution of behaviour that may result in alcohol or drug abuse. Although negative in its impact on human health, such adaptive behaviour can nevertheless 'fit the circumstances of a person's existence' (Dean 1997, p. 153) and prove to be beneficial in a social or collective context. Similar conclusions are given in our case study of heart disease among men in the Australian coalfields (see chapter 5).

Derrickson-Kossmann and Drinkard (1997) use the concept of an attractor to understand the dynamics of a psychological condition—dissociative identity disorder (DID). They note how therapists use cognitive interventions to perturbate the attractor for DID into an adaptive state more likely to increase internal communication and coherence.

The factors that influence health, taken as a whole, form nested sets of attractors (after Tarlov, in Byrne 1998, p. 108). These nested attractors operate in ways that we suggested in chapter 2 using the health hierarchy diagrams. Byrne suggests that there are three main domains where health attractors operate:

> The individual attractors are lifestyles—the product of the interaction of constraint and volition. The social attractors are the grand social forms which pattern the possibilities of lifestyles. Even these may be embedded within a wider Gaian biosphere level of possibilities . . . which is under serious perturbative assault from human industrial production and resource consumption (Byrne 1998, p. 116).

Table 3.1 is our attempt to list some of the attractors that influence human health across all levels of natural systems.

With an awareness of the main attractors and basins of attraction that influence human health, careful attention can also be focused on specific attractors that might operate in unique settings. Miller et al. (1998) identify specific attractors that shape the form of the system that is a family practice primary care centre. A particular centre has a vision of what its *modus operandi* or internal model will be. The core functions of the practice are created within the context of broad philosophies and policies of physician style, income generation, patient care, prevention services delivery, and organisational operations (Miller et al. 1998, p. 371). The various elements within the primary practice attempt to achieve these core functions by engaging in strategic actions to achieve the desired goal or end state. The end states or points are described as attractors and include an identified income level for its staff, patient care success rates, and the meeting of community expectations. After identifying these small-scale social system attractors, the next step in their analysis is to identify ways to influence the attractors so as to achieve desirable outcomes. They suggest three ways to change attractors:

1 *Joining*: enhancing existing attractors using the known internal models.
2 *Transforming*: changing an attractor or creating a new one.
3 *Learning*: increasing awareness of attractors and internal models.

(Miller et al. 1998, p. 373)

Table 3.1 The full scale of human health attractors

Scale of system	*Attractors and basins of attraction*
Microscopic and other types of pathogens	Selection pressures, fitness, genetic norms, favourable anthropogenic environmental changes (cooling towers, feedlots, intercontinental mass transport).
Organs	Genetic norms, heart infarcts and fibrillation, tumours, health, and death.
Body size, shape, and fitness	Cultural norms for body shape (perfectibility), fast foods and crash diets, sedentary lifestyle (computers), surgery.
Individual and small-group behaviour	Security, status, goals and values, expectations, levels and types of communication, professions, subcultures, health gurus.
Societal and institutional	Public and private health care and insurance systems, public policy, advertising, globalisation, mass media, transnational organisations.
Planetary systems	Enhanced greenhouse effect (global warming), ozone depletion.

There may be many more ways of influencing the range of attractors that operate at different scales. Some large-scale attractors may not be capable of being influenced by players operating in the small-scale (that is, local level) system. The primary practice is nested within larger scale systems such as the medico-industrial complex, the health insurance industry, the national health policy, and the biophysical environment. At these levels, different attractors exert their power and different ways of influencing them must be attempted. At the level of microorganisms, and the larger biophysical environment within which they evolve, pathogens such as the influenza virus can affect general practice in ways that simply cannot be influenced by agents in small-scale social groups.

3.3.1 Complexity and health: case studies and examples

Discoveries about the complexity of health issues come as no surprise to those prepared to think through the total picture in a systematic way. For instance, some disturbances that humans are enacting on long-stable cultural and ecological systems are manifested as epidemics of disease. An example of a small change to a system leading to a large effect is provided by Desowitz's case study of tractor-induced Japanese encephalitis in northern Thailand.

3.3.1.1 From buffalo to tractor attractors

> The traditional practice in Northern Thailand was to plough the rice paddies with water buffaloes and to keep pigs for food and market. Since *Culex tritaeniorhynchus* [the mosquito carrying the encephalitis virus] prefers steak to pork, the water buffaloes acted as a blotter, limiting viral transmission. Then, heeding the call of progress, the farmers of the region replaced their buffaloes with tractors. As the buffalo population declined, the mosquito(s) turned their attention to the pig and to man. Many pigs now became infected; the virus multiplied in the pigs; more and more mosquitos became infected; and, in turn, so did more and more humans. Hundreds died, and many of these victims were children (Desowitz 1981, pp. 21–2).

Desowitz's observations show the characteristic of interactive causality in complex systems, in this case among people, the mosquito, the virus, domestic animals, and introduced technology. As the landscape was changed by eliminating the buffalo attractor for the virus, the new tractor attractor created the circumstances where the system changed to favour humans as an end point for viral transmission. The next example provides further evidence of how perturbations to ecosystems can end up having unexpected health outcomes.

3.3.1.2 War and weather attractors

During the Korean War a mysterious disease emerged which affected thousands of United Nations troops and killed many. It was later discovered that the cause of the disease, known as Korean haemorrhagic fever, was a virus transmitted to humans via rodent urine and excrement (Hantaan or Seoul virus), as noted in chapter 1. The virus had remained dormant, perhaps for centuries, until heavy machinery and digging by soldiers disturbed the environment and exposed them to the pathogen through contact with soil and dust. Perturbation to a long-undisturbed natural system created the conditions for transmission of a new viral disease. Forty years later, the Seoul virus, possibly transmitted by adventurous rats aboard ships, is now endemic in major cities in the USA and is being detected in patients on the east coast (McAuliffe 1990; Garrett 1994).

Coincidentally, in 1992–93 a mystery virus struck at least eighteen people living on or near a Navajo reservation on the New Mexico–Arizona border, fourteen of whom died (CDC 1993). The pathogen was discovered to be a member of a previously unknown type of Hantaan virus, called *sin nombre* (meaning 'without a name'), and is a worrying example of what are termed 'emerging pathogens'

(Le Guenno 1995, pp. 30–1). What appear to be novel viruses may have existed for millions of years but have only come to light with contemporary environmental disturbances.

Le Guenno (1995, p. 32) asserts that the primary cause of most haemorrhagic fever outbreaks is ecological disruption which brings humans into contact with animal vectors. However, perturbations to ecosystems also result from natural disturbances. The emergence of *sin nombre* in the USA was the result of unusually heavy rain and snow in 1993 in the mountains and deserts of New Mexico, Nevada, and Colorado. The principal host of *sin nombre* in this area is the deer mouse, which lives on pine kernels. The high humidity resulted in an abundant crop; this created conditions suitable for an explosion in the deer mouse population which in turn coincided with the epidemic of *sin nombre*.

3.3.1.3 Bat attractors

The emergence of new diseases and unexpected renewed outbreaks of old diseases such as whooping cough and tuberculosis are becoming increasingly common in an era of increasing air travel, the development of tropical megacities, and the encroachment of humans into previously untouched natural environments (McAuliffe 1990). The outbreak of Ebola in Africa has been linked to the emergence of the virus from an as yet unknown reservoir that had previously been left undisturbed by the actions of humans (see Le Guenno 1995, p. 34). Deadly viruses that have fruit bats or flying foxes as their host have recently been identified. *Nipah*, carried by fruit bats, killed over 100 people in Malaysia in February 1999 and caused the death and forced culling of over 1 million pigs at a cost of $500 million to the Malaysian government, while another bat-borne virus, *Hendra*, claimed the lives of both people and horses in Australia in the mid 1990s. Humans are coming into more regular contact with these animals as the animals' habitat contracts under the pressure of agriculture and forestry. In Australia, carers—people who look after sick or injured bats—are most likely to come into contact with the new viruses, especially if they are bitten by their patients. That these viruses are capable of crossing species barriers makes their threat to humans and livestock very serious.

3.3.1.4 Factory farms and feedlots as attractors

A form of food production (social factor) with a notable impact on human health is factory farming. Many of our foodstuffs come to us from sources that are now widely known as agribusiness. Agribusiness treats food production much like any other form of production in a capitalist society: costs are minimised and maximum profit is sought. In the attempt to maximise output, producers have used a variety of techniques to enhance what could be produced by conventional farming methods. Genetic engineering, the use of antibiotics to control infection in intensive animal husbandry, and chemicals and drugs to control parasites and pests, are all well-established practices in agribusiness. So too are growth hormones and animal protein supplements used to minimise food costs in raising previously vegetarian animals for human consumption. All of these factors create a new basin of attraction with new attractors for both animal and human health. Feedlots and other types of factory farms can be conceptualised as dissipative structures, taking in the energy and materials (food, water, chemicals) provided by agribusiness and exporting enormous amounts of waste, both literally (effluent, nutrients) and metaphorically in the form of new disease.

The practice of protein supplementation has been implicated in Mad Cow Disease (MCD) in cattle and Creutzfeldt-Jacob Disease (CJD), the human equivalent of MCD, or BSE. In the mid 1980s, British veterinarians identified a new disease in cattle—Bovine Spongiform Encephalopathy (BSE). The symptoms of this disease of the brain include nervous and unpredictable behaviour, and extreme lack of coordination. The brain develops sponge-like holes as the disease progresses towards total degeneration of the victim's nervous system. In the last few weeks of the disease cattle are so badly affected by the destruction of their brain tissue that they appear mad, hence the popular name of the condition.

What was a serious disease in cattle, with the potential to cost the British beef and dairy industry many millions of pounds in lost production, became an issue of international concern when it was proposed in the early 1990s that BSE was capable of transmission to humans through the food chain. In other words, it is now thought that BSE and CJD are one and the same (Lacy 1996, p. 3).

Current research suggests that the best explanation of the origins of CJD is the prion hypothesis. According to Nobel Prize winning neurologist and biochemist Stanley Prusiner:

> the infective agents causing certain degenerative disorders of the central nervous systems in animals and, more rarely, in humans might consist of protein and nothing else (Prusiner 1995, p. 30).

Prusiner has called these abnormal infective proteins *prions*, and has claimed that they are capable of self-replication within the brain tissue of mammals. Prions are very robust and cannot be destroyed by normal cooking heat or by a wide battery of chemical agents. The causal link from animals to humans is still considered tentative; however, it is known that it involves the transmission of prions from one species to another.

One of the earliest known suspected prion diseases is scrapie, found in sheep and goats. Scrapie causes its victims to lose coordination and to itch, hence the appropriateness of the name, as infected animals scrape their wool or hair to relieve the itch. It was common practice in the United Kingdom in the 1970s and 1980s to use parts of sheep not used for human consumption as animal feed in intensive beef, veal, and milk production. The bone, offal, and flesh were ground up to produce a food supplement that represented the cheapest way to maximise protein input to commercial herds. It is thought that scrapie-infected sheep could have passed their infective prion to cattle, in which it manifested as BSE. Humans who consumed infected beef and dairy products could contract CJD.

The epidemiology of BSE suggested that this link was plausible. Since animal-based food supplements were banned for ruminants (that is, grazing animals such as sheep and cattle) in 1988, there has been a steady decline in the number of cases of BSE in the United Kingdom. The British Institute of Food Science and Technology (IFST) stated: 'The prohibition of the ruminant material from the animal feed, and the successive year-by-year reductions in confirmed new cases over recent years seem to demonstrate that the animal feed was a key factor' (IFST 1999). The annual figures of new confirmed cases in Great Britain were 36 682 animals in the peak year of 1992, and a steady decline to 3064 by 1998.

The evidence for the direct link to humans is less compelling, since it is possible that CJD has a very long incubation period, perhaps up to 30 years. However, as Lacy (1996) and others point out, there is at least one historical precedent of spongiform encephalopathy in humans that should have provided vital clues as to what was happening with CJD. Lacy observes that kuru, the fatal brain disease of the Fore people of Papua-New Guinea described in chapter 1, has a remarkable similarity to CJD. Kuru was a major health problem for the Fore people until the cause of the disease was discovered to be the eating of human flesh, in particular, the brains of kuru victims by their maternal relatives and their children.

Historically, CJD has a very low incidence. Prusiner notes that about one in a million suffer from it and it usually strikes at around 60 years of age (Prusiner 1995, p. 31). The numbers of cases of CJD in the United Kingdom is relatively small (eighty dead or dying by September 2000). A number of victims were dairy farmers who had direct contact with BSE in their herds. A disturbing trend, given the long incubation history of prions is the relatively young age (under 30) of some of the victims.

A further cause for concern is the discovery that cows can pass BSE to their calves, so the practice of destroying infected adult animals will not be sufficient to ensure that BSE is eradicated from the food chain. Moreover, because prions are so robust and cannot be destroyed by conventional means (including radiation), the fact that they can be transferred from mother to calf means that the infective prions must be able to pass from the central nervous system to the blood. Infective prions in the blood means that *all* beef products will be potentially infectious to humans;[4] this includes products such as gelatine which is used in an enormous variety of manufactured food products. The Nobel Prize for medicine was awarded to Stanley Prusiner in 1997, suggesting that there is now greater scientific acceptance that 'prions must be added to the list of well known infectious agents including bacteria, viruses, fungi and parasites' (Cooke 1998, p. 26).

3.4 Conclusion

The possibility that humans have created, through their agricultural practices (such as feeding animal protein to vegetarian ruminants for economic reasons), a health epidemic that will reach far into the future is a perfect illustration of how a seemingly small change in the attractors operating within a complex system can produce a very large effect. Understanding CJD requires insights from anthropological history, epidemiology, cellular biology, agricultural science, and neurology. Britain's IFST offers an important insight:

> In real life, simple 'single cause → single effect' relationships are rare, and it seems quite possible, or even probable, that BSE developed as a result of a number of coincidental factors coming into play in a combined circumstance (IFST 1999).

Such complexity of modern health problems has led Levins et al. (1994) to suggest that:

> In the end, it is likely that the classification of diseases into infectious, environmental, psychosomatic, auto-immune, genetic and degenerative will prove to be applicable only to a sample of cases where one factor overwhelms all others. The more accurate viewpoint will encompass full complexity of this network of factors that leads to recognisable disease (Levins et al. 1994, p. 55).

Chapters in part II demonstrate a number of the principles of complexity theory that we have covered in this chapter. In chapter 5, for example, we draw on complexity theory to analyse an 'epidemic' of heart disease among people in a coalmining community in New South Wales, Australia. Similar illustrations of complexity processes are highlighted in the ensuing chapters on the dynamics of the global pharmaceutical industry, infection control in hospitals, and HIV/AIDS in Africa. Our aim is to stimulate researchers to apply complexity theory to understanding the evolution of other complex health problems where the dynamic systems initiating or exacerbating disease patterns remain to be illuminated.

This chapter has extended our discussion of integrating theories and frameworks into arguably the most integrative theory currently available. Complexity theory's concern with non-linear relationships and interactions among causal factors and emergent properties of systems encourages the researcher to go beyond or transcend the boundaries set by conventional theories and frameworks. There are many ways in which a genuinely transdisciplinary health social science can be achieved and in chapter 4 we outline our basic framework for conceptualising health and taking action to improve it—transdisciplinary thinking.

Notes

1 We make no new claims about complexity theory; our intention is to summarise the main developments that we believe are applicable to a transdisciplinary view of human health.

2 See Lewin (1993, p. 12) for further explanation of the two strands of complexity theory.

3 See Kresh and Izrailtyan (2000) or http://husol.auhs.edu/com_man6.htm for more information about the heart as a complex adaptive system.

4 It is now clear that human blood products are capable of passing CJD from donor to recipient. A ban on blood donations from all those potentially infected with CJD is now in place in many countries.

4
Transdisciplinary Thinking in Health Social Science Research: Definition, Rationale, and Procedures

GLENN ALBRECHT, NICK HIGGINBOTHAM, AND SONIA FREEMAN

4.1 Introduction

The start of a new millennium is a good vantage point from which to see that humans have created global social systems that have transformed the natural world. Among other things, these relatively young social forms have overwhelmed cultural ecologies of Indigenous peoples and created human habitats highly dependent upon sophisticated technology and massive consumption of energy. Twentieth-century societies created the conditions whereby diseases that have plagued humankind historically are prevented or controlled. At the same time new and even more virulent forms of disease have emerged. The interaction of all these physical, biological, and social forces demands that we apply new ways of thinking that can understand and respond to an emerging reality that is more complex than ever before.

Transdisciplinary thinking is thinking that goes beyond (transcends) the boundaries of existing disciplines or fields of knowledge in order to more fully understand the complexity inherent in human existence in the natural world. We can no longer see ourselves as separate from the complex natural systems with which we interact. *Humans are now the major force acting on living and non-living systems on the planet.* We can no longer be content with disciplines and fields of knowledge that only attempt to dissect complex, adaptive systems into discrete and manageable parts. Postmechanistic thinking is creative and process-oriented, and searches for new, more integrative ways of knowing the world.

Transdisciplinary thinking about health strives to create the richest possible description of the context within which health and disease are situated. The pursuit of knowledge about a health problem demands, ultimately, a transdisciplinary mode of thinking. It demands a new way of thinking about how we can understand process and change. By hypothesising that complex adaptive systems in all domains have common structures and processes, we can envision a high degree of theoretical compatibility between the physical, biological, and social sciences. In addition, all complex adaptive systems will share the common property of uncertainty, hence, this too will be a principle held in common by all sciences. Prigogine outlines his case for the link between complexity, uncertainty, and transdisciplinary thinking:

> We come from a past of conflicting certitudes, be they related to science, ethics or social systems, to a present of considerable questioning, including questioning about the intrinsic possibility of certainties. Perhaps we are witnessing the end of a type of rationality that is no longer appropriate for our time. The accent we call for is one placed on the complex, the temporal and the unstable, which corresponds today to a *transdisciplinary movement* gaining in vigor (Prigogine quoted in Byrne 1998, p. 159).

The aim of this chapter is to provide a clear outline of the transdisciplinary approach to health research. In addition, we hope to offer persuasive reasons why health social scientists, health policy planners and managers, clinicians, and field workers in non-government organisations will wish to adopt transdisciplinary thinking as their basic strategy for understanding and seeking solutions to health problems. Finally, we list the steps required to perform transdisciplinary research, either in teams or as a solo investigator, and point out some of the implications we have observed in adopting this perspective.

4.2 From disciplinary to transdisciplinary insight

A useful means to define transdisciplinary thinking about health research is to compare it with other forms of thought in relation to the definition of health, the role of collaboration and conceptual frameworks, and how knowledge is applied. Table 4.1 compares the character of transdisciplinary approaches to health problems with that of single, multiple, and interdisciplinary approaches (Albrecht, Freeman and Higginbotham 1998).

Table 4.1 indicates that *single disciplinary* approaches use only the concepts of a single discipline to explain a health problem. Clearly, if the problem is more complex than a single domain, then discipline experts must act to maintain rigid boundaries of ownership around some part of the problem. A hierarchy of competing disciplines often emerges, with the most institutionally powerful discipline getting the most resources. Single disciplines tend towards 'specialised' knowledge

Table 4.1 Contrasting approaches to health problems

	Health problem/problem boundary	*Teamwork/collaboration*	*Role of conceptual framework*	*How knowledge is applied*
Single disciplinary	The health problem is what a single discipline thinks it to be.	None	Arises from a single discipline.	Production of 'specialised' knowledge and reductionistic accounts of problem or or intervention.
Multidisciplinary	The health problem is what several disciplines working independently think it to be; hard disciplinary boundaries are placed around the problem facets.	None or limited; disciplines work independently on distinct facets of a broadly conceptualised problem.	Mutually exclusive conceptualisations juxtaposed and broadly cumulative.	Interventions suggested by isolated, discipline-specific specific problem explanations.
Interdisciplinary	The health problem is what several disciplines working together agree it may be. Aspects of the problem from disciplines not included may be ignored. The health problem is defined by the totality of 'soft' boundaries between the various disciplines working together.	Collaboration using limited knowledge-bases. Different disciplines address inter-connected aspects of a specifically defined health problem, mainly bringing to bear their own theories and conceptual frameworks.	Isolated explanations of a problem from a limited number of disciplines are assembled and connections among them are sought.	Interventions sensitive to an explanation of the health problem informed by under-standing the connections among participating disciplines.
Transdisciplinary	Problem is defined as part of an open, dynamic system operating at multiple levels. Problem broadly expands to include all relevant disciplinary insights.	Open-ended collaboration. All disciplinary insights required to define the problem are assembled.	Common conceptual framework is sought which will be usable by any discipline, achieving an emergent new insight about the problem.	Interventions with the greatest possibility of success follow from a synthesis of knowledge from disciplinary collaboration.

and reductionistic accounts in both the biological and empirically oriented social sciences. They do not engage in understanding dynamic processes within and across systems.

Multidisciplinary researchers address a health issue by defining it in very broad terms so that different disciplines can work independently of each other on different aspects of the problem. The results are then pieced together at the conclusion of the research process. The health problem is characterised by a series of sharply defined discipline boundaries which, together, constitute the limit of our understanding of the problem. This approach is more committed to a wider perspective than disciplinary thinking. However, because it is affected by discipline hierarchies and rivalries, multidisciplinary efforts are resistant to the possibility that other perspectives may be relevant to the problem.

Interdisciplinary approaches encourage different disciplines to actively pursue the interconnected aspects of a health problem that is defined within the boundaries of the interacting disciplines. Each discipline brings its own discipline-specific insight to the problem, but is willing to see strict boundaries disappear. The health problem is defined by the totality of soft boundaries between the various disciplines working together. However, as with the multidisciplinary approach, power to explain the problem is limited to the disciplines assembled. It may be that other disciplines not even considered in the collaborative project are important. For example, world efforts to expand immunisation coverage of vaccine-preventable diseases were underway for over a decade before anthropological insights about how to encourage community acceptance of such vaccines were considered. Nevertheless, through an interdisciplinary approach, a limited *systematic* perspective of the problem is now possible.

The *transdisciplinary* approach, noted in table 4.1, is committed to fully exploring the boundaries of a health problem by 'drawing together disciplinary-specific theories, concepts and approaches' (Rosenfield 1992, p. 1351). It also promotes cooperation and coordination between disciplines and encourages the creation of multidisciplinary and interdisciplinary teams. As indicated in figure 4.1, it is possible to achieve a transdisciplinary outcome, commencing from all the approaches outlined above. There is no one pathway to the transdisciplinary understanding of complex health problems.

The goal of TD investigation is to examine a complex problem and discover a common element in all of the apparently disparate parts. The various strands of thinking about causal factors can coalesce into new conceptual frameworks. A 'common conceptual framework' (CCF) is a new way of understanding a problem which in some significant way unifies all the previously disconnected disciplines and fields of knowledge. Common conceptual frameworks can range from simple ideas, such as the concept of the earth being round, to complex ideas, such as evolution in biology or relativity theory in physics. We can add *complexity* and *emergence* as new types of CCFs that have been created in the last few decades. A CCF that achieves a high level of acceptance within the research community, and indeed the general public, may qualify as a paradigm (Kuhn 1970). A paradigm or whole new way of conceptualising the world is a rarely achieved breakthrough in empirical and conceptual thought. Such events transform or revolutionise all previous perspectives on an issue or problem. At the point of the creation of a new CCF, researchers can incorporate its explanatory power into all future work.

The idea of a common conceptual framework is important to understanding TD thinking as it is presented in this book. Clearly, with a conceptual framework that is held in common by researchers, previous boundaries around fields of knowledge disappear altogether or are transcended and a new or transdisciplinary explanation is created.

4.2.1 Transdisciplinary individuals or teams

Transdisciplinary thinking is primarily a process of assembling and mapping the possible interconnections of disciplinary knowledge about any given health problem until the fullest possible understanding of that problem emerges. The transdisciplinary model in figure 4.1 shows how it is possible to construct a transdisciplinary model of a health problem by the alternative pathways of single, multi and interdisciplinary insights. Figure 4.1 also notes that forming a new common conceptual framework that provides a new level of coherence for the causal influences may or may not be possible for a specific problem.

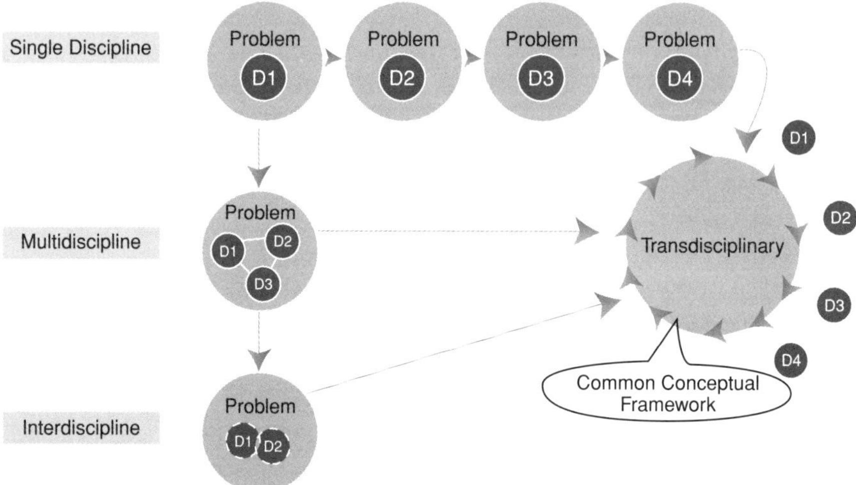

Source: Albrecht, Freeman and Higginbotham (1998)

Figure 4.1 The transdisciplinary dynamic

There are two ways of going about transdisciplinary thinking: one way is by an individual synthesising findings from a multitude of disciplines to provide a comprehensive explanation of a complex health issue; the other is by constructing a group or team who would bring their combined resources to focus on problem solving.

The first approach involves an individual researcher examining findings from a variety of disciplines (as shown at the top of figure 4.1, with the discipline circles moving from left to right). Using findings from single and interdisciplinary collaborations as a point of departure, the individual researcher transcends disciplinary boundaries by linking the disparate analyses into a coherent framework. In some cases this involves thinking *associationally* (Stephen Kunitz, personal communication, 1994) rather than in a narrow and reductionist fashion. In some circumstances an individual might enter a chaotic realm where creativity is maximised and new insights emerge. Robert Desowitz's work on people and parasites (chapter 3), Stephen Kunitz's examination of colonisation and disease (below), and Anthony McMichael's efforts to link climate and health (chapter 2) are clear examples of solo transdisciplinary thinking.

The second approach seen in figure 4.1 involves the collaboration of team members with backgrounds in different disciplines. Disciplinary boundaries are blurred as researchers work cooperatively to bring together into some unified framework the diverse elements of a comprehensive explanation, including the objective and subjective, the reductionist and holistic, and so on. This group-driven process is represented in the figure by the downward movement from single discipline to multidisciplinary and interdisciplinary action and then across to TD thinking. Under some circumstances, the effect of group members focusing on a particular problem is to create a CCF out of what were formerly disparate analyses. This is the process whereby discipline boundaries are transcended and a new or transdisciplinary way of explaining a problem emerges. Researchers cooperating within a complexity theory framework have a significant advantage in the task of combining disciplinary insights. For them, the search for relationships between attractors and perturbations in different domains and at different scales, as discussed in chapter 3, unites the transdisciplinary team.

A group of interacting researchers generating a critical mass of information derived from discipline and more expansive fields of knowledge will create the most favourable set of circumstances for the production of a new CCF. Such an outcome is consistent with our arguments in chapter 3 concerning the potential richness of interactions at the edge of chaos. The richer the interaction, the greater the information shared, the more likely it is that something new will emerge. To study a complex adaptive system, a TD team that itself displays the properties of such a system will most likely produce an account offering new insights into the problem.

4.2.2 Transdisciplinary analysis of the destruction of Indigenous peoples

The *individual researcher* approach to transdisciplinary thinking is demonstrated by Stephen Kunitz's analysis, 'Disease and Destruction of Indigenous Populations in the New World' (1997). The process underlying individual transdisciplinary research, rather than the substantive findings, is the main focus of our discussion. Between 1492 and the 1960s the Indigenous populations of South America dropped from an estimated 20 million to 10 million. In the Amazon region alone, the Indian population declined from approximately 1 million in 1500, to between 39 000 and 57 000 in the 1970s. What forces and processes have combined to bring about these significant declines? Stephen Kunitz, a medical doctor and anthropologist, examined the multiple elements interacting to bring about depopulation in the New World following European colonisation. The primary cause of depopulation appears to have been the spread of epidemics of acute infectious diseases such as measles and smallpox at initial contact. This generalisation marks the point of departure for Kunitz's broad synthesis of elements from single, multidisciplinary, and interdisciplinary studies that formed his transdisciplinary analysis.

First, Kunitz examined *single disciplinary* epidemiological findings, revealing that the introduction of acute infectious diseases had catastrophic effects for all Indigenous groups. However, in the Amazon region, rates of survival of the agricultural empires of the highlands were higher than survival rates for the hunter–gatherer cultivators of the forest lowland coastal areas of Brazil. Why such a difference? Clearly, the differential impact of colonisation on Indigenous peoples in the Amazon is too complex to be explained by a single discipline approach. However, in drawing together the insights from single disciplinary epidemiological and demographic studies, Kunitz was inspired to seek out knowledge from diverse areas to understand dynamic processes operating both within and across systems.

Second, Kunitz drew on various *multidisciplinary* insights relating to a broadly defined issue—the resistance of different Indigenous groups in Amazonia to infectious disease. Kunitz synthesised findings from history, geography, ecology, demography, nutrition, political economy, and anthropology to argue that isolation and mobility were crucial factors affecting the ability of tribal groups living in different locations to adapt to the changes brought about by colonisation.

Third, Kunitz drew upon *interdisciplinary* findings to examine a specific problem—the effect of acute infectious diseases on populations not previously exposed (that is, 'virgin soil populations'). Immunological and psychosocial research into virgin soil populations discusses whether, after European colonisation, high mortality rates in Indigenous peoples were the result of 'hereditary susceptibility' or 'social collapse'. Immunologists argue that in previously unexposed populations newly introduced diseases such as measles and tuberculosis are especially virulent because the victims have not been selected for resistance by epidemics that affected their ancestors. Other authors argue that dislocation, demoralisation, and social collapse accompanying colonisation exacerbate the effects of epidemics, leading to high case-fatality rates.

Interdisciplinary insights gained from combining immunology and social psychology cast light on the issue of virgin soil populations. However, other disciplines not yet included in this debate may add to our grasp of the problem. An anthropological study might reveal, for example, that the ability of particular groups to survive acute epidemics is related to the degree of social control imposed by leaders, or to the strength of religious beliefs. Nevertheless, interdisciplinary approaches do make possible a limited system-wide perspective of problems.

Finally, Kunitz employed a political-economy approach to tie together various elements contributing to a *transdisciplinary* analysis of the destruction of Indigenous peoples following colonisation. The Spanish conquerors came to plunder the wealth of the New World and treated the Indigenous populations as a servile labour force to be exploited. Relegation of Indians to the lowest social and political levels, combined with the generally low level of economic development in most South American countries, has contributed to a pattern of high infant mortality and deaths from endemic infectious diseases. Today, activities such as exploration and mining, road building, and ranching encouraged by the Brazilian government, multinational corporations, and the World Bank result in increased exposure to exotic diseases, violent clashes between Indigenous peoples and intruders, shrinking of Indigenous peoples' landholdings, destruction of the rainforest, and continuing population losses.

Kunitz's analysis is truly transdisciplinary; he has sought to fully explore all facets of the problem by transcending traditional disciplinary boundaries and allowing 'the problem to define the field' (Kunitz, personal communication, 1994). In complexity theory terms, his analysis works within two attractors that can also be described as the CCF of 'domination' and 'adaptation'. Kunitz observes that the sociopolitical domination that accompanied the introduction of epidemic diseases facilitated cultural domination in the form of destruction of traditional institutions, and also exacerbated psychological collapse from stress and demoralisation arising out of the colonisation process. *Domination* is the structural process imposed by colonial governments, while *adaptation* explains the dynamic processes occurring at the local level in response to continual change. In analysing the economic, sociopolitical, cultural, physiological, psychological, genetic, and ecological adaptation of various groups to the colonising experience, Kunitz reveals how a web of causal factors has resulted in such a diversity of outcomes that attempts

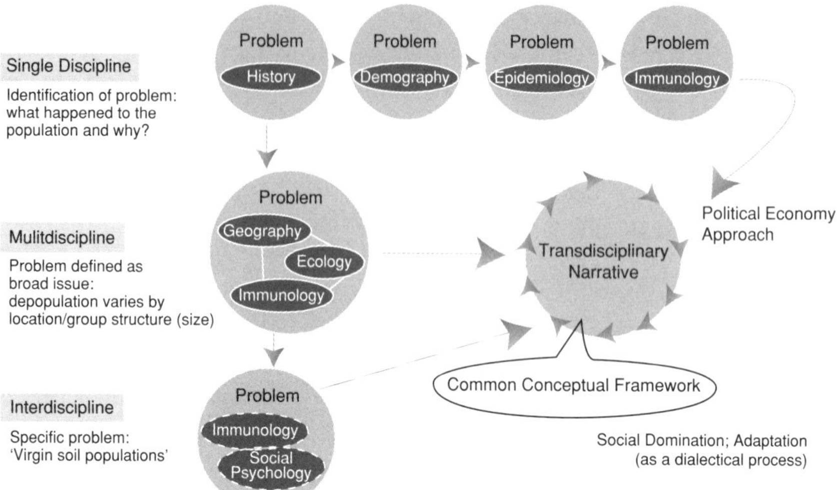

Figure 4.2 Kunitz's transdisciplinary analysis of colonisation and Indigenous populations in the New World

by any one discipline to explain the connections seem doomed to failure (Albrecht et al. 1998).

Figure 4.2 summarises the processes of individual transdisciplinary thinking Kunitz pursued.

4.2.3 Transdisciplinary teamwork examining the impact of colonisation of the Amazon on the spread of malaria

Patricia Rosenfield's (1992) pioneering article, 'The Potential of Transdisciplinary Research for Sustaining and Extending Linkages Between the Health and Social Sciences', illustrates the group or team approach to transdisciplinary thinking. Malaria and tuberculosis continue to contribute to the decline of populations in Amazonia. Rosenfield details a research project enquiring into this issue which over time led to a convergence of concepts and approaches necessary to transcend disciplinary biases. The project was carried out in Brazil by a team working on social economic research for the United Nations Development Program/World Bank/WHO Special Program for Research and Training in Tropical Disease (TDR/SER).

In 1979 the TDR/SER project set up a team of sociologists, economists, anthropologists, regional planners, and demographers together with malariologists, vector biologists, immunologists, and epidemiologists, to carry out transdisciplinary research on malaria in the Brazilian Amazon (Rondonia state). Project members came from several Brazilian university research units as well as from federal and state malaria-control offices. Initially led by a core group of social scientists, the team expanded to include medical colleagues, epidemiologists, and vector-control staff in order to have a direct impact on the Ministry of Health. The common problem they identified was the impact of colonisation on the spread of malaria. A comprehensive assessment of the problem, taking into account the 'perspectives of the migrant, the mosquito, the malaria parasite and the ministry of health', was related to the 'social and economic forces that bind these elements together' (Rosenfield 1992, p. 1351). Together, the members analysed how and where people were getting malaria, their attitude towards malaria and use of control services, the disease impact on their lives, and how all these factors coalesced to influence their attitudes towards colonisation projects (Rosenfield 1992, p. 1348).

From the beginning, the group members showed openness and readiness to consider and combine diverse concepts as well as to confer about methods and results. After this intense experience, they understood the common phenomenon they were analysing—migrants coping with a new disease. In a transcendence of traditional roles, sociologists dealt with the issue of prevalence-detection strategies, entomologists examined changing patterns of behaviour, and anthropologists confronted changed 'vectorial behaviours'. In the ensuing 8 years of face-to-face contact, the TD team was able to develop new approaches to disease control based on new social and medical science concepts. They redefined the concept and meaning of malaria in a mobile population and linked these insights with government resettlement policy. More practical ways of assessing and controlling malaria in a specific context were also developed so that eventually the team was able to analyse the problem 'from all systems levels at the same time' (Rosenfield 1992, p. 1351). An important finding was that, even when migrants had suffered multiple attacks and the death of family members from malaria, the perceived economic benefits offered by life in the new environment were a more important consideration. Other discoveries were that perceptions of fever were reliable indicators of malaria prevalence among the migrants, and that the control program was based on a false assumption—that transmission took place within the house (exposure was actually more likely during cultivation in the forest). Importantly, the project led to an intergenerational transfer of TD thinking by involving Masters and PhD students in the research group.

4.3 Doing transdisciplinary research

Kunitz and Rosenfield's research examples show clearly the exciting substance of transdisciplinary investigations. Yet, this style of research remains rare; little has been written guiding the would-be TD investigator. This section examines the main barriers to TD research and works through seven steps we have identified for pursuing a health problem following this perspective.

4.3.1 Steps in pursuing transdisciplinary research

From these research examples and others we present in this book, we have identified key stages in conducting transdisciplinary research. However, investigators may find themselves moving back and forth between stages in a non-linear and iterative process, rather than following a direct progression through these steps:

1. *Identify a problem*: An individual or a group of collaborating researchers identifies a health problem that merits action, is feasible, and is potentially fundable. (Often, funding agencies call for study proposals from research groups addressing agency-identified health priorities.)
2. *Assemble a TD group*: Sponsors or coordinators activate a network of researchers with the disciplinary and/or interdisciplinary skills that can contribute a perspective on the problem. Membership of this group or team may expand or change as new facets of the problem emerge or the problem definition changes as research proceeds.
3. *Review existing knowledge*: Exhaust all the disciplinary and interdisciplinary conceptualisations and explanations of the problem. Make a commitment to an expanded perspective whereby the assembled fields of knowledge jointly share their strengths and limitations in problem explanation.
4. *Design research enquiry*: Problems and questions that surface in stage 3 inform the researchers about the appropriate level and design of TD research that is needed. Depth of problem comprehension will determine whether research should be problem description, identification of causal factors, or clarification of the web of causal interconnections that link the explanatory variables from the different approaches (see the Preamble to part III).
5. *Implement research enquiry*: The TD team carries out the appropriate level of enquiry to produce the required knowledge and then moves to more advanced enquiry designs in pursuit of fuller TD problem explanation. Quantitative and qualitative methods are combined as necessary at each level of research enquiry. Knowledge emerging may suggest repetition of stages 4 and 5 to pursue promising themes or new questions.
6. *Synthesise data and explain problem*: Team members jointly review conceptual understandings and synthesise data sets. They search for a common conceptual framework that illuminates the problem and provides maximum explanatory

power. Some teams adopt complexity theory as their common conceptual framework, using non-linear thinking to identify patterns and regularities within the complex totality. Other researchers evolve alternative models.

7 *Specify location and type of intervention*: TD explanations enable the team, usually with an expanded network of local stakeholders, to identify points in the web of causal interconnections at which the most effective forms of intervention can be implemented in order to resolve the problem. Box 4.1 (below) gives an example of TD research steps arising from action to understand climate–disease interrelationships.

4.3.2 Barriers to transdisciplinary research

Given that a large number of disciplines and/or fields of knowledge must be engaged in a health problem in order to explain a complex and dynamic interaction of causal factors, it is not surprising that such engagements have yet to become commonplace. The resistance to such engagement is due to a number of barriers that work against transdisciplinary explanations. The first, as outlined in chapter 3, is *reductionism,* the attempt to reduce a complex whole into its constituent parts. For example, cardiologists reduce heart disease to the workings of arteries and valves or even further to changes at the cellular level in the walls of these arteries. A second barrier is *macro-reductionism* (DeWalt and Pelto 1985), the explanation of a problem exclusively in terms of its broadest possible context, as when investigators inappropriately use macro-level data (for example, city population) to interpret small-scale phenomena (for example, a couple's decision about contraception). Researchers following macro-reductionism would interpret a health problem—say, heart disease—using concepts that describe only the large-scale dimensions of its context, such as broad cultural beliefs or social class position. A third barrier, *discipline rigidity* and *super-specialisation,* is connected to the political economy of discipline competition within universities and other institutions. By controlling knowledge and developing professional bodies that accredit the practice and use of such knowledge, disciplines acquire power within institutions and societies. The quest for discipline autonomy promotes greater specialisation of individual workers within disciplinary boundaries at the expense of a fuller understanding of the problem. New fields of study rapidly assimilate themselves into the prevailing disciplinary political structures. The fourth barrier is the *complex and unpredictable* nature of health outcomes. Because of such complexity, health problems can emerge that could not be predicted, or readily understood, using causal models suggested by reductionism (micro or macro).

Box 4.1 TD teamwork to understand the climate–disease connection

A good example of scientists moving through the steps towards TD research comes from the birth of a new research field linking climate with the incidence and distribution of infectious disease (Colwell and Patz 1997).

1 *Health problem identified*
Global infectious disease burden exceeds several hundred million cases each year, accounting for one-third of human mortality. Epidemiologists have documented the seasonality of cholera, malaria, and other vectorborne and waterborne diseases, but the causal connections are not well understood.

2 *Assemble a TD team*
The American Academy of Microbiology convened a colloquium in 1997 assembling a full spectrum of disciplines possessing data and techniques that could confirm and clarify the link between climate, infectious disease, and human health.

3 *Review existing knowledge*
Epidemiologists linked up with climatologists studying the 1991–95 El Niño phenomenon to show the connection between this large-scale weather disturbance and rises in diseases such as malaria, Rift Valley fever, Ross River fever, and Hantaan virus pulmonary syndrome. An important discovery was the link between El Niño, higher seawater temperatures in the Bay of Bengal, and the increase in cholera cases in India and Bangladesh.

4 *Design and implement research enquiry*
In order to understand the causal connections, the participants in the colloquium brought together their respective insights into the relationships between climate and disease.

5 *Synthesise data towards a common conceptual framework*
Without formally adopting a conceptual framework, the scientists situated the problem in a complex ecology. They saw their common purpose as integrating information from long-term data sets, gathered from pathogen surveillance, field studies, and satellite measures, and testing computer models of the pathways connecting climate, weather factors, and disease transmission.

6 *Specify intervention*
The colloquium scientists advocated action to create a new interdisciplinary field to study the interface of climate and human health. Action components included new research centres and partnerships between existing institutions (for example, Centers for Disease Control and National Aeronautical Space Administration), strong leadership to unify interdisciplinary teams, and lobbying funding agencies to support long-term interdisciplinary projects. Also advocated was a major effort to communicate the findings of the new science among policymakers and the public, especially knowledge about weather conditions precipitating infectious disease outbreaks, so prevention can be planned.

4.3.3 Implications of transdisciplinary thinking

Our initial experience using a transdisciplinary perspective of health has led to several observations about the process. These are as follows:

- We know before beginning to study any health problem that it will involve many disciplines and fields of knowledge.
- An expanding team (that is, network) of researchers encompassing expanded fields of knowledge is the best way to understand the problem.
- Individual researchers can work in a transdisciplinary mode by discovering the limits of disciplinary boundaries; members of multidisciplinary and interdisciplinary teams can move towards TD research by making creative connections with others working on the same problem.
- The most effective group will most likely work face-to-face on a problem, allowing ideas to synergise and creativity to flourish over a period of time.
- We cannot predict in advance the result of transdisciplinary thinking.
- The process of exploring interconnections among influences at different levels of analysis is paramount; flow diagrams are useful, showing time and space linkages among variables and the evolution of the problem as a dynamic system.
- Transdisciplinary thinking is creative, and expansive, and may create new fields of study across sectors.
- Common conceptual frameworks enable all disciplines and fields of knowledge engaged in TD thinking about the problem to incorporate their insights and explanations into the same dynamic process. Concepts that have been used in this way include healthy cities, adaptation, mindlessness, health transition, social transformation, complex adaptive system, and attractors.

- For TD thinkers working within complexity theory, the search for disease and health attractors is a critical task.
- Transdisciplinary thinking informs problem-based curriculum development; it provides a systematic account of health problems from the point of view of all relevant disciplines and provides the logic for their interconnections.
- A transdisciplinary model is one that can be used to train health and social science researchers, health care professionals, managers, and policymakers, as well as those involved in environmental health generally, and engender a sense of a community of scholarship and research on the common problems of health and disease. Involve the community itself in research and knowledge acquisition.

4.4 The health social scientist

The TD approach can be used across all fields of research and intervention. In this book we focus on health social science contributions to TD research and in the final section of this chapter we consider the role of the health social scientist in relation to transdisciplinary thinking and teamwork.

4.4.1 Tasks and skills of a health social scientist

In our view, health social scientists need the knowledge and skills to carry out two critical tasks:

1 Apply transdisciplinary thinking to explain and help change human health problems.
2 Undertake transdisciplinary research by combining principles of quantitative and qualitative approaches.

In order to complete these tasks, a number of essential skills are required. In the section below, we provide an overview of the skills for applying TD thinking to health problems. In parts II and III of this book we expand this overview with a discussion of the concepts, methods, and strategies health social scientists can draw upon to fulfil their role as TD researchers.

Task 1
TD thinking applied to health problems includes the ability to:

- analyse a health problem from the limitations of existing fields of knowledge, then integrate problem explanations from other perspectives to provide an overall understanding and identify points at which the most effective forms of change can be used to break the process leading to the problem occurrence; such analyses are typically a group task, but can be successfully completed by individual researchers (see, for example, 4.2.2)

- use complexity theory as a potentially powerful tool for generating a common conceptual framework in TD teamwork
- identify and overcome interpersonal and institutional barriers to working successfully in TD teams
- identify theoretically grounded sociocultural and behavioural risk factors and outcomes, and be able to measure such variables in health research
- appreciate the alternative interpretive frameworks among social science disciplines and fields of knowledge, and devise strategies for selecting complementary approaches to analyse a problem
- use transdisciplinary principles to design health interventions, including ideas of community activation, participatory action research, and techniques for establishing or redirecting health-enhancing attractors.

Task 2

Health social scientists, whether trained in traditions of qualitative or quantitative research, need to acquire skills for combining research approaches. They can do this by expanding their own knowledge base or, more consistent with a TD approach, collaborate with colleagues to form an expanded skills-based team. From either foundation, health social scientists should be able to:

- extend the logic of basic epidemiology designs (for example, case-control study) to construct rigorous qualitative investigations (for example, qualitative case-control design)
- extend contextual knowledge of qualitative methods to construct valid measures of social and psychological variables and to improve interpretation of findings from quantitative studies (for example, use unstructured interviews to compile items for measuring health quality of life; use focus groups to understand survey prevalence rates)
- use intensive fieldwork methods, such as participant observation, interviews, and rapid ethnographic appraisals, to help plan, monitor, and evaluate health and behaviour change programs
- critically appraise the research methods used in either qualitative or quantitative investigations to determine whether the study findings are justifiable
- synthesise knowledge from different approaches and disciplines to construct a transdisciplinary narrative of the health problem and effectively promote the dissemination and use of study results among policymakers, organisations, and community members.

4.4.2 Resources for health social scientists: the transdisciplinary framework

By accepting that optimal health emerges from a complex and dynamic process of interacting influences, scientists need a new perspective capable of providing comprehensive explanations of the system within which health issues are situated. In essence, we require a transdisciplinary framework that can give multilevel explanations encompassing the viewpoints of community participants and researchers, reflect linear and non-linear thinking, as well as integrate qualitative and quantitative assumptions and methods. Such a framework would allow for interventions that are either researcher-initiated or the result of local action (for example, participatory action research). Further, it would enable health planners and administrators to frame policies that address the interdependent levels of health influences requiring resource mobilisation.

Researchers seeking a broader perspective of health complexity can draw on existing integrated conceptual frameworks reviewed in chapter 2. Prominent among these are the vertical reasoning models (for example, biopsychosocial model, health psychology), ecological frameworks (for example, biocultural, social ecology), political economy and globalisation theories, and health transition theory. Although these frameworks do not attempt to account for all of the interactions and processes surrounding a health problem, each offers multilevel analyses of the health context.

On the other hand, complexity theory, as we noted in chapter 3, offers a unifying theoretical framework with much potential for integrating health influences that operate across the full health hierarchy. Indeed, as we show in the case studies in part II, complexity analyses can be performed on problem explanations drawn from other integrated frameworks to gain a fuller interpretation of the problem context as a dynamic system.

Figure 4.3 presents a general framework for situating diverse ways of knowing and integrated conceptual frameworks (interdisciplinary fields of study) and their relationship to disciplines. The diagram shows dynamic processes leading to the heart of the model and the possibility of a common conceptual framework that draws together the major connections affecting health (Albrecht, Freeman and Higginbotham 1998). Significantly, TD thinking involves means for combining interpretive and structural reasoning, qualitative and quantitative methods, multilevel analyses, and non-linear expectations about relationships.

Before concluding this chapter, we raise two important issues about TD thinking. First, from figure 4.3 it is clear that transdisciplinary thought operates in an intellectual milieu comprising diverse theories of knowledge which span traditions of positivism to postmodernism. A sharply contested argument is whether such paradigms can (or should) be integrated.[1] While recognising the tensions between

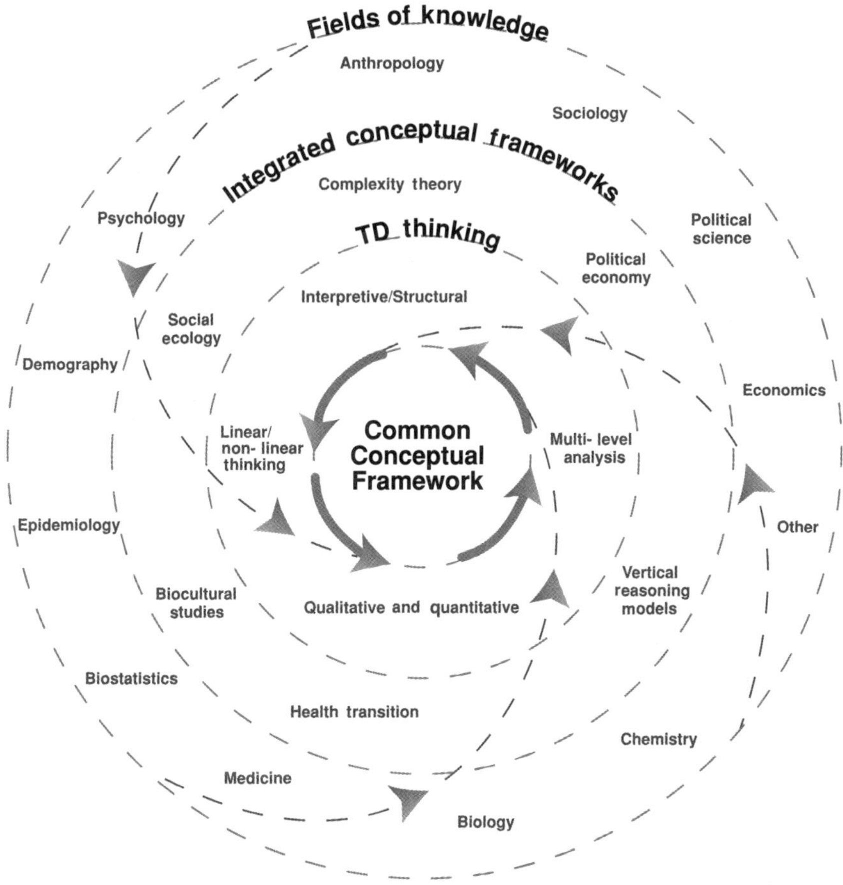

Source: Albrecht, Freeman and Higginbotham (1998)

Figure 4.3 The dynamic process of transdisciplinary thinking

paradigms, we concur with Greene (1994, p. 537) that it is possible to achieve 'dialectically enhanced inquiry benefits through a pluralistic acceptance of multiple ways of knowing'. Our explanation of transdisciplinary thinking proceeds from the assumption that reality is complex and convoluted and that truths about it will be revealed by a multiplicity of perspectives, of which modern science is but one. Our aim as transdisciplinary thinkers is to create a new perspective that connects this multiplicity of approaches so that differences are complementary rather than contradictory. Chapter 3 discussed complexity theory as a framework for pursuing such complementarity.

Second, transdisciplinary thinking implies epistemological tolerance, an ethics of inclusion, and an awareness that academics do not have a monopoly on knowledge of complexity. TD thought is open *a priori* to all theories of knowledge, including, as will be discussed in later chapters, lay and Indigenous theories of knowledge. If TD thinking is grounded in social science traditions that are sensitive to the role of all participants and stakeholders in processes of research and interventions, it can evolve reflexively as it assembles metatheory.

4.5 Conclusion

Transdisciplinary collaboration enables us to reveal health problems as the lived experience of morbidity and mortality among people and populations. These problems have historically been defined by the application of skills and knowledge in single disciplines (for example, epidemiology, anthropology, pathology). As researchers in single disciplines work to analyse the causes of the problem, they have connected with other disciplines at the limit of their own powers of explanation or expertise. In the last few decades, the need to engage in collaborative research to expand the explanatory power of health/disease related theory and action has generated whole new fields of study.

Collaboration enables researchers to creatively explore the intersections of assembled disciplines and approaches and create new interdisciplinary fields of study. A picture of the causal interconnections and elements of influence surrounding a health problem then begins to emerge. Conceptualising the elements of influence as a complex adaptive system involves looking for regularities and patterns that occur in the system. Regularities and patterns are then examined to identify a potential dynamic principle or common conceptual framework. For example, collaborative teams applying complexity theory search for health and disease attractors; they seek evidence of self-regulation within complex adaptive systems that may be stable or in a state far-from-equilibrium. Finally, researchers are able to identify the point(s) at which the most realistic and effective forms of intervention can be used to break the process that leads to the health problem outcome.

In summary, transdisciplinary thinking represents a realistic response to understanding and then assisting in the task of alleviating major health problems the world currently faces. It leads to interventions that use health resources more efficiently because they are allocated on the basis of a fuller knowledge of the sources of the problem and the most effective points of leverage for problem alleviation. At a minimum, transdisciplinary understanding suggests intervention avenues that would not make the problem worse, something that has occurred when culturally inappropriate or iatrogenic 'solutions' to health problems have been used (for example, misuse of antibiotics, Levy 1991).

This chapter has provided a justification for engaging in transdisciplinary thinking and practical guidelines for conducting transdisciplinary research. In part II of the text, we turn our attention to a series of examples demonstrating TD analyses of major health problems. The first case study, covered in chapter 5, explores the main cause of death in industrial societies—heart disease.

Notes

1 Greene (1994, p. 537) reviews contrasting views on this issue. She notes that Guba and Lincoln contest the mixing of enquiry approaches at the paradigm level. They argue that it is not possible for the researcher to simultaneously bring to bear both the 'objectivist detachment of conventional science' and the 'subjectivist involvement of interpretivism'. On the other hand, Patton (cited in Greene 1994, p. 537) argues that objectivist and subjectivist methods can be used together unproblematically, based on 'practical need and situational responsiveness rather than the consonance of a set of methods with any particular philosophical paradigm'.

Part II

Transdisciplinary Case Studies in Health Research

Preamble

Organisation of Part II

Part II contains case studies showing how a transdisciplinary framework can be applied to diverse health issues.

Our first case study, presented in chapter 5, tells the story of coronary heart disease in the Australian Coalfields and uses complexity principles to connect biological and social systems.

Chapter 6 explores the production, marketing, and use of pharmaceuticals as a major international health issue. Medicines are analysed from both political economy (structural) and cultural meaning (interpretive) perspectives; the evolution of drug resistance globally is shown to arise from connections between political economy and ecological and biological systems.

The case study in chapter 7 describes a successful TD intervention to improve infection control in hospitals by reducing the risk of needlestick injuries among nurses and doctors. This example draws attention to some keys to the success of transdisciplinary teams.

Efforts to halt the spread of HIV/AIDS in Africa are the focus of chapter 8, with case material drawn from Uganda and Zimbabwe. Chapter 8 concludes with general guidelines for devising transdisciplinary interventions.

The most comprehensive use of complexity theory in part II is given in our case study of the Coalfields heart disease epidemic. The other three chapters include a briefer complexity theory analysis of the problem, in addition to other forms of transdisciplinary analysis for those who are particularly interested in this approach.

5
Heart Disease in Transdisciplinary Perspective

NICK HIGGINBOTHAM, GLENN ALBRECHT, AND SONIA FREEMAN

5.1 Introduction

Transdisciplinary thinking was defined in chapter 4 and linked with complexity theory, a new scientific paradigm evolving across many branches of science. Complexity theory can be used to explain structure and order, as well as disorder and change, underlying complex dynamic systems, including diseases where aetiologies span many levels of the health hierarchy. Chapter 1 presented the story of John Knight, a heart attack victim from the Coalfields (Hunter Valley) of Australia, touching upon individual and cultural forces leading up to his illness and recovery. In this chapter we probe much deeper into the story of heart disease in the Australian Coalfields. Principles of complexity theory are applied to a body of transdisciplinary research on coronary heart disease in this region.

Our analysis deals predominantly with heart disease in males and reveals how the social is linked to the biological. Insights from this analysis support our argument that transdisciplinary thinking maximises understanding of the complexity of human health.

5.2 Pathways to coronary heart disease

Cardiovascular disease remains the leading cause of mortality in Australia (and other industrialised nations), accounting for about 45 per cent of all fatalities; more than half of these deaths were due to coronary heart disease (CHD) (Australian Institute of Health 1996). Non-modifiable risk factors for coronary heart disease have been identified as advancing age, male sex, and genetic heritage (see Johnson 1977; Berg 1983; Goldberg 1992). Primary preventable or modifiable factors are hypercholesterolemia, smoking, hypertension, and physical inactivity (see Kannel 1983; Gotto et al. 1990; Bijnen et al. 1994). Secondary modifiable factors include obesity, diabetes, excessive alcohol consumption, the contraceptive pill, and psychosocial factors such as socioeconomic class and status, education, and occupational stress (see Barrett-Connor1985; Friedman and DiMatteo 1989; Booth-Kewley and Friedman 1987; Kleinman et al. 1988; Dressler 1990; Plotnikoff 1994; Commonwealth of Australia 1994; Theorell and Karasek 1996). Risk factors are considered to work synergistically, that is, combinations of risk factors interact to produce a compounding effect rather than being additive. For example, results from the United States Pooling Project show that an increase in the rate of CHD associated with a rise of 100 mg/100 mL in blood cholesterol is three times greater in smokers with high blood pressure than in non-smokers with low blood pressure (Hetzel and McMichel 1987, pp. 83–4).

5.2.1 Non-modifiable risk factors

5.2.1.1 Sex

Plotnikoff (1994, chapters 1 and 2) has provided a thorough survey of CHD risk factors which we draw upon for sections 5.2.1–3. While CHD is a major concern for both males and females, there is a 10–15 year lag in the extent of atherosclerosis[1] in women compared to men up until about 50 years of age. Until menopause, women have a lower age-specific incidence of CHD than do men, but after this stage differences in CHD rates narrow. It has been hypothesised that the prevalence of CHD in females after menopause can be attributed to the reduction in the production of oestrogen, a hormone that exerts a beneficial effect on the cardiovascular system. Below the age of 50 years, men are six times more likely to suffer from CHD than women.

5.2.1.2 Age

It is considered that death rates from CHD rise in an essentially linear fashion with increasing age. There is a doubling of heart attack rates with each year of age increase for both men and women. However, researchers assume that the age factor simply represents the duration of exposure to other heart disease risk factors (Wolinsky 1979).

5.2.1.3 Genetics

A review of studies of family history of CHD (Goldberg 1992) concluded that CHD risk increases by 1–2 times with a parental history of the disease. However, the relative contributions of shared genes and environmental influences to the incidence of CHD in family groups have only recently been explored (Peyser 1997).

5.2.2 Primary preventable or modifiable risk factors

5.2.2.1 Smoking

Much research has been conducted into the links between cigarette smoking and CHD. A 1992 study has shown that smoking more than doubles the incidence of coronary disease, increases mortality from coronary disease by 70 per cent, and is directly responsible for 21 per cent of all mortality from heart diseases (Manson et al. 1992; see also Peto 1994).

5.2.2.2 Elevated blood cholesterol

There is evidence that elevated serum cholesterol is causally related to CHD. The effect of total serum cholesterol on CHD risk is mediated through low-density lipoprotein (LDL). High-density lipoprotein (HDL) has a protective effect. Diets high in saturated fats elevate serum cholesterol levels, directly increasing the risk of developing CHD. Other factors that influence serum cholesterol level and lipoproteins are advancing age, genes, hormones, alcohol, physical activity, and smoking.

5.2.2.3 High blood pressure

Elevation of blood pressure has been shown to predict the subsequent risk of CHD. Major factors which increase blood pressure are age, sodium, alcohol, and obesity. There is some evidence that dietary fats also increase hypertension.

5.2.2.4 Physical inactivity

Physical inactivity has been included on the World Health Organization list of primary risk factors. A meta-analysis by Berlin and Colditz (1990) conducted with findings from twenty-seven cohort studies concluded that physical activity produces a beneficial effect in terms of decreased risk of CHD. The association was strongest when highly physically active people were compared with sedentary ones.

5.2.3 Secondary modifiable risk factors

5.2.3.1 Obesity

Obesity has been linked to diabetes, levels of serum cholesterol, and high blood pressure. However, there are inconsistent results regarding the independent association of obesity with CHD.

5.2.3.2 Excess alcohol consumption

Excess alcohol has been shown to increase the risk of CHD among alcoholics and problem drinkers but evidence suggests that a moderate amount of alcohol provides protection against CHD.

5.2.3.3 Oral contraceptives

Women who use oral contraceptives have a 3–4 times greater risk of experiencing a myocardial infarction (MI). Advancing age, cigarette smoking, and hypertension are major factors which increase the chances of MI in women who take oral contraceptives.

5.2.3.4 Psychosocial risk factors

Various hypotheses have been put forward linking psychosocial factors and CHD. In studies conducted in many different countries, poverty and social disadvantage have been associated with CHD. In Australia, low socioeconomic status men and women are 54 per cent and 124 per cent respectively more likely to die from CHD than their higher socioeconomic counterparts (Commonwealth of Australia 1994). Nevertheless, a consensus has not yet been reached on the relationship between social factors and CHD.

It may be that stress associated with certain lifestyles, occupations, or low educational attainment is related to elevated mortality from CHD. William Dressler (1990) has developed the theory that education by itself is related to cardiovascular disease mortality. His research in several cultures suggests that lack of congruence between education and other circumstances in the individual's life create stress, resulting in elevated blood pressure.

Theorell and Karasek (1996) review research relating to the demand-control model of job strain which confirms that a combination of low job decision flexibility and high psychological and physical job demands—that is, the very long hours that people are now required to work, often without financial recompense—is associated with cardiovascular mortality (Theorell and Karasek 1996, pp. 10–12). Another suggestion is that work demands, especially time pressures, in certain occupations produce an 'occupationally enforced' Type A personality (Rosenman et al. 1975), that is, an independent risk factor for CHD. Type A people are those who 'chronically struggle against time, events and other people' (Plotnikoff 1994, pp. 2–18). Although more recent research reviews on the link between Type A personality and heart disease failed to confirm the association (Kaplan et al. 1993, pp. 417–27), personality traits such as competitiveness/aggression, anger/hostility, and depression have been linked to the disease. As yet the nature and mechanisms of these relationships are not fully understood.

While CHD remains a leading cause of mortality in Australia, it has declined by 65 per cent in the past 25 years. This is probably due to the lowering of modifiable population risk factors, notably smoking cessation, and changes in diet and exercise (Plotnikoff 1994). Dobson (1987) argues that the decline in cigarette smoking, systolic blood pressure, and cholesterol from the late 1960s to the early 1980s may account for an estimated 75 per cent reduction in the Australian CHD death rate among 40–59 year old females, and an estimated 40–50 per cent reduction in males of that age group.

These epidemiological findings underpin our examination of coronary heart disease in the next section. We present a case study showing transdisciplinary team research on heart disease prevention in the New South Wales Coalfields. The case study highlights the benefits of using complexity theory as a common conceptual framework for heart disease in particular, and as a tool for TD health research in general.

5.3 Heart disease in the Hunter Valley Coalfields

5.3.1 Epidemiology of a silent epidemic

In the early 1980s, a group at the University of Newcastle became a collaborating centre for the World Health Organization's Project to Monitor the Trends and Determinants of Cardiovascular Disease (MONICA). The MONICA Project confirmed earlier studies showing that, compared with other parts of Australia, the New South Wales Hunter Region in the 1980s had consistently high mortality rates from heart attacks (Leeder et al. 1983). The rate of death from coronary disease was especially high in the Coalfields area, which contains about 10 per cent of the Hunter Region's population. Furthermore, rates of non-fatal heart attack were more than 50 per cent higher in the Coalfields in 1993 than in the rest of the Hunter (calculated from data presented in Steele and McElduff 1995). Similarly, the standardised mortality rate for all causes of death is significantly higher in the Coalfields than in the rest of the Hunter (Page et al. 1990) and the state of New South Wales (Glover and Woolacott 1992). Deaths from heart disease are often talked about as being a 'silent epidemic' since, unlike mortality from cancers and road injuries, they occur almost unnoticed, as if they are the natural, expected, or even desired means of departure.

What are the dynamic processes that underlie the evolution of this silent epidemic in the Coalfields community? In order to answer this question, we combine principles derived from complexity theory and the findings from a large body of local research. Our aim is to construct a framework that can analyse the interconnections between a wide range of variables that influence the pattern of coronary heart disease in the Coalfields. Elliott (1995) demonstrates that relatively little research has been conducted on the aetiology and epidemiology of coronary heart disease in women. This is equally true in the Hunter Region. Consequently, our analysis deals predominantly with factors affecting coronary heart disease in men.

5.3.2 Transdisciplinary teamwork to explain CHD in the Coalfields

For nearly two decades, researchers at the Centre for Clinical Epidemiology and Biostatistics at the University of Newcastle have intensely examined the elements of influence contributing to the epidemic of coronary heart disease in the Coalfields (for example, Dobson et al. 1991; Higginbotham et al. 1999). The work began in an interdisciplinary spirit, bringing together the main disciplines that have something to say about heart disease. Epidemiologists, cardiologists, and biostatisticians shared their knowledge about the excess burden of CHD morbidity and mortality in the region, as well as the biological pathways and risk factors of the disease (for example, genetics, hypertension, atheroma, lipids). Team members trained in psychology, anthropology, health promotion, physical education, nutrition, and nursing shared insights about social and behavioural risk factors (for example, diet, smoking, food beliefs, social status) that predispose certain groups to greater disease burden, along with potential strategies for changing the community's risk profile. A series of team-driven collaborative studies were pursued, combining qualitative and quantitative research methods, and involving efforts to modify the risk factors of heart disease across personal, interpersonal, organisational, and societal levels of analysis (see Higginbotham et al. 1999). Gradually, a transdisciplinary orientation developed, informed by complexity theory as a common framework. Linear thinking about risk factor causes and disease incidence outcomes gave way to images of the community as an open, dynamic system (as described in chapter 3); unhealthy hearts were seen as byproducts of the historical interplay of social, economic, cultural, and biological forces.

5.3.3 The social context of Coalfields heart disease

In order to understand the emergence of heart disease within the dynamics of the Coalfields as an open system, the team had to bring together a range of social research findings. Three important areas were considered.

5.3.3.1 Socioeconomic indicators

When compared with many parts of Australia, the Coalfields are shown to have proportionally more people with lower levels of education and lower socioeconomic status. Traditionally, the main forms of employment have been mining and manufacturing, with a predominance of manual occupations (Australian Bureau of Statistics 1988). In the past 20 years unemployment has been exacerbated by the closure of all the coalmines (Deitz 1992; Kirkwood 1996). Epidemiological surveys generally have found that those in manual occupations have relatively higher rates of heart disease. Dobson et al. (1991) tested the hypothesis that the CHD rates in the Hunter Region could be explained by considering the area's occupational structure. These researchers found that mortality rates for ischaemic heart disease for different occupational groups were consistent with established differences associated with socioeconomic status. However, rates were higher for most occupational groups in the Hunter Region than for the same groups in New South Wales as a whole, so it was concluded that the region's occupational structure 'cannot alone explain the high death rate' (Dobson et al. 1991, p. 172).

5.3.3.2 Social history of discrimination against miners

A large percentage of people of Anglo-Celtic background live in the Coalfields region.[2] The sociopolitical environment has long revolved around coal mining and associated industries. In the nineteenth century in the coal regions of England and Wales, and from the early twentieth century in Australia, coal miners had to endure being spoken of in pejorative terms by mine owners, religious leaders, and other outsiders (ministers, educators, government officials) who endeavoured to ensure that the workers conformed to a sober, pious, and conscientious lifestyle. Andrew Metcalfe's (1988) ethnography and social history of the Coalfields, *For Freedom and Dignity*, is a major resource for understanding the stress and strain endured by miners and their families. Metcalfe (1993) also documents the institutionalised discrimination miners historically suffered from waves of outsiders who sought to reform what they regarded as an uncouth and brutal lifestyle. Metcalfe's theory is that sociopolitical, environmental, and cultural factors were influential in the formation of modes of thought and behaviour, which have implications for the acceptance or rejection of health messages. We could expect, therefore, that health promoters' messages to change 'unhealthy lifestyles' would provoke the same resistance historically reserved for outsiders when their actions are seen as paternalistic or interfering.

5.3.3.3 Social and cultural incongruity of health promotion messages

Heart health promotion campaigns are based on the assumption that the people exposed to the messages have an interest in preventing heart disease or will develop an interest once they are educated about heart disease risk factors. However, the way in which people respond to health messages is affected by their culturally constructed ways of understanding the world, their worldview. Worldviews are constantly being formed and modified in response to everyday experiences and wider socioeconomic issues. Health promotion messages advocating low-fat diets, cessation of smoking, or more exercise will be evaluated and accepted on the basis of their congruence with currently held worldviews. Worldviews may or may not include assumptions about health considered rational by health promoters. Calnan, for example, has shown that people do not subscribe to diets that are not in accordance with their beliefs (Calnan 1990). Thus, men who believe meat is essential to maintain their strength for physically strenuous work are not interested in low-fat diets.

It may be that reductions in heart disease gained overall in Australia have not benefited the people of the Coalfields because traditional heart health promotion messages lack social and cultural meaning in the local community. In other words, the standard health promotion communications, which have credibility among well-educated professionals and the urban middle class, are culturally inappropriate outside those contexts.

There are three strands to this argument:

1 Heart disease is not a priority community concern.
2 Health promotion campaigns have a low impact.
3 Heart disease views are a reflection of health ideology.

The first argument is that heart disease, and health in general, pales in comparison with other more immediate concerns of working-class communities such as work problems, housing, and opportunities for one's children. Hence heart health messages are ignored as irrelevant to current needs. The Newcastle team carried out a needs survey listing seventeen community and social problems. The survey was mailed to a random selection of Coalfields adults and a sample of adults from an upper middle-class area of Newcastle. Only 35 per cent of Coalfields and 27 per cent of Newcastle respondents endorsed heart attack as a 'High Worry' topic. Issues of major concern in the Coalfields were drugs, crime, and road safety (over 78 per cent endorsement) (Higginbotham et al. 1993).

Second, because heart health communications have low priority and are presented in ways that make little sense locally, we would expect them to have a low impact on people's awareness. This hypothesis receives support from other data collected in the needs survey. Table 5.1 shows Coalfields respondents' awareness of six health promotion activities in comparison with Newcastle, the largest city in the Hunter Region.

A third argument is that one's health ideology, with its origins in cultural beliefs and gender relations, forms the lens through which health promotion messages are filtered, responded to, or rejected. Gaynor Heading (1996) used a Health

Table 5.1 Comparison (%) of Coalfields and Newcastle respondents' awareness of six health promotion activities

	COALFIELDS			NEWCASTLE				
	Did not hear, heard, paid little attention	*Was interested, followed advice*	*Not stated*	*Did not hear, heard, paid little attention*	*Was interested, followed advice*	*Not stated*	*x21*	*P*
Men[a]								
Eat less fat	43	56	1	29	70	1	7.7	0.005
Free cholesterol test	55	33	2	57	42	1	0.2	0.69
Eat fruit and vegetables	45	54	1	33	66	1	6.4	0.012
Walk for pleasure	55	44	1	53	46	1	0.1	0.71
Quit for life	69	25	6	57	39	4	9.1	0.003
Healthy cooking	81	18	1	74	24	2	1.6	0.20
Women[b]								
Eat less fat	34	65	1	22	76	2	10.2	0.001
Free cholesterol test	52	47	1	47	52	1	1.2	0.28
Eat fruit and vegetables	41	58	1	27	72	1	12.4	<0.001
Walk for pleasure	54	44	2	42	57	1	8.2	0.004
Quit for life	68	26	6	51	45	4	20.9	<0.001
Healthy cooking	74	22	4	66	33	1	7.0	0.008

Notes
a For men, n = 170 (Coalfields), n = 243 (Newcastle)
b For women, n = 265 (Coalfields), n = 322 (Newcastle)

Source: Higginbotham et al. 1993

Ideology questionnaire to examine Coalfields residents' food and health beliefs, the reasons behind current eating patterns and health behaviour, and interest in heart disease prevention. Her sociological study provided insight into how health communications about diet are understood and acted on by groups of community members in the Coalfields. Heading's data reveal that it was not simply a lack of knowledge about heart disease that led some segments of the community to resist heart health promotion messages. Various groups had their own understandings and orientation to health risk that conflicted with the views of health promoters. Heading classified local residents into three groups.

The *resisters*, predominantly men, know about the relationship between lifestyle and risk factors but find this insufficient to undertake change. Also, they have come to disrespect medical advice. For this group, the social and cultural norms within their family, work, sport, and social communities, their focus on an immediate quality of life, and their distrust of health messengers, who appear to produce contradictory messages, are all reinforcers for their resistance.

A second group is the *pragmatists* for whom the cost and convenience of readily available foods, together with the pleasure and emotional satisfaction derived from consuming them, are the keys to food choice and barriers to selecting food that health promoters would recommend. Pragmatists, more likely to be younger people, are born into the hedonism of consumerism and a culture of fast, fatty food consumption habits promoted in the media.

A third group, the *acceptors*, most often women and older people, take on new health ideologies and as a result report lower levels of dietary fat consumption than the other two groups. However, this acceptance may be for reasons other than disease-specific fears, such as the desire to look good physically, cope better with stress, or an interest in body maintenance. Heading's survey revealed that those who were most resistant to heart health messages were more likely to have lower educational levels, and lower incomes, and be male. Nevertheless, this group had better knowledge about nutrition than those who accepted the validity of heart health messages (Heading 1996, p. 286).

5.4 Complexity theory and heart disease in the Coalfields

Our case study draws together findings about coronary heart disease in the Coalfields using complexity theory as a common conceptual framework to gain new insights about heart disease. We examine how the adoption of practices such as smoking, eating a diet high in saturated fat, and drinking excess alcohol can be traced to community members' ways of understanding the world. In turn, these worldviews are associated with historical processes such as immigration and economic exploitation, which have contributed to the formation of ideas and practices relating to both risk factors for CHD and risk imposition from environmental health hazards.[3] Different and opposing ideas and practices constitute the subcultures of the Coalfields, that is, organised values and ways of life of non-dominant groups (Albrecht et al. 1998).

The Coalfields is a locale of low economic status with a predominance of manual occupations, low educational attainment, and high unemployment levels (see Dobson et al. 1991). In this environment, characterised by many decades of class struggle and social discrimination, Coalfields miners and their families adapted[4] to the harsh conditions by cultivating a sense of community solidarity (cohesion) as a defence against outsiders. This sense of solidarity is a form of order which was self-generated by mining families to give meaning and coherence to their social environment.

5.4.1 The emergence of subcultures

Emerging from the tension between insiders and outsiders, and underpinning that process, was the cultivation of male solidarity both as a means of bolstering working-class masculinity and of retaining dignity under threat from social discrimination by outsiders. This resulted in a pattern of beliefs, values, and attendant way of life Metcalfe has named 'the larrikin response' (1988, chapter 6) and which we term the larrikin subculture. The idealised larrikin response[5] involves a celebration of behaviours outsiders criticise such as gambling, drinking, and fighting. It includes suspicion of religion, education, and law, and a refusal to labour beyond worker-defined limits (Metcalfe 1988, pp. 77–8).

Criticism from outsiders also provoked the emergence of an opposing worldview, which Metcalfe (1988, chapter 7) has labelled the 'respectable response'. This orientation, consistent with that of dominant economic, political, and religious groups, involved recognition by miners that their present lifestyle was unacceptable. While the respectables felt that they were the victims of circumstances, they were willing to change their ways. In recent years, the respectable subculture has included the belief that health can be maximised by reducing individual risk factors. The respectable group included both men—who endeavoured to adhere to the sober, hardworking lifestyles advocated by the dominant group authorities—and women, concerned that the lifestyle associated with the larrikin way was harmful to the health of their families.

The larrikin and respectable subcultures interacted to produce local behaviours and outcomes not predictable on the basis of analysing either pattern by itself. Those identifying with larrikin ways created group cohesion by opposing the views and lifestyles of dominant groups and their local followers. Maintenance of the local order of insider solidarity promoted negative feelings about educational opportunities and other cultural resources available in the wider community. This has implications for the tolerance of health education messages coming from outsiders and for the success of a heart health program which we have described below.

The larrikin subculture is produced and validated through cultural practices such as 'mateship', which are acted out within compatible Coalfields settings—the pub, social club, and football institutions. More generally, the worldview and attendant lifestyle of individuals is informed by perceptions of the everyday conditions of their lives, differing psychological and biological attributes, and household economic advantage or disadvantage. In a two-way process of causality, broad economic and political forces impinging on the Coalfields influence local interactions; local patterns feed back into the wider order and further unfold the complex dynamic social system.

In complex dynamic social systems, in which individuals make the most of prevailing circumstances, the tuning of interactions with others, both within and outside the group, results in the development of a form of order (see Lewin 1993, p. 59). Such order in the Coalfields has emerged out of the interplay between attempts by the respectable group to undermine the larrikin worldview, and opposition by the larrikins to any encroachment on their valued patterns of life. Forces implicated in the process include the transition from underground to open-cut mining, overall decline of the mining industry locally, the lack of technical and service-based jobs and subsequent unemployment, the advent of feminism, and the increasing influence of ecological thinking.[6]

Within this context, health promoters began efforts to reduce the incidence of heart disease morbidity and mortality among Coalfields residents in the early 1980s. Initially, women took on the role of change agents in response to warnings about the coronary heart disease epidemic. Their challenge was to alter facets of male culture such as eating large quantities of meat to gain strength for doing hard physical labour (Heading 1996, pp. 338–48), to discourage smoking and drinking with mates, and to bring home heart health education messages circulating in the wider community. However, the strength of the ethos of male solidarity, the formation of gender relationships based on male dominance,[7] and male resistance to the introduction of ideas associated with feminism have reduced women's ability to bring about change (see Heading 1996, pp. 295–8, 338–48).

Similarly, initial efforts to stimulate community action in response to the epidemic were woefully inappropriate. The release of research findings about the epidemic produced a backlash seized upon by the local print media. Newspaper stories citing the university findings were written to suggest that the researchers had characterised Coalfields residents as 'fatties' who needed to change their lifestyle to reduce the risk of heart disease (*Newcastle Herald*, 8–10 January 1986). Unwittingly, public health research aimed at stimulating prevention appeared to reproduce historical discrimination by outsiders and set up the lines of resistance by insiders.

In May 1990, the University of Newcastle TD research team, along with Coalfields politicians, organised a public forum designed to interest residents in forming a community coalition to develop local strategies for reducing heart disease. Although this attempt to engage broad community participation fell short of expectations, a Healthy Heart Committee was formed. Members of the committee included researchers, health professionals, and local government leaders, some of whom had been members of the previously active Healthy Heart Support Group. The support group had formed in response to publicity in 1986 about the elevated rates of heart disease mortality and combined active community people with a health worker who sought to raise awareness of the epidemic through talks to clubs, special meetings, and cholesterol-screening activities (Higginbotham and Titheridge 1993). Subsequently, the support group and new committee joined forces to establish the Coalfields Healthy Heartbeat and immediately commissioned a needs survey to gauge the depth of concern (or lack thereof) about the heart disease epidemic.

The 1991 needs survey revealed that a majority in the community believed that the individual, the family, and the medical profession—in that order—should be responsible for heart disease prevention. There was little support for the idea that the community should be responsible for health. Indeed, about half the respondents felt that community groups should get involved only rarely, if at all. Furthermore, as mentioned above, residents gave a relatively low ranking to worry about heart attack (that is, eleventh out of seventeen social issues) (Higginbotham et al. 1993, p. 317).

Among a spectrum of activities aimed at encouraging local organisations to adopt heart health strategies, the most successful interventions were undertaken by Coalfields primary schools.[8] Schoolteachers and principals and other outsiders have energetically acted as change agents. The schools promote healthy heart messages to children through integrated curricula, daily physical education, and nutritious food choices at the school canteen. In turn, children carry these messages back home to parents and siblings (Williams and Plotnikoff 1995).

Older Coalfields residents' reaction to heart health campaigns has been mixed. Heading's (1996) survey revealed that those who were most resistant to heart health messages were more likely to have lower educational levels and lower incomes, and be male. Nevertheless, this group had *more* heart-related food knowledge than those who accepted the validity of heart health messages. The reluctance of these men to act on their knowledge of heart health may be because the choice to align themselves with the views and activities of outsiders does not, as yet, have as powerful an attraction as maintaining ties within their immediate social group. This finding illustrates the way in which the interplay between competing worldviews shapes perceptions and affects action.

One group of Coalfields residents who *are* interested in changing their lifestyle to reduce heart disease risk factors are those who have already experienced heart attacks. The everyday experience of disability, and perhaps imminent threat of losing one's life, appear sufficient to tip the balance towards adopting lifestyle changes advocated by health professionals and the women in their families at the expense of their loyalties to mateship culture. With encouragement from Coalfields Healthy Heartbeat, a thriving peer support network is now in place offering counselling and a rehabilitation program to heart patients and their families (Hunter Branch, Heart Support–Australia Association). A list of Coalfields Healthy Heartbeat interventions and levels of participation is shown in table 5.2.

Table 5.2 Coalfields Healthy Heartbeat intervention strategies: levels of participation and years initiated

Awareness Raising and Public Relations
(began 1986)
Media releases
Public displays
Heart health promotions (for example, Heart Week)
Guest speaking at clubs, schools, worksites
FM radio broadcasts (ongoing)
Mobilising Community Resources (1990)
Local Management Committee
Rehabilitation research
Healthy Communities program
Community consultation meetings (yearly)
Incorporating heart health into community events: fun run, motorcycle race, agricultural college events, Tidy Towns program, high school Health Expo
Heart Health Rehabilitation (since 1992)
Heart Support—Australia, branch office (40 regular members)
Rehabilitation exercise program (150 users)
Telephone counsellors trained (>45 counsellors)
Promoting Healthy Lifestyles
Cooking classes (since 1993; 200 users)
Low-fat cooking class
Healthy cooking for families
Healthy cooking demonstration
Supermarket tours (nutrition education)
Weight Control (1994; 20 users)
Regular classes
Classes targeted at the obese
Gentle Exercise (1993; >200 users)
T'ai chi classes
Promoting Healthy Lifestyles (cont.)
Gentle Exercise (cont.)
Regular classes with childcare provided
Walking for pleasure—walking trails book published
Anti-smoking programs (1994)
QUIT
Adolescent QUIT
Institutional and Environmental Development
Walk-in Heart Health Resource Centre (opened 1993)
Schools (launched 1992)
Healthy Heart Schools Network (15 primary and two high schools)
Health Promoting Schools (alcohol awareness, sun protection, quit smoking programs at three high schools)
Restaurants, Clubs and Retailers (1993)
'Healthy Eats' restaurant program (10 clubs and restaurants)
Fast food outlet accreditation (six shops)
Reduction in access of minors to cigarettes campaign
Industry Programs (1991)
Aluminium smelter
Garment manufacturing
Mobilising Institutional Resources
University research and educational resources (1990)
Regional Assistance Scheme funding (began 1994)
CHHB ongoing funding by New South Wales Health Department (1996)

Source: Albrecht, Freeman and Higginbotham (1998)

5.4.2 Conceptualising the unfolding of subcultures: the spiral diagram

Figure 5.1 displays the unfolding of two opposing subcultures related to heart disease in the Coalfields as described above.

This complex diagram, read from left to right, contains five components. Interactions within the Coalfields social system are represented as two spiralling lines, which move from the left to the right. Six opposing swirls arising from the

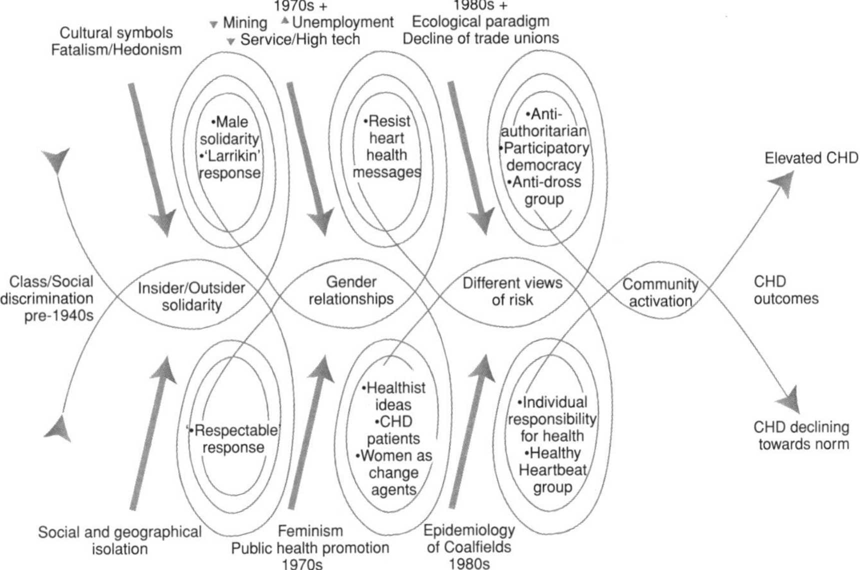

Figure 5.1 Evolution of subcultures related to CHD

spiralling lines represent the historical emergence of subculture components. Four central ellipses, created by the interaction of the two spiralling lines, represent areas of change and flux in the system which stimulate the formation of subcultures. Six black arrows pointing towards the central ellipses show external influences precipitating change to the system.

Figure 5.1 conveys the evolution of the larrikin and respectable subcultures across time using complexity theory principles. Identifiable aspects of these two subcultures are conceptualised in complexity theory terms as *social attractors*, identifiable sets of shared beliefs and practices which give the social system an emergent order at different historical moments.[9] A feature of non-linear systems is their possession of more than one attractor depending upon historical continuity and present environment.

Thus the complex Coalfields social system is viewed as two spirals of interacting forces which, from time to time, crystallise into identifiable components of a subculture (that is, social attractors). Figure 5.1 presents opposing social attractors that have emerged since the 1920s. The first set of opposing spirals are the larrikin and respectable subcultures, while the subsequent opposing spirals present elements of these two subcultures at later points in time: male solidarity and women as change agents, acceptance or rejection of health promotion campaigns, and individual versus community responsibility for health.

Complexity theory claims that spontaneous order and organisation can come from flux and disorder in natural systems. In figure 5.1, social attractors spiral out from either side of the central set of ellipses representing change in the system. Change is the catalyst for people to adopt a position, to formulate a view, or to align themselves in relation to others. Outside influences both precipitate and are subsequently affected by these changes. Coalfields social attractors have emerged from flux and disorder caused by the clash of views of insiders and outsiders, by differing interpretations of gender roles and relationships, by the dissemination of alternate ideas relating to health risk, and by differing opportunities to participate in community groups.[10]

The most recent example of social attractors, shown in figure 5.1, is the mobilisation of community groups. Evolving from the respectable subculture is the institutionalisation of heart disease prevention in the form of the Coalfields Healthy Heartbeat shopfront office in the Coalfields Community Centre. The office has two employees, undertakes a large number of activities guided by a local management committee, and operates under the auspices of a well-established charitable foundation. Although locally managed, the program embodies an outward orientation, seeking support, ideas, information, and working relationships with a variety of educational, medical, research, and community organisations.

A contrasting social attractor takes the form of a community group mobilised in 1994 to fight the development of an aluminium dross smelter close to homes and schools. Objections to the dross plant arose because its byproducts were considered hazardous to health. Like the Healthy Heart Committee, the anti-dross group was mobilised to protect and maintain health. However, for opponents of the dross smelter, the emphasis is less on individual responsibility for health than on industry and government responsibility towards the community.

Clashes between the anti-dross group and those supporting the smelter development have been intense and frequent. Protests have taken the form of public meetings, written submissions to the city council, rallies and marches, letters to the newspaper, lobbying state government ministers, and encouraging school children to write letters of protest to the government (Miller 1994, p. 1). Prior to its completion in 1996, the dross plant had received support from a range of outsiders, including business groups, planners, and state government departments and ministers (*Newcastle Herald*, 3 April 1996, editorial, p. 16). Similarly, local supporters include some city councillors, the business council, and residents who believed the plant would reduce unemployment in the region (Sorenson 1994a, p. 1). One councillor suggested that the anti-dross protesters were 'a vocal minority compared with the 15 000 plus people who live in the township' (Sorenson 1994b, p. 1). Clearly, though, the views of the anti-dross group follow closely those of the larrikin subculture and the sentiments expressed by the pro-dross group are compatible with the respectable strand.

Significant insights from the pattern of social attractors as shown in figure 5.1 are that historical characteristics of subcultures underlie the formation of present-day perceptions in the Coalfields and determine the form of community action adopted. An enduring theme in the larrikin subculture is an anti-authoritarian rejection of outsider-imposed threats to lifestyle.[11] This is a prominent concern of the anti-dross campaigners. Another campaign element with historical connections is concern for the environment.[12] The 1991 needs survey found that 61 per cent of Coalfields residents felt that the environment was an area of 'worry' and, along with local pollution, ranked highly as a problem (Higginbotham et al. 1993, p. 317).

For most of the twentieth century trade unionism and socialist ideologies were prominent in the Coalfields (Turner 1979; 1983). A downturn in mining, reduction in blue-collar jobs generally, and rising unemployment has eroded the membership and thus the influence of trade unions. Given these declines, and the preexisting concern for the environment, it is not surprising that the anti-dross campaigners have adopted the ecological paradigm to press home their argument that Coalfields residents must mobilise to fight against outsider-imposed threats to their lifestyle. While this activism is directed towards a health-related issue, connections with earlier industrial struggles are apparent. One Coalfields resident explicitly linked the current fight against the proposed dross plant to a famous industrial conflict nearly 70 years earlier: 'The fathers and grandfathers [of both towns] fought at Rothbury[13] against oppression. Why are we not united against pollution?' (Wright 1994, p. 7)

In the same manner that trade unionists' struggles were aimed at increasing participation in decision-making affecting their lifestyles, contemporary activists continue the call for participatory democracy to replace imposed decision-making.

> The people of [the Coalfields] have demonstrated great courage and tenacity in their bid to stop the progress of an industry that they believe will be detrimental to their health and lifestyle. Politicians, whether they are of local, State or Federal persuasion, should remember that they represent the people (Johnson 1994, p. 6).

Further emergence of a clear pattern is seen in the involvement of former prominent mining union leaders, some of whom are in their 70s and 80s (*Newcastle Herald*, 13 October 1994, p. 3). A smooth transition has been made from leading the miners in industrial disputes against mine owners and allied politicians, to leading community activists in their struggle against the owners of the proposed aluminium plant and politicians in favour of the development. Indeed, the number of socialists and communists embracing environmental concerns has led their opponents to label them watermelons: green on the outside, red on the inside.

Despite the protesters' best efforts, the dross smelter was approved in 1996 and continues to operate. However, the strength of the social attractor of community protest is such that the group remains active, collecting evidence of pollution from the dross smelter and nearby aluminium-processing plant, and pressuring politicians to police environmental regulations. Indeed, the divisions between the pro- and anti-dross groups persist, as predicted by our complexity diagram and reflected in a newspaper editorial:

> There is something unsettling about this long-running and bitter dispute which must lead observers to wonder whether the decision of any disinterested umpire will ever be accepted by such intransigent warring parties (editorial, *Newcastle Herald*, 3 April 1996, p. 16).

The paradox of the Coalfields community's apparent indifference to reducing a major health problem (CHD) while mobilising strongly in response to perceived health threats from the dross plant is also part of an historical pattern. In the past, mining communities in the Coalfields have taken responsibility for their own health by mobilising to provide health care facilities and associated support services for the sick and injured.[14] The extremely dangerous conditions in coal mines was one of the prime motivations. In 1900, for example, the mineworkers' accident fund was set up to pay a small allowance to victims of mining accidents. In its early days, miners contributed half of the scheme's funds, with the remaining costs being shared by the government and mine owners (Metcalfe 1988, p. 231). Since the mid 1980s, miners' lodges in the Hunter Valley have levied their workers to provide donations to the Hunter rescue helicopter service that transports seriously ill patients to the major teaching hospital in the area. Threats to replace this service with a private commercial operation from outside the region resulted in the Miners' Union signing up helicopter operators as union members so that industrial action could be taken if necessary to protect the service.

Ongoing medical care was also a shared concern in the Coalfields. In the early part of the twentieth century, miners' lodges introduced a medical scheme that employed salaried doctors to treat mining families free of charge (Metcalfe 1988, p. 117). Mining lodges, miners, and mining communities in the Newcastle and Hunter Valley areas were also responsible for pooling their resources to establish local hospitals.

Clearly, there is a strong cultural heritage of local community responsibility for providing treatment for the ill and injured—of looking after your own. This is very different to having to cede control of decision-making concerning health matters to outsiders. By contributing to the establishment and ongoing ownership of medical services, Coalfields families feel that it is their right to use those services when necessary. Ironically, the same communitarian spirit, ethos of participatory democracy, and male solidarity which underpinned the evolution of the larrikin subculture, and which prompted some to reject the heart health promotion messages of outsiders, has also underpinned the creation of grassroots health services.

In review, complexity theory provides a framework for identifying dynamic processes that form two contrasting subcultures in the Coalfields. It offers us insights into the emergence of this complex social system through an analysis of the interplay of industrial history, heart disease risk factors, gender relations, and community responses to the epidemic, as well as to the health promotion campaigns aimed at its alleviation. The recurrence of patterned forms of order seen in the spiral concept suggests future directions for heart health interventions in that region. One inference to be drawn from these recurrences is that action to reduce coronary heart disease among high-risk groups, who may be identified with the larrikin heart subculture and resistant to outsider interventions, will be most successful if it involves self-generated action similar to that undertaken to protest against the dross plant. A health project can unleash energy available in this community if it develops as a local response to health needs insiders perceive as relevant on the basis of their preexisting worldviews. In contrast, it is futile to approach the larrikin heart with an outsider-imposed disease control program; the anti-authoritarian feeling underlying the larrikin tradition rejects authoritarian solutions, no matter how well-intentioned they may be.

5.5 The larrikin heart

The concept of a dissipative structure that we introduced in chapter 3 provides a useful analogy for the way in which the embodied self maintains integrity by interacting with the environment. As seen in figure 5.2, the larrikin response is viewed as a way of transforming disorder, arising from social discrimination (a form of perturbation), into order via the construction of supportive social relations and a positive self-image. *Social entropy* is exported to the environment through disrupting work patterns, antagonising respectables, and refusing to live a rational lifestyle. However, a byproduct of this process is an increase in biological entropy. The human body takes in energy from social relations and from products made meaningful by those social relations (for example, camaraderie, mateship, drinking, eating certain foods such as meat, smoking, gambling, risk taking, and masculine bonding). However, unless the waste products of this process (cholesterol, stress, obesity, addiction) can be exported (through exercise, diet, drugs, relaxation, or therapy, for example) they are stored in the body, increasing the risk of cardiovascular disease or other losses to self-regulation.

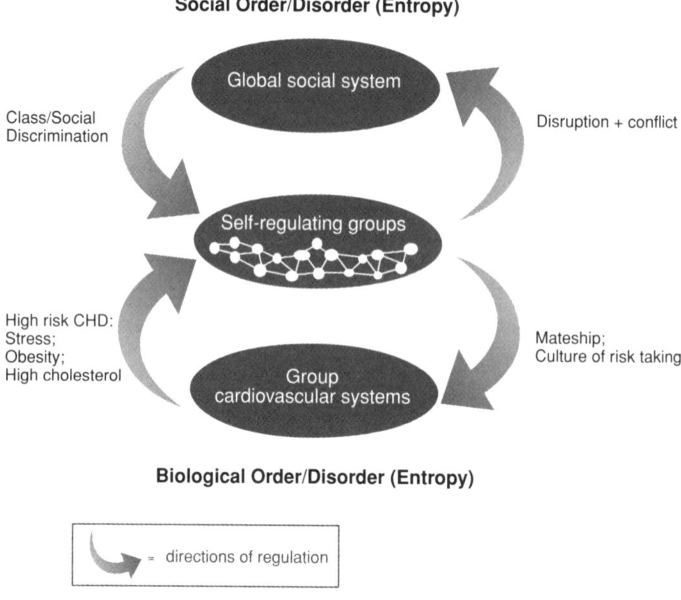

Source: Albrecht, Freeman and Higginbotham (1998)

Figure 5.2 The larrikin heart as a way of transforming disorder

In essence, self-regulation towards coherence and order in the social system produces an opposite process in the biological system: a disruption in biological self-regulation towards the disorder of heart disease. Is this a unique dynamic found in the Coalfields or a process underlying other health problems in other local environments? We believe that the Coalfields example shows how well complexity theory can be used to explain health problems.

5.6 Conclusion

Our case study of CHD provides an elaborate example of how TD researchers, travelling in transdisciplinary space, were able to address the leading cause of death in postindustrial societies. The TD team juxtaposed biomedical findings about the causes of CHD with insights from ethnographic fieldwork describing lay notions of the disease and its prevention. Similarly, epidemiological data on risk factors and the incidence of CHD were understood in the light of historical analyses and political economy theories of imposed risks. Complexity theory explained the evolution of connections between these seemingly unrelated bodies of knowledge and how non-linear relationships characterise community health. In particular, the analysis drew power from our conceptualisation of the Coalfields as a dissipative structure, through which energy is exchanged between biological and social systems, resulting in elevated rates of CHD among Coalfields men. By encouraging the use of a full range of logics or ways of reasoning (including lay beliefs and rationales), complexity theory became a valuable learning resource and common conceptual framework for the team. It enabled the TD researchers to understand the dialectical relationships emerging between themselves and the study community, and stimulated new avenues for research.

Notes

1 The most important type of arterial disease is arteriosclerosis, characterised by hardening and loss of elasticity of the arterial walls, and narrowing of the channel, which reduces the flow of blood. Most arteriosclerosis is associated with atherome, which is a deposit of greasy material, mainly cholesterol, in the lining of the artery (Wingate and Wingate 1988, p. 47).

2 A large percentage of Coalfields residents are descended from United Kingdom and particularly Welsh miners who immigrated to Australia in the early part of the twentieth century (Metcalfe 1988, p. 7). It has been hypothesised that because many people in the Coalfields are descended from relatively small areas of Wales and northern England there may be an unusually high prevalence of recessive genes associated with heart disease risk (Malcolm 1993, p. 103).

3 We have by no means exhaustively examined all elements of influence impacting on CHD. Areas for further research include whether or not the construction of self influences decision-making relating to CHD and the possible impact of workplace stress on CHD (see Knutsson et al. 1986 and Siegrist et al. 1990 for examples).

4 The concept of adaptation is highly contested. In this context we use Alland's 'mini-max' model of adaptation as a useful construct for describing the responses of a population to the cultural dynamics operating at local, national, and international levels. Some researchers define adaptation to mean 'perfect fit', an 'ideal adjustment', or a 'solution without problems'. However, according to Alland, at best, an adaptive strategy miminises risks and maximises benefits. But rarely are risks avoided altogether (Alland 1970; McElroy 1990, p. 381). In adapting their worldview and lifestyle to achieve 'fitness', that is, making the most of the sociopolitical circumstances, Coalfields residents have adopted strategies that increase their risk of contracting heart and other diseases.

5 We do not intend to suggest that these views are attributable to individual miners. Metcalfe (1988, p. 76) has emphasised that the larrikin–respectable categories are ideal types, drawn from cultural models which miners created to make sense of their lives. Individuals can draw on aspects of either or both responses, selectively mobilising a range of ideas which do not necessarily appear rational or consistent to outsiders.

6 Influences such as this are known as perturbations to the system in complexity theory (Goerner 1994, p. 48).

7 According to Metcalfe, 'Aggressive masculinity became an expression of miners' solidarity, and misogyny could double as a mark of loyalty to workmates' (1988, p. 181).

8 Freeman et al. (1990) have reported that children living in low economic status areas are likely to have higher levels in childhood of factors associated in adults with risk of CHD. Barker et al. (1989;1992) have suggested that adult disease (including CHD) may have its origins in foetal and childhood experiences.

9 A social attractor is conceptual rather than a mathematical device to assist in the description of patterns that become apparent after iterations of an apparently random system. In the Coalfields, social attractors are empirically described patterns that emerged from triangulating data from historical archives, participant observation, needs, and attitude surveys and statistics from the MONICA Project.

10 Bak and Chen's discussion of self-organised criticality (1991, pp. 26–33) is relevant to the process of interactive evolution illustrated by the spiral diagram.

11 This is best illustrated by miners' participation in trade unions and an acceptance of socialist and communist ideologies (Turner 1974, p. 352; 1979; 1983; Metcalfe 1991).

12 From the 1920s the environmental concerns of miners in the Coalfields were expressed as 'ecological socialism' (Metcalfe 1988, p. 204).

13 In 1929, an attempt by coalmine owners to reduce miners' wages in defiance of a court ruling led to a lockout in the northern Coalfields of New South Wales which lasted 15 months. The re-opening of a mine at Rothbury with non-union labour precipitated a riot between miners and police during which one miner was killed. This incident was followed by a period of extreme industrial turmoil in the Coalfields, and left a legacy of bitterness among mining families (Turner 1974, p. 412).

14 Balance sheets of the Richmond Main Lodge at Kurri Kurri for the years 1934, 1950, and 1959, for example, show that the lodge raised regular levies for Kurri Kurri District Hospital and for funeral, medical, and sick leave funds (Metcalfe 1988, p. 117).

6
Pharmaceuticals in Transdisciplinary Perspective

LINDA CONNOR, NICK HIGGINBOTHAM, SONIA FREEMAN, AND GLENN ALBRECHT

'The power behind your doctor'

Chances are your GP sees, on average, two drug company representatives a week, meeting each, on average, three times a year and spending 11 minutes with each. The GP will spend about 80 minutes each week reading medical newspapers and journals largely funded by drug company advertisements, spend 14 minutes reading drug company mailings, and attend several meetings a year, mostly organised by drug companies.

'Future shock'

If we turn our gaze backwards two or three generations to the beginning of the twentieth century, we are shocked by the primitive nature of the treatments being offered to those suffering from illness. Even one generation back, at the beginning of the 1960s [*sic*], the idea of routinely prescribing medicines to pregnant women was still common—an idea which today would bring gasps of horror from most medical practitioners. One cannot help but wonder what the inhabitants of this planet will think 100 years from now when they, in turn, look back at the medicine of the late twentieth century.

Will they be appalled at the mishandling of antibiotics, which led to the spread of microbial resistance and perhaps, as some commentators have suggested, so assaulted the human immune system that scourges such as acquired immune deficiency syndrome (AIDS) were able to take root?

Will they feel outrage that even in remote jungle outposts the coolers existed to keep sugar-laden soft drinks chilled, but the cold-chain of freezers essential to keep measles vaccines at the right temperature was missing, resulting in some two million preventable deaths of young children each year?

Will they be shocked to discover that the pain killer dipyrone, which was described by the American Medical Association (AMA) in 1977 as 'obsolete' provided some 5 per cent of the turnover of a leading research-based drug manufacturer in 1987, despite the existence of equally effective and safer products on the market?

Will they be stunned by the hard-sell promotion for an anti-arthritic product, benoxaprofen—which triggered enormous sales in its short market life, and a series of unfortunate side effects—and the paltry sum which victims of the drug received in compensation?

Will they be dismayed by the practice, widespread for a generation, of starting men and women on the road to drug dependence through the incautious prescribing of benzodiazepine tranquillisers in place of sound counselling and support?

Will they be staggered by the poor quality of many of the drug toxicology tests and clinical trials performed, such as the study which found that one product caused no more cancer in chickens than a placebo, but which failed to report that half the chickens died of heart failure?

Will they be amazed that in 1980 the World Health Organization (WHO) said that the antibiotic neomycin 'should never be used in the treatment of acute diarrhoea', yet 7 years later, 14 per cent of anti-diarrhoeals on the market in developing countries contained neomycin?

Will they laugh or shake their heads sadly at the promotion of pizotifen in Western Europe for the prevention of migraine headaches with a caution that it may cause slight weight gain in some patients, while in several developing countries the same product promises rapid growth and effective appetite stimulation among malnourished children?

Will they conclude that the inappropriate use of medicines was one of the factors which transformed the hope of the WHO strategy for 'Health for All by the Year 2000' into a hollow dream?

The preceding excerpts from Ann Casey (1993) and Andrew Chetley (1990) draw attention to the realm of medicinal products and the question of how they can be distributed fairly, at a reasonable price, and be used beneficially rather than harmfully in a global market economy. While Chetley highlights problems in the provision, supply, and use/abuse of pharmaceuticals over the past century, Casey focuses on the promotional role of pharmaceutical companies and their agents. In this chapter, we will explore how transdisciplinary thinking can be applied to the production, marketing, and use of pharmaceuticals, integrating different types of analysis to provide a more profound understanding of the health issues at stake.

6.1 Introduction

In chapter 2 we provided an overview of the hierarchy of health influences and the disciplines that are traditionally associated with different levels of the hierarchy. We presented theories and frameworks that integrate a variety of disciplines with the aim of providing a fuller understanding of health problems. In chapter 3, we outlined the potential of complexity theory as a highly integrative framework that can be applied to issues in health. In this chapter, we integrate theories and approaches from different disciplines to investigate the ways in which pharmaceuticals are an issue of importance in international health.

Health social science researchers have examined pharmaceutical issues from both the *structural* and *interpretive* perspectives. Structural analysis operates on a macro scale. Company reports, parliamentary proceedings, policy documents, media sources, and many other data are examined to see how political and economic forces shape the production, distribution, and consumption of pharmaceuticals. 'Structures' are defined as patterns of social interaction between people or institutions, for instance, networks of capital investment, relationships between management and workers, and interactions between international agencies and national governments. These are all social creations but they are argued to be powerful and constraining, and not easily changed.

Interpretive perspectives usually operate on a micro scale. Local and community interactions are studied to see how people talk about their use of medicines and how they act in cases of illness. Health provider–patient interactions, retail advertising and sale of drugs, and health care within households and local communities are studied by interview and participant observation. The aim of interpretive research on health and healing is the 'understanding and reconstruction' of the symbolic world that people create (Guba and Lincoln 1994, p. 113).

In this chapter we first use political economy, a structural theoretical approach, to examine the World Health Organization's (WHO) Action Program on Essential Drugs (usually abbreviated to Drug Action Program, or DAP). An analysis of events surrounding the formulation of this policy at World Health Assemblies (WHA) since 1978 offers an insight into the competing interests of groups with differing economic and political agendas (Hardon 1992). Controversy has surrounded attempts by developing countries to implement WHO recommendations. In a detailed example, we explore how the introduction of the Bangladesh National Drug Policy (NDP) has been shaped by global processes as well as by political and economic constraints at the national level.

To complement the structural perspective, we address the cultural meaning of medicines through interpretive analyses. The rationale for combining structural and interpretive perspectives is provided by Van der Geest (1985, p. 144). He has urged anthropologists to 'study linkages among international, national, regional and local processes' so that global power relations can be contextualised and given meaning in terms of the knowledge of particular groups in specific historical circumstances. This is, in fact, recognition of the value of a transdisciplinary approach to the health issues connected with pharmaceuticals and of the importance of moving between levels of the health hierarchy in addressing health problems.

In the final section of the chapter, we move across more levels of the health hierarchy in our attempt to understand the evolution of drug resistance on a global scale. In addressing this problem, we show linkages between the political economy of pharmaceuticals, and ecological and biological levels of the health hierarchy.

6.2 Structural analysis: political economy or modernisation theory?

The theoretical foundations of *political economy* were established in the eighteenth and nineteenth centuries. The transformation of European society by capitalism and industrialisation led to an interest in the relationship between the production of wealth and the activities of the state by writers such as Karl Marx. Political economy approaches to the analysis of social life were particularly popular among social scientists in the 1960s and 1970s in the context of civil rights movements and anti-colonialism. This use was in part a reaction against conservative structural-functionalist theories, including modernisation theory, which dominated social science in the 1950s and 1960s.

Political economy is concerned with the relationship between social classes (most simply, between those who have capital to invest and those who work for wages), the role of the state in supporting or regulating the economy, and the way the imperative of profit affects other areas of social life. Political economy is an example of a *critical theory* which seeks to transform society by understanding the oppression and exploitation of workers and less powerful groups, such as rural people in developing countries (Guba and Lincoln 1994, p. 113). A basic assumption of this kind of theory is that there are conflicts of interest between manufacturers and workers, and between rich countries and developing ones. For this reason social theorists label it as a type of conflict theory.

An opposing structural analysis is that of *modernisation theory*. Although this is also a macro level theory, it makes the opposite assumption—that there can be agreement among groups, no matter how different their power and wealth, about the form of the social policies designed to bring about further development. For this reason it is labelled as a type of *consensus theory*. This theory examines processes by which less-industrialised societies achieve modernity, based on the assumption that modernisation on the pattern of Western industrial society is the inevitable and desirable pattern for all societies to imitate.

Modernisation theory focuses on patterns of diffusion of innovations and the characteristics of people adopting the innovations. It is assumed that the impact of modernisation is 'inherently beneficial and progressive' (Stock 1985, p. 117). Economic reform is seen as an integral part of modernisation; it is noticeable that world policy debates are now dominated by expert recommendations of economic liberalisation and structural adjustment—that is, the reduction of services provided by governments and the increase of their provision by the free market. These policies have implications for the provision of pharmaceuticals.

Modernisation theory assumes that all societies and all people share an interest in and a desire for economic development. In contrast, political economy suggests that there are conflicting interests in national societies and internationally, between nations. It focuses on social and economic inequality and argues that what is beneficial to large corporations and their profits may be at the expense of small business, local people, and the environment. Studies which use a political economic framework examine inequalities of power, the interdependence of government and commercial enterprise, and how political structures affect social policy and health. Political economy appears to us to be the more compelling theory for understanding the pharmaceutical industry on a global and national scale.

6.2.1 Dependency theory

Dependency theory extends the concepts of political economy to look at the relations between Western capitalist nations and developing countries. The most well-known exponents of dependency theory are Andre Gunder Frank and Emmanuel Wallerstein.[1] Dependency theory is sometimes called *world systems theory* or the *development of underdevelopment* approach. In terms of dependency theory, the *core* or *metropolitan* countries—industrialised countries with high capital reserves—are exploiters of the *periphery*—the ex-colonies (usually termed developing and, until recently, Third World nations) which provide cheap raw materials, labour, and mass markets of consumers. The peripheral countries have weak state regulatory bodies which do not inhibit processes of capital accumulation. As some critics of dependency theory have pointed out, this scenario has been complicated by the rise of the newly developed economies of Asia, such as Korea and Taiwan. However, the economic crisis of the late 1990s in Asia suggests that these economies are still subject to the economic domination of Europe and the USA.

Rather than viewing Western development in technological innovation as leading to progress, dependency theorists view such innovations as contributing to the disempowerment and impoverishment (termed *underdevelopment*) of developing countries and economies. It is considered that the penetration of peripheral countries by metropolitan economic interests, cultural influences, and technology fosters underdevelopment rather than prosperity.

The breadth of analysis of studies drawing on political economy and dependency theory makes them well-suited to incorporation into a transdisciplinary framework of problem solving. They are typically characterised by synthesis and interpretation of existing sources of information rather than the undertaking of more narrowly conceived empirical studies. A criticism that is often made of dependency theory is that it is too deterministic, meaning that it is primarily concerned with the structures of society, leaving little or no scope for understanding the initiatives or agency of subordinate groups or individuals. The breadth of analysis often overlooks the fine-grained detail of social and cultural practices, implies that individual actors have no choices, and that they are at the mercy of global forces. A transdisciplinary approach allows us to overcome these limitations by combining more interpretive micro studies with the macro studies of global and national structures. First, we look at an example of an analysis from the political economy point of view which is of vital importance in the health of the world's people.

6.3 Political economy of the pharmaceutical industry

Thomas Bodenheimer used dependency theory to analyse the transnational nature of the pharmaceutical industry (1984, pp. 187–215); the basic terms of this argument continued to be used by researchers in the 1990s (Silverman et al. 1992; Chowdhury 1995). Bodenheimer argues that there is conflict between the core countries (locus of capital accumulation) and those peripheral nations whose resources are exploited to produce capital profits through the mechanisms of cheap labour, low taxes, and transfer pricing.[2] Research and development are generally concentrated in the world's affluent core countries while the assembly of medicines is increasingly being carried out in low-wage, low-tax peripheral nations.

In this view, the potential for chemical and biological discoveries to reduce suffering and promote health for the world's people has been only partially realised due mainly to the actions of transnational companies who treat potentially life-giving scientific advances as vehicles for creating immense profits. The world pharmaceutical market is dominated by a small number of transnational companies based mainly in the USA, Switzerland, Germany, the United Kingdom and, more recently, Japan. In 1992–93, the top twenty companies controlled more than 50 per cent of global sales (Chowdhury 1995, p. 1). Bodenheimer describes the development of technological innovation and monopoly patents as a means of maintaining high profit levels. Sponsorship of research in universities and medical schools is viewed as contributing to biased and profit-motivated research. The aggressive promotional activities of detailers (salespeople), including the bribing of physicians and health officials, are cited as further ways by which transnationals and their agents maximise profits at the expense of the health of the world's people.

Much criticism is directed towards the activities of the transnational corporations in less developed countries (Hardon 1992; Silverman et al. 1992; Chowdhury 1995). Unsafe drugs are marketed in the periphery after they have been banned or limited in industrialised countries. Stereotypic images of women and their pharmaceutical needs are used to market drugs such as tranquillisers and tonics. Some social groups are used in drug experimentation studies that may be of little relevance to their health. Aggressive marketing in developing countries has resulted in some countries spending up to 40 per cent of their health budget on drugs, draining funds needed for basic health services (Bodenheimer 1984, p. 194; Weerasuriya and Brudon 1998, p. 32). One result is increased indebtedness to transnational banks that are often closely interlocked with the pharmaceutical industry. Furthermore, linkages between industry and government regulating agencies in both Western and undeveloped countries may act as barriers to action on the perceived abuses and excesses of the pharmaceutical industry (see section 6.4.1).

This analysis does not go unchallenged by proponents of the free market and of modernisation theory. For example, David Taylor (1986, pp. 1141–9) writes on behalf of the Association of the British Pharmaceutical Industry that the multinational drug industry is being inappropriately scapegoated for the failures of local élites. Similarly, excessive government regulation will lead to the rigidity characteristic of all command (that is, highly centralised and regulated) economies. In general, Taylor argues that competition and consumer choice will lead to a better health system than government monopolies and socialised medicine. In a more recent analysis, health economist Patricia Danzon states that national regulatory policies for pharmaceuticals 'should be designed to balance the desire to control costs with the health concerns of individual patients today and the need to preserve incentives for innovation to develop the drugs for tomorrow' (1997, p. 92). Danzon does not engage with arguments of the pharmaceutical industry's critics who argue that most research and development expenditure is not directed towards the development of new and urgently needed drugs (see, for example, Silverman et al. 1992; Chowdhury 1995), but is thinly disguised promotion or research on copy-cat drugs that will increase market share.

6.3.1 Globalisation and the pharmaceutical industry

Dependency theory provides a useful analytical tool for explaining the worldwide evolution of the political economy of pharmaceuticals. However, in the past 20 years, globalisation of the world economic system, including the establishment of international trade organisations, regulatory bodies, and lobby groups, has blurred distinctions between the notions of core and periphery. Two global organisations playing key roles in the evolution of the global pharmaceutical system are the World Trade Organization (WTO), established in 1995, and the World Health Organization.

The trend towards globalisation has profound implications for both developed and developing countries, opening up the possibility of changes in cultural mores, agricultural practices, social and political relationships, and the health of populations. Supporters claim that globalisation 'will produce the best possible outcome for economic development' (Velasquez and Boulet 1999, p. 288). However, the United Nations' *Human Development Report* for 1997[3] warns:

> Globalisation has its winners and its losers. With the expansion of trade and foreign investment, developing countries have seen the gaps among themselves widen . . . Poor countries often lose out because the rules of the game are biased against them, particularly those relating to international trade (cited in Velasquez and Boulet 1999, p. 288).

Recent global developments in trade regulations support this view. The Agreement on Trade-Related Property Rights (TRIPS), introduced under the auspices of the WTO, provides globalised control over intellectual property rights in areas such as copyrights, trademarks, and patents, including patents for pharmaceuticals and agricultural products and processes. Velasquez and Boulet (1999, pp. 288–91) note a number of adverse effects for developing countries brought on by the TRIPS Agreement, which:

- reduces the autonomy of state governments by curbing their ability to determine their own patent laws
- inhibits the development of Indigenous pharmaceutical industries
- limits the ability of fledgling state companies to improve technological and manufacturing skills by graduating from producing copies of drugs developed elsewhere to researching and developing new formulas

- reduces the possibility of reverse engineering, that is, the process by which research on drugs is copied and adapted to suit local conditions
- skews research and development by multinationals towards the most profitable patented drugs, rather than towards those which will be of most benefit nationally
- limits access to less expensive generic drugs
- promotes monopoly control over biotechnology through patenting seeds, plants, and non-biological and microbiological processes, including the production of Indigenous medicines (for example, herbal medicines).

However, improvements in pharmaceutical systems have been achieved in several developing countries through global initiatives by the World Health Organization's Action Program on Essential Drugs. In the next section we describe the introduction of DAP, its effect on the global pharmaceutical system, and its potential to improve access to drugs in the developing world.

6.4 Political economy at the global level: WHO Action Program on Essential Drugs

By the 1980s many developing countries had multiple problems around the supply of drugs. In terms of consumption, poor people had limited access to appropriate pharmaceuticals, while there was a proliferation of unnecessary and often harmful brand-name medications including vitamins, tonics, cough medicines, restoratives, antacids, and psychotropic drugs (Chowdhury 1995, p. 3). Large numbers of drugs were purchased, including many types of antibiotics, predominantly without prescription (Reich 1994, p. 130; Saradamma et al. 2000). While there was a large range of outlets for drugs, most retailers had little education and there were economic incentives for all drug providers, including doctors, to prescribe multiple drugs, with little fear of regulatory control or litigation (Reich 1994, p. 131; see also Kamat and Nichter 1998). The distribution of medicines was also a problem. In many public facilities, drugs were supposed to be free but they were never available; private clinics had greater supplies but they were not affordable for most of the population. There was no public control over drug prices or private dispensing. A high proportion of drugs were imported, costing governments foreign exchange which was in short supply. Also, though many countries had a small domestic production capacity, local factories did not have very good quality control (Reich 1994, pp. 131–2).

The Essential Drugs concept was introduced by WHO in 1978 after considerable pressure and resolutions by the non-aligned countries of the world at their 1976 conference (Chowdhury 1995, pp. 38–9). Essential Drugs policies were developed to ensure 'the availability of a regular supply to all people of a selected number of safe and effective drugs of acceptable quality at lowest cost' (Lee et al. 1991, p. 51). DAP was established in 1981 and was later extended to provide objective information about drugs to health workers and the public. In 1986 the WHA approved a revised drugs strategy which added 'rational use' of drugs to the distribution of essential drugs as an element of DAP (Lee et al. 1991, p. 52). At the time of writing, DAP remains active, publishing the *Essential Drugs Monitor*, a biannual newsletter.

Proposals to implement DAP in the private sector have met with vigorous opposition from the pharmaceutical industry, with one spokesperson claiming that such lists 'would have a very adverse impact on the practice of medicine, the level of competition in the pharmaceutical industry, the rate of pharmaceutical innovation and the overall cost of illness in human and economic terms' (cited in Lee et al. 1991, p. 52). However, proponents argue that the adoption of an essential drugs program offers the opportunity for developing countries to limit drugs to those considered essential, promote generic rather than brand names, and reduce the cost and toxicity of drugs.

Essential drugs programs have been successfully implemented in a number of countries. In local health units of the Democratic Republic of Yemen's public health system, an essential drugs program ensured ample supplies of necessary drugs, and rational prescribing was promoted, with fewer injections, less antibiotic prescribing, and fewer drugs per prescription (Lee et al. 1991, p. 52). The benefits of regulating the private market were demonstrated early in Sri Lanka, which in 1972 reduced the number of drugs imported from 2100 to 600 by removing all unsafe and cost-ineffective drugs from its private market and extending the use of generic names to the private sector. These measures enabled the State Pharmaceutical Corporation to effectively undertake bulk purchasing and save on foreign exchange by 40 per cent in the first 6 months after implementation of the program (Mamdani and Walker 1986, p. 193; Chowdhury 1995, pp. 28–36). In Guinea, which first adopted an essential drugs policy as part of a major government-sponsored reform of the health sector in 1986, health indicators have risen and the affordability of drugs has increased over the 10-year period between 1986 and 1996 (Timmermans 1996, pp. 7–8).

One of the ways in which essential drugs programs have been implemented is through the centralised bulk buying of essential drugs on the open market through international tenders. Centralised purchasing in Egypt has helped to keep the prices of pharmaceuticals constant for 10 years and has also created a favourable climate for the development of a strong local industry. Centralised purchasing enabled Costa Rica to make savings of £17.6 million in 1978 alone, and increased its ability to meet people's drug needs from 46.8 per cent in 1970 to 81.5 per cent in 1976 (Mamdani and Walker 1986, p. 194).

Such measures do not provide the whole answer. Many developing countries are still paying very high prices for drugs, in spite of buying drugs through competitive tender (Chowdhury 1995, pp. 17–20). This is partly due to the limited information available regarding alternate supply, quality and costs of products, bureaucratic delays, transfer pricing, and the availability of foreign exchange when the tender is accepted (Mamdani and Walker 1986, p. 194).

It is increasingly being recognised that donor-supported essential drugs programs may be paternalistic and fail to recognise the existence of local production capabilities which could be initiated into the program. Also, donors tend to want high-profile programs that yield benefits quickly. This often results in centralised programs that discourage coordination among sectors within the country and hinder local involvement. Essential drugs programs need to address the issue of fostering self-reliance rather than dependency. It has been suggested that policy makers need to broaden these objectives from drug procurement from abroad to a more general program that includes local production, quality control capability, and local packing and management of distribution (Munishi 1991, p. 13).

Another major problem is that developing countries have attempted to introduce changes without the necessary administrative and legal frameworks. Many developing countries have weak regulatory mechanisms for enforcing national drug programs. Furthermore, commitment to an essential drugs program requires a strong political will, a commitment often lacking in politically unstable developing countries. However, even when the necessary political will exists (and this may be associated with authoritarian regimes), national governments in developing countries may have to battle with opposition from multinational pharmaceutical companies, Western governments, and international financial institutions who are striving to ensure the freedom of the private pharmaceutical industry to maximise its profits. According to Mamdani and Walker, the policies embodied in the DAP are likely to be only partly successful unless they are accepted by the top six drug-producing nations (France, Germany, Italy, Japan, the UK and the USA) who also contribute over half the total annual WHO budget (1986, p. 1913).

6.4.1 Power, conflict, and the Action Program on Essential Drugs

The political economy approach impels us to focus our attention on the issue of power. For example: Who are the main beneficiaries of policies and practices relating to the pharmaceutical industry? Who makes the decisions? What is the role of international groups and agencies? What is the relationship between the private and public spheres? What types of knowledge are seen as privileged or legitimated? What sort of ideology underpins the health system? To whom are health workers responsible?

For conflict theorists, power and authority are the key to the control of scarce resources. Those who hold power have an interest in maintaining the status quo, while those who do not, often have an interest in change. The world is thus defined in terms of potentially conflicting groups (Litva and Eyles 1995, p. 9). Hardon (1992, pp. 49–64) has documented how attempts by WHO in the early 1980s to formulate and implement an Essential Drugs Policy to increase the availability of safe, effective, and affordable drugs in developing countries resulted in conflict between consumer and producer groups manifested at public forums, notably WHA.

WHO's role in formulating an Essential Drugs Policy was opposed by the International Federation of Pharmaceutical Manufacturers Association (IFPMA), by conservative political groups in developing countries, and by the governments of some Western countries. WHO's initiatives have been supported by consumer groups, including Health Action International (HAI), a coalition of about fifty non-governmental organisations from twenty-seven countries active in public health issues related to health and pharmaceuticals. WHO initiatives have also been welcomed by the governments of some developing countries. Lobbying at World Health Assemblies by representatives of producers and consumers in alliance with various government delegations has had a vital effect on the success or otherwise of proposals for implementing essential drugs policies and for monitoring the pharmaceutical industry.

Following the introduction of the DAP in 1981, the pharmaceutical industry and US representatives at the World Health Assemblies put pressure on WHO to confine essential drugs policies to the public sector in developing countries. Any recommendations to regulate the private sector activities of multinational pharmaceutical companies were strongly resisted. To head off a proposal by WHO to introduce a regulatory code on pharmaceuticals, and in response to the growing organisational strength of consumer groups, IFPMA introduced its own marketing code in March 1981. The code was criticised by HAI which argued that the provisions and procedures for interpreting, monitoring, and enforcing breaches were inadequate. HAI resolved to continue calling for a 'proper code of practice through WHO, UNCTAD[4] and/or other appropriate parts of the United Nations System' (HAI 1982, p. 3, quoted in Hardon 1992, p. 51). Nevertheless, WHO 'welcomed' the IFPMA code and decided to refrain from pursuing its own code for a 'trial, but unspecified period' (Mamdani and Walker 1986, p. 191).

To date, pressure from the pharmaceutical industry and certain Western governments has been successful in preventing WHO from developing a code or even strong guidelines on the marketing, distribution, and use of pharmaceuticals in developing countries. However, the struggle continues. Consumer groups cooperating with HAI continue to lobby government representatives, national policy makers, and the public in both developed and developing countries. They have succeeded in heightening public awareness of the issues involved and have called on public support for their national essential drugs policies covering both private and public sectors.

6.5 Bangladesh: conflicts over national drug policy

The controversies which took place at the World Health Assemblies highlight the broad areas of conflict surrounding essential drugs policies at the global level. The following case study of the implementation of an essential drugs policy in Bangladesh provides insight into the interaction of global and national power relations.

6.5.1 The Bangladesh essential drugs policy

In 1982 Bangladesh became the first developing country to introduce a National Drug Policy (NDP), a policy aimed at boosting domestic production of essential drugs with strict controls on which drugs could be manufactured and marketed in the country. There were to be no royalty agreements with overseas companies unless they had a factory in Bangladesh, raw materials were to be purchased on the basis of competitive world prices, transfer pricing was to cease, and products were to be made under acceptable quality control procedures. In addition, there was to be a phased withdrawal of almost 40 per cent of the drugs then available on the market: products that were harmful, products that were irrational combinations or unnecessarily expensive, and products labelled as either useless and unnecessary or 'famous brand name products' made under licence (Silverman et al. 1992, pp. 130–1; Chowdhury 1995, pp. 45–62).

Within a decade, the value of local production of drugs increased by more than 217 per cent, with production of essential drugs increasing from 30 per cent of local production in 1981 to 80 per cent in 1991. Prices of raw materials and retail prices were held in check. In 1981 eight multinational companies controlled 65 per cent of the local market but by 1991 local companies controlled more than 60 per cent of local production (Chetley 1993, pp. 10–11). Losses to the eight pharmaceutical companies were estimated to be in the millions of dollars (Silverman et al. 1992, pp. 142–3; Chowdhury 1995, pp. 98–105).

6.5.2 Threats to the policy

From its inception, the Bangladesh NDP has come under unceasing attack from representatives of the international pharmaceutical industry and their governments, from the medical establishment in Bangladesh, which was concerned about

A large proportion of local business élites opposed the NDP. In developing countries, drugs imported at relatively high prices are often subjected to further substantial mark-ups by local distributors and businessmen. A 1977 Bangladesh Ministry of Health report found that these mark-ups accounted for up to two-thirds of the retail price (Kanji 1992, pp. 2–3). The financial interests of professional groups and property owners in the production and sale of pharmaceuticals made it predictable that they would oppose measures which threatened their profits (Kanji 1992, p. 85).

Both supporters and opponents of the NDP acknowledge that it did succeed in raising the proportion of drugs used from the essential list. A 1992 survey of drug use at primary care level revealed that 78 per cent of drugs were prescribed by generic name and 85 per cent were from the Essential Drugs List (WHO 1993, p. 20; Chowdhury 1995, pp. 98–108). This survey of the effects of the essential drugs policy in the public sector provides insight into why the pharmaceutical industry opposes its extension to the private sector: the policy would make the bulk of the pharmaceutical industry's brand-name products obsolete. Also, centralised procurement through international tender would undermine the industry's ability to negotiate deals with influential individuals and professional groups (Kanji 1992, p. 74). However, the local pharmaceutical industry, which had initially been opposed to the NDP, changed its position. The increased market share for local drugs and the opportunity to get UNICEF contracts was a benefit to local pharmaceutical manufacturers (Reich 1994, p. 135).

In 1992 the Bangladesh NDP came under pressure in the context of pre-negotiation actions being carried out by the Industry and Energy Unit of the World Bank's resident mission in Bangladesh. This surfaced at the time when the World Bank was introducing the Fourth Population and Health Project, worth US$600 million. The impression was created that funding of the new 5-year project was linked to recommended deregulation of the drug industry, including the introduction of new products by using free sales certification, lifting all controls on pricing, removal of control over advertising from the drug licensing authority, removal of existing restrictions on foreign firms regarding the choice of products they can produce, and allowing pharmaceutical companies to import their inputs freely.

Health agencies (WHO, UNICEF) and donor nations funding the Fourth Population and Health Project formally requested that the World Bank review its recommendations for drastically changing the drug policy. In the face of these challenges, the World Bank revised its position. It affirmed its support for the NDP objective of increasing supply of essential drugs and making these available at affordable prices, while at the same time seeking to alter the controls which were deemed cumbersome and discretionary.

The opposition to the Bangladesh NDP by Bangladesh professional groups and economic élites, the transnational pharmaceutical industry, and allied Western interests was mainly due to concern about the potential loss of profits and flow-on of this policy to other countries. These interest groups rationalised their stance as adherence to the ideology of the free market (Kanji 1992, p. 74). The struggles over this issue highlight the complex interrelationships between political, economic, and social issues. In Kanji's political economic analysis, the drugs policies of a country cannot be separated from its strategy of development aimed at improving health through raising living conditions generally. As well as being determined by local cultural, political, and economic imperatives, the development aims of such countries are subject to international forces, particularly when they are dependent on aid, including loans for pharmaceuticals (Kanji 1992, pp. 88–9).

Many consumer groups see the Bangladesh NDP as representing 'what should be done in all countries to control the private sector, especially multinationals, for pharmaceuticals and other products as well'. Members of IFPMA see it as 'what should not be done in any country, especially the adoption of an essential drugs list in the private sector' (Reich 1994, pp. 135–6). Some support for the essential drugs concept for the public sector stems from the potential to market pharmaceuticals to those who were previously unable to afford them; however, this support from private and professional interests depends on keeping access to the private sector open. Chowdhury documents the ongoing struggle in the 1990s to maintain the integrity of the NDP under persistent attack by powerful transnational pharmaceutical companies (1995, pp. 145–63). There is still a multitude of products on the market and there may be a perception that brand-name drugs are superior.

6.6 Interpretive studies on the use of pharmaceuticals

Structural analyses of the pharmaceutical industry highlight how its transnational character allows better control of the market, transfer pricing, dumping, and other practices that enhance profits. Attention is paid to the effects of the patent system, the transfer of technology, biased information on drug use, and promotional activities by sales representatives. But as Nichter and Vuckovik (1994, p. 331) point out, investigating the structure and practice of the pharmaceutical industry does not necessarily make its existence and successes intelligible. What is needed is information about the context in which drugs are promoted and sold in developing countries in ways that allow the continuation of dubious marketing practices and the maximisation of profits at the expense of health concerns.

Once a national drug policy has been implemented to improve distribution and regulation of essential and beneficial therapeutics, we might assume that rational use of drugs will prevail. However, the concepts 'need', 'irrational', and 'essential' are part of the culture of biomedicine, not of the local culture (Van der Geest et al. 1990, p. 185). The actions of pharmaceutical distributors, prescribers, and consumers themselves are often irrational from the point of view of those experts who help design the national policies. It is commonplace to find essential drugs being prescribed inappropriately: when they are not indicated, in doses that are not beneficial, or in combinations that are contraindicated. To understand the way in which pharmaceuticals are actually used in local communities around the world, we must turn from the structural orientation we have drawn on so far, to more interpretive or *meaning-centred* approaches in medical anthropology.

6.6.1 The cultural context of pharmaceutical use

Understanding why certain prescribing and consumption patterns persist despite the best intentions of policy makers requires examination of the cultural context of pharmaceuticals. Anthropologists have recently begun to analyse patterns of pharmaceutical-related behaviour and the cultural interpretation of medicines in different settings (Van der Geest and Whyte 1988; Etkin and Tan 1994). Nichter and Vuckovik (1994), for example, describe how the proliferation of medicines changes people's perceptions of health, how they are used to create illness identities and express social relations, and, through self-medication, how medicines may become a source of empowerment or an instrument of dependency.

Information about pharmaceuticals passed on through the oral transmission of instructions or via self-help networks is given meaning through being 'culturally reinterpreted' by the receiver (Van der Geest et al. 1990, p. 183). Cultural meanings ascribed to drugs are extremely important in shaping usage patterns. Taking medicines involves more than the 'embodiment of substances'; embodied also are 'ideas about self, illness causality, responsibility, the meaning of sickness and perceptions of entitlement' (Nichter and Vuckovik 1994, p. 288). For instance, in West Africa, Hausa people say that injections are particularly effective because the needle penetrates the body to the source of the illness. Thus injections are often specifically requested by patients at health care facilities. Commercial drug dealers also cater to this demand by selling injections to anyone willing to pay for them (Stock 1985, p. 130). Drugs can also be classified as 'hot' or 'cold' according to local humoural medical theories and in many cultures particular substances are thought to be suitable for certain people, such as herbal tonics for the elderly (Van der Geest et al. 1990, p. 184). Culturally specific knowledge of this type is of crucial importance in understanding medicine use in local communities.

6.6.2 Drug proliferation and health perception

An important link between global and local dimensions of pharmaceuticals is the effect of drug proliferation on perceptions of health and illness (Nichter and Vuckovik 1994, p. 287). In Nigeria, for example, there was a forty-fold increase in pharmaceutical imports between 1969 and 1981. This growth was made possible by increased petroleum revenues in the 1970s. All levels of government increased funding to the health care sector, resulting in the establishment of new facilities (Stock 1985, p. 132). The effect was that Nigerians began using more pharmaceuticals, particularly the more specialised and expensive products (Stock 1985, p. 121). As in many developing countries, patent medicine shops and licensed pharmaceutical outlets are concentrated in large towns. According to Stock, this reflects the greater level of demand and purchasing power in those areas: 'Urban consumers generally are more aware of a greater range of pharmaceutical products and are more likely to be able to afford costly drugs' (Stock 1985, p. 125). While much of the expansion in the numbers of pharmaceutical outlets in Nigeria is attributable to the growth of the health care system, it is also a consequence of consumers' increased capacity to purchase drugs from retail outlets (Stock 1985, p. 121).

6.6.3 Consumer demand, marketing, and drug promotion

A complex link exists between consumer perceptions of drugs, consumer demand, and the marketing and dispensing of drugs. Significant factors are political decision-making, the growth of the health care system, and the subsequent increase in public familiarity with pharmaceuticals. However, a crucial aspect is the role of the pharmaceutical industry in promoting the sale of its products. Extensive promotion helps to stimulate public demand and convinces physicians and official buying agents to purchase drugs which may be of marginal utility in developing countries, or to choose expensive brand names rather than their generic equivalent (Stock 1985, p. 132). One of the aims of WHO's DAP is to replace expensive brand-name pharmaceuticals with generic drugs. However, Nichter and Vuckovik question the public's willingness to accept generic medications in a context where commodity fetishism—the status of commodities—affects perceptions of the efficacy of medicines (1994, p. 287), and more expensive imported drugs may be associated with the status of élite groups.

Modern and traditional values may be embodied and communicated to others through particular types of promotion. The consumption of commercial drugs affiliates the consumer with modern values and lifestyles (Nichter and Vuckovik 1994, p. 288). On the other hand, a return to herbal medicines affiliates the individual with traditional or alternative values and may signal dissatisfaction with the values and concepts of the Western medical system (Nichter and Vuckovik 1994, p. 289), or indeed of the West and modernity itself.

6.6.4 Medicine as prevention

The distinction between curative, preventive, and promotive health is the product of a biomedical conceptualisation and may have little relevance in the developing world. For many people, preventive health means preventing poor health from becoming worse by taking or purchasing medicine. On the other hand, curative medications are used for what Western observers deem to be 'irrational' purposes, such as promoting a general sense of well-being or as 'talismans to ward off illness' (Nichter and Vuckovik 1994, p. 292). In many developing countries the growth of the health care system has led to increasing numbers of people becoming accustomed to Western drugs either in combination with, or in preference to, traditional remedies (Cosminsky 1994). Injections are often the most valued form of Western medicine. This is due in part to the success of past mass campaigns against diseases such as smallpox and sleeping sickness, but is also due to perceptions of the value of injections for preventing or curing sexually transmitted and other diseases (Stock 1985, p. 123).

6.6.5 Commoditisation

As medicines are highly valued, they often escape the formal distribution systems that would confine and regulate them in developed countries. Formal regulatory mechanisms in developing countries are often not highly developed so a flourishing parallel market system grows up. The informal trade in medicines by non-qualified prescribers compensates for shortages in the public sector. Shops, kiosks, market stalls, and itinerant pedlars often retail supplies with little labelling or instructions. These include essential drugs, such as antibiotics, that find their way from the public health system onto the market (Van der Geest et al. 1990, p. 183).

In some countries, entrepreneurial traditional healers in urban settings have responded to the growing market for modern drugs by preparing and bottling their own traditional medicines for commercial sale. The production of these bottled remedies has helped to 'blur the distinction between Indigenous and Western medicines in the minds of consumers' (Stock 1985, p. 132) and contributed to the commoditisation of all health care. The commercial appeal of traditional remedies may be enhanced though their scientisation using advertising which features charts and graphs, excerpts from scientific journals, and testimonials by a doctor. By associating with these drugs, practitioners and patients alike appear scientific while still being associated with natural, non-commoditised processes (Nichter and Vuckovik 1994, p. 298).

6.6.6 Drugs and social control

Medication may be a contributing factor in inhibiting organised political activity. From an interpretive perspective, workers may take medicine such as amphetamines or narcotics in the hope that they will gain some measure of control over or relief from deteriorating life conditions. However, from a structural perspective, the availability of medicines for such purposes may also serve to 'shift the onus of blame and responsibility for health to the individual such that responsibility comes to entail purchase of products that produce health' (Nichter and Vuckovik 1994, p. 292). In Nigeria, people who immigrate to the city are able to purchase a range of drugs for the treatment of illness as well as for non-medical purposes. Stimulants such as amphetamines are used by immigrant labourers to increase their capacity for heavy work, to ameliorate feelings of hunger, and to stay awake long hours. The workers quite often develop an addiction to these substances and so must find a way of sustaining their drug habit if they return to the village (Stock 1985, p. 131).

6.6.7 Self-treatment and the quick fix

There is a need to establish the extent to which taking medicine as a quick fix diminishes the importance of knowledge about bodily symptoms that may previously have guided health behaviour. Popular medicines may mask signs that were once monitored as criteria for assessing illness severity. The result may be that seeking health care is delayed, with possibly disastrous consequences for the individual and the community at large. For example, white capsules are very popular with prostitutes in Nigeria as a cure-all for the prevention of venereal infection. But by taking over-the-counter medications when they suspect they have an STD, the prostitutes remain a risk to the community (Stock 1985, p. 132). Self-treatment is likely to involve not only the use of common patent medicines but also antibiotics taken on a regular basis as a cure-all (Stock 1985, p. 132). The practice of taking low-dose antibiotics fosters drug resistance, again placing the prostitutes and the broader community at risk (Nichter and Vuckovik 1994, p. 291). Such practices are viewed by regulating bodies as inappropriate use of drugs, but in many countries regulatory mechanisms are weak and the dissemination of information to consumers scarce (Van der Geest et al. 1990, p. 184). Health practitioners themselves may prescribe according to the quick fix principle in order to ensure patient satisfaction rather than the long-term interests of the patient or the community.

6.6.8 Efficacy

In considering the inappropriate use of drugs we need to take into account that efficacy is defined quite differently by Western-trained professionals and by the lay public. It is important to keep in mind Arthur Kleinman's statement that 'efficacy, itself, is a cultural construct' (Kleinman 1973, p. 210). Rather than evaluating drugs exclusively in biomedical terms of effectiveness, lay people may evaluate effectiveness in terms of whether therapy allows them to cope with their job and manage relationships with families, friends, and the authorities (Higginbotham and Streiner 1991, p. 74s).

All medicines are evaluated in terms of specific knowledge people have about drugs, which may differ significantly from biomedical knowledge. Different coloured medicines may be viewed as stronger than others, different tastes more effective, and injections more powerful than oral medications (Higginbotham and Streiner 1991, pp. 74s–5s). Those monitoring essential drugs programs in developing countries point to the need for consumer education to counter inappropriate drug prescribing and use. However, Nichter and Vuckovik point out that 'social processes are at play in the health marketplace which will not be offset by education based on clinical or economic logic alone' (1994, p. 299). They suggest that there is a need to 'look beyond rational drug use to rationales for using drugs' (1994, p. 300). Van der Geest, Hardon, and Whyte (1990) argue that the use of drugs is an area in which people are actively observing and experimenting. In an area of rapidly changing practices, education may play an important role, especially when government systems are not capable of strict regulation. They point out that information is easier to supply for a limited range of essential medications. This is a strong argument for extending essential drugs policies into the private sector.

6.7 Towards a common conceptual framework

So far in this chapter we have looked at pharmaceuticals in terms of a macro or structural perspective and a micro or interpretive perspective, moving across different disciplines and different levels of the health hierarchy. While it is useful to delineate between structural and interpretive perspectives, the forms of social life they refer to are dialectically related. In other words, there is a reciprocal process whereby individuals create and change social structures, and social structures inform systems of cultural meaning. This dialectic parallels the complexity theory principle outlined in chapter 3: that local interactions in a dynamic system produce emergent global patterns. In an evolving reciprocal process, global patterns then influence local interactions (Lewin 1993, p. 12). The example in box 6.1 gives

Henderson and Fischer's (1999) explanation of how structural and interpretive levels of the political economy of pharmaceuticals were intricately connected to generate the antibiotics market in China from the 1980s.

Box 6.1 Globalisation and pharmaceuticals: the Chinese antibiotic market wars

Henderson and Fischer (1999) found that between 1980 and the late 1990s the market for pharmaceuticals grew in China within an environment of contrasting views about what should be the most appropriate structure for health care delivery in that country. Furthermore, prescribers' and consumers' perceptions of antibiotics (in particular, cephalosporin antibiotics[6]) influenced competition for a share of the Chinese pharmaceutical market by domestic and foreign producers. Henderson and Fischer identified four key factors influencing Chinese usage of antibiotics.

Characteristics of the drug category—Cephalosporins had an edge over other antibiotics because they were rated as 'broader spectrum' (kill a broader range of bacteria), had fewer side effects, could be administered though intramuscular injection or intravenously, and the older generation cephalosporins were less expensive than some of the newest imported antibiotics.

Perceptions of the drug—Chinese consumers have faith in the power of injections and believe that foreign brand goods are more efficacious than generic equivalents produced domestically. Similarly, prescribers perceived that 'the injectible market is where the money is in China' (Henderson and Fischer 1999, p. 6). These views were tempered by the opinion of some physicians that there is an overuse of injectibles.

Characteristics of the market—The sales and marketing strategies of foreign companies focused on a handful of large cities, including the major coastal areas, insured patients, and the wealthy. In contrast, domestic companies tended to target uninsured poorer people in rural areas, relying on the market advantages and protectionism of local distribution networks. Both commercial groups had to operate within state regulatory policies involving licensing agreements for imported drugs, process and product patents, price controls for health services and products, and health insurance regulations, including essential drug list formularies that governed reimbursement for drug charges.

Perceptions of the market—The strategies of domestic and foreign companies and the policies enacted by the Chinese government to regulate the pharmaceutical system evolved in the context of two potentially conflicting perceptions. The common view of both foreigners and Chinese was that China was a nation of many markets, each of which had to be addressed 'almost independently' due to inadequate infrastructure, interprovincial rivalries, duplication of industrial assets, and a tradition of self-reliance. Many Chinese and foreigners also believed that domestic companies were 'incapable of brand-building' on a national scale, were only competitive because of state subsidies, and would be 'swept away in the face of foreign competition'. By 1999, Henderson and Fischer observed that the 'entire structure of market-making is in the midst of great flux in China' and 'cultural perceptions held by both Chinese and foreigners were being subjected to a renewed reality test' (1999, p. 2).

6.8 The dialectic of power

Henderson and Fischer's observations in China demonstrate the complex interlinkages between local and global levels of the pharmaceutical system. One of the dynamics by which these interlinkages are articulated is the operation of power. The concept of power is critical to understanding all social life. Sociologist Max Weber (1968) defined power as 'the probability that one actor within a social relationship will be in a position to carry out his [*sic*] will despite resistance regardless of the basis on which this probability rests'. Political economists and other structural theorists have questioned this definition of power, because it does not take account of the structural relationship of classes or other social agents that may be independent of the will of individuals.

Medical anthropologist Gregory Pappas sought to develop a more differentiated theory of power that could bridge the 'structure/agency' dichotomy. He delineated the concepts of autonomy, dependency, domination, and exploitation (1990, pp. 199–200). Whether in a nation-state, a class, or an individual, *autonomy* refers to the capacity of a social agent to control the course and outcome of action, while *dependency* refers to the constraint on autonomy that results from certain connections with other processes, actors, or agents. Dependency may be linked to relations of *domination*, in which there are unequal resources in interactions. Domination becomes *exploitation* where unequal access to resources is used to the advantage of the resourced agent at the expense of the unresourced. These concepts—power, autonomy, dependence, domination, and exploitation—can illuminate the dialectics of local and global events and processes surrounding pharmaceutical production, marketing, and consumption, as each of these processes involve social relationships.

In the first part of the chapter we reviewed the arguments about the exploitative relationship of the global pharmaceutical industry with disempowered groups in developing countries. International relations of economic dependency between countries become the foundation for policies that further advantage powerful nations. Attempts to redress this situation by multilateral agencies such as WHO result in power struggles with other powerful international organisations, national groups, and transnational corporations and their lobbyists who are beneficiaries of the current global order.

At the level of behaviour, the power of a social agent is often felt most acutely during times of sickness. Individuals may purchase Western pharmaceuticals to bypass family members or members of the community who may react to the individual's sickness with social sanctions, or labelling as 'sick', thereby imposing the constraints of ritual and socially based therapies that may be used to affirm the patient's place in family and society, by reinforcing relations of dependency and domination. Whyte views medicine taken in this way (that is, the clandestine purchase of Western medicine) as a liberating force that enhances the sufferer's autonomy (cited in Van der Geest 1988, p. 340).

Likewise, the purchase of medicines over-the-counter may enhance the sufferer's autonomy, enabling the purchaser to elude physicians as agents of domination. The desire to escape social control is often greatest when the sickness is embarrassing or when a person's reputation is at risk, as in the case of sexually transmitted infections (Van der Geest 1988, p. 340). In these cases, self-treatment involving over-the-counter pharmaceuticals may be viewed as resistance to medicalisation; the sufferer rather than a medical authority figure wields the power to define and treat the illness.

The availability of medicines in non-pharmacy shops and from street vendors has the potential to alter the power relations of health care. The ready availability of over-the-counter medicines may influence prescribing practices because doctors may be more inclined to give in to the demands of patients if they know that the patient will go elsewhere if refused. Also, the importance of family members' support and advice may be reduced if individuals can manage their own illness through over-the-counter purchases (Nichter and Vuckovik 1994, p. 299). The relativities of power in gender relations may change, as they did in northern Ghana, for example, where women bypass elder men who are traditional herbalists and use Western pharmaceuticals for themselves and their children (Bierlich 1999, p. 322).

Just as accessibility to pharmaceuticals may be an indicator of autonomy, inability to access needed medicines may be a sign of dependency. An examination of the meanings of medicine use in households may reveal that unequal access to material goods, including pharmaceuticals, is determined by patterns of authority, duty, and affection which are reproduced in the home. Expenditure on pharmaceuticals for a particular family member may be an indicator of the sufferer's position within the household, with inequalities most evident in terms of age and gender divisions (Nichter and Vuckovik 1994, p. 295).

It has been argued that self-care of common illnesses increases self-reliance and self-control. But is the idea of choice and self-control illusory if it is based upon the marketing claims of pharmaceutical companies? The well-documented encouragement to consumers to purchase inappropriate or dangerous medications for the economic benefit of manufacturers is an example of exploitation and points to structural level power relations between multinational companies and national élites which benefit economically from unregulated distribution and advertising.

When discussing pharmaceuticals we need to take account of the social agents, such as community members, political élites, or corporations, who construct discourses about health that have wider political effects (Nichter and Vuckovik 1994, p. 288). This is clearly evident at the structural level in the struggles over the implementation of the Bangladesh NDP, where rhetoric about the efficacy and availability of pharmaceuticals could not be separated from proponents' own prospects of economic or political gain. As discussed in chapter 5, resistance to the dominant health promotion discourse of outsiders was evident in the Coalfields among males who acted out larrikin values associated with a more general orientation of resistance to political domination. Health promotion discourses that are used by health authorities to emphasise individual responsibility for health care may divert attention away from environmental and occupational conditions that affect social groups, not just individuals (Nichter and Vuckovik 1994, p. 292).

The production and consumption of traditional medicines may also be highly politicised. Support of traditional medicines by governments has been employed not only as an economic imperative, but also as a means of resistance to forms of colonialism and as a grassroots strategy to foster cultural identity during times of social transformation. The People's Republic of China's Barefoot Doctor program in the 1960s incorporated all of these reasons, as has, more recently, the promotion of traditional healing by the Tibetan government-in-exile (see, for example, Janes 1995). The construction of health knowledge and the taking of medicines are 'powerful means of both regulating the body and embodying political values' (Nichter and Vuckovik 1994, p. 288).

Figure 6.2 summarises our understanding of the dialectics of power in the pharmaceutical sector. In this figure, the large arrows circling the system demonstrate how power (that is, domination or exploitation) acts as a mediating factor or common conceptual framework linking relationships and resources that make up the global pharmaceutical system.

In the following section, we use complexity theory to explore the linkages between the political economy of pharmaceuticals, and ecological and biological levels of the health hierarchy.

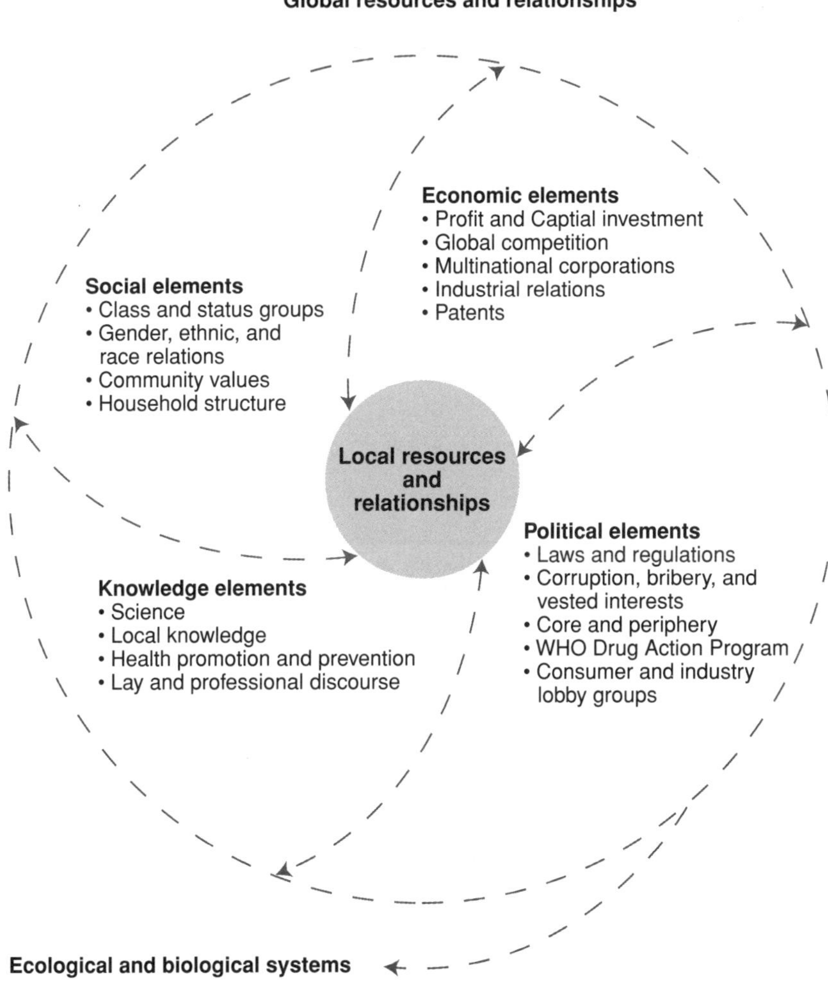

Figure 6.2 Power as a mediating factor in resources and relationships associated with the global pharmaceutical system

6.9 The evolution of drug resistance and the health hierarchy

The political economy of the pharmaceutical industry is an important component of a larger evolving system whereby pharmaceutical products have been created, produced, distributed, and consumed over the past 50 years. Complexity theory and transdisciplinary thinking enable us to view this evolving system as a whole. The health hierarchy shown in chapter 2 (figure 2.1) located the subsystem of political economy within the domain of social systems. The social system within the hierarchy is influenced in varying degrees by behavioural, biological, ecological, and physical subsystems. Optimum health, it will be recalled, requires the provision of essential resources from all levels in the hierarchy. We can see the inter-relationship among all these subsystems in the realm of pharmaceuticals by examining the growing failure of antimicrobial agents to deal with infectious diseases.

We have witnessed in recent years the emergence of strains of bacteria dangerous to human health and resistant to almost all forms of antibiotic drugs (Levy 1998; Collignon 1999). We face the possibility that in the near future certain bacterial infections will not be treatable by any known antibiotic (Levy 1998); antimicrobial resistance is now a concern worldwide. Multidrug-resistant strains of micro-organisms such as *Staphylococcus* and vancomycin-resistant *Enterococcus* have the potential to cause epidemics of infectious disease which have no effective means of treatment. Old diseases, such as tuberculosis, which were arrested in the late 1940s and throughout the 1950s with the introduction of life-saving antibiotics, have now evolved multidrug resistance and are once again responsible for increasing deaths worldwide.

The total environment within which organisms that produce human illness evolve has radically altered in the last two centuries. As humans became more numerous, lived closer together, and created new types of physical environments, they influenced the selective pressures on the evolution of micro-organisms. With the introduction of antimicrobial agents, another new factor in the fitness landscape of micro-organisms emerged. The loss of effective pharmaceuticals occurs because of a number of mutually reinforcing factors within the health hierarchy. They can be conceptualised in the following way.

6.9.1 Physical systems

We start our examination of health hierarchy subsystems related to antibiotic resistance by first considering physical systems. The rate of infections acquired in hospitals has increased throughout the developed world. In the USA alone, according to the Centers for Disease Control and Prevention, about 2 million

Table 6.1 Health hierarchy factors contributing to antibiotic resistance

Health status	*Factors in antibiotic resistance*
Body	• Invasive treatment (for example, heart surgery)
	• Invasive technologies (for example, catheters)
Behaviour	• Lack of hand-washing and poor hygiene
	• Sharing needles among injecting drug users
Social systems	• Patient pressure for fast-acting drugs
	• Overprescription of antibiotics by doctors
	• Overcrowding within the hospital system
	• Excessive promotion of antibiotics by drug companies
	• Failure of national and international drug policy to achieve rational use of antibiotics
	• Cultural beliefs about dosage, efficacy, and self-treatment
Biological and ecological systems	• Rapid evolution of micro-organisms
	• Routine use of antibiotics in intensive agriculture
	• Rapid growth of the fast-food industry
Physical systems	• New invasive technologies used within medicine
	• Design of medical buildings (for example, airconditioners)

people annually develop an infection from their hospital treatment. Of these patients, 90 000–100 000 die as a result of their infections (see Boodman 1997; CDC 1998). In many cases, death is directly linked to exposure to bacteria that are resistant to at least one commonly used antibiotic. A key causal factor is the failure to practise basic infection-control sanitation, such as hand washing (discussed below). However, building design and the use of new technologies also contribute to the spread of drug-resistant bacteria within the physical environment of the hospital.

A favourable physical environment within which organisms can live and reproduce is a key factor in their evolutionary success. In complexity terms, the modern intensive care hospital can be seen as a new fitness landscape containing new attractors for the successful reproduction and evolution of new strains of micro-organisms. Hospitals are specifically designed to treat and care for people who are ill. It is not surprising that when a large number of sick people, many with surgically produced open wounds, are placed in close proximity to one another, cross-infection takes place. Hospital technologies designed for human comfort, such as airconditioning systems, become the sites of colonies of infectious disease. Other technologies, such as latex gloves, designed to protect the health worker from infection, are implicated in the spread of disease between patients if staff fail to don a fresh pair of gloves for each new patient contact. In addition, the moist, nutrient-rich environment of the skin inside the glove can be an ideal source of ongoing infection (see Fridkin and Gaynes 1999). Intensive care equipment, built for efficient use, may have substances and surfaces that are impossible to clean without lengthy sterilisation. They present nutrient-rich environments for organisms to thrive and be passed from one patient to another. The system taken as a whole, despite the attempt by hospital administrators to reach a high level of predictable order, is in fact poised at the edge of chaos. There are many new possibilities capable of emerging from the interaction of all the variables, including antibiotic-resistant organisms. Such a situation can lead to epidemics of infectious disease within the hospital setting, with consequent loss of human life. Health attractors within the system are opposed to disease attractors evolving within the very same system.

6.9.2 Biological and evolutionary factors

WHO describes the basic biological causes of antibiotic resistance:

> Microbes (bacteria, fungi, parasites and viruses) are responsible for infectious diseases and antimicrobial agents (such as penicillin, erythromycin, and many others) have been developed to combat the spread and severity of many infections. However, the use of these agents for any infection, real or feared, in any dose and over any time period, forces microbes to adapt or die ('selective pressure'). The microbes which survive are those that carry genes for resistance to antimicrobial agents and, in the medical setting, a resistant microbe is one which is not killed by an antimicrobial agent after a standard course of treatment. Antimicrobial agents are also used in agriculture such as livestock and crop production, as well as in fish farming and to treat and control animal diseases and enhance growth and yield. All of these uses increase the total selective pressure exerted on the microbial world and encourage the emergence of resistance (WHO 1998).

Evolution in the natural world can be viewed as a race between the relative fitness of organisms competing for resources within the same environment. When that environment is the human body, the race is between the body's ability to respond to attacks on its integrity via the immune system and the ability of micro-organisms to evolve ways of defeating the immune system and to reproduce.

When a micro-organism uses the evolutionary strategy of rapid cross-infection of the host population, sickness and ultimate death of the host is not a problem for that organism because its reproductive strategy has been to newly infect as many new hosts as possible. With diseases such as influenza or smallpox (see chapter 2), we can see just how successful an evolutionary strategy this blitzkrieg system of infection can be for the virus that transmits the disease. The co-evolution of host and virus is a natural part of evolutionary history. Clearly, since the species *Homo* has been around for about 2 million years, the battle between health and infectious disease has been such that the result, on balance, has enabled the human species to continue to expand its population and geographical range. However, if we continue to act in ways that give micro-organisms an evolutionary edge over our immune systems, we just might tip the balance in such a way as to place our own future in jeopardy.

The development of drugs to combat potentially fatal infectious diseases such as pneumonia, malaria, tuberculosis, and HIV/AIDS, introduces these new agents into the evolutionary environment for the organisms concerned. They respond by evolving in standard ways to the new threat to their existence. Stuart Levy describes how organisms' resistance to the agents designed to kill or retard them can occur in a number of ways:

> Bacteria can acquire resistance genes through a few routes. Many inherit the genes from their forerunners. Other times, genetic mutations, which occur readily in bacteria, will spontaneously produce a resistant trait or will strengthen an existing one. And, frequently, bacteria will gain a defence against an antibiotic by taking up resistance genes from other bacterial cells in the vicinity. Indeed, the exchange of genes is so pervasive that the entire bacterial world can be thought of as one huge multicellular organism in which the cells interchange their genes with ease (Levy 1998).

A relatively new environment within which micro-organisms can rapidly evolve is the socially created physical system of intensive food production. In chapter 3 we discussed how new ways of producing food in beef cattle feedlots and factory farms (chickens, pigs, turkeys) involve, among other things, the routine use of antibiotics to increase growth and reduce cross-infection in intensively housed populations. A new basin of attraction is created for food production with a powerful new attractor influencing system evolution. The goals of maximum system profitability and productivity change the nature of the system as a whole and introduce new possibilities for the creation and transmission of disease. In relation to this method of food production, George Khachatourians argues that:

> Antibiotic-resistant bacteria arising from agricultural practices enter human environments and move about with people and goods, thus creating transborder resistance. Not until recently did we suspect that the broad agricultural use of antibiotics could lead to widespread resistance in bacteria and the attendant effects on patients in health care settings and, after their discharge from institutions, the community at large (Khachatourians 1998).

With the rapid social development of fast and convenience food industries (see chapter 3), the potential for newly evolved drug-resistant bacteria to enter and spread in the human food chain is greatly amplified. One particular microorganism, *Salmonella*, illustrates just how effectively our socially created environment of food production and consumption can favour drug resistance in an organism dangerous to human health. Khachatourians offers this description:

> Multidrug-resistant *Salmonella typhimurium* definitive type 104 (DT 104) initially emerged in cattle in 1988 in England and Wales and was subsequently found in meat and meat products from other domestic animals, as well as unpasteurized milk from other locations. Human illness occurred through contact with farm animals and consumption of beef, pork sausages and chickens. The number of DT 104 isolates from humans in Britain increased from 259 to 3837 between 1990 and 1995. The proportion of antibiotic-resistant Salmonella associated with human infections rose from 17% to 31% of isolates between 1979/80 and 1989/90 and the proportion of Salmonella isolates exhibiting antibiotic and multidrug resistance to ampicillin, chloramphenicol, streptomycin, sulfonamides and tetracycline increased from 39% to 97% in the same period (Khachatourians 1998).

Hence, ironically, the synergistic effects of inappropriate use of antibiotics in both medical and agricultural contexts leads to the very problem that generated the need to develop drugs in the first place—potentially lethal disease. It is estimated that some 2–4 million people in the USA contract *Salmonella* infections each year (Angulo 1998) and, as humans consume food contaminated with *Salmonella*, some come into contact with antimicrobial-resistant strains. Such systematic contamination of the food chain creates potentially life-threatening infections that require complicated treatments.

6.9.3 Social system factors and policy failures

Cultural and social factors influencing the use of new drugs can either enhance or retard the ability of micro-organisms to evolve resistance to antimicrobial agents. As argued above, consumer pressures for a rapid cure, social and economic barriers hindering access to appropriately trained prescribers, and preference for self-treatment (in which a full course of the drug is seldom taken), not to mention fear of progressing illness, combine to promote the misuse of antibiotics, considerably increasing the opportunity for resistant strains to flourish (see Saradamma et al. 2000).

Where public institutions such as nursing homes and prisons are involved in treating large populations of infected people, it is possible for the community involved (the elderly, prisoners) to be given less than optimal treatments for particular infectious conditions. When best evidence-based treatment is not adopted for economic (budget cuts) or social reasons (discrimination), there the possibility exists for the further development of drug-resistant strains of bacteria or viruses. These types of institutions act as attractors for particular disease outcomes based on the levels of care and the intensity of interactions taking place between 'inmates' and, ultimately, the general public.

The latest treatment for HIV-infected people uses combination therapy of protease inhibitors and non-nucleotide transcriptase inhibitors. If these drugs are prescribed incorrectly (only one drug, an inappropriate combination) or are inadequately administered (wrong dosage or failure to follow food requirements), then HIV resistance to one or more of the drugs is likely (Rabkin and Chesney 2000, in press). Maddow (2000) warns that some HIV-infected prisoners in the USA may not be receiving best-practice treatment for this disease as manifest in the following ways:

- prisoners with HIV/AIDS are unable to comply with strict food schedules associated with the taking of medications
- prisoners are not being prescribed the most efficacious combination of antiviral drugs
- there is failure to get frequent and accurate viral load tests so as to ensure optimum drug combination and strength.

Consequently, the chances of the evolution of multidrug-resistant strains of HIV are increased, with the possible result that the prison population may become a source of untreatable strains of HIV. Such drug-resistant strains of HIV will not only kill people inside prisons, but will emerge from this environment to infect the wider population and render ineffective, in the public domain, the current hard-won array of antiviral pharmaceuticals used for the treatment of HIV/AIDS (Maddow 2000).

The pressure from patients directed at doctors for immediate antibiotic treatment even when it is contraindicated for the condition (as in the case of viral infections), also leads to the increased incidence of drug resistance (CDC 1998). Overprescribing, combined with public policy failure to either develop or ensure adoption of evidence-based treatment guidelines, can create a dramatic decrease in the effectiveness of specific drugs. In Finland in the late 1980s, for example, there was an increased incidence of strep bacteria resistant to the antibiotic erythromycin. A campaign restricting the use of this drug produced a drop from 19 per cent strep erythromycin resistance in 1993 to 9 per cent in 1996 (Schwartz 1997). Morton Schwartz, writing in the *New England Journal of Medicine*, observed, 'This is an impressive example of how an enlightened national policy on antibiotic use can become an effective health measure' (1997, p. 492): when policymakers and professional bodies resist the move towards regulation of antibiotic use, this becomes a factor in promoting resistance in the organisms we are trying to control.

Hospital understaffing and downsizing are other institutional factors exacerbating the spread of drug-resistant bacteria through failure to maintain sterility. When a situation of hospital understaffing is compromised further by, for example, a major epidemic or a disaster that overloads the intensive care system, the spread of drug-resistant disease within hospitals (nosocomial infection) increases (see Fridkin et al. 1996).

6.9.4 Behavioural factors

An example of behaviour implicated in disease transmission and the exacerbation of antibiotic resistance is the failure to perform basic hand-washing. With multidrug-resistant bacteria now endemic in the health care environment, the point of physical contact between health care professional and patient is a critical source of transmitting drug resistance. The CDC summarised the results of several studies in the USA from which CDC revealed that only 14–59 per cent of doctors and 25–45 per cent of nurses regularly wash their hands between patients (Boodman 1997). In combination with the other factors that create the problem of antibiotic-resistant bacteria, professionals' resistance (or inability) to practise frequent hand-washing is now thought to be a major factor in rendering antimicrobial agents less effective than they ought to be.

6.9.5 The body

The body has become a site for invasive and at times heroic attempts to prolong life and recover health. Operations involving human to human organ transplants, xeno transplants (involving organs from a species other than humans, for example, pigs), and other complicated surgery (for example, multiple bypass heart surgery) have now become common and the technologies used to enter the body have become increasingly sophisticated. Catheters and breathing tubes, for example, are often associated with the transmission of infections to patients whose health is already compromised (for example, dialysis, organ transplant, and heart operation patients). Animal-to-human organ transplants may also be associated with the cross-species transmission of drug-resistant strains of micro-organisms.

In summary, organisms that are resistant to our best efforts of drug treatment arise from the unintentional provision of new fitness landscapes or environments for the microbiological evolution of such resistance. New attractors within fitness landscapes such as new antimicrobial drugs, weak pharmaceutical use regulations, intensive care units, medical technologies, prescribing habits, sanitary behaviour, rubber gloves, fast food, and intensive agricultural production all play a role in the creation of microbial resistance. The evolution of antibiotic resistance occurs within an evolutionary setting for micro-organisms largely of our own creation.

Resistance by those with vested economic interests against exercising appropriate controls over these new attractors, and the socially designed and constructed environments within which micro-organisms flourish, is the root cause of the entrenched antimicrobial resistance we now face in the institutional and clinical setting. We view this outcome as a classic case of our failure to understand the full complexity of a system that has interacting components from the micro (microbiological) to the macro (political economy) level. The use of transdisciplinary methods for studying the interconnections between the elements of such interrelated complexity is essential for understanding the pharmaceutical industry in relation to the biological world it has attempted to control.

6.10 Conclusion

The aim of this chapter has been to create an integrated framework for combining political economy and more interpretive, anthropological perspectives on pharmaceuticals. Such an analysis shows how a transdisciplinary perspective illuminates the relationship between macro and micro as well as structuralist and interpretivist approaches to understanding health problems, drawing on power as a common conceptual framework. However, not all research questions pertaining to pharmaceuticals will be answered by reference to this particular framework. Thus the chapter often considered pharmaceuticals in relation to physical systems as well as biological and ecological systems. A complexity theory analysis of the problem of resistant antibiotics allows us to extend our understanding to other levels of the health hierarchy. A fuller understanding of questions concerning the production, distribution, and consumption of pharmaceuticals in an increasingly globalised world can be achieved by drawing on concepts and methods from social, biological, ecological, and physical science disciplines, integrated by common conceptual frameworks.

Notes

1 Further reading on dependency theory and health systems can be found in Lynn Morgan 1987, 'Dependency Theory in the Political Economy of Health: An Anthropological Critique', *Medical Anthropology Quarterly*, vol. 1, no. 2, pp. 131–54.

2 Transfer pricing involves artificial manipulation of prices to take advantage of low-tax policies in developing countries. For example, a multinational drug company supplies raw materials for drugs to a subsidiary in a low-tax country at an artificially low price. The subsidiary then sells the finished product back to the parent company at an artificially high price. As a result, the parent company's books show low profits from these transactions so the company pays less tax. The subsidiary's books show low costs for raw materials and high income from sales. The subsidiary then repatriates the profits back to the parent company (see Chowdhury 1995, pp. 17–20).

3 United Nations Development Program 1997, *Human Development Report 1997*, Oxford University Press, New York, p. 82.

4 United Nations Conference on Trade and Development (Mamdani and Walker 1986, p. 189).

5 Zafrullah Chowdhury, a physician, is the author of *The Politics of Essential Drugs. The Makings of a Successful Health Strategy: Lessons from Bangladesh* (Zed Books London, 1995) which is a detailed account of the Bangladesh National Drug Policy.

6 Cephalosporin antibiotics are 'a type of antibacterial agent' which has 'the same basic structure as the penicillins'. They can be used as 'empiric therapy' for 'suspected infections', either alone or in combination with other drugs, and are also used to prevent surgical infections (Henderson 1999, p. 3).

7
The Problems and Potential of Transdisciplinary Teams

CARLA TRELOAR AND NICK HIGGINBOTHAM

7.1 Introduction

Effective transdisciplinary analysis of a health problem usually requires a team of collaborating researchers who bring together the right mix of disciplinary and interdisciplinary skills and ideas to fully understand the issue and create an appropriate intervention. However, historically, good teamwork and effective collaboration in the health research field have been rare—more the exception than the rule. If this is so, what then are the barriers to working successfully in TD teams? How can these barriers be overcome for health social scientists wishing to perform TD research? What can we learn from successful TD collaborations? What working conditions should TD team leaders seek to put into place to maximise creativity and the chance for a breakthrough?

In this chapter we answer these questions by identifying some principles that underlie the social and institutional organisation of interventions based on transdisciplinary teamwork. Initially, we look at barriers to TD teamwork observed by Rosenfield (1992) and Sewell (1989). Then we present Carla Treloar's Care Aware case study which highlights factors contributing to a successful TD intervention in a hospital setting. This project used *social marketing* techniques in an education program to prevent health care workers from being exposed to HIV infections through workplace accidents. Social marketing applies principles of commercial marketing to influence behaviour in relation to social issues, such as family planning, drug abuse, and road safety. Collaboration between HIV/AIDS physicians, a hospital infection-control consultant, and two health psychologists led the team to question the orthodox beliefs surrounding the causes of hospital accidents and choose a new direction for the intervention.

In chapter 6 we described how the concept of power can be used as a unifying principle to explain the relationship between structuralist and interpretivist approaches to analysing the pharmaceutical industry. In the Care Aware program, the concept of 'mindlessness' was developed to link the insights of clinical medicine, infection control, and health psychology/behavioural medicine.

Although the Care Aware program was primarily aimed at behavioural change, the team was able to widen the scope of the investigation by including multiple perspectives. Their analysis was informed by Winett et al.'s (1989) multilevel framework for integrating psychology and public health concepts and methods. The key principle is that interventions must follow from consideration of the connections between causal influences existing at different levels of analysis. Identifying and explaining factors existing at multiple levels of influence is an important part of the generic TD framework presented in chapter 4. In the last section of this chapter, we analyse the success of the Care Aware project using complexity theory principles.

7.2 Obstacles for TD teams

Patricia Rosenfield's influential article, 'The Potential of Transdisciplinary Research for Sustaining and Extending Linkages between the Health and Social Sciences' (1992), draws upon her experience working on tropical and diarrhoeal disease programs to identify the factors contributing to the success or failure of a transdisciplinary project. She concludes that 'The institutional and financial obstacles impeding the progression of knowledge and theory are far more stubborn than the conceptual ones' (1992, p. 355).

Similarly, William Sewell, a participant in interdisciplinary social psychology between World War II and the 1960s, reflects on the decline of that so-called golden age. Although the contexts are different, the authors outline a number of common organisational barriers to the effective operation of TD teams. These barriers, outlined in the following section, are often interdependent and accumulate to oppose the TD process (see figure 7.1).

7.2.1 Threat to traditional structure of universities

Attempts to establish and maintain transdisciplinary teams may be hindered by the limited funding and resources of structural units in universities, such as departments or schools. Transdisciplinary teams may create unwanted competition. As a result, institutions may not support transdisciplinary efforts and overtly or covertly make it difficult for the work to begin or continue.

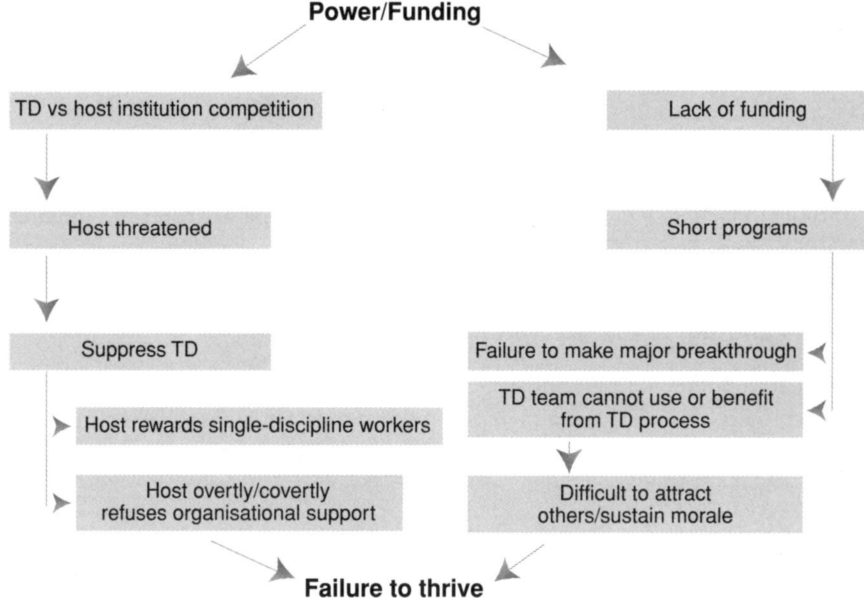

Figure 7.1 Influence of power and funding on the formation and operations of a TD team

7.2.2 Satisfying career opportunities

Teaching achievements and research publications will most likely be rewarded by promotion and tenure if they follow paths in established disciplinary or interdisciplinary fields of knowledge. Institutions have the power to suppress transdisciplinary teams by ignoring their achievements in favour of other members who devote themselves wholly to work in established areas of study. It may be easier to have discipline-based research published in established journals.

7.2.3 Lack of adequate and appropriate funding

Funding for TD work tends to be inadequate and available only for short-term projects. Project follow-ups are usually limited; the opportunity to cultivate greater insights and understanding of the issue that can be obtained through long-term involvement is lost. Further, team members who work on short-term projects are prevented from exploring the transdisciplinary process in a more detailed and personal way. The ability to move into transdisciplinary thinking comes through face-to-face team contact over time (Rosenfield 1992, p. 1345).

7.2.4 Lack of major breakthroughs

Short-term TD projects have a lower potential for making a major theoretical or conceptual breakthrough. The lack of a stimulating outcome restricts the TD team's ability to attract new members and funding, and may drain the team's momentum. In contrast, teams with long-standing experience in one area are able to attract new members and maintain or expand the group's activities and funding.

7.2.5 Advances in research methods may not produce a better understanding of the health problem

Sewell found that despite the lack of a major theoretical breakthrough, the research skills of the TD team members did improve, which is an achievement in itself. However, more advanced research skills without major conceptual advances will not sustain a TD relationship in the long term (Sewell 1989).

7.2.6 Relationships between fields of study

A number of difficulties of transdisciplinary research have their origins in the relationships between the fields of study involved. Disciplinary scepticism, limited knowledge of other fields, and an inadequate mix of disciplines within a TD team can all work to undermine its effective functioning (Rosenfield 1992, p. 1344). Team members need to talk freely and openly about their ideas of the problem. Sewell observes that many ideas may originate from a field of study outside those usually associated with the subject (1989, p. 4). The success or failure of transdisciplinary work, even with adequate funding and institutional support, is very much dependent on the types of issues, disciplines, and people involved.

7.2.7 Personal qualities of transdisciplinary researchers

Certain personality traits can enliven transdisciplinary collaboration. In her own work, Rosenfield observed that because of the many factors which contribute to the disruption, stagnation, and possible failure of a transdisciplinary team, members of that team need to be 'intellectual risk takers' (1992, p. 1354).

7.2.8. Reliance on key individuals

In the face of these obstacles, the existence of a TD team may depend on the driving force, commitment, and political power of a few key individuals. Unfortunately, the team may not be able to exist without these leaders; heavy reliance upon a leader may result in one field of study becoming dominant, thereby limiting the TD nature of the project.

7.3 Successful transdisciplinary research: the Care Aware program

The Care Aware program aimed to reduce exposure (that is, physical contact) of health care workers to HIV infection through minimising hospital accidents such as needlestick injuries and blood splashes (Treloar et al. 1996). Although the course of the project changed substantially from its outset, the project produced an enhanced understanding of worker accidents and a successful educational intervention using social marketing principles. The team was successful not only in designing an effective intervention, but also in constructing an open forum for discussion unconstrained by disciplinary traditions.

7.3.1 Accidental exposures among health care workers

In December 1984 the first HIV infection acquired in a workplace was reported in Britain. The transmission of the virus occurred when a nurse accidentally stabbed herself with a needle immediately after drawing blood from a patient (*Lancet* 1984). These types of needlestick injuries and other accidental exposures, such as blood splashes and blood spills, are common in the health profession. Yet it is only since the early 1980s, when the risk of acquiring HIV infection through such accidents was realised, that prevention of exposures have become a priority.

Blood-to-blood contact is also possible if blood is spilt onto the broken skin of a worker or comes into contact with mucous membranes (eyes, inside the nose and mouth). For health workers the most hazardous means of contact is a needlestick injury. The chance of transmission of HIV infection as a result of a single needlestick injury is approximately 0.3 per cent (Henderson et al. 1990).

It is difficult to count the number of health workers who have contracted HIV through workplace incidents. Some researchers stated that as many as sixty-four new occupationally acquired HIV infections occur per year in the USA (Jagger and Pearson 1991). In less developed countries the number of health care workers who have been infected is not known. The high prevalence of HIV/AIDS coupled with the lack of resources and infection control measures in many places mean that it is likely to be high.

Transmission of HIV is only one consequence of accidental exposure. Each year 200 health personnel die in the USA as a result of occupationally acquired hepatitis B (Beekmann et al. 1990), and 18 000 new cases of hepatitis B are caused annually by needlestick injury (CDC 1987). Some researchers suggest that workers may be exposed to as many as twenty pathogens from a single needlestick injury (Tandberg et al. 1991), including hepatitis C and others yet to be identified. Studies estimating the cost of needlestick injuries range from US$135–749 per puncture (McCormick et al. 1991; Short et al. 1991).

7.3.2 The cue to action: definition of the problem and formation of the TD team

The Care Aware program originated with a discussion held on a street corner outside the teaching hospital where the program was later based. A member of the clinical staff of the HIV/AIDS unit had recently suffered a needlestick injury. A senior physician and an infection-control consultant encountered each other, by chance, on the roadside.

Infection control consultant: 'I heard about the latest one. What can we do to get them to follow the guidelines?'
Medical specialist: 'I just don't know.'

The medical specialist (A), however, was also a PhD scholar at the Centre for Clinical Epidemiology and Biostatistics at the University of Newcastle, where transdisciplinary teaching is promoted. He discussed an idea to apply for a Commonwealth grant to conduct an education program improving compliance with the Universal Precaution guidelines and decided to speak to a health psychologist (B) who was interested in trialling academic detailing education (see 7.7.1) in a clinical setting. The physician also spoke to a colleague, an HIV/AIDS medical specialist (C), who had worked closely with the infection-control consultant (D) in establishing the HIV/AIDS unit at the teaching hospital and providing HIV education over many years. Subsequently, after a successful grant application, a recent psychology graduate (E) interested in behavioural medicine was appointed to the position of project officer (and enrolled as a PhD student).[1] Hence, the transdisciplinary team was formed through existing formal and informal relationships as shown in figure 7.2.

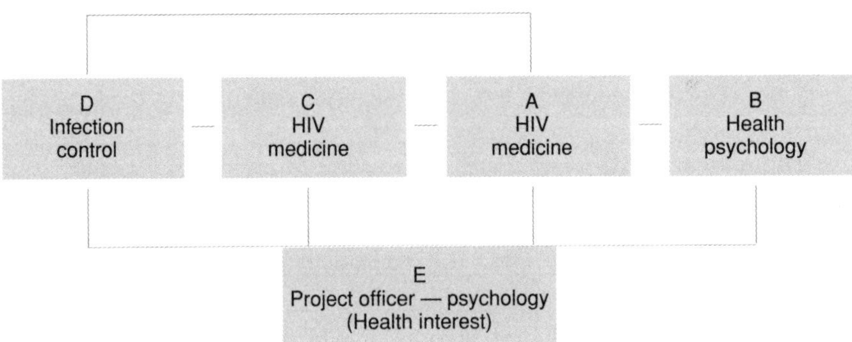

Figure 7.2 Formation of the Care Aware TD team

7.4 Initial course of the project

The team received a grant from the Commonwealth AIDS Workforce Information program to develop and evaluate an academic detailing education program in order to increase the compliance of health workers with the Universal Precautions infection-control guidelines. The initial team meetings were designed to build a common understanding of the problem and introduce the non-clinical team members to the issue. To achieve this the team members familiarised themselves with the standard methods employed to avoid accidental exposure, undertook a literature review, held weekly research meetings in the HIV/AIDS unit, and interviewed a number of workers who had sustained accidental exposures.

7.4.1 Universal precautions to prevent accidental exposure

The Universal Precautions model of infection control was promoted to protect health employees by recommending that all patients and their body substances be treated as if they were infectious with HIV and other viruses (CDC 1987; 1992). This approach aims to protect workers from both diagnosed and undiagnosed infectious agents. The Universal Precautions model recommends that personnel adopt barrier precautions when they anticipate contact with blood or other body substances. These precautions include the wearing of gloves, gowns or aprons, eye protection, masks, and other devices depending on the medical procedure to be performed. To prevent needlestick injuries, needles and other sharp instruments should not be recapped, bent or broken by hand, removed from disposable syringes, or otherwise manipulated by hand, and should be placed in puncture-resistant containers for disposal. These containers should be located as close as possible to the work area (CDC 1987).

Since the publication of the Universal Precautions model, interventions to prevent accidental exposures have assumed that they are caused by non-compliance with the guidelines, and that strict adherence to the guidelines would reduce, if not eliminate, exposures (for example, Hadley 1989; Verrusio 1989; Courington et al. 1991). Initially, the Care Aware team also believed that compliance with Universal Precautions was the best method of preventing exposures.

7.4.2 Literature review

A review of the HIV/AIDS literature enabled the psychologists to become familiar with the clinical and epidemiological aspects of the problem (physiology of HIV/AIDS, risk factors for transmission, magnitude of problem, prevention strategies). Similarly, reviews of social marketing and academic detailing studies gave the whole team an appreciation of how these techniques could be applied locally. The literature revealed the widespread belief that accidental exposures were the result of non-compliance with guidelines. Most investigations were descriptive studies of injury type; only a few reported interventions to promote compliance with the Universal Precautions guidelines.

7.4.3 HIV/AIDS unit's weekly research meetings

Attendance at the research meetings presented the project officer (PhD student) with opportunities to become a recognised member of the HIV/AIDS unit and establish personal relationships with the members of the clinical team who would become key informants in the process of developing education materials.

7.4.4 Qualitative interviews: a multilevel form of investigation

The project officer conducted interviews with thirty-eight people who had sustained accidental exposures (Treloar et al. 1995). These interviews enabled her to become familiar with clinical terms and develop a new vocabulary to discuss and understand the problem. She also gained a deeper appreciation of the emotional impact of these injuries on the workers and their families as they came to terms with the fact that they were dealing with a life-threatening virus.

7.5 Changing the study focus

As work began, new information came to light that changed the direction of the transdisciplinary project. Data from the indepth interviews with thirty-eight injured staff identified potential risk factors and precursors to exposure. The interviews allowed the participants to describe in detail how the accident happened. Surprisingly, the team found that only ten people (26 per cent of the sample) were non-compliant with the Universal Precautions guidelines at the time of the exposure. Needlestick injuries account for the majority of reported accidental exposures; recapping of needles is often singled out as a prohibited and highly dangerous practice (Sellick et al. 1991; Whitby et al. 1991). However, the ten incidents of non-compliance included only one instance (3 per cent) of exposure due to recapping.

It has only been since the identification of HIV that the infection control guidelines have mandated that needles not be recapped after use. Prior to this, recapping was taught to both medical and nursing students as a way to prevent jabs from unprotected needles. However, data from the region's two largest hospitals over the previous 2 years revealed that less than 5 per cent of all reported exposures were due to recapping of needles.

The needle disposal containers (burn bins) in five wards of a regional hospital were then monitored over an 8-week period to estimate the prevalence of needle recapping. This exercise was conducted under the supervision of the team's infection control consultant to ensure safety. Of the approximately 6800 needles counted in the needle disposal bins, 1556 (23 per cent) had been recapped. However, no needlestick injuries were reported from the areas audited during the course of the study, despite identification of over 1500 opportunities for needlestick injury due to recapping.

A literature review showed that, although recapping did account for some needlestick incidents, the majority of injuries occurred after use of the needle and before disposal, confirming our observations that a small proportion (in a range less than 20 per cent) of reported needlestick injuries are from needle recapping practices. The Care Aware team's preliminary study results were integrated and compared to the literature's conclusion that compliance with the Universal Precautions guidelines would protect health care workers against accidental exposure. Using various methods and data sources (triangulation) we came to the conclusion that:

> Compliance with the Universal Precautions infection control guidelines is necessary but not sufficient to protect health care workers against accidental exposure.

7.5.1 Focus group discussions to explore the new conclusion

The team initially planned to run focus group discussions to explore the behaviour of health care workers and evaluate the variables in the theory of social behaviour. However, the focus of these discussions changed in the light of the conclusion from our preliminary studies. If our initial assumptions were wrong, then what factors would improve protection for health workers? Interviews with health employees identified factors at the organisation level—low staffing levels, being rushed or busy—that were common across a number of accidents. However, these factors were not amenable to change in a program of limited funding.

The group leader presented figure 7.3 to participants in focus group discussions and asked them to comment on the findings, discuss their own experience, and their perceptions of the causes of accidental exposures.

A participant in the first focus group described her experience of accidental exposure by drawing an analogy with motor vehicle accidents. She said that she had heard that the majority of accidents occur on the journey home from work, so drivers had been advised not to travel the same route home every day. On considering this, the health psychologist connected this anecdote to the phenomenon

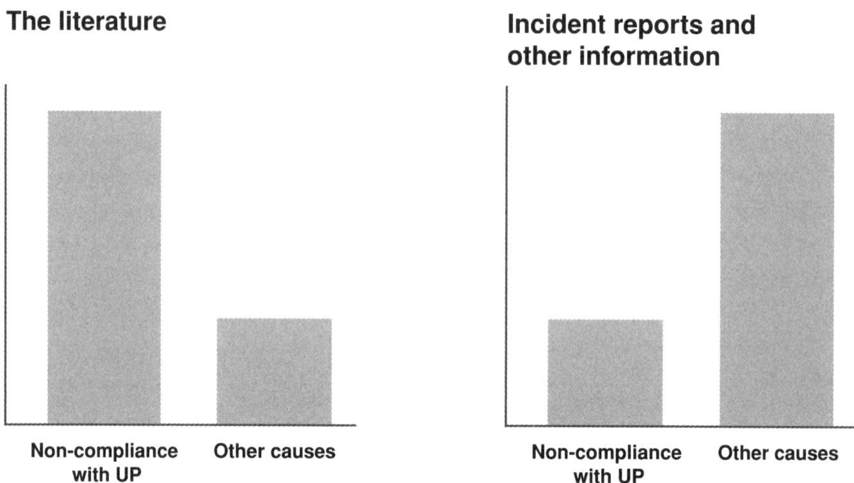

Figure 7.3 The relative impact of non-compliance with Universal Precautions (UP) guidelines on the cause of accidental exposures according to the literature and those recorded on hospital incident reports

described as 'mindlessness' in the psychological literature. This led to a thorough review of the data already collected in interviews and group discussions. Health care workers often described how they work 'ahead of themselves', 'thinking 2000 miles ahead, thinking about what they had to do next', and working as if they were 'on automatic pilot'.

7.6 Mindlessness as a common conceptual framework

The initial phase of the project had two TD objectives. First, the non-clinical members of the team became familiar with the vocabulary, environment, and culture of health care workers. Second, the data collected through interviews, literature reviews, and focus group discussions were presented and discussed at weekly TD team meetings to provide the foundation for the development of the intervention program. Identification of automatic pilot, or mindlessness, as a significant influence on accidental exposure was a major breakthrough that enabled the TD team to function at a higher level of cohesion. The non-clinical members of the team were now able to explain the theoretical basis of mindlessness and explore with the others its potential application as a framework for a hospital intervention.

The psychological literature abounds with articles concerning automatic pilot, mindlessness, cognitive errors, action slips, and more (see, for example, Reason 1979; Norman 1981). These phenomena manifest in a variety of ways among otherwise healthy people—putting shaving cream on a toothbrush, placing a dirty plate in the refrigerator and the butter in the dishwasher, being unable to remember why you went into a room—these are all symptoms of automatic pilot.

We actually need mindlessness to guide our behaviours. First attempts at driving a car are often punctuated by unnatural lurches and jumps; as skill develops, there is less need to concentrate on coordinating all the various movements. Mindlessness itself is not observable, only its outcomes. We realise that we are driving mindlessly when we find ourselves on the familiar route home rather than on a planned detour. Mindlessness is the stereotypical use of information and is a problem of experts and not novices as, by definition, it develops with repetition of a behaviour (Langer 1989).

With regard to the transdisciplinary approach, the psychologists explained these concepts to the clinicians and asked them to evaluate the merit of this idea with regard to accidental exposure. We had achieved a stage where we could discuss the project without disciplinary boundaries.

A phenomenon described by both the project team and our interview participants led to the development of a model of mindlessness that became the team's common conceptual framework and guided our intervention. Health workers described their motivation or alertness as being generally low. However, when an exposure occurs, awareness of the dangers in the environment peaks (see figure 7.4). This dramatic upswing in awareness is often aided by the concentrated effort of the hospital's infection-control educators. As time passes other activities become priorities and make greater demands—hazard awareness slips to pre-exposure levels. We felt that the education program should prompt and maintain a heightened awareness, at least during dangerous procedures.

The cognitive conservation model of mindlessness (figure 7.5) was based on this observation. The model assumes that people try to minimise the cognitive capacity involved when performing a behaviour. In this state, we can function

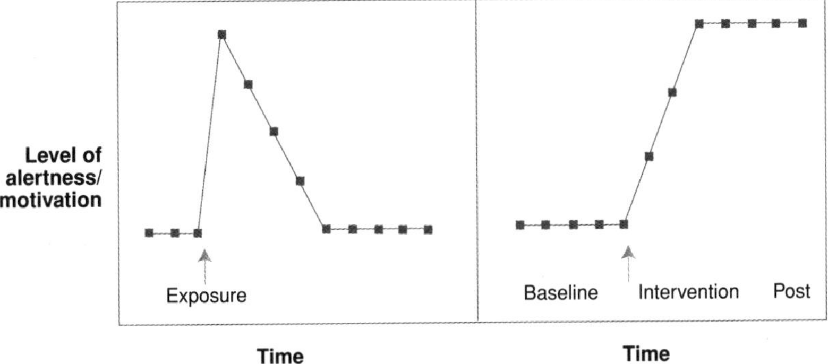

Figure 7.4 Representation of the levels of alertness stimulated by a nearby needlestick accident, and by the planned Care Aware intervention

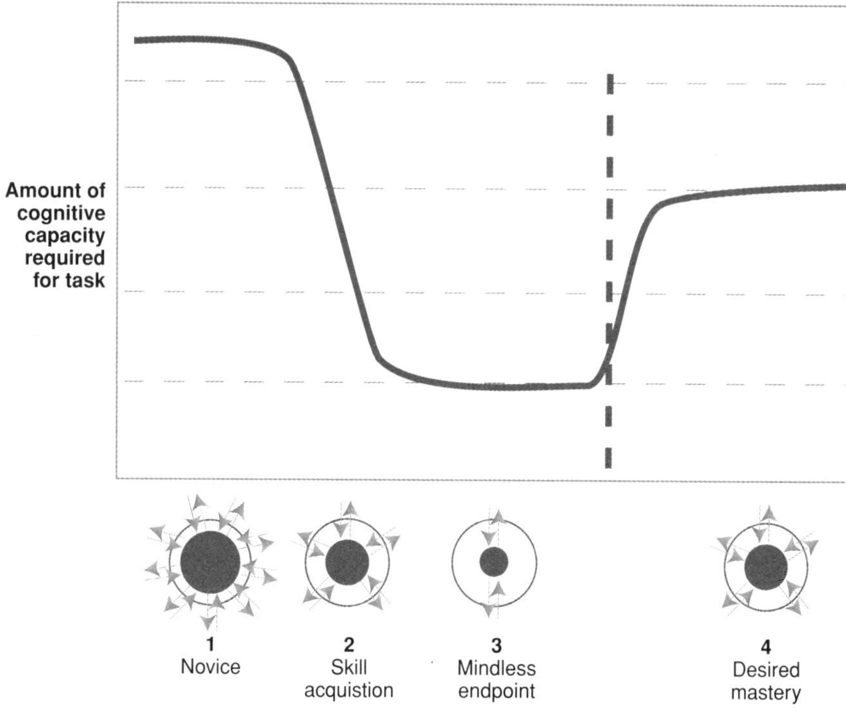

Figure 7.5 The cognitive conservation model of mindlessness

without directing obvious attention to our actions and exert little effort towards feedback and monitoring these behaviours.

The initial three stages of the model show the process of decreasing cognitive capacity. First is the *novice* stage, in which high levels of cognitive capacity are required in learning a skill. Behaviour is continually monitored and adjusted. The second stage, *skill acquisition*, is temporary: the skill is performed with some degree of mastery but requires a moderate amount of cognitive capacity to perform, monitor, and provide feedback.

The third stage, the *mindless endpoint*, uses minimal cognitive effort to perform and monitor behaviour. Stage 3 behaviour is typically inflexible; behaviour runs according to pre-programmed scripts. Sensitivity to changing goals of the behaviour or demands of the environment is reduced. Once a behaviour is started it is difficult to modify, given the minimal amount of attention directed to its monitoring (Reason 1984). Action slips or cognitive errors are common in this state of reduced cognitive effort. Stage 3 functioning is usually the endpoint in learning any behaviour.

The Care Aware intervention sought to promote Stage 4 functioning that requires the same cognitive capacity efforts as Stage 2. An adequate amount of cognitive capacity is directed towards ensuring that the behaviour is mindfully controlled, adaptive to environmental demands, and sensitive to changes in behavioural goals. Mindless experiences would occur less frequently in Stage 4 compared to Stage 3 functioning, as greater amounts of attention guide the target behaviour.

Social cognition research suggests several ways to encourage Stage 4 functioning. First, mindlessness occurs in judgment situations which are not cognitively demanding (for example, Fiske and Neuberg 1990). Second, altering the way that an object is defined linguistically encourages people to use that object creatively (Langer and Piper 1987). Mindlessness is decreased when objects, people, or events are defined ambiguously, so that people have to use some effort to decide how they should be classified (de Bono 1992). These principles were used to compose the Care Aware education messages.

7.7 Using social marketing techniques for health interventions

The TD team experimented with a number of intervention messages before using four steps to stimulate the move from Stage 3 to Stage 4 functioning in the cognitive conservation model:

1 Compliance with Universal Precautions guidelines alone is not sufficient to ensure safety in the workplace.
2 Health care workers often describe themselves as being on 'automatic pilot'.
3 Being on automatic pilot can lead to accidents.
4 A checklist (figure 7.6) can be used to guard against automatic pilot, increasing work practice safety and awareness.

The checklist is used to redirect attention: staff are encouraged to not only comply with the Universal Precautions guidelines, but also to perceive their work environment as a dynamic, ever-changing system (that is, a mindful definition of the work environment).

The TD team explored many ways of delivering these messages. Buddhist meditation was explored as a potential technique for highlighting the effects of mindlessness on everyday activities. An anthropologist with an expert knowledge of meditation techniques known as 'Quietening the Mind' and 'Developing Single-Pointed Concentration' discussed the incorporation of these techniques in the Care Aware intervention. The clinical members of the TD team acknowledged the theoretical application of these techniques but did not feel that the situation would allow sufficient time to recruit and teach health care workers how to meditate.

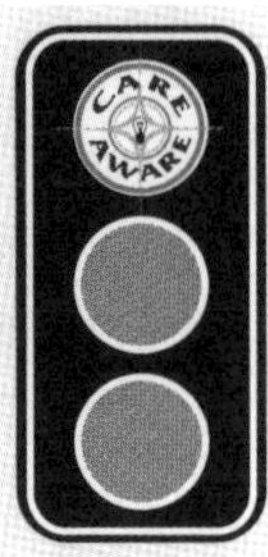

What am I doing?

- Could this be dangerous to me?
- What steps are involved?
- What infection control precautions must I take?

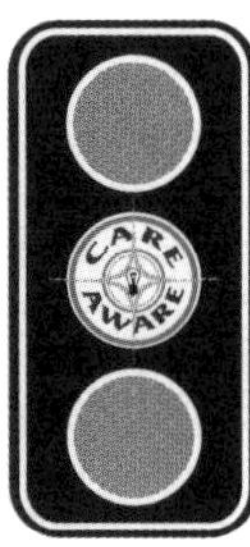

What can go wrong?

- What are the hazards in my environment?
- Does the equipment work?
  Is it conveniently placed?
- What about distractions?
  Could I be bumped?
  Is the patient cooperative?
  How do I feel? Tired, worried, sick, bored?

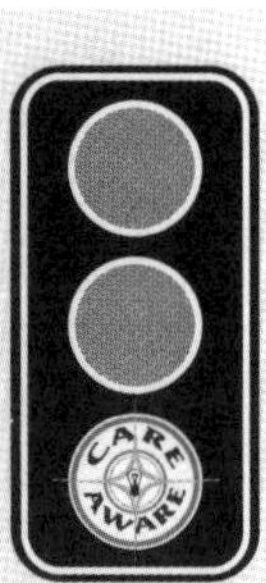

What can I do about it?

- Think ahead.
- Be prepared.
- Know what to do if something goes wrong.

Figure 7.6 The Care Aware checklist

7.7.1 The Care Aware academic detailing program

Academic detailing was chosen for delivering the intervention messages. 'Detailing' refers to strategies pharmaceutical company representatives use to persuade a physician to prescribe a certain brand of drug. These principles were modified for the needs of this program. Soumerai et al. (1989) have demonstrated the impact of these techniques compared with traditional education programs. Academic detail techniques that have proven useful are shown in table 7.1 (Soumerai and Avorn 1990, p. 549).

Table 7.1 Effective academic detailing techniques

1	Conduct interviews to investigate baseline knowledge and motivations for current prescribing patterns.
2	Focus programs on specific categories of physicians as well as on their opinion leaders.
3	Define clear educational and behavioural objectives.
4	Establish credibility through a respected organisational identity, referencing authoritative and unbiased sources of information, and present both sides of controversial issues.
5	Stimulate active physician participation in educational interactions.
6	Use concise graphic educational materials.
7	Highlight and repeat the essential messages.
8	Provide positive reinforcement of improved practices in follow-up visits.

Academic detailing involves brief one-to-one educational visits to physicians by specially trained pharmacists or physician counsellors. Soumerai and Avorn (1990) note that the most important aspect of this technique is its flexibility, allowing the encounter to be tailored to the specific requirements of each person.

7.7.1.1 Social marketing

Social marketing uses the principles of commercial marketing, such as definition of target adopters, and attractive and appropriate packaging of the product as a vehicle to stimulate behaviour change (Kotler and Roberto 1989). However, social marketing is *consumer*—rather than profit—oriented, and aims to produce outcomes which are of benefit to the consumer rather than the marketeer. A successful social marketing intervention must be meaningful to the population and based on their concerns, beliefs, and experiences (Kotler and Roberto 1989).

7.7.2 Consultation and cooperation

The TD team wanted to ensure that the education materials were seen as credible by the notoriously sceptical health workers and so relied heavily upon the social marketing research process. This included critical feedback from key informants, especially the highly experienced nurse specialists in the HIV inpatient units. Multimedia which could be incorporated into the detailing encounter were required. An advertising agency was commissioned to produce a package of materials linked with a logo and theme. An iterative communication process among the advertising agency, the project team, and the group of key informants continued until a consensus was reached about the relevance of intervention messages.

A similar process was used in the development and rehearsal of the academic detailing visit. A coherent, polished, 5-minute script was required for the academic detailing interview. The team worked with the educator in producing an outline of the main messages of the program and the strategies to deliver these messages. The detailing encounter was trialled with a number of key informants and videotaped, allowing the educator to polish and refine his performance.

The team's primary concern was that the program be credible and not overly intrusive. We sought to achieve a balance of informative, relevant messages to be delivered in a manner that was interesting and non-threatening to staff. The techniques derived from the social marketing literature assisted in achieving these goals.

7.7.2.1 Care Aware program outcome measures

Although lack of compliance with infection-control Universal Precautions is not the major contributor to accidental exposures, we chose to measure compliance as a key outcome. Compliance with the guidelines is necessary (but not sufficient) to avoid accidental exposure; it is the first defence against exposure. An increase in compliance levels measured after the education program would indicate that staff were more aware of the dangers in the work environment and had changed their work practices to avoid that danger. Outside the Universal Precautions criteria, the incidence of other unsafe practices (OUP) was also measured, as such acts still carry a risk of exposure. In brief, we hypothesised that the Care Aware program would significantly increase health care workers' compliance with the Universal Precautions guidelines, that the incidence of other unsafe practices would decrease, and that the program would be well-received by the participants.

7.7.3 Care Aware program intervention methods

The intervention was conducted in the Intensive Care Unit (ICU) and Emergency Unit (EU) of a 533-bed tertiary referral hospital in New South Wales, Australia, with a full range of specialist and allied health services (see Treloar et al. 1996 for more details). The project team hosted a number of informal sessions for the staff of each ward to introduce the program, provide a timeline, and emphasise that the program was funded by the Commonwealth government not by the hospital administration. This clarification was important to establishing the program's credibility and minimising suspicion of the project's aims and objectives.

A nurse observer was present in each unit for approximately 14 hours per week to observe health care workers' procedures and record their compliance before the education was introduced. The 8-week observation period included an initial 2 weeks (the familiarisation period) during which unit staff could adjust to the presence of an observer and the observer assigned individual code numbers to staff members. Following the pre-education period, there was a 1-week break in observations to launch the education program in each unit, then observation data were collected for 6 weeks.[2]

The observer also recorded whether any OUP occurred during observed procedures and noted information about the patient (age and sex), the urgency of their problem, activity indicators, time of day, day of the week, ward busy-ness, and occupation of the health care worker.

7.7.4 Content of the academic detailing visit

The educator approached staff members individually asking if each one would participate in a short interview. The educator introduced himself as part of a program to prevent accidental exposures in hospitals and presented the results of preliminary investigations. He explained that most injured workers were compliant with the guidelines at the time of exposure and that they felt as if they were working on automatic pilot.

The intervention subjects were asked to describe the possible role that automatic pilot may have had in an exposure they had experienced. Participants who had not experienced an exposure were told that the program was designed to maintain their good safety record. All participants were told that the project team had developed a method for preventing exposures—the Care Aware checklist.

The three steps of the checklist were explained and subjects were asked to use the checklist to direct their own behaviour through a routine procedure. For those who indicated that the checklist was too complex to use routinely, the educator suggested that they use it as a cue to switch off automatic pilot during dangerous procedures. Finally, the educator asked whether staff had noticed any unsafe aspects of the work environment and thanked the participants for their time.

A number of materials were developed to reinforce the messages delivered through the detailing interviews. The Care Aware booklet contained the primary safety messages and was used to guide the subject through the interview. The educator placed Care Aware posters and stickers in each unit and rotated the posters at least every 3 days to ensure that they did not become invisible. A poster presenting the checklist was positioned behind the lavatory door in each unit. This poster was expected to attract comment and graffiti.

7.7.5 Multiple levels targeted

The Care Aware program primarily sought to change individuals' habits by asking them to consider influences on their behaviour. However, the TD team acknowledged the significance of organisational influences that were outside the scope of the program and beyond the control of the individual staff members. The academic detailer collected the participants' perceptions of the main hazards in their work environment and presented these to the nursing and medical managers of each unit as a stimulus for policy change.

7.7.6 Results

The team examined the Care Aware program's impact on adherence of staff to UP guidelines and incidence of other unsafe practices, as well as staff perception of the usefulness of the program. Overall, the results showed that the program was successful in changing health workers' safety behaviour and enhancing staff and management awareness of workplace injury.

7.7.6.1 Effect on compliance behaviour

The majority (>75 per cent) of full-time and part-time staff were invited to participate in the intervention. The pre-education and posteducation compliance scores of eighty staff were compared to examine the effectiveness of the intervention. Posteducation compliance scores increased by 16 per cent compared to pre-education scores ($p = .006$).

7.7.6.2 Effect on other unsafe practices

The incidence of OUP for these eighty participants fell from 5.8 per cent in the pre-education period to 1.9 per cent in the posteducation period ($p = .01$). The most frequently observed OUP involved leaving a contaminated piece of equipment in an inappropriate place or failing to replace a full contaminated waste container.

7.7.6.3 Participants' evaluation of the program

Thirty-four participants were asked what they liked about the program and what could be improved. They had four main reactions, with most endorsing the first two:

1 The program was good, worthwhile, and had an impact on work practices or attitude towards work practices, such as being 'more aware' or 'more careful'. In some cases new actions were taken, such as wearing gloves more often.
2 The program contained 'nothing new' but acted as a reminder. Some staff described themselves as 'stale' and the program served to bring them up to the required standard of awareness.
3 A small number felt that the program was 'nothing new' and had little impact but it neither irritated nor excited staff.
4 Even fewer said the program had obvious areas for improvement: it dragged on for too long, was shallow, and could have addressed more specific issues for the unit.

7.7.6.4 Organisational hazards in units

The five most frequently mentioned organisational hazards are listed in table 7.2, with poor-quality gloves being the top one. Staff complained that even with minimal use their fingers tore through the end of the gloves. The next three most common complaints in ICU (taps, valves, and blunt needles) related to the use of alternative techniques to reduce the use of needles and sharp instruments. This equipment was available in the unit but acceptability and use among staff was low. A few wanted to have sharps disposal bins on trolleys that would be wheeled to the bedside. For Emergency Unit staff (as well as from quality and size of gloves) there was danger seen in understaffing of the work environment. Staff were also worried about the insufficient number of needle disposal bins. As a result of bringing this to the attention of EU management, disposal bins were installed next to each bed in this unit.

Table 7.2 Five most frequently mentioned environmental/organisational hazards in each unit

Intensive Care Unit		*Emergency Unit*	
Poor-quality gloves	20	Poor-quality gloves	24
Need more three-way taps	14	Unit needs more staff	11
Need more one-way valves	6	Gloves are not available in all sizes	6
Need more blunt drawing-up needles	5	Unit needs more disposal bins	3
Sharps bins should be on trolleys	3	Unit needs more inservice/education	2

7.8 Factors contributing to the success of the Care Aware project as a TD collaboration

Sewell (1989) and Rosenfield (1992) painted an uncertain future for TD research. Competition for scarce resources and the unpredictable nature of the personalities involved in TD groups were identified as threats to the establishment, maintenance, and ultimate success of TD research. The Care Aware project combined the fields of clinical medicine, infection control, and health psychology in its quest to better understand and prevent accidental exposures to infectious disease among health workers. This program succeeded both as an intervention and in constructing a TD understanding of accidental exposures.

7.8.1 Some keys to success

Some keys to the success of the Care Aware project, and how they relate to the problems of power and funding encountered by earlier TD researchers, are now discussed.

7.8.1.1 Openness of medical specialists to other disciplines

Traditionally, medicine perpetuated disciplinary élitism. In contrast, the two medical doctors in the Care Aware team had previous training in other areas (sociology and biochemistry) and were very interested in collaborating on an equal basis with other disciplines.

7.8.1.2 Experience in AIDs care

The field of AIDS clinical care tends to follow a holistic approach to patient care that incorporates many fields of knowledge. In addition, behavioural and social approaches are highly regarded because they hold the key to prevention.

7.8.1.3 Strong leadership

The principal investigator of the TD team was an intellectual risk taker who assertively defended the project when threatened by hospital administrators and funding agencies.

7.8.1.4 External funding

The funding for the program was secured from the federal government, enabling the program to pay its own way and not rely on the resources of the host departments.

7.8.1.5 Career advancement

The team members ensured that the project produced publications that helped all members' careers. Papers were accepted by clinical medicine, health psychology, and infection-control journals.

7.8.1.6 Team motivation

In essence, this program was action research, as members of the research team were caring for HIV/AIDS patients. The ideas generated by the project team were immediately tested on the hospital wards by other professionals (for example, nurse specialists).

7.8.1.7 Prior relationships

It was useful that the team was established through existing relationships between team members. Thus, the team was founded in a climate of cooperation and without the need to establish disciplinary dominance.

7.8.1.8 Commitment to the TD process

Each member of the team felt that his or her own field of knowledge had something to offer the team. Team meetings were dynamic and exciting as ideas were debated with little regard for their disciplinary origins.

7.8.1.9 Accessible TD conceptual framework

The team jointly discovered the social psychological process of mindlessness as the common conceptual framework for the TD education intervention. This framework is highly accessible: most people can grasp the concept quickly and provide examples of their own automatic pilot experiences. Mindlessness is a compelling approach to understanding complex behaviour and easily translates across domains of knowledge.

7.8.1.10 Dedicated staff time

The Care Aware project was the full-time responsibility of the PhD student who was also the project officer. This position was externally funded; her time for the project could not be taken up by demands from either institution (hospital or university). This dedicated position ensured continuity and ongoing momentum for the project.

7.8.1.11 Specialised roles

As well as their particular expertise, members brought to the TD team their status and position within each of the parent institutions. When negotiations with external agencies were needed, team members were able to take on responsibility for handling such negotiations based on their department's prior alliances and relationships with these agencies.

7.9 Care Aware and complexity theory

The transdisciplinary thinking guiding the Care Aware program encouraged hospital staff to not only adopt the Universal Precautions guidelines more effectively, but to see their workplace as a dynamic, ever-changing system as well. Crucial factors influencing health professionals' actions were *personal disorganisation,* in the form of mindlessness, exacerbated by *institutional disorganisation,* in the form of hectic working conditions. Complexity theory enables us to understand why the Care Aware change strategies targeting personal disorganisation were successful.

Hospitals and clinics, and the professionals who work within them, can be viewed as complex adaptive systems with the ability to self-organise and evolve. Miller et al. (1998, pp. 369–76) argue that these small-scale social systems operate according to internal models or rules that forge pathways of activity towards the achievement of specific endpoints (that is, attractors). We can think of a hospital's internal models as its central activities and stated mission such as funding priorities, patient care policies, and staffing policies. Local (internal) and global (external) attractors interact with one another to influence the evolution of the hospital system. Local attractors include income goals and standards of patient care, infection control, and occupational safety (Miller et al. 1998, p. 371). Prominent among the global attractors affecting the organisation are government regulation of the health sector, consumer expectations, demands of professional bodies, and patient support groups as well as the unexpected arrival of infective micro-organisms, such as CJD prions and the Ebola virus, for which the local health system is unprepared (see

3.3.1.3 and 3.3.1.4). Equally important global influences are popular philosophies of clinical practice, including evidence-based medicine and patient empowerment. Also significant are global pressures on the health system arising from the political economy, such as government requirements that public services become competitive, restructure their operations to maximise efficiency, and adopt corporate management styles.

The key agents in a hospital—doctors, nurses, administrators—enact the organisation's internal models. These blueprints of thought and behaviour inform individuals about how things work in a particular situation; internal models help people to anticipate and predict events and respond to changing situations (Miller et al. 1998, p. 371). Examples include institutional values—making money, ethics, organisational commitment, teamwork—as well as understandings of relationships and management of resources. The unique shape (that is, pattern of performance) of a health institution, as an adaptive system, arises from the interactions among the groups of agents as they grapple with both local and global forces. For example, the arrival of HIV/AIDS precipitated a worldwide overhaul of hospital infection-control precautions; a similar disturbance has followed the accidental spread of CJD prions through surgical procedures (*Sydney Morning Herald*, 4 May 2000, p. 3). In essence, the hospital's attractors derive from its professionals' patterns of action as they strive to follow the organisation's internal models within a changing environment.

How can we relate these concepts to the change strategies adopted by the Care Aware project? First, the project aimed to alter an internalised way of acting that was hazardous (operating on automatic pilot or mindlessness). Second, the project identified the need to change policies promoting the disorganised working environment, including low staffing levels. However, political realities and funding constraints meant that an intervention targeting institutional disorganisation was beyond the scope of the project.

Having identified the problem, the Care Aware project applied academic detailing techniques to improve safety in the workplace. Why were the methods successful? Miller et al. (1998, pp. 373–4) describe three successful change strategies for health organisations based on complexity principles: transforming, joining, and learning. *Joining* involves 'enhancing existing attractors' and is successful only when the methods are consistent with the internal models of the individual or the institution. *Transforming* involves 'changing an attractor or creating a new one'. One form of transforming, *wedging*, involves pushing a system to the 'edge of chaos', which may precipitate realignment to new attractors. *Learning* involves teaching staff to be aware of internal models and how those internal models may be limiting them. In the light of this knowledge, decisions can be made to either maintain or change allegiance to relevant attractors.

Joining strategies were used in three ways in the Care Aware project. First, the notion of mindlessness was targeted after health care workers themselves identified it as a problem. Mindlessness is an internal model through which individuals self-organise. Second, social marketing messages targeting mindlessness were meaningful to the health care staff because they were grounded in their concerns, beliefs, and experiences (Kotler and Roberto 1989). A process of feedback from key informants ensured that social marketing messages had high credibility with health care professionals. Third, the Care Aware intervention reinforced the value system of busy hospital workers. It was delivered in a non-punitive way and acknowledged the professionals' commitment to patient and colleague safety and care. In other words, strategies were devised which were compatible with preexisting attractors.

The Care Aware project used learning strategies by assisting hospital staff to be aware of the operation of internal models and raising the sense of discrepancy between habits and values. In the case of mindlessness, the discrepancy arises from the awareness that while mindless behaviours are necessary they are dangerous in the hospital environment. Health care workers were prompted to recognise this discrepancy to ensure that behaviour is mindfully controlled in situations of high risk.

Transforming is a rather drastic way of forcing change through coercion, deliberately creating a disturbance in a system in order to force a re-organisation (Miller et al. 1998, p. 374). This strategy was not used in the Care Aware project. Neither the institution nor individual health care workers would have responded positively to this method. However, transforming is taken up in the next chapter as potentially relevant to interventions in African communities to prevent sexually transmitted HIV infection.

The success of the Care Aware program came from providing individuals with resources (for example, reminders, posters, cognitive checklists), and establishing relationships between hospital staff and Care Aware team members that assisted the participants to self-regulate in response to various internal and external inputs and changes. Self-regulation towards a safer personal and group environment was achieved by controlling mindlessness. Personal integrity was maintained in the face of continuing stressful working conditions, by involvement in an intervention that projected views compatible with the preexisting attractors, such as maintenance of professional knowledge, and expertise and workplace safety.

7.10 Conclusion

Obstacles to the success of TD projects are numerous and often arise from institutional and financial concerns. This chapter presented a project that managed to overcome these obstacles and reach a TD understanding of accidental exposure to HIV infections and other pathogens among hospital workers. It did so through good luck as well as commitment from team members to the TD process. The Care Aware project also shows how the organism-like quality of a hospital setting can be understood as a complex adaptive system using complexity theory.

The intervention described in this chapter took place in a clinical setting in an industrialised country. In the next chapter we present several case studies of interventions in community settings in developing countries. At the conclusion of the next chapter we draw on the case material presented in both chapters to highlight some key principles for guiding a TD intervention.

Notes

1 This chapter was written by (B), the health psychologist, and (E), the PhD student.

2 A compliance score for each procedure was obtained by calculating the ratio of compliant behaviours to opportunities for compliance and expressing this as a percentage. Pre-education and posteducation compliance scores were calculated for each subject by averaging their scores in each period.

8
Transdisciplinary Research in the Community

NICK HIGGINBOTHAM, DENNIS WILLMS, AND NELSON K. SEWANKAMBO

8.1 Introduction

Health social scientists draw upon a spectrum of concepts, methods, and strategies to improve health. While some interventions focus on modifying individual or group behaviour within various settings, others seek to bring about structural change within community environments, including the health system itself. In chapter 7 we read how transdisciplinary insights informed a behaviour change program within a clinical setting. In this chapter we explore the philosophies and practical applications of interventions involving community mobilisation and participatory action research using a transdisciplinary perspective.

8.2 Community-based interventions

Winett et al. (1989, pp. 125–31) observe that community-based interventions usually have the ultimate aim of changing the health-related knowledge and behaviour of individuals. But they also target organisational change (for example, workplace practices), environmental change (for example, providing community facilities), and policy change (for example, laws or regulations). A major rationale for community-based interventions is the belief that reliance on individual approaches is unlikely to produce improvements in health status indicators nationally or even locally. This is because, as we have seen, health problems have multiple and complex causes. Winett et al. point out that these causes operate at the individual-psychological level, the interpersonal social level, and the community system level.

participation may simply involve the contribution of money or labour to a donor- or government-initiated project and there is little or no input by the community into planning the intervention. This kind of community participation usually fails to promote a sense of community ownership if the felt needs of the community have not been incorporated; community participation becomes equated with complying with the demands of the project managers. For example, it became clear during the 1970s that up to half of the improved water systems in developing countries had stopped working within 5 years (Elmendorf and Isely 1983, p. 195). A common finding was that villagers did not maintain the water systems even though it was within their capacity to do so. Rondinelli writes, 'The primary factor' in the breakdown or misuse of water supply systems in developing countries has been 'the lack of effective institutional arrangements for community management' (Rondinelli 1991, p. 417). Elmendorf and Isely further note:

> it's become overwhelmingly clear in fact, that the main obstacle to the use and maintenance of improved sanitation systems is not the quality of technology, but the failure in qualified human resources and management and organisation technique, including a failure to capture community interest (1983, p. 195).

These problems are also found in community-based health promotion campaigns in industrialised countries. After reviewing several community-based heart disease prevention programs in the USA, Winett et al. (1989, p. 125–42) concluded that community activation offers the greatest opportunity for successful long-term community participation. When project organisers actively involve community groups in both the design and implementation of the projects, it will:

> enhance program delivery and reach, improve the likelihood that individual and organisational behaviour change will be maintained, and encourage the ownership and eventual control of interventions by the community (Winett et al. 1989, p. 14).

The aim is to eventually have the sponsors and experts withdraw from positions of authority, while the community itself supports the program. This model is referred to as a 'collaborative intervention model', in contrast to a 'professional/technical' approach (Winett et al. 1989, pp. 49–50).

Collaborative models involve a change of emphasis from 'do-to' or 'do-for' strategies to 'do-with' interventions in which the project managers and the community cooperate to ensure the success of a jointly agreed-upon program (see Wass 1994, pp. 143–4). Participatory action is an example of do-with research in which the traditional power relationship between the researcher and the subject is reversed, or at least equalised.

8.3 Participatory action research

Participatory action research can take several forms. In its most democratic form, participatory action research is conducted solely by the participants. Kemmis and McTaggart defined this approach as

> collective self-reflective inquiry undertaken by participants in social situations in order to improve the rationality and justice of their own social and educational practices, as well as their understanding of these practices and the situations in which these practices are carried out (1988, p. 5).

Patricia Nickson (1993) described a participatory action intervention that took place in Boga, a rural health zone in Swahili-speaking northwestern Zaire, where she worked as a senior nurse in a church-sponsored hospital. The zone contained a seventy-five-bed hospital and seven health centres providing a full range of primary health care activities such as maternal and child health care, control of endemic diseases, health education, home visits, and basic curative care. However, traditional remedies including herbal therapies, spiritual healing, and the use of fetishes were also popular.

From 1982 a development project with committees in each village promoted the training of village health workers and traditional birth attendants. Originally voluntary, by 1983 the cost of the visiting health workers was being shared equally by the health zone, the local district Collectiv[1] and each respective village. This system resulted in an improvement in the use of basic health care services throughout the 1980s. By 1988, however, it was apparent to health workers and community leaders alike that the primary health care services were well used but the living conditions and general health of the population was not improving. Malnutrition and preventable diseases remained common.

A small study team formed to analyse this paradox. It consisted of two nurses, a community health worker, the Chief of the Collectiv of Boga, and a village leader. The health study team soon realised that the health services were based on external rather than local conceptions of health. In order to change this, the team held indepth discussions with local people (for example, women's church groups, village development committees, social gatherings) to learn their understanding and definition of family health.

Emerging from these discussions was the cultural notion of *obusinge*. Beyond its literal meaning of health, this concept was seen as the right of everyone to health, including harmony and an absence of misfortune in personal relationships. Each village in the district then formed a committee that considered its local version of *obusinge* and what goals and strategies they would adopt to improve people's living conditions. In one village, people constructed schoolrooms, then planted coffee which they could eventually sell to earn enough for a teacher's salary; village women could then have a basic education and their children would be less likely to suffer malnutrition. Knowing it would take several years for the coffee plants to yield a harvest, the committee approached the Collectiv for a loan to tide the village over. This prompted the Collectiv to establish a loan fund for the benefit of all villages. Another village decided that it was more important to devote energy and resources to constructing a road to make the villagers less isolated, even though health workers considered that clean water was the first priority (Nickson 1993).

Nickson points out that the expertise of health professionals who were part of the health study team formed a resource for local community initiatives, but the decision-making power belonged with the people and their traditional authority structures. In 1988, as the health study team was forming, the Chief of the Collectiv also created a tradition reform committee made up of elders who were charged with examining health traditions in the light of contemporary development issues. The Chief also convened weekly meetings of a Collectivé Action Group made up of community-elected village leaders as well as the leaders of development resource groups (such as the school headmaster and water engineer) to discuss community development. The meetings provided a forum for the discussion of problems, with the elected representatives expressing the concerns of their respective groups and relaying information back to them.

The consultative processes described above led to a sense of community ownership of decisions for improving the health of each community. The result was a strengthened commitment at village level to implementing decisions and community disapproval of those who would not cooperate (that is, self-regulation).

The Boga, Zaire, project exhibited several transdisciplinary principles. It opened lines of communication between stakeholders, which led to new understandings of health and the ways in which it could be improved. Conceptual frameworks were created which moved beyond scientific notions of health to include health-related local knowledge (for example, *obusinge*). These local conceptions became the source for action by community groups. Interventions, such as the one addressing child malnutrition, were not based on formal theoretical frameworks or strategies, but, nevertheless, clearly showed a commitment to address health issues at multiple levels as proposed by Winett et al. The Boga groups worked to improve the health of their people, not just in terms of individual bodies (for example, malnutrition), but also in terms of key community and institutional structures (for example, lack of education facilities and community organisation to finance projects).

Another form of participatory action research involves professional researchers working with community groups on the interests and issues of that group. This kind of research requires a 'profound respect' for participants' experience and a 'profound trust in their judgments about what is in their interests' (Wadsworth 1993, p. 2). Dennis Willms and Nelson Sewankambo provide an example of this approach, in which transdisciplinary teamwork led to a culturally appropriate HIV/AIDS intervention in a rural Ugandan community. In their case study, which is described below, the compelling nature of the problem itself determined how the study would unfold; an innovative intervention discourse evolved from insights gained during participatory action research. Epidemiological and anthropological understandings were integrated with Indigenous knowledge to develop a framework for interpreting risk. As in the Boga example, this new set of understandings then became the source for developing interventions to improve quality of life.

8.4 Dialogue between epidemiology, anthropology, and community voices: an HIV/AIDS intervention in Uganda

Medical anthropologist Dennis Willms and clinical epidemiologist Nelson Sewankambo formed a successful research collaboration transcending disciplinary boundaries. Together with people in a Ugandan rural community hard-hit by the AIDS epidemic, they developed a highly innovative approach to confront the devastating disease. The project began in 1992 in Rakai district, Uganda, in a town that had developed as a trading centre and truck stop along the infamous trans-African highway. The team chose this town because it was deemed a hotspot for commercial sex and the associated risk of HIV/AIDS.

They began work with an ethnographic phase that would allow later development of a culturally appropriate HIV/AIDS intervention. The collaboration necessitated a flexible and evolving research design, a process familiar to qualitative researchers. There was also careful consideration of the most appropriate ways of recovering various forms of evidence, both qualitative and quantitative. The participatory philosophy adopted for this project was such that even the word 'intervention', with its top-down, hierarchical connotations, was considered inappropriate so was replaced by the concept of 'enabling resources'. This decision followed the realisation that sustainable interventions require ongoing community participation, continuing dialogue and ownership, and a combining of all available resources. The following section describes the genesis of the project.

8.4.1 Epidemiological and anthropological perspectives

In Uganda, epidemiological research has established the prevalence of HIV and the profile of factors associated with the risks of this infection (see Ntozi et al. 1997), yet epidemiologists are confronted with the problem of how to fully understand and interpret the relationship between these factors. This problem prompted epidemiologist Nelson Sewankambo to query if there were other sets of evidences, besides that currently used by epidemiologists, that would help explain these risks and the determinants of these risk behaviours.

Experience working as a physician counselling clinic patients suffering from sexually transmitted diseases (including HIV/AIDS) also led Sewankambo to question the effectiveness of current programs which seemed to be working too slowly, if at all. It was his practice to talk through the clinical intervention differently, based on his reading of the kind of person he was counselling. In other words, he shaped the messages according to interpersonal evidence gathered in the clinical encounter. The question arising from these encounters was: Why did certain people, when they seemed to know the cause of HIV/AIDS, continue to place themselves at risk? Sewankambo felt that one way to find out was to look at how patients understood their risk of HIV. He hypothesised that if he learnt from such patients how they talk about their risk this would provide data that could be used to strengthen the effectiveness of clinical interventions. To assist him in getting this kind of information Sewankambo turned to the social sciences.

Anthropologists and others using ethnographic research are interested in the rates of morbidity and mortality generated by epidemiologists, but also address the sociocultural environments in which risk events occur. In addition to epidemiological understandings of risk, qualitative ethnographers seek to understand ways of knowing which may be different from quantitative scientists' explanations. For example, medical anthropologists have outlined a number of ways that people understand risk, including fatalistic, spiritual, and sociostructural (Davison et al. 1992). These understandings may overlap only partially, if at all, with epidemiological concepts of risk.

Pooling their combined knowledge, Willms and Sewankambo discussed how they might go about studying the individual experience of risk and collective representations of risk. It was decided that ethnographic methods would be particularly effective for shedding light on the contextual determinants of risk behaviours—allowing the researchers to talk to people about their illness, sickness, and disease experiences. Eliciting stories from people about these illnesses (illness narratives[2]) would uncover the meanings of risk, the risk situations that occur for them, and their risk reality (the environment or sociocultural background). By enquiring about risk in this way, the researchers hoped to map local understandings of risk onto epidemiological concepts and discover the impetus (whether conscious or unconscious, deliberate or coerced) for risk behaviours.

8.4.2 Study design

Willms and Sewankambo's study was prompted by the belief that most HIV/AIDS interventions in Africa do not produce sustainable behaviour change. They cite the following problems encountered in intervention designs:

- Community participants are usually not involved in designing health promotion interventions.
- When interventions are in place, evaluation designs are inadequate in determining whether behaviour change is the result of the intervention.
- Sexual health promotions have had difficulty overcoming the obstacle of effectively moving people from an awareness of the risks of HIV/AIDS to a state of mind where they feel vulnerable, and then to situations where they intentionally change their behaviour to eliminate the risk of HIV.
- Sociological and psychological studies, largely quantitative in design, aim to explain the knowledge, attitudes, and practices (KAP) of groups at risk for HIV/AIDS. While able to demonstrate the extent of high-risk sexual behaviours, KAP studies provide inadequate information about the range of local cultural practices and therefore do not provide sufficient evidence for developing culturally compelling HIV/AIDS interventions (see below).

Willms and Sewankambo decided to involve community participants in every stage of their study design, dissemination, and evaluation. Participatory action research methods were used to overcome the obstacles cited above and to identify Indigenous means for confronting these problems in cooperation with government and non-government agencies. The research integrated epidemiological, ethnographic, and Indigenous knowledge systems with the aim of understanding problems comprehensively. It was hoped that the knowledge generated would lead to interventions that are enabling resources for the communities concerned (that is, appreciated, compelling, and actually result in a demonstrated reduction in risk behaviours).

8.4.3 Methods

The initial ethnographic fieldwork took place in a trucking town located in southern Uganda's Rakai district over a 4-year period beginning in 1992. Epidemiological research in Rakai district has highlighted risk factors for HIV/AIDS and identified the groups which are most at risk. Results from longitudinal studies indicated that the infection rate is highest in trading centres along major trucking routes. In 1988 blood serum studies done in the study town revealed that 76 per cent of bar hostesses sampled were HIV positive (Carswell et al. 1989). Using this information the team decided to study long-distance truck drivers, bar hostesses who are commercial sex workers, and sexually transmitted disease patients.

Methods included indepth interviews (structured and semi-structured), informal focus groups (chance discussions or discussions with natural groups), and participant observation. Four Ugandan research assistants, living and working in the trucking town, began with an ethnographic investigation of the town itself including such factors as population, political economy, social organisation, and religious life. Over time, each research assistant moved from general descriptions of town life to specific details of the life of representative individuals of these risk groups (that is, truck drivers and bar hostesses). Each person was interviewed on a number of occasions. The evidence generated was non-numerical and experiential: life stories, illness narratives, and observation of critical events (for example, rituals observed at funerals of people who died of AIDS). Validity was obtained through saturation sampling (that is, interviewing to the point where the same understandings, metaphors, and expressions emerged over and over again (Willms and Johnson 1996)). The researchers felt that they had uncovered 'authentic representations of what is real, true and evident' in the lives of the sample group.

8.4.4 The interpretive framework

The team developed an interpretive framework based on emergent understandings of risk, risk profiles, risk situations, risk events, and risk realities. The framework was used to interpret data relating to three major risk groups—long-distance truckers, alcohol sellers/bargirls, and STD patients (see also Sewankambo, Spittal and Willms, in press).

8.4.4.1 Risk profiles

Case studies were written on individuals (for example, truck drivers, commercial sex workers) which communicated their HIV/AIDS understandings and experience. A risk profile is defined as a distillation of many life histories from people at risk who are situated in a particular risk reality.

8.4.4.2 Risk situations

Risk situations were defined as social events where a convergence of precipitating factors, sexual imperatives, and individual dilemmas compels the actors caught in these circumstances to participate in high-risk sexual activity. The examples in boxes 8.1 and 8.2 provide rich examples of risk situations described by Willms and Sewankambo (1994). The first shows how divorced women in the trucking town, who feel they have no choice but to support their families by selling alcohol from home, are placed at risk of HIV/AIDS by customers' demands for sex before they will pay for the alcohol. The second example describes how long-distance truck drivers incorporate multiple sexual partners into their occupational role, which accelerates the spread of HIV.

Box 8.1 Risk situation example 1: alcohol sellers and drinking places

It is not uncommon in these trucking centres for women, because of varying but similar circumstances, to find themselves living in town, literally besieged by hunger. This happens, in particular, during seasonal drought. Often in dire straits to feed families, they feel they have no choice but to enter into occupations that either directly or indirectly make them vulnerable to HIV infection.

Many young women explain that serial divorces, which characterise contemporary polygynous unions, with subsequent adoption of the children of the previous marriage by the new stepmother, lead to situations of neglect. This neglect will force a girl to leave home and seek asylum with relatives in town. As a consequence, early marriage is almost inevitable. Dire circumstances, including perceived lack of support, or not receiving essential items such as food, salt, soap, sauce, and lead these young women to enter into situations of serial monogamy (that is, married for some time to one man and then moving on to another). Sometimes, in a place where infection rates are high, a young girl may unknowingly, or even knowingly, be with a man who is already symptomatic.

The single-room mud-and-wattle row housing is typically where women concurrently raise their families and eke out a living. Alcohol selling, whether it be making and selling *omwenge* for the drinking hut or selling crude *waragi* illegally out of their home must, to be successful, be linked inevitably to sexual pressure. Men will actually threaten to sabotage a woman's endeavour by either refusing to drink or drinking on credit, then refusing to pay if she does not comply. Men from the community (for example, policemen, medical workers) and men passing through (for example, trailer and lorry drivers, army men) frequent these places. Often they come looking for women to sleep with. The woman propositioned may already have 'daily men' or even a 'permanent partner', so she will go to her other friends, typically alcohol sellers, to make the arrangement. Often women who sell alcohol out of their homes lament that they deplore it. It means having visitors who are often drunk, rude, even physically abusive in their homes, and if too drunk they will sleep there.

Complicating this risk scenario is the fact that mobile markets are lucrative places for women selling alcohol. A woman may have relationships with men in town, but the markets become a venue for increased support by men/traders (see box 8.2 below).

In terms of intervention, the challenge of this risk situation is twofold. First, the alcohol seller's risk environment mirrors that of the frequently targeted bargirl. That is, she too depends both on daily men and permanent partners to live and continue in business. The difference is in the number of children produced in these relationships; condom use is very questionable for the alcohol seller, unlike the bargirl who is able to negotiate condom use with daily men. For the permanent partner, who may have a wife and children at home, failure to use a condom is not associated with a desire to sire more children, but with trusting that the alcohol seller is being faithful in the union, faith to the man supposedly guaranteed by his continued support (Willms and Sewankambo 1994, pp. 9–10).

Box 8.2 Risk situation example 2: mobile traders, truckers, and makeshift markets

The stricture to provide for family (in AIDS-affected areas, this means harbouring the orphans of those lost to the disease), combined with the cash demands of a modern economy, means that many men must move for weeks or months at a time from village to urban centres to find work. Many men engage in trade-oriented activities that take them long distances and across borders; in country, they work in mobile markets buying, selling, and transporting their wares. These patterns of mobility, combined with beliefs surrounding the problem of abstinence, almost guarantee that these men are at extremely high risk for infection. *Magendo* (typical businessmen) have the money to buy sex in the market centres in rural areas or truckstops along the main transportation routes. With multiple partners the norm in this business, many traders become seduced by these men's *magendo* status, yet, recognising the nature of their sexual liaisons, become increasingly fatalistic.

The night before market days, which usually occur bi-monthly, rented lorries loaded with wares (cattle, drugs, cloth, dry goods) and traders, both men and women, arrive to set up makeshift shops in spaces guaranteed them by market associations. Typically, the same group will travel together for the duration of a particular market week. Many equate the environment in the markets to a wedding or a bachelor party. A temporarily constructed socioeconomic situation, the makeshift market assumes the atmosphere of an entertainment centre. On good market days, women traders, feeling the effects of alcohol will, in some cases, be willing to engage in sex for exchange. Willing or not, they find themselves increasingly intoxicated, while bargaining in kind to get on a lorry, or to buy a meal. Prolonged separation from home and the prevailing attitude that 'women are like buses, whoever has a ticket is free to board the bus up to his destination', only adds fuel to the fire. The situation is like that of the long-distance trailer driver who frequents trading centres. A man may find a woman for a small part of the day—in the bush or 'hotels' erected for this temporary arrangement—while at the same time be committed to a 'permanent partner' in the market (even sharing a tent) and wife/wives/children back home.

For the long-distance trader/trailer driver, the conditions of the road or a ban on night driving require that they put up for the night in the truckstop or trading centre. Bars, hotels, discos, and drinking huts cater to this kind of transient commercialism. A man will typically keep a woman (bargirl, alcohol seller, waitress) in each of the stops along the way. She may even be responsible for washing and pressing his clothes for the next time he passes through. Her situation and felt needs cause her to take on more than one safari man, resulting in complex interpersonal dynamics between the woman and the men in her life.

Condom use is not easily addressed in these relationships; to do so acknowledges that other sexual partners exist in the same vicinity or in places elsewhere. Yet in some instances, men eventually marry the women they meet along these routes. The geographical network of HIV transmission illuminated here is astounding, and the risk scenario makes it an important stage of intervention (Willms and Sewankambo 1994, pp. 12–14).

8.4.4.3 Risk events

The critical moment in a risk situation when individuals take a course of action or make a choice is termed a *risk event*. For example, the moment when a man makes sexual demands on a partner, insists on not wearing a condom, and the partner agrees.

8.4.4.4 Risk realities

A person's risk reality comprises the physical setting in which risk events occur, as well as the cultural trends and pressures that lead individuals to those settings. Risk reality also includes a phenomenological description of the context of risk. For example, the ethnographic descriptions revealed that, due to the ravages of the AIDS epidemic, people in the town believe that they are all walking dead. Identifying this ethos of hopelessness has profound implications for the kind of intervention possible in this area.

8.4.5 Tailoring culturally appropriate HIV/AIDS interventions

One of the strategies of the study was to open up a meeting place called 'Talking About AIDS: The Town Study Group'. Researchers joined with members of the community in talking about the disease and attended AIDS funerals almost daily. It became obvious that this kind of research strategy was in and of itself a kind of intervention, since the telling of stories and illness narratives is therapeutic, enabling community participants to clarify their relationships, their options, and their choices. The researchers hypothesised that talking with others helped participants 'transcend their life experiences' and critically evaluate and rationalise their present situation (see Spittal et al. 1997 for a full description of this process). A challenge facing the researchers was to evaluate qualitatively the extent to which the telling of stories (illness, disease, and sickness narratives) helped people come to terms with their life circumstances or prompted them to alter sexual practices that place them at risk of HIV transmission.

The relationships that developed between researchers and participants during the qualitative ethnographic phase laid the basis for the design of a participatory intervention. Identifying risk situations that became evident through case studies and drawing on their ethnography of risk in the trucking town fuelled attempts by the researchers to generate culturally compelling programs as enabling resources. These terms are explained below.

8.4.5.1 Culturally compelling programs

The terms 'culturally sensitive' and 'culturally appropriate' are often used to describe interventions that accommodate cultural context in their design and delivery (Higginbotham 1984). Yet, such interventions do not necessarily result in behaviour change. While community members receive program messages in the idiom of their cultural experience, they may *still* not feel vulnerable or at risk of illness.

Culturally compelling programs are co-developed in partnership with members of the community and are designed to enable people to alter not only their beliefs, but also their behaviours (in this case, the sexual behaviours which put them at risk). Researchers do not impose concepts that they bring into the community. Programs are developed with the community; knowledge is negotiated between the community and the researchers. The culture's own resources of metaphor, narrative, analogy, and vernacular expression are tapped. Community members can easily recognise and own the problem as one which affects them and which they can have a part in solving.

8.4.5.2 Enabling resources

Enabling resources are resources that help individuals to make healthy lifestyle choices. Resources may be both within themselves (for example, fortitude, values, will, intention), or outside of themselves (for example, models, health care services, medicines). In cooperation with community members, the challenge is to construct possibilities for accessing both kinds of resources.

In the Rakai trucking town project, the team is developing, in partnership with influential community members, culturally appropriate enabling resources that are tailored to persons constrained by risk. Such enabling resources contain the following ingredients:

- participating in a problem-solving exercise that addresses the issue of income generation (for example, alternative occupations for alcohol sellers)
- helping people think through how they might reason, evaluate, and make informed lifestyle decisions—an exercise in moral reasoning that affects them as sexual partners, spouses, and parents
- modelling the process of communicating risk (safe sex) to children
- lobbying relevant funding agencies for external resources for other felt needs (for example, clinical facilities for women and children, specific mobile facilities for targeted risk groups, income-generating credit facilities for women, etc.).

8.4.6 Barriers and constraints to community change

The ethnographic study highlighted a number of barriers and constraints that needed to be addressed in order to develop culturally appropriate interventions.

First, the ethos of the citizens is one of hopelessness and despair. The difficulty is in devising ways of enabling people to take deliberate health-promoting steps when everyone thinks they are dying. The prevailing environment of AIDS-related suffering and desperation requires a rethink of the usual assumptions underlying intervention design.

Second, the study revealed that multiple intervention strategies are required, some of which will address the problems of the AIDS epidemic in an indirect way. Willms and Sewankambo began with the notion that it was best to develop a primary prevention model for HIV/AIDS. Experience with the community revealed that a combination of intervention strategies was more appropriate. Essential components included clinical care, especially for women and children, HIV testing facilities complemented with counselling, and income-generating projects for risk groups such as women in single-parent families who currently need to survive by selling alcohol (and providing sex) to truck drivers. The challenge was to decide how these interventions could be accomplished in a manner that is efficient and accountable and involves the different groups concerned.

In summary, this transdisciplinary study highlights a reflexive approach to an intervention that developed over several years, taking into account emergent understandings from collaborations with community participants. Original objectives were reconsidered during the course of the study. One of the original objectives was to develop a counselling program targeted at bar hostesses and STD patients attending the health centre in the Rakai trucking town. However, the researchers came to believe that this particular intervention, although worthwhile, was based on their initial assessment of the problem. Early findings during the study showed that the proposed intervention did not seem to address the complex situational requirements and actual *needs* of people at risk of HIV in Rakai. The team decided that while counselling is required, this kind of intervention demonstrates only a narrow interpretation of program requirements. Willms and Sewankambo argue that a more comprehensive approach, which represented both a long-term and a practical response to needs, was required.

8.4.7 A participatory workshop with traditional healers in Zimbabwe

Before teasing out several complexity theory implications of the study described above, it is useful to briefly describe a comparable HIV/AIDS prevention project in Zimbabwe. In this second study, Willms and his colleagues applied similar principles to design an education workshop for African healers to help stem the risk of HIV transmission in their *matare*, or traditional surgery (Willms et al. 1996). Zimbabwean healers are traditionally consulted about social, psychological, spiritual, and physical complaints and they play a major role in the counselling and support of the large number of AIDS sufferers. However, their traditional methods of intervention—such as scarifying with knives, biting out diseases, or manually cleaning out the uterus after delivery, all involve contact with bodily fluids and carry potential risks both for the healers themselves and for their clients. Healers also include circumcision, ear piercing, and midwifery in their range of services, activities that involve exposure to unsterilised instruments and bodily fluids. Instructing traditional healers on the dangers of these practices—from a Western medical point of view—had proven ineffective, if not alienating, in previous education campaigns. The healers felt their ancestors would protect them from AIDS and took no steps to minimise transmission of the virus.

The HIV/AIDS education workshop, which drew on the results of 2 years fieldwork (1992–94) employing participant observation, indepth interviewing, and focus groups, set out to treat the healers as autonomous professionals and develop a partnership for negotiating a merged understanding of the health problem (Willms et al., in press). In the 3-day workshop traditional materials (medicine containers, bones, scarification knives), oral and performance skills, invocation of the spirits, and a structure akin to the traditional healing process were used to maximise the healers' participation. In this way, the healers came to identify and own the problem of HIV/AIDS infection. Having expressed it in language that drew on their previous conceptions of disease augmented with new understandings, they began to develop strategies for preventing the spread of infection. Willms and colleagues found the participatory workshops highly successful in reorienting the healers who attended, within their own framework of knowledge about the AIDS epidemic. They observed that these changes found expression in the participants' conversations with local chiefs and healer colleagues when they returned home.

8.5 AIDS prevention and complexity theory

Complexity theory can deepen our understanding of the system-wide changes required to prevent the spread of the HIV virus as found in the Uganda and Zimbabwe case studies. Miller et al.'s complexity theory framework (1998) explains successful interventions according to three key processes: *joining, learning,* and *transforming*. We saw in chapter 7 that the clinic-based Care Aware project successfully applied learning and joining strategies. This also occurred in the Uganda community-based intervention. The strategy of opening up a community meeting place called Talking About AIDS promoted the process of learning; it enabled residents of the trucking town to clarify their relationships, their options, and their choices. In other words, they were helped to understand how their internal models of sexuality may be limiting the way they evaluated and reacted to their present situation amid the AIDS epidemic. This action was successful because it resulted in some people altering sexual practices placing them at risk of HIV/AIDS.

Willms and his colleagues' HIV/AIDS prevention workshops with the traditional healers in Zimbabwe moved from a learning mode to a joining mode of intervention. Joining works by enhancing existing attractors and is successful only when the methods are consistent with the internal models of the individual or the institution. In the education workshops, new understandings of HIV/AIDS were created among the participants in a way that reinforced the traditional healers' professional pride and standing. The workshops also reinforced the healers' attraction to preexisting values and methods by using traditional materials, oral and performance skills, invocation of the spirits, and a structure akin to the traditional healing process. The joining process was successful because, while HIV/AIDS was presented as a new disease which needed new strategies, these strategies could be understood and carried out within the healers' own framework of knowledge.

In complexity theory terms, learning and joining strategies take advantage of existing attractors (for example, preexisting values) to direct the action of a dynamic system. However, there may be circumstances in which the key attractors shaping the problem need changing or need to be replaced by new attractors. For example, while the residents of Rakai district who currently do not have AIDS may be drawn to the attractor of HIV/AIDS risk prevention, those who already have the disease or feel themselves unable to escape exposure, may feel compelled to follow whatever action can fulfil their basic survival needs. For this latter group, such as the woman selling liquor to feed herself and her children, safe sex is not an option. Change in this situation is more likely through the dramatic process of transforming; an intervention that aims to either change or establish new attractors.

Transforming is a drastic way of provoking change by deliberately creating a disturbance in a system (through 'hammering' or 'wedging'), or by the non-intentional experience of a shock to the system (Miller et al. 1998, p. 374). Transforming via wedging is done by gradually intensifying perceptions of a discrepancy (between how things are and how they should be) in a manner that pushes a system towards the edge of chaos (Miller et al. 1998, p. 374). The edge of chaos is where complex adaptive systems are most creative and new or hidden attractors can emerge. Lewin (1993, p. 20) described this process as 'the pattern of innovation at the point of change'. While wedging precipitates internal transformation, hammering is intentional coercion from an outside agent to change attractors. An example of hammering would be the government health ministry imposing new clinical practice guidelines for management of a diarrhoeal disease in children.

8.5.1 Transforming a system at the edge of chaos

The HIV/AIDS epidemic in Africa has created a disturbance in the existing pattern of beliefs and behaviours in society. This is akin to a perturbation in a complex adaptive system and, as shown in Kenya and Zimbabwe, has led to new patterns of knowledge and behaviour in response to HIV/AIDS. The trucking town residents felt that the epidemic was an inescapable fate; the healers felt that it was a new disease that had nothing to do with traditional healing practices. The aim of a transforming intervention (a kind of counterperturbation) would be to create a set of attractors in competition with those that gave rise to the epidemic (low status of women, unprotected sex with multiple partners) as well as its consequences (for example, pervasive hopelessness and a sense of being the living dead).

A complexity perspective suggests that African societies adversely affected by the epidemic are poised at the edge of chaos.[3] Systems on the edge of chaos display several properties:

> Perturb such a system, and you might get some small response. Perturb it again, with the same degree of disturbance, and the thing might collapse completely. Perturb it many times while poised at a critical state, and you'll get a range of responses which can be described by a power law; that is, big responses are rare, small responses are common, and intermediate responses fall in between (Bak, cited in Lewin 1993, p. 61).

Guastello (1995, p. 52) notes that a system on the edge of chaos cannot be altered by 'natural selection, or an organisational or political policy operating on only one feature of the system'. Systems on the edge of chaos are able to 'slip in and out of a chaotic regime through self-organisation' (Guastello 1995, p. 52). Attempts to change one feature only will cause the system to 'mutate and evolve to compensate for the environmental insult' (Guastello 1995, p. 52). Guastello claims that the 'secret of real system change' is to 'locate the dynamical key that supports and unravels the entire system'. If the stable elements of the system are 'scrambled' the system will then reconstruct itself around a 'new dynamical key' if those elements are allowed to 're-organise in a new fashion' (Guastello 1995, p. 52). The process of self-organisation is the complexity principle whereby a system in a state of chaos 'reorganises its elements to produce a more stable structure and a less *resource* costly existence' (Guastello 1995, pp. 57–8). This is the challenge for people trying to alter the HIV/AIDS epidemic in Africa and elsewhere.

8.5.2 Highway truckstop as a dissipative structure

Another use of complexity theory to understand the dynamics of the AIDS epidemic in Africa is represented in figure 8.1. Here we conceptualise the Trans-African truckstop town (for example, in the Rakai district) as a *dissipative structure* interacting with the wider environment. Changes taking place in the external environment have generated a dramatic influx of energy into a previously quiet rural village along the Trans-African Highway. This increase in energy originates from the globalised economic imperatives that have prompted the steady army of truck drivers and traders to move their goods up and down the continent. Male drivers seek out the truckstop as a place to satisfy their commercial as well as social (entertainment, companionship, networking) and biological (food, drink, sexual) needs. Women from outlying rural areas are drawn to service the drivers' and traders' needs as a means of making their own living and obtaining the resources to look after their children and families. The vulnerable economic and social position of divorced women and those living without the support of their kin groups is a motivating force for their joining this setting. The mixing of outsiders and locals generates a culture of consumption dominated by the gratification of needs. Unfortunately, unprotected sex with multiple partners is a feature of the truckstop culture and an ideal opportunity for transmitting HIV.

A byproduct of the culture of consumption is the culture of despair. The cause is a feeling of being unable to evade the prevailing cycle of exploitation, disease, and death. The women selling alcohol to truck drivers feel they have no choice but to have unsafe sex. Unsafe sex has resulted in an epidemic of HIV/AIDS. The

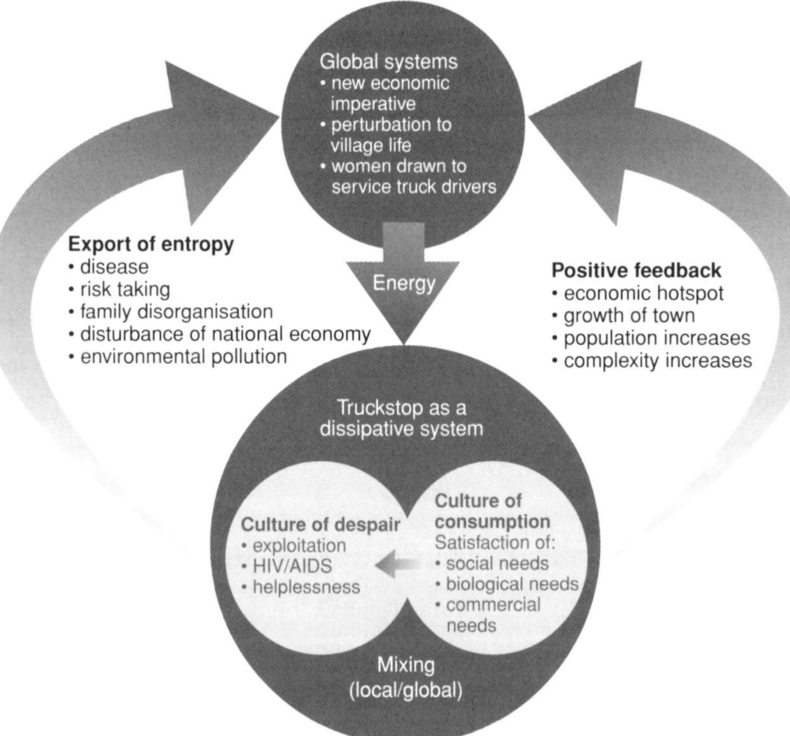

Figure 8.1 Truckstop as a dissipative system

pervasive deaths from AIDS began in the mid 1980s; the sense of inevitable doom among those left behind further engenders a perspective of helplessness and loss.

The truckstop as a dissipative structure generates growth that has both constructive and destructive consequences. On the one hand, greater complexity and order is generated in the form of more business opportunities, increased population, thriving commercial development, improved town infrastructure, and a boost to the regional economy. On the other hand, the dissipative structure feeds back into the external environment greater infection of the HIV virus among the most economically productive age group in the society. In addition, at the local level, negative impacts include destroyed families, older children required to serve as parents for younger children, an unstable workforce, greater hardship and poverty, and pollution of the environment. If this feedback continues, it will ultimately destroy the dissipative structure because the wider environment (for example, national economy), which cannot continue to absorb such entropic waste, will collapse.

Our analysis of the truckstop as a dissipative structure draws attention to the profound economic impact that follows the rapid expansion of HIV-infected people within the wider African environment. The globalisation process that has promoted economic development in Africa (such as truckstop towns) may disconnect from the continent. Capital inflows could decline dramatically because of rising costs of health care insurance, loss of employees to HIV/AIDS, and the continuing need to recruit and train new workers (Brown and Halweil 1999). Local businesses of all descriptions will find it hard to survive.

The magnitude of the HIV/AIDS perturbation in Africa requires an equally powerful transformation of existing attractors that enable the virus to flourish. Given that economic globalisation and its local effects are the most influential attractors in the system (and indirectly underlie the spread of HIV), then strategies to stop the virus must be connected to all efforts towards economic development and every form of commercial transaction. For example, all aid efforts, regardless of sector, should integrate HIV/AIDS prevention action. Grants, loans, and other forms of assistance from aid agencies (bilateral, multilateral, NGOs), as well as investment from national governments themselves, could be tied to efforts by the recipient group to prevent the spread of HIV.

Companies and corporations could gain tax concessions and priority for tenders by safe sex promotion among their workforce. Rural areas could gain priority in infrastructure projects (roads, reforestation, water projects) by putting in place active AIDS campaigns. The aim would be to saturate the message of safe sex and institutionalise safe practices throughout society by integrating it into all facets and levels of the country's economic life. Without such dramatic measures, the future of that economic life itself is in doubt.

8.6 Guidelines for transdisciplinary interventions

Insights gained from the clinical and community intervention studies outlined in this and the previous chapter (that is, the Care Aware, Boga, Uganda, and Zimbabwe case studies) allow us to offer guidelines for transdisciplinary interventions:

1 Try to consider all the elements of influence having an impact on the health problem.
   - Pursue leverage on the problem at all levels of analysis that are both strategic and practical (that is, multilevel interventions from micro to macro perspectives, and incorporating both structuralist and interpretivist viewpoints).
   - Allow the problem itself to drive the formation of a transdisciplinary team.

2 Compose preliminary research questions based on the initial interpretation of the problem but remain open to change. Be prepared for objectives to change in the light of knowledge gained during the study.
   - Willms and Sewankambo's early ethnographic data suggested that their initial plan to set up an AIDS counselling service in Uganda was woefully inadequate.
   - The objectives of village development committees in Boga were formulated after an initial process of defining health.

3 Consider all the options for obtaining the information (evidence) needed to initiate the intervention (for example, qualitative, quantitative, researcher-driven, participatory action).

4 Try to break down barriers relating to knowledge.
   - Willms and Sewankambo incorporated insights from anthropology, epidemiology, and Indigenous knowledge systems.
   - The Care Aware team combined theoretical insights on infection control from clinicians and psychologists with the experiential knowledge of health workers.
   - Indigenous knowledge systems of the Boga villagers were combined with the knowledge and expertise of outside resource groups including health workers, veterinary assistants, water engineers, and agriculturalists to implement interventions.

5 Move beyond disciplinary-bound concepts and assumptions towards a common conceptual framework.
   - Willms and Sewankambo drew on anthropological, epidemiological, and lay knowledge to arrive at the concepts of culturally compelling programs and enabling resources.
   - The Care Aware team used the common conceptual framework of mindlessness to address workplace injuries transcending the boundaries of biomedicine, health psychology, immunology, and infection control.

6 Allow emergent understandings to guide the intervention.
   - The framework of risk based on ethnographic fieldwork fuelled the Ugandan intervention.
   - Emergent understandings of the importance of mindlessness enabled the Care Aware team to use social marketing as the intervention method.
   - In Boga, local cultural beliefs about the complex nature of health (*obusinge*), involving harmony in personal ties, led to innovative interventions to improve health through economic and social change.

7 Seek to break down barriers between the formal research stage and the intervention stage.
   - In the Ugandan study, informal consultation with community members to learn about their experiences of HIV/AIDS later became a recognised part of the intervention strategy—Talking About AIDS.
   - In Boga, interventions were incorporated into the everyday social and political life of village communities.

8 Rethink the orthodox wisdom about how to design interventions, even to the point of using a different term.
   - The need to develop diverse and indirect multilevel solutions to the complex health problems faced by the Ugandans led Willms and Sewankambo to coin the term 'enabling resources'. This distinguished their collaborative participatory action model from top-down hierarchical programs.
   - The Zimbabwean healers' workshop created a mixture of traditional and Western methods to draw on participants' own knowledge, values, and spiritual beliefs rather than attempt to educate healers using alien notions of infection control.
   - Preliminary research in the Care Aware program led the team to rethink the orthodox belief that needlestick injuries were caused by workers' failure to comply with infection-control guidelines. Subsequently, a unique academic detailing intervention was crafted, drawing upon expertise from the field of commercial marketing.
   - Participatory action research in Boga, Zaire, led to innovative structural level interventions such as building schools to educate mothers and planting crops to pay for these facilities in order to improve child survival.

9 Break down the barriers between researcher and program participants by developing new lines of communication and collaboration.
   - The participatory action research strategy in Uganda established personal ties between subjects and researchers which empowered both to consider innovative strategies for collaboration.
   - The Zimbabwean healers were treated as equal partners in the HIV/AIDS workshop process; their models of understanding disease transmission were drawn upon to find solutions.

- In Boga, lines of communication were kept open between village development committees, health workers, and resource groups through addressing the felt needs of the study group members as well as the basic needs. To remain viable over the long term, the group needed to reconcile the competing priorities of professional and lay participants.
- The Care Aware program originated from concerns of hospital staff about the lack of communication with the health department hierarchy over infection-control measures. The study promoted cooperation between the research team and hospital workers to communicate workers' concerns about appropriate ways of dealing with infection-control procedures and infected staff to hospital authorities.

10 Identify the barriers and constraints that need to be overcome before interventions can be implemented.

- Willms and Sewankambo's insight that those at risk of HIV thought they were already dead led to a rethinking of traditional assumptions about what motivates people to change behaviour.
- The Zimbabwean traditional healers' understanding that AIDS was due either to immorality or to outside influences meant that the dangers of some practices were not appreciated.
- The Care Aware team identified institutional barriers preventing effective implementation of infection control education programs (for example, breakdowns in communication between staff and hospital authorities, economic constraints, orthodox beliefs about the causes of injuries).
- Economic constraints and problems accessing technical resources were identified as constraints in achieving improved health status in Boga.

11 Recognise that the benefits of interventions are not always quantifiable; acceptance of this possibility may alter the type of intervention chosen.

- In Boga, Nickson found that the process of empowerment was more important to the health of the community than objective measurement of results.
- The Uganda study team knew intuitively that the telling of stories was therapeutic. It may not be possible to evaluate rigorously the results of this strategy. The inability to quantify or even qualitatively assess beneficial events does not mean that such effects do not exist.
- Qualitative interviews with health workers about the importance of discussing workplace safety issues resulted in the Care Aware team recommending that several small group discussions should be incorporated into future trials of the program.

12 Identify opportunities where carefully introduced disturbances (perturbations) to the existing situation can allow self- or community-generated change to take place towards a new safer or healthier state through incorporating new

knowledge, practices, and modifications to the environment. In complexity terms, this is the strategy of transforming an adaptive system by changing attractors or creating new ones.

8.7 Conclusion

This chapter reviewed several instances where community-based interventions and participatory action methods were used to involve people in changing aspects of their lives which impact on their own health. We do not suggest that these are the only useful forms of research. As outlined in chapter 2, some disciplines and interdisciplinary fields of knowledge have developed sophisticated causal models or understandings of symbolic systems that are powerful research tools. However, TD thinking encourages us to see many contemporary diseases as embedded in multilayered webs of causality operating on different levels. For such problems, community action research may prove to be especially appropriate because the transdisciplinary teamwork accesses people's own conceptual framework and social structures as well as the material and biological context of the disease. Changes in the comprehension of the problem, phrased in language which makes it accessible to the participants, is most likely to lead to the ownership and implementation of changes, and to create synergistic effects in the social and biological structures which are necessary to improve people's health. Like the perturbation which sends waves of change through an unstable open system, a disturbance in conceptual structures about health and illness can lead to ongoing and self-organising changes. These are changes that can spread and hopefully enhance people's social worlds.

Notes

1 A collectiv is the lowest level of civic administration and is led by a chief who governs a population of approximately 10 000 (Nickson 1993, p. 44).

2 Personal illness narratives and life histories are discussed in greater detail in chapter 12.

3 Per Bak notes that the principle of 'self-organised criticality' (the principle that dynamical systems evolve towards a critical state) is the same kind of phenomenon as edge of chaos (cited in Lewin 1993, p. 60).

Part III

Transdisciplinary Methods in Health Social Science Research

Preamble

Organisation of Part III

Part III offers a framework that TD researchers can apply to select study designs and methods as they work their way through a health problem. Using this framework, the introduction and four chapters in part III show how various tools of quantitative and qualitative enquiry can be appropriately combined to gain a health research perspective across three levels of TD enquiry (problem description, identifying the elements of influence, and clarifying causal links in a dynamic system).

Chapters 9 and 10 describe some fundamental designs and methods of epidemiological and qualitative approaches respectively, and discuss their relevance for TD research, while chapters 11 and 12 suggest possibilities for hybrid research designs applied to cross-sectional surveys and case-control studies. These hybrid designs incorporate the strengths of both qualitative and quantitative methods and approaches.

The final section in chapter 12 explains how the case study method can draw together diverse knowledge from many sources to communicate and connect sufferers' and TD researchers' emergent insights about the dynamic nature of a health problem.

The conclusion discusses the health problems that could dominate the twenty-first century and the ways a transdisciplinary health social science is prepared to meet those challenges.

Levels of enquiry in transdisciplinary research

The four chapters in part III explore methods for performing transdisciplinary health social science research. To gain a TD health research perspective, investigators need to combine quantitative and qualitative research techniques. For this purpose we offer a general framework that TD researchers can apply to generate knowledge about a health problem. It shows how to select research designs and techniques that are appropriate for the level or stage of understanding that researchers have achieved about the focal problem. The framework makes two assumptions about the nature of TD research. First, researchers require different kinds of knowledge as they move from initial and partial comprehension of the problem towards analyses of its multiple determinants, culminating in a more comprehensive TD understanding. Second, at each level in the TD research process, the key questions can be answered by a combination of qualitative and quantitative ways of knowing.

For practical purposes, we can identify three levels or stages of comprehension that TD researchers move through in the course of their work. *Level I* research involves gathering basic descriptive information about the issue from different disciplinary and interdisciplinary fields of knowledge. Key questions include: Who says the problem exists? How is it defined? What is the nature of a case according to different observers? How many people, groups, or communities are affected and who are they? How severe or disabling is the problem? How many new cases occur over time? For whom is the problem a priority? How many economic and social resources are devoted to the issue? In other words, Level I requires description of the shape of the problem from all relevant sources. The early information identifying the presence of a heart disease epidemic in the Coalfields of Australia (chapter 5) is an example of Level I enquiry.

Level II research moves beyond a description of the problem to identification of all potential elements of influence or causal factors that operate in the problem context. Relevant disciplines contribute knowledge about potential problem determinants. The key questions at this stage include: What characteristics of person, place, and time are associated with onset of or changes in the problem? That is, what variables, operating at different levels of the health hierarchy, are linked in some way to expressions of the problem according to evidence of TD researchers? Willms and Sewankambo's identification of risk situations and risk realities experienced by Ugandans caught up in the HIV/AIDS epidemic (chapter 8) suggests Level II knowledge of socially situated causes of the disease.

Level III TD research takes the elements of influence and critically evaluates their role in the emerging causal web. Intersections and interactions are explored among the causal factors operating at different levels and across time. The researchers look for patterns that occur in the problem context viewed as a dynamic, open system. Matrices and flow diagrams are often used to portray the workings of the system (figure 5.1). The main questions are: How do the variables combine and interact to determine the characteristics of the problem? Is there an underlying principle or common conceptual framework suggested by the comprehensive analysis of the problem? Where can the system be entered with alternative elements of influence to bring about desired changes? An example of Level III research is Treloar's TD Care Aware intervention, promoting hospital infection control, which conceptualised workplace injuries as arising from a pattern of mindlessness set up by hospital routines (chapter 6).

Selection of study designs and methods for a transdisciplinary investigation

The second dimension of the TD research framework is the construction of study designs—quantitative and qualitative—that will answer the key questions addressed at each level of the TD research process. Choice of research methods always follows a statement of the research question under consideration or, more generally, reference to the types of information that are most needed and most useful in a given situation (Patton 1990, p. 196). As TD researchers move from Level I through to Level III research, they draw upon two equally valued traditions for investigating the problem:

1 quantitative designs and techniques
2 qualitative enquiry along a spectrum of less structured to more structured approaches.

TD thinking requires investigators to move between quantitative and qualitative ways of knowing at each stage. Consequently, a number of new hybrid designs, purposefully combining elements of both traditions, have been developed by TD researchers. Hybrid designs in TD investigations characteristically employ the rigour of experiments and quasi-experiments, such as set rules for subject selection (for example, randomisation) and control of exposure or treatment, with the concern for contextual factors that emerges from qualitative techniques. A good example is the qualitative case-control design described in chapter 12.[1]

Table PIII.1 presents a TD research methods framework, suggesting designs and techniques that can be applied at each level of enquiry. Level I problem descriptions are often drawn from cross-sectional surveys which are strengthened by adding insights from use of qualitative techniques such as epidemiological case reports, focus group discussions, free-listing tasks defining domains of cultural knowledge, and open-ended interviews. Cognitive laboratory techniques, such as the think-aloud protocol, are a hybrid method for improving survey questions (see chapter 12). Similarly, case-control or cohort studies, the quasi-experimental methods for identifying elements of influence at Level II, can be improved through combination with methods such as direct observation of the problem context, life histories, and long interviews with selected patients or other individuals. Hybrid designs at this level include qualitative case-control and contrasting groups techniques as well as epidemiological case series. At Level III causal links can be analysed by combining the strongest causal evidence from the quantitative tradition (randomised controlled clinical or field trials) with the insights about the workings of the problem context as a whole, arising from indepth ethnographic designs using participant observation and case studies. Level III hybrid designs include ethnographic studies of treatment decision-making (Young 1981), qualitative evaluation of health interventions (for example, Greene 2000; Patton 1987), and case studies which have combined both qualitative and quantitative methods.

Table PIII.1 Levels of enquiry in transdisciplinary research and corresponding designs and methods*

	Level I: Problem description	*Level II: Identify elements of influence*	*Level III: Clarify causal links*
Quantitative	• cross-sectional surveys	• case control design • cohort studies • ecological designs	• randomised controlled trials • clinical and field trials • community intervention
Hybrid designs	• case series • cognitive laboratory techniques	• qualitative case control • contrasting groups	• case studies • ethnographic treatment decision models • qualitative program evaluation
Qualitative	• epidemiological case reports • open-ended interviews • free listing • focus group discussions	• semistructured interviews • direct observation • life histories	• ethnography using participant observation and prolonged engagement in the field • illness narratives

* There are other types of designs and methods—we have confined this typology to types of enquiry discussed in part III of this book.

TD investigators developing hybrid designs to study a health problem are guided by principles of *triangulation* and other strategies to ensure trustworthiness of data and interpretations. Chapter 10 introduces a range of strategies within the social sciences for enhancing validity of knowledge as well as linking research styles and methods across different disciplines. Hence, familiarity with the procedures that enhance the quality of information and interpretations is highly useful for TD researchers wishing to systematically capitalise on the strengths of multiple perspectives of the problem, multiple sources and methods of providing information, and a collaborative team of investigators.

Note

1 Patton (1990, chapter 5) refers to such hybrid designs as a type of mixed form design, using experimental framework, qualitative data, and content analysis.

9
How to Perform Transdisciplinary Research: Epidemiological Study Designs

JULIE BYLES, NICK HIGGINBOTHAM, AND RICHARD HELLER

9.1 Overview of epidemiological studies and levels of enquiry

Transdisciplinary health social science research draws upon quantitative and qualitative ways of knowing in order to explain and resolve health problems. Chapter 9 outlines the contribution of epidemiological methods to TD research.[1] Epidemiology is grounded within a philosophy of science that values highly systematic rules for generating and verifying evidence about phenomena and causality (Rothman 1998). We accept these values in our demonstration of the importance of epidemiological designs for TD health research, but it is necessary to acknowledge that this perspective offers a partial understanding of the complexity of health and illness. It generates necessary but not sufficient knowledge that must be juxtaposed and synthesised with other partial understandings in order to more fully comprehend this complexity.

Epidemiology is 'the study of the distribution and determinates of health related states or events in specified populations and the application of this study to control health problems' (Last 1995). The results of epidemiological investigation are useful to understand the natural history of diseases and opportunities for prevention or therapy, to estimate the demand for health services, and to evaluate the effectiveness of preventive measures and treatments. The principal function of epidemiology though is to understand the causes of disease (Kelsey et al. 1986, p. 3). In this regard, it shares with other quantitative sciences a concern to establish causal pathways that are as certain as possible.

Knowledge of the causes of disease can lead to the development of strategies to prevent disease. Cancer, for instance, is one of the most common causes of death in the developed world and is becoming more common in countries undergoing demographic transition.[2] In 1964, the World Health Organization estimated that most cancers (now estimated at approximately 90 per cent) were due to behavioural or environmental risk factors and were potentially preventable (Doll and Peto 1981). Tobacco smoking, for example, accounts for 30 per cent of cancers; this knowledge has spurred the development of methods to prevent uptake and encourage cessation of smoking (Newcombe and Carbonne 1992). Other potentially avoidable behaviours associated with cancer include solar radiation and excessive use of alcohol. Of course the complexities of the determinants of exposure to these factors are less well understood. As we noted in chapter 2, health status emerges from interactions within and between the many levels of the health hierarchy, involving body, behavioural, social, biological, ecological, and physical systems.

How was the causal pathway between a human behaviour such as smoking and an outcome such as cancer identified? These causal pathways are never completely certain. Smoking does not always result in lung cancer and people who develop lung cancer are not exclusively smokers. The clue to the causal link is the scientific observation that the probability (or risk) of developing lung cancer is higher if you smoke than if you do not (around twenty times higher in fact). The epidemiological term for the relationship between two outcome probabilities is *relative risk*: relative risk represents the risk in the exposed divided by the risk in the unexposed. A relative risk greater than 1.0 indicates an increased risk or probability of disease in the exposed population.

A key idea underlying this probabilistic approach to studying cause and effect is the *null hypothesis*. The null hypothesis is a statement of belief to which data can be applied in order to test that belief. If the data show the statement is not true then the hypothesis is rejected. In the smoking and lung cancer example, the simple hypothesis might be:

There is no difference between the risk of lung cancer for smokers and non-smokers.

Data showing that there is a twenty times higher risk among smokers of developing lung cancer than the risk among non-smokers disprove this hypothesis.

From an epidemiological perspective, the best source for such data would be a randomised controlled trial (RCT), where all variables are theoretically equal except for the study factor (smoking) and the outcome factor (cancer). However, humans are not passive laboratory subjects to be subjected to scientific manipulation. The ethics of research into human health and disease place appropriate restrictions on what can be done. Nevertheless, questions concerning human health can ultimately only be answered by research involving human beings, research which may require non-experimental and naturalistic methods of enquiry as well as RCTs (see chapter 10).

lung cancer, are increasing dramatically in the Asia–Pacific region and elsewhere and will dominate as the major causes of the burden of disease in the not too distant future (Murray and Lopez 1996; Higginbotham 1999).

9.2.1 Case reports, case series, and case studies

The simplest observational study is the case report. A case report describes a single unusual case that stands out from what is commonly observed to be true. Unlike most epidemiological study designs, the case report and case series are essentially qualitative methods—their value is dependent on the rich description of a problem in the fullest possible clinical context.

A case series describes a number of cases of the same or related unusual observations. The series stands out against what is commonly understood to be normal for that particular population. Case reports and case series are important means by which unusual diseases or unusual patient symptoms are brought to the attention of the medical community. These studies may be our only means of surveillance for rare clinical events, may make us aware of unusual manifestations of a disease, may serve as a trigger for larger and more decisive studies examining the relationship between certain exposures and subsequent disease, or can describe the mechanism of a disease process by reporting the results of highly detailed clinical and laboratory studies in a small number of patients (Henekens and Buring 1987, pp. 106–8). In terms of sampling strategy, case reports and case series are non-probability samples (see 10.3 for further discussion).

Box 9.1 Case-series points to cause of railway deaths

Of 224 railroad-related deaths occurring in North Carolina from 1990–94, 128 cases (57 percent) involved trespassers. Trespasser fatalities typically involved unmarried male pedestrians 20 to 49 years of age with less than a high school education. Eighty-two percent of incidents occurred in the trespassers' county of residence, indicating that few deaths involved transients. Seventy-eight percent of trespassers were killed while intoxicated (median alcohol level, 56 mmol/L [260 mg/dL]) (quoted from Pelletier 1997, pp. 1064–6).

Although neither case reports nor case series can be used to test hypotheses, both can be important sources of information and may provide the first clues in the identification of a new disease or the side effects of a new drug. For example, the initial 'discovery' of AIDS, the effects of the drug Thalidomide, and the realisation that drinking alcohol during pregnancy can have a harmful effect on a foetus's development (for example, foetal alcohol syndrome) were all based on either case reports or a small case series.

A major limitation of case reports and case series is the lack of an explicit control or comparison group to allow possible associations to be tested and quantified. In the railway example above (box 9.1) it seems reasonable to assume that the likelihood of being drunk is higher among the rail accident victims described than among the general population, but is their prevalence of intoxication higher than might be expected among unmarried males in this age group? While epidemiologists use case reports to draw attention to unusual health conditions, the case study design is applied for natural enquiry to explore relationships between variables (that is, Level III analysis) as described in chapter 12.

9.2.2 Cross-sectional surveys

In epidemiological research, cross-sectional surveys are most useful for answering questions about the proportion of a population experiencing a given problem at any one time (prevalence). In fact, the cross-sectional study is the only study design for this purpose. Cross-sectional surveys may be administered in a face-to-face encounter between interviewer and respondent, by self-administered questionnaires, or by telephone interviews. Questions about prevalence can only be answered if you know both the numerator (the number of people affected) and the denominator (the number of people in the population). Consequently, cross-sectional studies fundamentally require the administration of a questionnaire or health examination to the entire population (a full census) or, more efficiently, a representative sample of the population. The use of a random (probability) sample allows for statistical techniques to be used to generalise from the sample data to the entire population.

For example, we may wish to estimate the proportion of women aged 18–70 years who have had a screening test for cervical cancer within the last year. Assuming we had a reliable and valid way of determining a woman's screening status (that is, were able to accurately and dependably discriminate between those who had and those who hadn't been screened), we could obtain such an estimate by surveying a representative random sample of 500 women. From these women, we could estimate the proportion of women in the entire population who had been screened within the previous year. However, if we wished to say something special about a particular subgroup of women, say, those with low incomes, we may need to specifically sample and survey women belonging to that group.

Other examples of prevalence surveys include work by INCLEN health social scientists. Kasniyah (1992) estimated the proportion of caretakers in Central Java who have taken eligible children for measles immunisation, while Saradamma et al. (2000) investigated the proportion of antibiotic medications that are acquired without a prescription from private pharmacies in Kerala state, India.

Cross-sectional studies are also often used to answer questions about relationships of association. In the cervical cancer screening example, we may also want to collect data to determine the sorts of knowledge and attitudes that are associated with use of screening. By comparing the level of knowledge between screened and unscreened women, we may begin to understand some of the psychological factors that influence women to screen.

Participants in cross-sectional studies are selected to be representative of the population without reference to exposure or outcome. Unlike cohort and case-control studies (see below), cross-sectional studies collect all the data about exposure and outcome simultaneously. Each person is interviewed or examined only once, although study participants may be asked to recall past exposures or behaviours (for example, number of pregnancies, childhood sun exposure, and so forth). Chapter 11 demonstrates how to enhance the validity of cross-sectional studies by using techniques from cognitive psychology and anthropology.

There are advantages and disadvantages of cross-sectional studies as discussed below.

9.2.2.1 Advantages of cross-sectional studies

- Cross-sectional studies may be used to study several exposures and outcomes simultaneously.
- They enable control over selection of subjects.
- They enable control over measurement.
- They are of relatively short duration.
- They are a good first step for a cohort study.
- They provide prevalence estimate (see 11.2.3 for sample size calculations).

9.2.2.2 Disadvantages of cross-sectional studies

- Cross-sectional studies do not establish sequence of events since both the outcome and the exposure occurred prior to the study.
- There is a potential bias in measuring exposure (since the outcome is known at the time of the survey).
- There is a potential survivor bias (since only people still living can be included in the study and since people with disease of long duration are more likely to be counted than people who recovered quickly or who have died).
- Their use is not feasible for rare conditions or exposures since large numbers of unaffected people will need to be surveyed to obtain enough cases for reasonable prevalence estimates.
- They do not provide any measure of incidence (see below).

Chapter 11 provides indepth coverage of cross-sectional surveys. Included are discussions of survey design, measurement, sampling, sample size, and how questionnaires can be strengthened using methods from cognitive psychology and anthropology (hybrid designs).

9.3 Level II: identifying the elements in the causal web

In Level II investigations, quantitative techniques are used to identify all the important variables that appear to influence the health problem. The main concern here is to identify potential causal influences that operate across different levels of analysis (for example, biological, individual, social) so that the key features of the causal web become visible. Cohort, case-control, and ecological designs are useful in Level II quantitative research.

9.3.1 Cohort studies

Cohort studies differ from cross-sectional studies in many ways. First, individuals are selected according to whether they have been exposed to the study factor (exposed) or not (unexposed). The second major difference is that cohort studies measure the incidence rate rather than prevalence. Whereas prevalence is an index of the number of cases (both new and old) as a proportion of the entire population, incidence refers only to new cases. The incidence rate is the number of new cases developing among the population at risk within a specified time period.

In a cohort study (also known as longitudinal, prospective, follow-up, or incidence study), exposed and unexposed groups who are initially free of disease are followed in time during which the incidence rate (risk) of the outcome is measured. The relative risk can then be calculated.

If we take the example outlined in box 9.2 (see below), we may wish to know whether women who are widowed are more frequently admitted to hospital than are married women of the same age. To answer this question we can observe and quantify the number of admissions occurring among widowed women over a fixed time period, say 1 year. This value would be the *incidence rate.*

$$\text{Incidence rate for hospital admission for widowed women} = \frac{\text{number of hospital admissions for women in the cohort for 1 year}}{\text{number of widowed women in the cohort for 1 year}}$$

Note that each new admission for each woman is considered to be a new incident. In contrast, an estimate of prevalence would count only women who were actually in hospital at the time of our survey. We can also calculate the incidence rate by hospital admission for the married women in the cohort.

Having calculated these two admission rates, we can then compare them and estimate the relative risk of hospital admission for widowed women compared to married women of the same age.

$$\text{Relative risk of hospital admission} = \frac{\text{Incidence rate for widowed women}}{\text{Incidence rate for married women}}$$

A special type of cohort study is a historical or retrospective cohort study in which the group, such as employees in a particular industry, are enrolled from company records many years before and the outcome is measured in the present. As long as information on exposure (for example, petrol fumes, noise, radiation) is available and the people available for follow-up, similar kinds of estimates can be made as in prospective studies without the necessity of waiting many years for the outcomes (Kelsey et al. 1986, p. 9).

9.3.1.1 Advantages of cohort studies

- Cohort studies ensure that the exposure has definitely preceded the outcome.
- They allow the establishment of absolute risk (incidence).

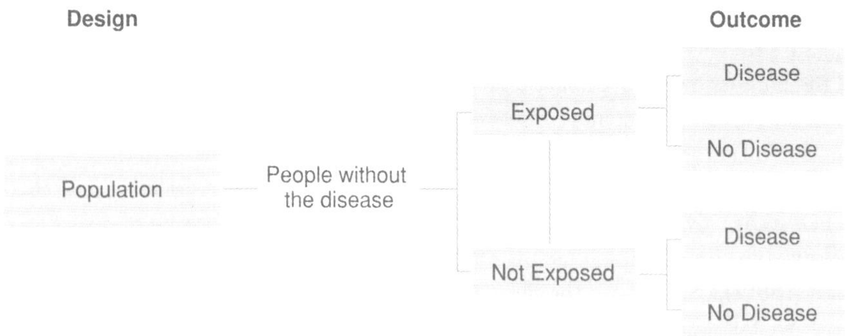

Results

		Outcome	
		Present	Absent
Exposure of Interest	Yes	a	b
	No	c	d

Direction of Study →

Figure 9.1 Outline of a cohort study

- They ensure that exposure can be measured without bias because at the time of the study the outcomes are not known.
- They can assess multiple outcomes.
- They enable other factors (for example, smoking) to be measured.

Box 9.2 The qualitative–quantitative interface in a longitudinal study of widows

The *Australian Longitudinal Study on Women's Health* includes a large cohort of women aged 70–75 years at baseline. The plan is to follow these women for another 20 years or until their death, to explore the impact of biological, psychological, social, and environmental factors on their health, morbidity, and mortality.

Loss of spouse is a major life event that affects many older women. At the time of first survey, 35 per cent of the cohort were widowed, and cross-sectional analyses showed that the recently widowed women had lower mean health-related quality of life scores than other widows and married women in the cohort.

Longitudinal analysis will help determine whether widowed women's health-related quality of life improves with time, and to document the change in health status for women widowed between baseline and follow-up (3 years later).

But the quantitative analysis can only describe the experience for broad categories of women, and the depth of insight into their needs and experiences is minimal. By combining quantitative and qualitative approaches the researchers have been able to draw an expanded picture of the women's needs and experiences. First, women's written comments on the questionnaire were analysed at baseline to help to explain and illustrate the statistical associations. These comments provided insight into the women's needs that could not be extrapolated from the quantitative data and these insights were used to define domains and items for a further survey of recently widowed women. This next survey confirmed the themes identified from the women's comments, and quantified the prevalence of each need or situation. More specific open questions relating to each theme revealed little new data, indicating that saturation of information had been reached.

Key elements identified through this combined approach have been incorporated into the follow-up survey (Byles et al. 1999).

9.3.1.2 Disadvantages of cohort studies

- Cohort studies are not efficient, as very large numbers will be needed for an uncommon outcome.
- They are expensive because of the resources needed to follow up people over a long time.
- Their results are not available for a long time; by the time the results are available, the problem may have no relevance.
- They are usually restricted to study of exposures which are measured at the start of the study; increase in knowledge may reveal far more important exposures which were not known at the time.

Another major limitation of cohort studies is the problem of confounding.

Confounding occurs when a third factor, called a confounder, distorts the apparent effect of a study factor on the outcome. There are many examples of confounding in published scientific research, and this problem is highly troublesome for epidemiologists (see 12.2.3.4). Take, for instance, the association between the use of hormone replacement therapy (HRT)[3] and the reduced risk of hip fracture observed from a cohort study. The truth of this association is distorted by the fact that women who use hormone replacement therapy tend to be of a particular

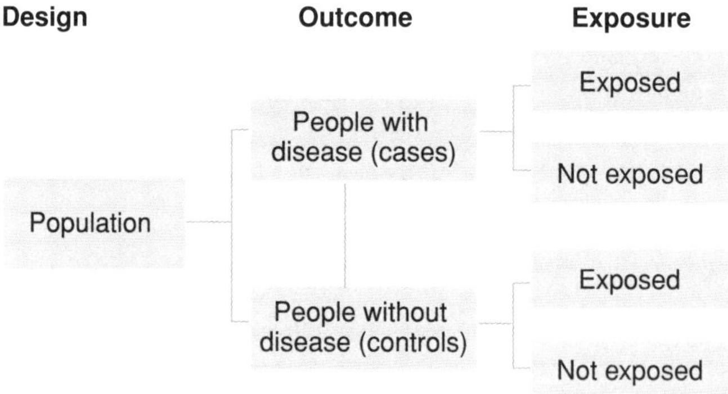

Results

		Outcome	
		Present	Absent
Exposure	Yes	a	b
	No	c	d

Direction of sampling ↓

Figure 9.2 Case-control studies

economic group and are often very health conscious. These women are also more likely to exercise and have better diets, and they are less likely to use alcohol to excess. These confounding factors may be the cause of reduced hip fracture risk rather than the HRT.

9.3.2 Case-control studies

The case-control study is the most efficient way of assessing association when the outcome is rare. In this study type, the researcher begins with a group of people who have the outcome (cases) and a comparable group of people who don't have the outcome (controls). The researcher then obtains information regarding past exposure to the study factor. A statistical association exists if the exposure is more common among the cases than controls. The strength of this association is calculated in terms of the odds ratio (the odds of exposure in the cases relative to the odds of exposure in the controls) and is comparable to the relative risk statistic that can be calculated from a cohort study.

Box 9.3 Understanding late diagnosis of breast cancer

To understand the influence of socioeconomic and cultural factors on the late diagnosis of breast cancer, researchers at the Leo Jenkins Cancer Center in the USA compared women who had presented with late stage disease (cases) and women with early cancer on demographic factors and attitudes and beliefs. Importantly, the researchers matched the controls to the cases in terms of area of residence. If they hadn't the study could have been severely limited by selection bias if women with advanced disease were referred in from outlying areas while women with early disease were managed locally.

One problem the researchers could not avoid was the retrospective measurement of beliefs and attitudes. It is quite possible that the women's beliefs were biased by the treatment options and prognosis. The structured interviews used in this study were based on preliminary indepth interviews by a cultural anthropologist. Here is another example of complementary qualitative and quantitative research methods (Lannin 1998, pp. 1801–7).

Nonetheless, efficient case-control studies are very difficult to conduct properly. The greatest difficulty is in identifying controls that are similar to cases in all respects except for the presence of the outcome and, potentially, the history of exposure. It is impossible to make any valid deductions from case-control studies unless the controls come from the same source population as the cases and have been selected independently of the exposure of interest. For example, in a case-control study of stroke patients, with hypertension as a potential exposure of interest (that is, risk factor), neighbours of the stroke victim who are similar in age and sex can be chosen as controls. Knowledge of the neighbours' hypertension status should not be known in advance.

The second problem is assessment of an exposure which has occurred in the past and may be subject to recall bias or other bias. For instance, in a case-control study of the relationship between bowel cancer and having a family member who has bowel cancer (family history), it is reasonable to think that the person with bowel cancer may have sought out such information from their family members, whereas the unaffected control may not have found out this information. Case-control studies will be explored in greater detail in chapter 12.

9.3.2.1 Advantages of case-control studies

- Case-control studies are valuable for studying rare conditions.
- They are of short duration.
- They are relatively inexpensive.
- Only a relatively small number of subjects are required.
- They yield odds ratio (usually a good approximation of relative risk).

9.3.2.2 Disadvantages of case-control studies

- Case-control studies are limited to one outcome variable.
- There is a potential bias from selection of cases and controls.
- They do not establish sequence of events.
- There is a potential bias in measuring exposure.
- There is a potential survivor bias.
- They do not yield absolute risk (incidence) estimates.

The case-control design is taken up again in chapter 12 where we demonstrate how it can be combined with qualitative methods to create the hybrid qualitative case-control study.

9.3.3 Ecological studies

Ecological designs are based on the comparison of two geographic areas (or other common ecologies) where one is thought to have a high degree of exposure or outcome and the other a low degree. The unit of analysis is the group rather than the individuals within the group. These two populations are then compared with respect to the incidence, or prevalence, of the outcome of interest (see Susser 1994). Ecological designs have led to interesting associations between the diets of people in China and Eastern Europe and the incidence of cancer of the oesophagus (Streiner and Norman 1996, p. 67; see also mention of clinical ecology research findings in 2.4.2). However, care has to be taken in attributing causality to such an association; just because there are associations on a population basis does not mean that the individuals who were exposed (for instance, to a particular dietary chemical) have the outcome (the disease being examined).

In figure 9.3 each data point on the scatterplot represents a geographical area. As the prevalence of the exposure to dietary fat increases (moving along the horizontal axis) the incidence of prostate cancer increases (moving up the vertical axis).

9.3.3.1 Advantages of ecological studies

- Data are obtained from published sources or government statistics, which reduces the cost.
- Ecological studies are useful for generating hypotheses about causality.

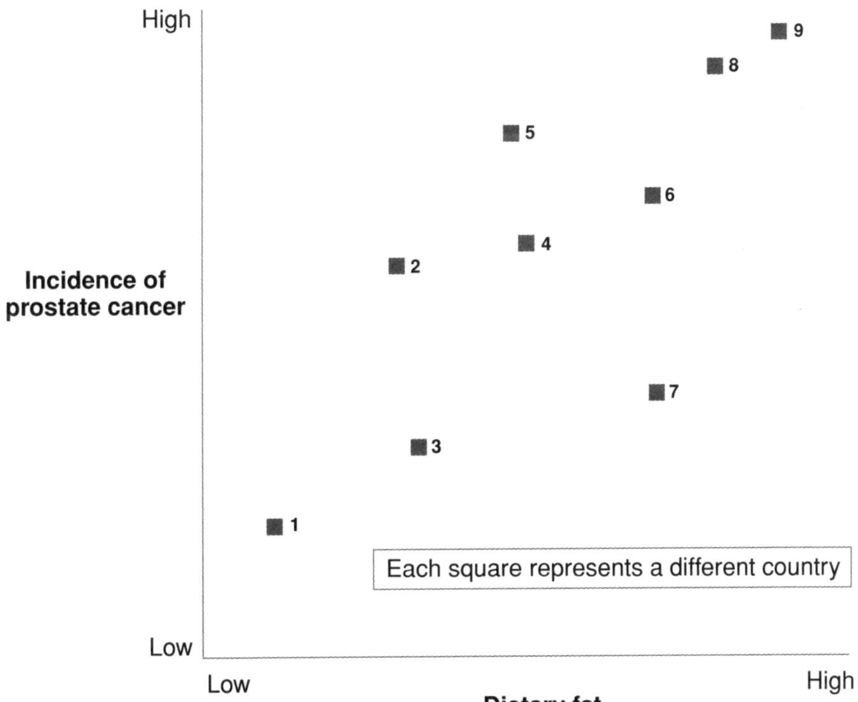

Figure 9.3 Scatterplot of ecological relativity between dietary fat and incidence of prostate cancer

9.3.3.2 Disadvantages of ecological studies

- Correlations from ecological studies are usually much higher than for studies which examine the exposure and outcome in the same individuals. High correlations can lead to a misleading assumption about causation—the study does not actually tell us whether the individuals who have been exposed are the ones who developed the outcome. Making the incorrect assumption that an ecological correlation represents a causal relationship is called the *ecological fallacy* (see Schwartz 1994).
- The time sequence for the association between exposure and disease is distorted.
- Insufficient data are available to control for confounding.

An ecological fallacy is easiest to see when it produces a counterintuitive result. For instance, a famous study in the 1930s showed that areas with large immigrant populations had a high correlation with high rates of literacy. Individual studies would show that the migrants themselves were more likely to be illiterate, but they settled in cities which had large populations of literate people (Robinson, cited in Streiner et al. 1989, p. 43). Other suggested ecological correlations, such as proximity to nuclear power stations and incidence of childhood leukaemia (Hocking et al. 1996), are still being debated.

9.4 Level III: clarifying causal links with experimental studies

Transdisciplinary research at Level III brings together all that is known about the causal web surrounding a health problem (from Level II studies); each element of influence is critically evaluated to assess its role as a causal factor. Importantly, the overall pattern of interactions among the variables is made visible through flow diagrams with the anticipation that some underlying principle may become evident.

Analytic techniques in epidemiology, formulated to determine causality of disease states, mortality, and various health indicators are essential for Level III TD investigations. Epidemiological design and measurement principles can be applied to evaluate the rigour of a study and decide how much we can trust the study's results, especially the relationship between the independent and dependent variables (that is, the study's internal validity). Behavioural epidemiology takes one step back along the causal path of disease outcomes to identify the psychosocial and behavioural variables leading to risk factors for the disease in question (see, for example, Sallis and Owen 1998): What, say, is the effect of peer pressure on initiation of smoking among adolescent boys, or the role of female literacy on birth spacing in rural Africa?

Following on from the analysis, however, epidemiological studies are still largely open to interpretation. Researchers must present their results within the context of other research (including relevant qualitative data) and relative to the causal model. Hill (1965) has provided a set of rules that can assist the researcher in weighing up the evidence before them. These rules include:

1 the strength of the association in terms of the relative risk or odds ratio
2 the consistency of the association from setting to setting and across studies
3 its specificity (that is, cause leads to only one outcome, and one outcome results from that cause)
4 the temporal relationship (cause precedes effect)
5 the biological gradient (dose–response relationship)
6 biological plausibility (a credible mechanism of action)
7 coherence (postulated causal relationship should not conflict with what is generally known about the disease)
8 evidence from experimentation (that is, randomised controlled trials).

All eight criteria are rarely satisfied, but we could infer causality if our study design allowed us to demonstrate some of the eight. The more criteria that are satisfied the stronger the evidence that a specific factor forms part of the causal pathway for the condition in question.

9.4.1 Randomised controlled trials

An investigation in which similar groups of individuals are allocated at random by the investigator to receive or not to receive a therapeutic or preventive intervention is termed a *randomised controlled trial* (RCT). Participants are observed for the occurrence of outcomes of interest. The RCT is the mainstay of Level III investigations.

The importance of randomisation is not in achieving balance between the groups in terms of known confounders but in evenly distributing unknown confounders. Given sufficient study participants, all factors should be evenly distributed between the groups before the experimental intervention begins. Differences in outcome can then be reasonably judged to be the result of the intervention.

The following hypothetical example shows the problem that RCTs are designed to solve. Hysterectomy is one of the most common operations performed on women. The operation involves removal of the uterus (womb) and sometimes the ovaries as well. The most common reason for performing this operation is for heavy bleeding that has no known pathological cause (called dysfunctional uterine bleeding). Hysterectomy prevents the bleeding but can introduce new symptoms and can lead to new physical problems such as prolapse of the vagina. Even in the short term, there are risks associated with the procedure.

Imagine a surgical meeting where one surgeon (let's call her Dr Slick) presents a new procedure called endometrial ablation that removes the problem of bleeding but leaves the pelvic structures intact and therefore has fewer problems with prolapse. Dr Slick presents her results from 200 women she has treated with this procedure and from 400 patients she treated using hysterectomy. The 200 women offered the new procedure were private patients since the public hospital where Dr Slick worked would not allow the new procedure to be performed on its patients.

After Dr Slick has presented her results, Dr Bland comments that he too has been experimenting with this new procedure. He has been offering the procedure to those wacky feminist women who question the need for hysterectomy. He has noted that these women tend to do better overall and are less likely to return for further procedures.

Dr Trad disputes these results, saying he has always found hysterectomy to be the best approach. He's been trying the new procedure for the past 5 years and now finds women are much more likely to come back with menopausal symptoms and seeking hormone replacement therapy. He blames the new procedure for this effect and is considering reverting to the traditional approach.

What do you think of the evidence presented by these surgeons? It is clear that in this case there are substantial differences (in social status, number of births, clinical condition, time of presentation) between the groups of patients to whom the two different treatments were applied. In these circumstances, it is difficult to be certain that one operation is better than the other. The good outcome observed by the clinician may be caused by the other factors in which patients differ (that is, confounding factors). Dr Slick, for example, may really be observing the relationship between having had fewer children (her private patients) and prolapse. The outcomes observed by Dr Bland may be influenced by the attitudes of his patients. And Dr Trad may be confusing secular trends (that is, general changes in society that affect everyone) with the effect of his operation. Studies are not true experiments if they fail to use a protocol that attempts to minimise the variation between the groups.

The best way to minimise confounding factors and to increase certainty about causality is randomisation of treatment and control groups. In this case, the three clinicians would have to decide what indications require surgery and then randomly allocate all their patients who correspond to this protocol to hysterectomy or ablation without regard to their insurance status, the severity of their condition, or the subjective judgment of the doctor about which operation is more effective. There would have to be a substantial area of doubt about the value of both operations to convince the clinicians, their hospital ethics committee, and the patients that it was ethical to do this investigation. It is easier to randomise patients when a promising new operation is being introduced and it can be compared with the standard treatment. Drug treatments can be *double blinded* (neither patient nor experimenter knows who is receiving the active drug or the placebo pill), but this is not possible with surgical or social interventions. If the intervention is seen as a desirable option (such as enhanced midwifery care), special measures to ensure that patients are not steered into one or other group (such as allocation by a central registry) are necessary to preserve the value of the study design (Oakley 1992).

Despite the difficulties, RCT designs are the most convincing evaluation of an intervention. The control group may receive no intervention, a placebo, or the currently accepted intervention. For ethical and sometimes administrative reasons, allocation of subjects to intervention or non-intervention status by randomisation may not be possible. This situation does not mean that useful research cannot sometimes be carried out but, in general, the inherent biases in the way people have been allocated to intervention/non-intervention mean that any results need most careful scrutiny.

Field trials differ from clinical trials in that the subjects are usually healthy and receive a vaccination or a health education package. Community intervention trials

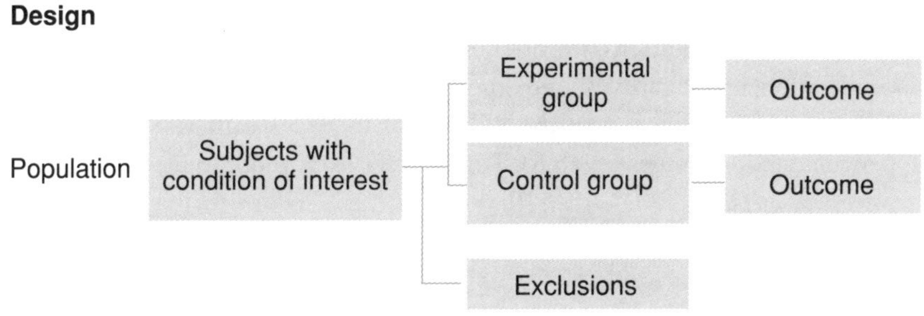

Results

		Outcome	
		Present	Absent
Exposure of interest	Yes	a	b
	No	c	d

Direction of sampling →

Figure 9.4 Randomised controlled trials

are similar to field trials but allocation is made to groups rather than individuals (for example, allocation of fluoridation to certain districts of a country). Such designs are known generally as group randomised trials and are commonly used in evaluation of health promotion strategies using schools or workplaces as intervention sites (Murray 1998).

9.4.1.1 Advantages of randomised controlled trials

- With randomisation, comparability of groups is very likely for both known and unknown confounders since the groups are derived from the same source population and should differ only by chance.
- Experiments provide the best chance of obtaining strong evidence of a cause and effect.
- Randomised controlled trials allow standardisation of eligibility criteria, the manoeuvre, and outcome assessments.
- Randomised controlled trials allow the use of statistical methods, which have few inbuilt assumptions.

9.4.1.2 Disadvantages of randomised controlled trials

- Randomised controlled trials may be expensive in terms of time, money, and people.
- Many research questions are not suitable for ethical reasons, problems with cooperation, or the rarity of outcome.
- To a greater or lesser extent the RCT tends to be an artificial situation, thus, patients who volunteer for an RCT may differ from those to whom the results would be applied.
- Standardised interventions may be different from common practice.

9.5 Critical appraisal

Sifting through the evidence for causation can be a complicated and confusing business. Several studies on the same topic may produce differing results. Which study is to be believed?

Scientific standards can rarely provide conclusive proof. Nevertheless, there are ways to determine the relative strength of the evidence presented by a particular study. This property is known as *study validity*. It is useful to develop a system and skills in gauging study validity. Several guides to interpreting or critically appraising research designs are available and here we reproduce a generic guide that we have found to be particularly useful (table 9.1). The guide identifies those key features of the study to look out for, and how to interpret the results in view of the approach, measures, and methods used in relation to the study question. In the next chapter, a comparable guide is offered for systematically appraising studies that use qualitative approaches to data gathering.

Table 9.1 Guide for critical appraisal of epidemiological studies

Can you find the information in the paper?	*Is the way this was done a problem?*	*Does this problem threaten the validity of the study?*
1 What is the research question and/or hypothesis?	Is it concerned with the impact of an intervention, causality, or determining the magnitude of a health problem?	
2 What is the study type?	Is the study type appropriate to the research question?	If not, how useful are the results produced by this type of study?
3 What are the outcome factors and how are they measured?	**a** Are all relevant outcomes assessed? **b** Is there measurement error?	**a** How important are omitted outcomes? **b** Is measurement error an important source of bias?
4 What are the study factors and how are they measured?	Is there measurement error?	Is measurement error an important source of bias?
5 What important potential confounders are considered?	Are potential confounders controlled for?	Is confounding an important source of bias?
6 What is the reference population and source population? What is the sampling frame and sampling method?	Is there selection bias?	Does this threaten the external validity of the study?
7 In an experimental study, how were the subjects assigned to groups? In a longitudinal study, how many reached final follow-up? In a case-control study, are the controls appropriate?		Does this threaten the internal validity of the study?
8 Are statistical tests considered?	Were the tests appropriate for the data? Are confidence intervals given? Is the power[4] given if a null result?	Do the conclusions drawn follow logically from the results of the analyses?
9 Are the results clinically or socially significant?	Was the sample size adequate to detect a clinically/socially significant result?	
10 What conclusions did the authors reach about the study question?	Do the results apply to the population in which you are interested?	Do you accept the results of this study?

Source: Darzins, Smith and Heller (1992, pp. 389–94)

9.6 Conclusion

In this chapter we have provided a broad introduction to the epidemiological designs and techniques that contribute to gathering information for TD research. These basic designs each have their own role in building an understanding of a particular problem or state. Transdisciplinary teams pursuing Level I problem description can apply case study, case series, and cross-sectional designs; those engaged in identifying elements influencing a health problem (Level II) can make use of cohort, case-control, and ecological designs. Experimental procedures involving randomised trials are used in Level III studies to evaluate the causal role of different variables implicated in health and disease. TD teams immersed in the problem context work their way from Level I through Level III investigations. However, as described in the preamble to part III, it is when this process of discovery through epidemiological methods is intertwined with knowledge gained through qualitative methods used in other disciplines that the fullest transdisciplinary understanding emerges. Such an understanding allows us to see clearly the problem context, identify significant elements of influence shaping the problem, and recognise the complex interactions (linear and non-linear) among influences and outcomes.

Notes

1 For the purposes of this chapter, we illustrate the positivist spectrum of epidemiology methods, favouring numerical, quantitative, and experimental or quasi-experimental techniques and procedures. Certainly, many contemporary epidemiologists incorporate qualitative methods in their investigation of disease processes in human populations. However, it is the quantitative expertise of the discipline that we review to provide a fundamental tool for transdisciplinary researchers.

2 Demographic transition is the shift from a high birth rate and short lifespan, to lower birth rate and greater longevity. The result is a population with more older people and fewer young people (Doll and Peto 1981).

3 Hormone replacement therapy is a general term to describe oestrogen and/or progesterone supplements. The therapy is commonly used for symptoms experienced around the time of menopause or to prevent conditions such as osteoporosis and heart disease.

4 The probability that the null hypothesis will be rejected statistically if it is indeed false.

10
How to Perform Transdisciplinary Research: Qualitative Study Designs and Methods

LINDA CONNOR, CARLA TRELOAR, AND NICK HIGGINBOTHAM

10.1 Introduction

The discussion of useful methods and designs for transdisciplinary research continues in this chapter. Complementing the epidemiological methods reviewed in chapter 9 are qualitative approaches commonly used in social and behavioural research. In this chapter we discuss the logic of enquiry underlying qualitative research, including the role of the researcher, the evolution of research projects, and sampling strategies. We briefly summarise main qualitative methods and approaches, and some techniques of analysis. Issues of triangulation and criteria for assessing the quality of qualitative research are discussed. The chapter concludes with an examination of ways in which qualitative methods can be related to the three levels of TD research.

There are many ways in which qualitative research methods and designs can be incorporated into larger programs of TD research. This chapter is intended as a foundation for the discussion of hybrid designs. Readers who are already familiar with the characteristics of qualitative research may wish to briefly review this chapter and then move on to chapters 11 and 12 where hybrid designs for TD research are introduced.

10.2 Characteristics of qualitative approaches

The formal properties of qualitative research designs are somewhat different from those of quantitative designs used in epidemiology because the purpose and

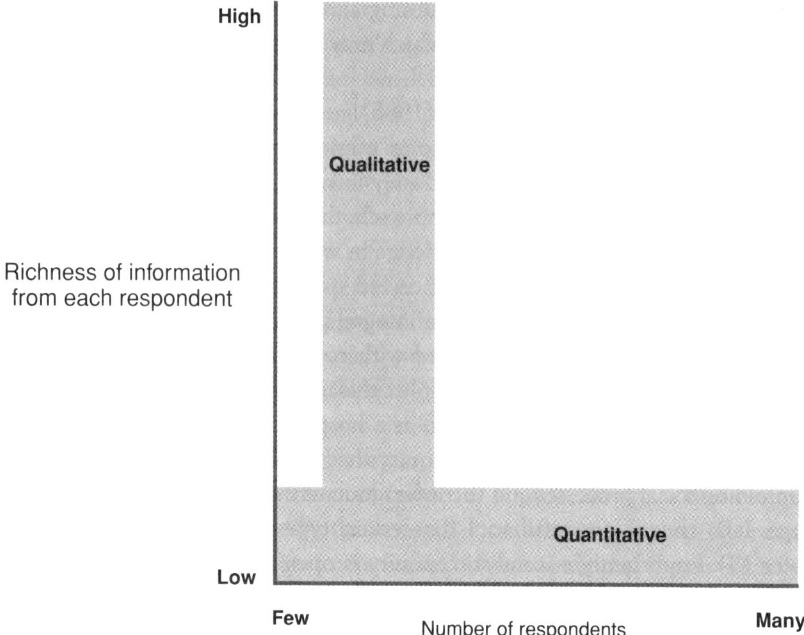

Figure 10.1 Comparison of the characteristics of qualitative and quantitative research

10.2.1 The researcher as instrument

A major difference between quantitative and qualitative approaches concerns the role of the researcher in the research process. In qualitative research, particularly of the more naturalistic type, the researcher's own personal attributes are explicitly recognised as an important element of the research process. The researcher is thus a research instrument (Lincoln and Guba 1985). In quantitative research, the researcher is ideally considered to be a neutral element in data collection. The research instruments in quantitative research are likely to be a set of previously validated questions, a structured survey questionnaire or measurement scale. Any influence exerted by the researcher in interactions with subjects of the study is considered a source of 'non-sampling error' or 'bias' and essentially to be avoided (see Stone and Campbell 1984 and box 11.4.2 for an example). The more structured types of qualitative research, such as those described in chapter 12, also try to avoid researcher influence on data collection as much as possible.

In naturalistic approaches, such as participant observation research by anthropologists in unfamiliar cultural settings, the novice fieldworker may be given particular social roles by virtue of gender, age, ethnicity, and marital status. These roles will influence the ways in which certain groups of people are accessible as subjects of study. In highly gender-segregated societies, for example, male fieldworkers may have limited access to social interaction with women. Young unmarried researchers may not be given certain information because of their perceived immaturity by members of the group they are studying. Personal characteristics and experiences of researchers will affect the way they seek out, filter, and interpret information, as Erving Goffman's study shows (see box 10.1).

How do qualitative researchers, using themselves as a research instrument, properly calibrate themselves (Mechanic 1989, p. 149)? To a major extent, the interpretation that emerges depends on the researchers' weighting of some data relative to others in a larger organising framework. Borman et al. (1986) point out that this is one of the most controversial aspects of qualitative designs. They suggest that researchers using more structured quantitative designs criticise qualitative data as 'too intuitive, personal and individualistic', because it is the researcher who acts as both 'filter for and interpreter of the data' (1986, p. 43). This criticism has some validity but it neglects to consider the methods by which properly trained qualitative researchers ensure that their data have reliability.

Lincoln and Guba (1985, pp. 301–31) have discussed in some detail the ways in which qualitative researchers establish the trustworthiness of their research data. The research process is carefully documented so that the steps taken can be scrutinised by others. Qualitative researchers typically set the goal of understanding a problem or issue from the point of view of those being researched and continually refer their findings back to subjects to establish whether this goal has been met. As discussed below, researcher insights can be strengthened by the use of triangulation and other strategies. It is also important to note that some research problems on sensitive topics (for example, highly personal issues or illicit activities) depend on personal attributes of the researcher for the study to be carried out at all. A famous example of this is the sociologist Howard Becker's participant observation study 'Becoming a Marihuana User' (1953). Becker, himself a former professional musician, used his own personal networks as entrée to subjects with whom he conducted observations and unstructured interviews about the process by which one learns to smoke marihuana and perceive the effects as enjoyable in a way that fits in with other members of the peer group. It is difficult to imagine how this sensitive and groundbreaking study could have been carried out in a more tightly structured way given the difficulty of establishing trust and rapport with subjects engaged in illicit recreational drug use in the 1950s.

An example of a famous and theoretically influential participant observation study where the researcher's role as research instrument is apparent is Erving Goffman's study of mental hospitals.

Box 10.1 Erving Goffman's study of mental hospitals

In his book *Asylums* (1961), Erving Goffman portrayed mental hospitals as degrading places that stripped individuals of their identity and self-esteem and induced deviant adaptations as a response to institutional life. But Goffman, as a participant observer who worked as an assistant to the athletics organiser in a mental hospital, brought his own personal biography and assumptions that shaped how he saw events. As a middle-class, independent academic who valued personal autonomy and the right to be eccentric, the regimentation of the mental hospital must have appeared very repressive. Later in his life, after having lived through an episode of mental illness involving a person close to him, he is said to have stated that if he had written *Asylums* at that time it would have been very different (Mechanic 1989, p. 148).

It is notable that studies on the experiences of mental patients by Linn (1968) and Weinstein (1979; 1983) using patient surveys have failed to replicate Goffman's view of the patient's experience. The surveys do provide evidence of the stigma associated with mental illness but not in the profoundly negative way depicted by Goffman. As the medical sociologist David Mechanic has noted, Goffman's study appears credible despite disconfirmation by surveys because readers find his analysis 'meaningful and convincing when they view themselves as the hypothetical patient in the context he describes' (Mechanic 1989, pp. 148–50). The study has remained one of enduring theoretical significance in sociology, perhaps because of the awareness of nuances of social interaction in the mental hospital that Goffman's self-calibration was able to produce.

Because qualitative methods encourage the evolution of understandings about the information collected and give recognition of researchers' subjective experiences in producing scientifically useful knowledge, there is a need to plan coordination of TD teams working with these methods so that team members can share insights as they emerge and share evolving design decisions. Members of TD teams will be calibrated in different ways as research instruments because of their own biographies, personalities, sociodemographic characteristics, and disciplinary training. This is a form of researcher triangulation that is discussed below; it can add a rich dimension to the research as investigators learn from their differences. This is one way in which a TD approach provides the multiple perspectives necessary to comprehend many aspects of health-related problems. Some of the problems encountered in the organisation of TD teams have already been addressed in chapter 7.

10.3 Designing a qualitative study

An obvious difference between much qualitative and quantitative research is the extent to which the design is specified in advance. It is a prerequisite of quantitative research that hypotheses, sampling procedures, instruments to be used, and methods of analysis should be specified in advance. Not to do so would subject the research to the suspicion of data dredging—running through statistical tests with the hope of finding significant relationships between variables. This level of specification means that timetables, personnel, and end products are all much more predictable for quantitative research than for qualitative methods (Lincoln and Guba 1985, p. 221). It is also the case that the flexibility required to undertake naturalistic enquiry (as opposed to more structured qualitative research) is usually more available to the lone researcher or small team undertaking fieldwork than it is to the often large research teams that may be involved in quantitative studies. Nonetheless, qualitative research can provide important elements in larger TD research projects, not least because of its powerful capacity to illuminate the wider context of a health problem from the subjects' points of view.

Qualitative researchers, whether using naturalistic or more structured approaches, usually intend to spend a long period of time on data collection and their results often depend on establishing rapport with the people they are researching. Hence, considerable thought is given to ways of entering the research setting, whether it is geographically remote such as a cultural group in another country, or just unfamiliar, such as a hospital or illness support group meetings. Careful consideration is also given to the relationships that will be established and the best way of leaving the field (Janesick 1994, pp. 211–15).

10.3.1 Setting out the focus and purpose of the enquiry

Determining the focus of an enquiry establishes the broad boundaries for the study (for example: What makes people decide whether to have their children immunised?). Decisions have to be made about where the boundaries of interest lie—perhaps in a geographically localised community, a group of people with particular attributes, a process, or an historical period—so that relevant material can be collected. However, as qualitative researchers may not initially know precisely what data will be important, the focus of the enquiry may change as data are collected. This process, which would be considered a major flaw in an epidemiological study, is expected in the more naturalistic qualitative designs (Lincoln and Guba 1985, p. 225).

Decisions about design, methods, analysis, and reporting flow from the purpose of the research. The importance of a study's stated purpose in making decisions about methods becomes evident from examining alternate purposes. Expectations and audiences, reporting and dissemination approaches vary for different purposes. The researcher must be clear at the beginning which purpose has priority. Patton (1990, pp. 150–2) outlines five primary types of research according to purpose, which may overlap in practice. These types are:

1 *basic research* to contribute to fundamental knowledge and theory
2 *applied research* to illuminate a societal concern
3 *summative evaluation* to determine program effectiveness
4 *formative evaluation* to improve a program
5 *action research* to solve a specific problem.[2]

With clarity of focus and purpose, the researcher can proceed to make specific design, data gathering, and analysis decisions to meet the priority purpose and address the intended audience. The next step is to frame the research questions.

10.3.2 Framing the research questions

Should a small number of questions be examined in depth or a larger number of questions in less depth? Naturalistic researchers approach a study with an open-ended set of research questions. The study must therefore go through several stages: looking for what is salient, finding out about it, checking findings, and formulating new questions on the basis of these findings (Lincoln and Guba 1985, chapter 8). Those undertaking more structured qualitative research may already have quite specific initial questions using well-defined concepts.

A review of relevant literature is important in focusing the study, avoiding unnecessary duplication, and in framing initial questions. This allows the researchers to think about the information emerging from the study and the literature in an iterative or cyclical way: the empirical information drives the researchers to certain literatures, which in turn suggest further possibilities for data gathering and analysis. During this iterative process, research questions as well as analytical categories may be refined or refocused as a consequence of new data emerging, or further literature review, or both.

10.3.3 Sampling in qualitative studies

Once the focus and purpose of the research have been established and the initial research questions have been formulated the researchers must decide how the data will be collected. This section briefly discusses the principles of sampling in qualitative studies.

Selection of subjects is a major consideration in a study aimed at identifying social aspects of a health problem. In epidemiological studies, the overall research design—for example, cohort, cross-sectional, case control—determines which subjects are selected and how (see chapter 9). Usually, *probability samples* are sought using one of the basic probability sampling techniques of random sampling, stratified sampling, or cluster sampling. The power of probability sampling comes from a statistically representative sample that permits generalisation from the sample to the source population (the *external validity*). Probability sampling in relation to epidemiological study designs and cross-sectional surveys is discussed in chapters 9 and 11.

Probability sampling is also quite common in qualitative studies. It may be preferred for the same reason as are epidemiological studies: the power of generalisation that it offers. If the researchers are working in a small community such as a village or an institution and they want to generalise to all members of that community, then it may be quite feasible to devise a good probability sample. Even with larger populations it is possible to achieve a fair degree of representativeness with manageable sample sizes using techniques such as stratified and cluster sampling that are discussed in chapter 11 (see also Bernard 1994, pp. 80–94).

10.3.3.1 Non-probability sampling strategies

Despite its low external validity, qualitative researchers often use *non-probability sampling* for a number of reasons:

- Pilot studies to test interview questions and scales may not require a representative study.
- Subjects may be chosen for case studies because of particular attributes that they possess. For example, one can learn a great deal about social aspects of a health problem, such as myocardial infarct, if one intensively researches the lifestyle and resources of carefully selected persons with this condition, rather than using a standard survey of the whole community or posting a questionnaire to sufferers. As discussed in chapter 9, case studies of rare disorders may require non-probability sampling.
- Other research units, such as communities, may also be chosen because of their special attributes. The Oceanpoint community discussed in chapter 12 was

chosen because of its geographical distinctiveness and certain sociodemographic characteristics that made it interesting for an ethnographic study.
- There may be problems in identifying a *sampling frame* for the population one wishes to study; certain people (for example, injecting drug users) may be difficult to find.
- Research on sensitive or illicit topics is likely to require the establishment of rapport between researcher and subject in the context of participant observation that would not be possible with a probability sample. Howard Becker's study of marihuana users is an example of this.
- Research on social networks usually requires a non-probability sampling strategy such as snowball or chain sampling (discussed below); the information of interest is how subjects are known to or interact with one another.

There are a number of terms to refer to non-probability sampling, some of which overlap. Some methodologists, such as Patton, refer to all non-probability samples as 'purposeful' sampling (1990, pp. 169–83). This is broadly synonymous with the term 'theoretical sampling' used in the grounded theory framework of Glaser and Strauss (1967, p. 48). Bernard refers to four types of non-probability sampling—'quota', 'purposive', 'snowball', and 'haphazard' (1994, p. 73). Non-probability sampling techniques usually have the following characteristics:

- they are not specified or drawn in advance but in a serial fashion (that is, the information from the previous sampling unit influences the way in which the next unit is chosen)
- the criteria for sampling may change as the study progresses
- sampling is typically terminated when no new information of significance is obtained from more sampling units (a situation of informational redundancy) (Lincoln and Guba 1985, pp. 201–2).

As Patton points out (1990, p. 169), it is important to distinguish between the logic of quantitative and qualitative sampling; they differ markedly in terms of method of case selection and assessment of the appropriate size of sample. One type of sampling should not be judged by the standards of the other. A well-chosen qualitative sample is as satisfactory for its purpose as a properly calculated random sample.

Some non-probability sampling strategies are more systematic than others. At the non-systematic extreme (one might say at the opposite end of the sampling spectrum to random sampling) are the strategies known as *haphazard sampling* and *convenience* (or *accessibility*) *sampling*. Using these types of sampling, people are selected for study because they are easily available (university students or hospital patients), not because they have been deliberately chosen to yield the richest data for the study's purposes. Some people think that if randomisation is not necessary, any group of interviewees will do. This is very far from the logic of qualitative research. Haphazard or convenience sampling are not recommended strategies. They may be used at the initial, exploratory stage of research, but these strategies will yield data of the lowest validity or generalisability (Patton 1990, p. 183; Bernard 1994, p. 96).

The following examples are some of the most commonly used strategies of non-probability sampling in qualitative research.[3]

Quota sampling

As in stratified probability sampling, the population is divided into subpopulations and then the proportions of each subpopulation are determined. The Oceanpoint study discussed in chapter 12 used quota sampling for interviews to achieve proportions of each subpopulation according to gender, age, and socioeconomic status that reflected as closely as possible their proportions in census data for this coastal suburb. Unlike stratified sampling, the characteristics of respondents are not specified in advance but are chosen in serial fashion (Bernard 1994, pp. 94–5).

Snowball or chain sampling

Subjects are asked to recommend others they know for the researcher to contact. This may be useful in studies of social networks or social influence, or in difficult-to-find populations. If enough enquiries are made, a list of names which are frequently referred to may be compiled. This strategy is useful for reaching people with publicly acknowledged expertise. However, using this strategy in the personal domain, say, for enquiries about poor health or sexuality, may cause ethical problems because confidential information about third parties is revealed to the researcher in advance of the subject's consent. This can be avoided by the use of indirect means of contact between researcher and potential subjects.

Critical case sampling

Sampling can be designed to select cases that will allow a generalisation that has wide applicability. Its effectiveness depends on an understanding of the most important attributes that influence an outcome. For example, the initiators of a new community program may decide to test its feasibility in a community where significant resistance to the program is expected. The results of the intervention would provide a critical case for the feasibility of the program—'If it works in this community, it will work in most communities' (Patton 1990, p. 174).

Maximum variation sampling

This strategy involves selecting a small sample with maximum variation in defined attributes (age, education, gender, type of illness). It can be used for two purposes. The first is to highlight the experiences, themes, or outcomes which these maximally varied sampling units have in common. If there is wide variation within the group, then common themes (such as in the experience of hospital care) are obviously important. This type of sampling can be used to document unique experiences as well as shared patterns (Patton 1990, p. 172).

Extreme or deviant cases

More information about social processes or the effects of particular variables may be obtained from cases at either end of a continuum or from unusual cases than by researching a typical case or a randomly selected one. In her study of child health in Yemen described in detail in chapter 12, Cynthia Myntti selected samples of mothers who ranked highest and lowest on a previously administered score of child health to investigate the critical variables that contributed to children's health in this community.

Criterion sampling

This strategy is employed to sample cases that meet a criterion of importance to the study such as membership of a particular group or participation in a type of program. Criterion sampling may be undertaken as a follow-up to a survey study when the researchers want to identify particular subjects for indepth analysis (Patton 1990, pp. 176–7).

Box 10.2 Sampling strategies used in the Care Aware project

A variety of sampling strategies may be used in complementary ways to strengthen transdisciplinary research. For example, the Care Aware project (chapter 7) used different sampling strategies at various stages. Initial focus group discussions were conducted with staff of the hospital unit that cared for people with HIV and AIDS, who constituted a criterion sample. These health workers were considered to have the greatest level of skill, knowledge, and awareness of accidental exposure to needles in the work environment. The issues raised by this group were posed to other groups of health workers in the second phase of the investigation. Other wards in the hospital were sampled and nurses were invited to attend focus group discussions. These health workers from non-infectious disease wards were considered to be critical cases for the intervention in terms of their level of awareness and knowledge about accidental exposures. For the final stage, when the Care Aware intervention was conducted, all workers in two hospital wards were invited to participate to maximise the sample size for quantitative analyses. The two wards,

> Intensive Care and Emergency, were chosen because of their high rate of procedures performed on patients. These wards provided the best opportunity to measure health workers' compliance with safety guidelines (that is, criterion sampling was used).

10.3.3.2 Sample sizes in non-probability sampling strategies

Unlike quantitative random sampling which aims to achieve a measurement of outcome (or prevalence estimates) within a specified *confidence interval* (see 11.2.2.4), qualitative sample size is not mathematically determined. Just as the choice of subjects is determined by what the researcher wants to know, so the number of people included is a matter of judgment. This number may be five or several hundred, depending on the topic and the resources available. Qualitative analysis can be carried out on a single case if it is sufficiently information rich. It is important, however, not to overgeneralise from non-probability samples and not to use them as if they were probability samples.

The fact that 'there are no rules for sample size in qualitative enquiry' can be a source of anxiety (Patton 1990, p. 184). Most authors recommend that data collection should continue until no new information is received. This is termed 'the point of theoretical saturation' in the grounded theory approach of Glaser and Strauss (1967), or 'the point of redundancy' in the words of Lincoln and Guba (1985, p. 202). Preparation for qualitative research, such as funding applications, may require arguing for a minimum expected sample size but reserving the option to change this during the research process. Documentation of the rationales for sample size, as well as sampling strategies, is an important aspect of the write-up of qualitative studies.

10.4 Overview of qualitative methods and approaches

There is a range of qualitative methods and approaches that can be combined as building blocks in various TD research designs. The epidemiological research designs discussed in chapter 9 have quite standardised formats. Qualitative research designs are typically more fluid and open-ended. While the more structured qualitative research may follow a strictly standardised design format, less structured research evolves in serial fashion as new insights that suggest new methods and approaches are gained. Thus, the methods discussed in this section are not necessarily part of fixed designs but can be used in the process of carrying out a qualitative study. The most commonly used qualitative research methods are briefly summarised here.

10.4.1 Interviews

Interviews could be considered the foundation of social research. Many texts have been written on the subject of interviewing (see Spradley 1979; Babbie 1990; Oppenheim 1992; Bernard 1994). The essence of the interview is the direct interaction of interviewer and respondent, either in face-to-face contact or via media such as the phone, video, or email. There are many types and styles of interviews, varying from structured interviewer-administered questionnaires to unstructured indepth interviews. Interviews may also be formal or informal, planned or opportunistic, depending on both the nature of the research question and the social milieu in which that research is taking place. Main types of interviews are summarised below. Aspects of interviewing technique and their effects on the data collected are discussed in chapter 11 (see 11.4.1).

Structured interviews

In *structured interviews* such as interviewer-administered questionnaires, the researcher follows a standardised guide for the interview and discourages the respondent from providing any extra information. This sort of interviewing is undertaken in the more structured types of qualitative research, and the aim is to maximise the standardisation of the procedures and the comparability of the data collected from respondents.

Semi-structured interviews

With *semi-structured interviews* the researcher has a list of specific topics to be covered but is flexible in the order and wording of questions. This format can obtain comparable information from a large number of subjects of a type that is more complex or sensitive than a structured survey interview can produce. Some researchers, such as Bauman and Adair (1992, pp. 10–11), refer to this type of interview as a *structured indepth interview*, referring to both the researcher-specified focus on specific topics and the flexible format that encourages the respondent to use their own words to address issues in their own order. This type of interview can also be used to pretest questions using probes and 'think-alouds' (see chapter 12).

Unstructured indepth interviews

Unstructured indepth interviews enable the interviewer to select the topic but have no preset questions or order to follow. These interviews can be quite lengthy, often taking more than an hour. Interviewees select the order and control the themes and areas covered in order to express their own understandings. The style is conversational although the interviewer may probe for more information. Interviewers can analyse these sorts of data to establish the scope of reactions, the content, and the variety and depth of feeling of people's responses (see Bauman and Adair 1992, p. 10).

Ethnographic interviews

The *ethnographic interview* is a particular form of the indepth interview developed in anthropology to elicit specific forms of cultural knowledge from respondents or informants (this latter term usually used by anthropologists). It is relatively unstructured and non-directive, but uses particular types of questions (descriptive, structural, and contrast; see Spradley 1979, p. 60). The form of the ethnographic interview explicitly acknowledges the role of the informant or interviewee as the cultural expert from whom the interviewer is seeking particular sorts of cultural knowledge. The ethnographic interview requires a good level of local language competence on the part of the researcher, whether the language used be a foreign language or a local dialect or idiom derived from the ethnographer's own native language (Spradley 1979, pp. 17–21).

Free-listing techniques

Free-listing techniques are often used at the beginning of the research process when the researcher is interested in defining the boundaries of the research area from the point of view of the research subjects. Many qualitative studies start by asking interview subjects to list as many words as possible that refer to a broadly described topic. An important rationale for qualitative approaches is to achieve sensitivity to subjects' understandings of a problem. As well as discovering the boundaries of a particular cognitive domain of knowledge, inferences about what is significant or salient for respondents can be made from the frequency and order of their responses. Weller and Romney (1986, p. 9) have referred to free-listing tasks as the mapping of a semantic or cultural domain. The domain of interest might be names of diseases or methods of infant feeding, for example.

Group interviewing

This refers to a situation where several people respond to topics or questions posed by an interviewer or facilitator. Although a number of group data collection techniques exist (delphi groups, brainstorming), *focus group discussions* are more commonly used in health research. Like other interview situations, the group interview may be more or less structured. The advantage of group interviews is the richer information that may emerge from participants' interactions with each other as well as with the interviewer. In focus groups, discussion is triggered and guided by a set of questions or a prompt such as a description of a child's illness, or film, or video. Wilkinson (1998) has identified five main uses of focus groups in health research:

- studies of lifeworlds and health beliefs
- assessment of health status and health care needs
- health education and health promotion
- participatory and social action research
- evaluation and marketing of products and services.

10.4.2 Direct observation

Direct observation refers to the range of activities in which a researcher watches and records information about people or an event but does not have interaction with the people or situations being observed. Observations may be structured or unstructured, or become more narrow and focused as the study proceeds and the issues of interest become clearer. Observation may be continuous or conducted at random, involving 'spot sampling' (Bernard 1994, p. 321). Observations may be made of people, social situations, or inanimate objects. As an example of the latter, the Care Aware study (chapter 7) observed the proportion of recapped needles in needle disposal bins in a number of hospital wards to determine health workers' compliance with safety guidelines.

The observer can be obvious to those being observed or disguised or hidden in some way. For example, an observer might stand at the edge of a school playground with a clipboard and pen and record close contact among children in a study of the transmission of infectious disease. In this case, the children would be aware of the observer but the observer's presence may have little effect on the behaviour of children involved in playground games. In a contrasting example, an observer might take an inconspicuous place in a public area such as a health care clinic to observe waiting times, types of drugs dispensed, or the number of mothers attending with young children. The people present in this area would be unaware of the observer and hence unaware that they were participating in a study.

Technological advances such as inconspicuous audiotaping and videotaping equipment may make observational data easier to collect and less reliant on copious hand-written field notes. However, direct observational methods where the subjects are unaware that they are being observed, and in fact are acting as participants in a study, raise numerous ethical issues, including invasion of privacy (Adler and Adler 1994). In some situations involving direct, unobtrusive observation of sensitive, illegal, or gender-based activities, the safety of the observer is of greater concern than in studies where the researcher has permission to be present or has obtained the consent of the participants.

In practice, very few projects or published articles rely only on observation methods. Observations are limited to describing, in some way, *what* people do, but cannot provide any commentary on *why* they do it (Bernard 1994). Reports of observation studies rely on the observer's own interpretations and assumptions (Adler and Adler 1994). Further, participants may change their behaviour if they know they are being observed and if they know the particular issue of interest to the observer. These limitations of the observation method raise concerns about its reliability (or consistency of observation)[4] and validity (the interpretations made from the observational data). Observations are used more as an 'integrated' rather than 'primary' method (Adler and Adler 1994, p. 389).

10.4.3 Ethnography and participant observation

The first-hand study of a small community, with its own characteristic culture or way of life, is referred to as *ethnography*. *Participant observation* is the term most often used to describe the main methodological approach of ethnographic studies. Participant observation is not so much a formal technique for working in the community as much as a general approach or state of mind. This approach is especially characteristic of the work that anthropologists do in small-scale societies, but it has also been employed in enclaves or *subcultures*[5] of industrialised countries, such as alternative lifestyle groups. Robert Park and other members of the Chicago School of urban sociology relied heavily on participant observation in research such as W.F. Whyte's *Street Corner Society* (1955) about the street life of the inhabitants of an Italian slum in Chicago. Sociologist Erving Goffman's 1950s study of a mental hospital (see box 10.1) used a participant observation approach.

Participant observation is an approach to research in which the investigator is not merely a detached observer of the lives and activities of the people under study, but is also a participant in their round of daily activities. By becoming an active member of the community, the researcher of community life may become a trusted friend and associate of the people in the community. By doing, as far as possible, whatever the people the researcher is studying are doing, the researcher can attain a better understanding of what such activity means to the people themselves, in the context in which it occurs. The researcher must explore the relationship of observed behaviour to verbal accounts and interpretations by members of the group under study. Participant observation is the key method by which the researcher can discover the relationships between people's knowledge, attitudes, and practices. Interviews and self-administered questionnaires only provide the researcher with information about what people say they do, which has a variable relationship to what they may actually do.

Participant observation is not the same as casual observation. Participant observation studies involve a relatively lengthy period of engagement with the field site, whether this be in a foreign place or a part of the researcher's own society. It may be necessary to learn one or more foreign languages, or unfamiliar dialects or idioms. Participant observers undertake fieldwork, which means the research is conducted in the social and physical environment of the target group, which in effect becomes a host to the researcher. Participant observation research usually involves stages of entering the field, developing rapport with subjects or informants, acceptance and cultural familiarity, and leaving the field.

The researcher has to develop a methodical way of recording observations. Temporary notes in a portable notebook provide the basis for more permanent notes which, for contemporary researchers, are likely to be word-processed. Researchers need to be versatile in a variety of recording techniques, including wordlists, mapping, and making diagrams, drawings, charts, and indexes.

Field researchers undertaking participant observation will generally try to observe and talk to as many different kinds of people as possible in the group they are studying (varying according to variables such as age, sex, leadership, and wealth). There may also be a small number of individuals from whom the researcher obtains a large amount of detailed information about particular topics or the general life of the community. Such people are generally referred to as 'key informants'. *Key informant interviewing* is used to best advantage when it is closely linked to participant observation or other methods. The researcher needs to be able to assess the informant's situation within the group under study.

Sometimes it is said that the key informant, because of special personality characteristics or social situation, chooses the researcher, not vice versa. Some field researchers emphasise that the key informants should be carefully chosen on the basis of their position in a particular setting and their knowledge of that setting. Key informants may be chosen for their specialised knowledge (for example, healers, political leaders) depending on the topic of research. For example, the researcher studying Indigenous health beliefs may want to know what the difference is between laypersons' and specialists' knowledge of Indigenous medicine (see Romney et al. 1986). Researchers may stratify their interviewees and select key informants to represent groups of particular interest regarding the research question. If possible, it is useful to have more than one representative of each critical group as key informants.

The selection of individuals in field studies is, therefore, a different procedure from the selection procedures associated with random sampling in survey research. In field research key informants are non-randomly selected for their knowledge which may complement the researcher's observations and point towards further investigation that needs to be done. However, researchers seeking to maximise data generalisability may wish to identify a sampling frame of knowledgeable individuals and then select informants for intensive interviewing at random.

Many community health researchers now recognise that ethnographic data are essential in the implementation of programs. However, given the shortage of time and budget resources for health programs, it is often necessary to gather qualitative data in a relatively rapid manner. One technique that has been developed to meet this need is *rapid assessment procedures* (RAP), which is usually undertaken in the context of applied research projects and prior to interventions (Scrimshaw and Gleason 1992). Data from RAPs cannot provide a thorough analysis of local socio-cultural systems, but do offer basic information about attitudes and approaches to health care services and cultural practices in relation to disease. RAP can be a valuable tool in the analysis of critical relationships and causal processes in relation to health problems. Manderson and Aaby describe RAP as useful for examining 'understandings of the relationship between the biological and social worlds' and the 'salient indicators for a given disease' (1992, p. 49). Good quality RAP is usually carried out by an anthropologist who already has a high level of linguistic and cultural knowledge of the target group.

10.4.4 Analysis of documents and images

Written materials such as government records, letters, memoranda, minutes of meetings, reports, newspaper items, and articles in the popular press can be used as data for a qualitative study. Images such as photographs and drawings may also provide valuable information. It is important to recognise that such documents may not necessarily be accurate or without bias, despite the often presumed objectivity of written or published materials. The rationale and criteria for sampling need to be carefully specified. These sorts of data are often used in conjunction with other methods such as interviews.

Media analysis of health reporting can be a valuable source of information for public health and social science researchers. Deborah Lupton (1995), for example, analysed front-page health reporting in a major Australian metropolitan daily newspaper over a 1 year period. From a total of 140 stories in 117 issues, Lupton found that despite the diversity of stories appearing, the overall coverage was 'predominantly conservative, giving greater voice to élite groups than less powerful groups, such as advocacy, activist and community groups, and to men rather than women' (1995, p. 501). The socioeconomic and political contexts of illness were underreported compared with illness as an individualised phenomenon (1995, p. 506).

Archival records may be relevant for some health research topics. Examples include:

- service records (for example, information about clients attending a medical facility over a certain time period)
- maps and charts of the geographical characteristics of a place

- lists of names
- survey data (for example, old census records)
- personal diaries, calendars, and so forth.

The usefulness of archival records will vary for different studies. It is important to realise, however, that most archival records were produced not only for a specific purpose, but also for a particular audience. The conditions under which the record system evolved and the purpose for which it was developed need to be fully appreciated when drawing inferences from these types of data as they have their own forms of bias or distortion (Yin 1994, p. 82).

10.5 Analysis of qualitative data

While quantitative approaches typically emphasise the importance of testing for the patterns of associations operating in the sample as a whole, qualitative strategies typically seek to explore the differences between people (or other units of analysis, such as health teams or communities) in an attempt to understand these differences within a broader social context. In addition, as discussed in 10.2, qualitative analyses can be either deductive (based on a framework derived from prior theory) or inductive (the theory is derived from the data collected during the course of the

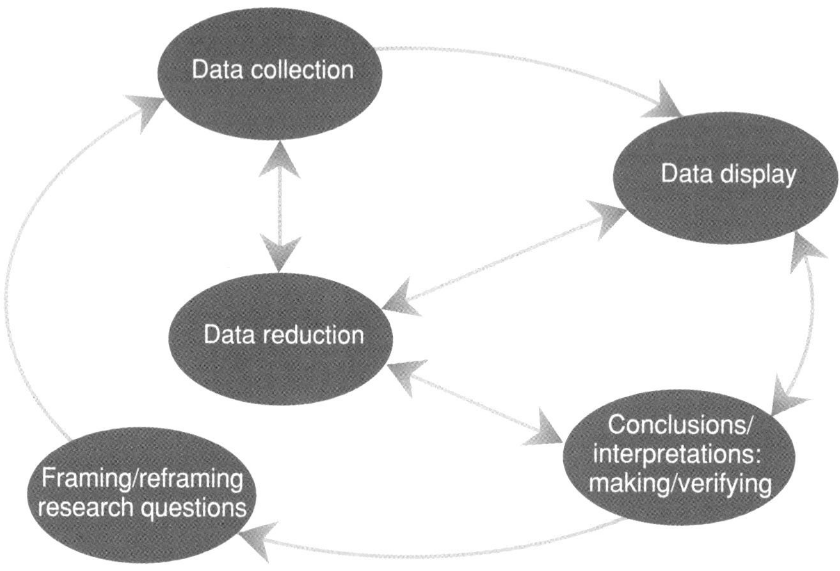

Source: Adapted from Miles and Huberman 1994

Figure 10.2 Components of data analysis: interactive model

study). Quantitative analysis is characterised by systematic progression from hypothesis generation through to data collection and data analysis. This may also occur in the more structured types of qualitative data analysis, but we are more likely to find an iterative process in which the development of theory, data collection, and data analysis can take place simultaneously, as figure 10.2 (adapted from Miles and Huberman 1994, p. 12) shows.

This iterative process enables information gathering to be continually improved during the course of the qualitative study. The emphasis is not so much on the reproducibility of the data gathering exercise as it is on developing the best method to address research questions that may be evolving in order to best serve the overall purpose of the research.

Grounded theory, an early and influential model of an inductive and iterative process of qualitative research, was developed by Glaser and Strauss (1967) and has more recently been discussed by Strauss and Corbin (1990; 1994). Data (usually notes or transcripts) are first coded using open (as opposed to pre-determined) categories; the categories are referred to as 'saturated' when the data yield no new categories. The constant comparative method is used to look for similarities and differences between codes. This process produces preliminary hypotheses and leads on to 'axial coding', a second order coding where connections between categories are made. 'Selective coding' is a more theoretically oriented form of coding that integrates core categories of data sets. By the repetition or iteration of components of this process, a theoretical scheme is produced, which is then tested against the data.

10.5.1 Processes of analysis

Most forms of qualitative analysis involve some type of *content analysis* and *coding* whether it be of words, phrases, or ideas derived from interviews, group discussion, fieldnotes, traditional folklore stories, political speeches, poems, images, or the mass media. Proponents of the less-structured or naturalistic types of qualitative research hold that data analysis procedures cannot be rigidly specified in advance. In the words of Patton, 'there are no absolute rules except to do the very best with your full intellect to fairly represent the data and communicate what the data reveal given the purpose of the study' (Patton 1990, p. 372). According to this view, reports of data analysis procedures should provide enough detail for evaluation by other researchers. As discussed in chapters 11 and 12, however, more structured qualitative research does have formalised guidelines for analysis.

Miles and Huberman (1994, pp. 10–12) have outlined the generic steps that most qualitative researchers go through in the process of analysis. These steps are represented in figure 10.2. Very briefly, they are as follows:

- *Data reduction*: This requires that researchers select, focus, and simplify the data to a manageable level. This process occurs continuously and often at the same time as data collection. It may involve summaries and memos as well as *coding*. A code is a tag that can be applied to a chunk of data. This chunk of data is later retrieved (with all other like-coded chunks) so that the researcher can compare and contrast like-coded chunks with each other or with other chunks.
- *Data display:* The researcher seeks to organise and compress information with the aim of moving to the final stage of drawing conclusions. Most data are initially displayed as text (or images). As analysis proceeds, data display may move to more compact and accessible forms such as matrices, charts, lists, tables, graphs, network diagrams, or typologies. These are tools that the researcher uses to highlight and document the important associations between the data.
- *Conclusion drawing and verification*: This process, which incorporates theorising about the data, actually occurs from the start of data collection. Initial interpretations of the data may be open and vague, leading to new or reframed research questions. Interpretations become more focused as data collection and analysis proceed. The final conclusions should be explicit and grounded within the data. The conclusions drawn should be verified and a number of methods can be used in this process (for example, checking with research subjects, going back to original fieldnotes, review by colleagues).

10.5.2 Coding

In qualitative data analysis, a code is a word, phrase, abbreviation, or symbol which is applied to an image or segment of text which may be a word or phrase, a sentence, some paragraphs, or pages. Codes provide the researcher with a way of categorising the data.

Each writer in the area of qualitative data analysis has a slightly different way of conceptualising the types of codes that are created by the researcher systematically working through text data. More structured qualitative researchers often use predetermined codes in data analysis. These can be contrasted with inductively derived codes generated from the data (as in Glaser and Strauss's grounded theory model). Some researchers work with both these types of codes for analysing their data. There is also the use of codes at different levels of inclusiveness, such as the distinction made by Willms and Johnson (1996, p. 80) between hierarchical and non-hierarchical coding. Codes can incorporate different levels of theoretical abstraction, as in Miles and Huberman's distinction between descriptive and pattern codes (1994, pp. 57–61), or Strauss and Corbin's typology of open, axial, and selective codes (1990, pp. 61–142).

10.5.2.1 Labelling codes

There are a number of ways of labelling codes. Numeric labels can be used. Ethnographic researchers working in a foreign language or trying to become familiar with a subcultural idiom or native language, may be interested in using Indigenous labels as codes because of the difficulty of making translations at this level of data analysis. In *The Ethnographic Interview* (1979, pp. 17–24), James Spradley discusses the importance of native language terms in ethnographic research.

It may be necessary for researchers to make up their own terms in order to avoid premature stereotyping of the data into established categories of analysis. Strauss and Corbin (1990, pp. 67–9) write about this process and its advantages. It is also possible to use terms from the existing literature in the researcher's field of study (Strauss and Corbin 1990, pp. 48–56). This is necessary in the more structured precoding designs, and may facilitate comparative analysis with others' research, but goes against the principle of inductively derived codes which is important to more naturalistic research projects.

The process of coding is part of data analysis, but it has to be complemented by critical reflection about the connections between the data and their meaning. Coding alone cannot produce or test theory.

10.5.3 An example of data display: typologies

One example of data display is a typology. In many ways devising a typology is simply a way of clarifying the major issues on which contrasting groups compare and differ or, in the words of positivist social scientists, a way of summarising 'the intersection of two or more variables' (Babbie 1998, p. 188).

Typologies can be derived from the subjects' own words or concepts, or may be derived from the researcher's interpretation of those concepts. For example, in a hypothetical study examining the sociocultural factors influencing mothers' participation in a child immunisation program in rural India, we may be interested in examining the relationship between program participation and practice of traditional preventive health measures.[6] The typology of mothers' immunisation practices we construct could then look like:

Table 10.1 Immunisation typology

	Immunisation	*No Immunisation*
Traditional care	Protectionists	Traditionalists
No traditional care	Modernists	Non-protectionists

Note the 'sample' has been divided up into four groups of mothers:

1 *Protectionists* use both the immunisation program and traditional methods.
2 *Traditionalists* use traditional methods only.

3 *Modernists* use the immunisation program only and no longer rely on traditional methods.
4 *Non-protectionists* use neither traditional methods nor the immunisation program.

Comparing and contrasting the emerging themes arising from these four groups may lead to important insights into what factors are important determinants of subsequent health behaviour. For example, women adhering to traditional measures may cite distrust of needles or indicate their reliance on the advice of traditional healers or senior female relatives more often than women participating in the immunisation program. Such factors may provide the basis for developing a theory that not only explains their behaviour, but also differentiates between women who do and do not participate.

Consistent with the iterative process inherent in qualitative data analysis, such typologies can be used both as endpoints in themselves (by acting as a means to summarise results) and as a means of identifying subgroups of interest that can then be involved in further qualitative enquiry, for example in the contrasting groups design discussed in chapter 12. Using the above typology, the researcher may decide to undertake more interviews among only traditionalists and modernists, or among only protectionists and non-protectionists. Alternatively, the researcher may undertake purposive sampling to further identify and explore issues among one particular subgroup.

10.5.4 Computer-assisted data analysis

A qualitative research project on a medium to large scale (say, by one or two researchers collecting data full time over a period of several months to a team research project over a period of years) may yield vast amounts of textual data. Qualitative data have to be written down (visual data aside). As Pfaffenberger has pointed out:

> to analyze this textually captured data is to engage in a paper-pushing enterprise of monstrous proportions. If the job is to be done properly, the researcher is in for such tormenting jobs as manually searching thousands of pages of notes for an obscure passage, recoding all the field notes to suit a newly discovered framework of coding categories, and rewriting the notes to flesh out events from memory (1988, p. 12).

Such cumbersome tasks of data analysis were also the fate of quantitative researchers until liberated by computer statistical packages in the 1960s (Pfaffenberger 1988, pp. 12–13). Now, large data sets can be readily analysed with the assistance of programs such as Statistical Package for the Social Sciences (SPSS).

There are now a number of qualitative data analysis programs widely available which may have a similar revolutionary effect on the producers of large-scale qualitative data sets. For maximum efficiency, the decision to use a data analysis program should be taken before data collection begins so that the text (long version of fieldnotes, transcripts) can be directly word-processed.

The advantages of using computer programs for qualitative data analysis have to be balanced against the disadvantages. Computer programs do not replace the labour-intensive process of familiarising oneself with the primary data, which is the foundation of all good qualitative data analysis. The programs may be time-consuming to learn, which has to be weighed against the amount and type of data to be managed. The more complicated programs may require technical back-up that is not available under field conditions. Some methodological approaches may not require extensive sorting, searching, and retrieval of information. It is important to keep the potential of these programs in perspective—whatever their benefits, they do not do the thinking for the researcher.

Many qualitative research textbooks now contain surveys of the available qualitative data analysis software (see, for example, Miles and Huberman 1994, pp. 311–17), although by the time such publications are printed they are often not up-to-date on the latest developments.

10.5.5 Statistical analysis

In general, it is not appropriate to apply statistical techniques used in purely quantitative studies (the calculation of odds ratios, attributable fractions) in a qualitative research design. However, simple descriptive statistics can be applied to the results derived from content analysis. For example, using the typology described previously, we might say that 85 per cent of women adhering to traditional methods felt they should only follow their mother-in-law's advice about what to do to keep their baby healthy compared to 55 per cent of women who participated in the immunisation program. See Weller et al. (1987), Romney et al. (1986), and Dey (1993, pp. 27–8, 48) for further discussion and examples of the use of statistical analysis of qualitative data.

10.6 Triangulation

In keeping with the growth of new knowledge perspectives in recent decades, triangulation has evolved from a strategy grounded in the notions of validity, reliability, objective truth, and bias, to a broad-ranging strategy which also encompasses the qualitative concerns for depth, multiple perspectives, and complex meanings. During this evolution, there has been much debate on philosophical and epistemological issues, including the extent to which qualitative and quantitative paradigms can be combined, the nature of reality, and whether the aim of triangulation is to enhance validity or some alternative (Denzin 1978 and 1989; Patton 1980; Lincoln and Guba 1985; Silverman 1985; Fielding and Fielding 1986; Rizzo and Corsaro 1995).

In this section we move from a discussion of triangulation as a strategy for achieving quality in the more structured qualitative studies to the criteria that can be used in less structured qualitative research. In TD research, where quantitative and qualitative methodologies are often combined in various ways, it is possible to use the whole spectrum of criteria and strategies for ensuring quality (see 10.8). Some of these designs and the ensuing issues are discussed in chapters 11 and 12.

10.6.1 Triangulation and TD validity

The term 'triangulation' derives from the navigation and military strategy of using multiple reference points to locate an object's position. According to the principles of geometry, multiple viewpoints allow for greater accuracy. Similarly, it is argued, researchers can improve the accuracy of their judgments by collecting different kinds of data bearing on the same phenomena (Jick 1983, p. 136):

> Triangulation is a strategy for ensuring that a study's findings are not the artefact of a single method, a single source, or a single investigator's biases. It is, therefore, a means of increasing confidence in the validity or authenticity of the data and its interpretation (Willms and Johnson 1996, p. 5).

Triangulation is not a method in itself but, as Willms and Johnson indicate above, a methodological strategy.[7] Insofar as different disciplines tend to utilise certain methods in preference to others, learning the skills (and hazards) of triangulation is essential to a TD approach. Willms and Johnson (1996, p. 5) give a clear explanation of the types of triangulation encountered in social research.[8]

10.6.1.1 Triangulation of data sources

This involves comparing the consistency of different pieces of information. Examples include:

- comparing public and private comments
- checking for consistency in people's behaviour
- comparing information obtained through interviews and observations with that from written documents.

10.6.1.2 Researcher triangulation

Researcher triangulation involves using more than one person to collect and analyse data, and is therefore a feature of all TD team research. Examples include:

- using several interviewers so that results cannot be attributed only to a particular interviewer's style or personal characteristics
- several people making observations of the same phenomena
- several people independently analysing the same qualitative data set and comparing their findings
- inviting the subjects of the study to review the findings.

10.6.1.3 Methods triangulation

Methods triangulation involves the use of more than one method to collect data. Examples include:

- comparing data from one or more qualitative methods with data from one or more quantitative methods
- using several different qualitative data methods (focus groups, indepth interviews)
- using a number of different sampling strategies.

In TD research, the process of drawing information from many sources and methods and examining data from multiple researcher perspectives as the process moves through the three TD levels generates a deeper understanding of the health problem and generates useful knowledge for interventions. The following example from the Care Aware project described in chapter 7 shows how processes of triangulation can work in TD research.

Box 10.3 Triangulation in the Care Aware project

The Care Aware project provides an example of TD triangulation in research about influences on accidental exposures to needlestick injuries among health care workers. The TD team used a variety of methods and data sources to build a profile of the occurrence of accidental exposures including interviews with health workers who had sustained accidental exposures, audits of needle disposal bins to count the numbers of recapped needles, focus groups with health workers, and examination of routine exposure surveillance data collected in local hospitals.

The team found that the majority of people were compliant with safety guidelines at the time of their exposure. There were over 1500 recapped needles in the needle disposal bins with no report of recapping injury. Less than 5 per cent of reported needlesticks were attributed to recapping practices. These findings were in disagreement with the published literature which claimed that non-compliance with the safety guidelines, particularly the act of recapping needles, was the major contributor to accidental exposure. This discrepancy was posed to focus group discussions of health workers for their comment. Analysis of these discussions led to the identification of mindlessness or automatic pilot as a determinant of accidental exposure among health workers.

The Care Aware team had collected evidence through preliminary phases of the research with health workers that automatic pilot was understood and acknowledged as part of working life. Other informal information gathered throughout the course of the project validated the understanding gained through formal data collection and analysis. Notably, on the first day of intervention, before any Care Aware materials had been distributed, team members noticed one health worker in the target group wearing a humorous badge that said 'On automatic pilot'.

The transdisciplinary nature of the Care Aware team meant that processes of researcher triangulation were built into all of the team's activities. As discussed in chapter 7, the team planned and discussed each step of the project. New insights were examined from each member's disciplinary perspective. In essence, the multiple theoretical and disciplinary perspectives of the Care Aware team members resulted in each new piece of data being examined in terms such as 'Does this make sense to me?' and 'Does this make sense in relation to the other data I have seen?' The process of involving all members of the team was particularly important when concepts from the social psychology literature (such as mindlessness) were introduced as the basis of possible educational interventions. The non-psychologists (two physicians and one infection-control nurse consultant) in the Care Aware team gave immediate feedback on whether these concepts would be credible and accessible to health workers. Further, the team developed a shared understanding of occupational exposure that emerged from the activities of the project and that was not dominated by any one disciplinary perspective.

10.6.2 Limitations of triangulation

Willms and Johnson (1996, p. 5) claim that triangulation is 'a means of increasing confidence in the validity or authenticity of the data and its interpretation'. However, with the growth of new, non-positivist knowledge paradigms, critiques of triangulation have emerged. For example, Shadish argues that 'validity is a property of knowledge claims, not methods' and 'no method guarantees validity' (1995, p. 420). Although it seems sensible to use a range of triangulation strategies, there is still no guarantee that this will produce high-quality research. Fielding and Fielding have criticised multiple triangulation on the basis that:

> Theoretical triangulation does not necessarily reduce bias, nor does methodological triangulation necessarily increase validity . . . We should combine theories and methods carefully and purposefully with the intention of adding breadth or depth to our analysis but not for the purpose of pursuing 'objective' truth (1986, p. 33).

Norman Denzin is a prominent exponent of triangulation whose formulations have evolved over the years in the light of the debates about whether the aim of triangulation is validity or some other alternative. In early formulations, Denzin (1978, p. 304) characterised the aim of methodological triangulation in the following terms:

> methodological triangulation involves a complex process of playing each method off against the other so as to maximise the validity of field efforts.

A decade later, taking account of various critiques and discussions of his earlier formulation, including those of Fielding and Fielding (1986), Denzin's position had changed. Denzin, like other qualitative researchers, had become more receptive to the new paradigms and perspectives of scientific knowledge that developed in the 1970s, rejecting positivism in social research. This has led to the development of a broader range of criteria for assessing the quality of qualitative research:

> The goal of multiple triangulation is a fully grounded interpretive research approach. Objective reality will never be captured. In depth understanding, not validity, is sought in any interpretive study (Denzin 1989, p. 246).

Most researchers now agree that triangulation in itself should not be viewed as a guarantee of the validity or truthfulness of a study. Fielding and Fielding argue that the value of triangulation resides in its effects on the researcher:

> Triangulation puts the researcher in a frame of mind to regard his or her own material critically, to test it, to identify its weaknesses, to identify where to test further doing something different (1986, p. 24).

These goals can be achieved in a number of ways, and in the next section we present some criteria for assessing the quality of qualitative research. These criteria can be used in the implementation of new research projects as well as the critical appraisal of others' research. The criteria have greater generality than triangulation strategies, and can be applied to research from a range of knowledge paradigms and perspectives (Treloar et al. 2000).

10.7 Assessing the quality of qualitative research

Qualitative and quantitative researchers pose the same fundamental question about their studies: Can we trust the data and the inferences drawn from them? The quality of a quantitative study, conducted using positivist or postpositivist[9] paradigms of scientific knowledge (Guba and Lincoln 1994), such as the epidemiological study designs discussed in chapter 9, is judged by assessing its validity and reliability. Conventional standards for reporting (for example, Begg et al. 1996) and assessing (for example, Darzins et al. 1992) quantitative studies provide a framework for evaluating quality and some guidelines for the generalisability of the results.

Qualitative research is informed by a variety of knowledge perspectives. These may include positivism and postpositivism, but also interpretivist and postmodern perspectives.[10] Each of these perspectives has its own criteria for assessing quality (Denzin and Lincoln 1994, chapter 6). The more structured types of qualitative research are more likely to be informed by positivist perspectives. Practitioners are likely to use strategies for ensuring quality that are also found in quantitative studies. As the style of research moves towards the less structured, it is more likely to draw on the knowledge perspectives of postpositivism, interpretivism, and postmodernism. From these perspectives, the richness of the data and their ability to generate theory, their empirical groundedness in wider contexts of social life, their incorporation of multiple subjective understandings, and the reflexivity of the researcher are all-important criteria of quality.

In quantitative research, specified criteria exist for assessing the validity or trustworthiness of the data (Darzins et al. 1992). However, qualitative researchers draw on a range of perspectives that inform their studies. This makes writing a prescriptive set of guidelines difficult. We have attempted to synthesise the main issues across different perspectives and highlight where differences exist.

The checklist was devised for assessing the quality of written research reports (similar to the process of critical appraisal used widely in quantitative research). These guidelines can also be used to plan and conduct research to meet the anticipated criteria of quality.

10.7.1 Is the purpose of the study clearly stated?

A clearly stated purpose is critical to the reader's understanding of a research report as it provides a context and generates a set of expectations for evaluation of the report (Knafl and Howard 1984). The researchers should state how the purpose of the study was initially formulated. They should also indicate the nature and direction of any alterations to this purpose as the research developed (Cobb and Hagemaster 1987, p. 139). Likewise, when undertaking qualitative research, clarity of purpose is the first step in the development of a useful and high-quality project (see 10.3.1 above).

10.7.2 Is an appropriate rationale provided for using a qualitative approach?

The rationale for using a qualitative approach should detail why and how well the method(s) can address the study purpose, why the chosen approach is better than other approaches (Banister et al. 1994, p. 3) and how the approach relates to the existing knowledge concerning the study purpose (Davies et al. 1995, p. 265). Box 10.4 explains how qualitative methods were chosen for evaluating India's National Pulse Polio Immunisation program, which was administered to 120 million children twice in 1997.

Box 10.4 INDIACLEN National Pulse Polio Immunisation Program Evaluation

The government of India implemented a National Pulse Polio Immunisation Program involving the mass administration of trivalent oral polio vaccine to children 0–5 years of age. Each cycle of immunisation took place on two National Immunisation Days 6 weeks apart, with vaccine administered to 120 million children on each occasion. Extensive mobilisation of social and logistical resources was required to staff and equip over 6 million immunisation posts and to ensure that targeted children attended. During 1997–98, the All-India Institute of Medical Sciences and the Indian Clinical Epidemiology Network evaluated the polio program using qualitative methods (Arora, Lakshman, Patwari et al. 1999). The study covered twenty-four districts across fifteen Indian states and involved highly diverse cultural and geographical settings.

The evaluation designers believed that indepth interviews and focus group discussions were the most appropriate methods to identify successful features in the program's management, intersectoral coordination, and social mobilisation. Opinions were gathered from 2163 respondents ranging from the prime minister and other central and state policy makers and bureaucrats, to key informants involved in regional and local planning, to mothers and other users of community services.

The evaluation concluded that the effects of the polio eradication on the health system had mostly been positive, but that there were 'threats' that had to be recognised explicitly and dealt with preemptively. The investigators indicated that the polio eradication had strengthened management capacity, improved social mobilisation, and increased confidence in the health care system. Nonetheless, better planning was required to minimise the disruptions to the service systems caused by the National Immunisation Days.

10.7.3 Do the researchers clearly outline the conceptual framework (if any) of the study?

Some researchers will seek to analyse the data deductively, that is, from an existing conceptual framework (for example, Treloar 1997) whereas others will generate theory from the data in a more inductive or grounded manner (Strauss and Corbin 1990). Qualitative reports should clearly state whether the interpretation emerged from the data (in the grounded theory tradition) or from a planned theory-testing investigation. Some health research has a more descriptive purpose and does not aim to use, develop, or test a particular theory or conceptual framework.

Evidence of iteration (a systematic procedure for cycling between data, interpretation, and theory building) should be presented (Stiles 1993, p. 605). In TD team research, the iterative process may be particularly fruitful where researchers from different backgrounds are able to broaden the scope of literature review, and initiate new questions, methods, and analytical procedures.

If the research used a more deductive or theory-testing approach, a review of relevant literature should be included as well as a discussion of how the framework has shaped the analytical categories used as well as the interpretation of data (Cobb and Hagemaster 1987). Researchers using this approach must also be attentive or alive to data which may disconfirm or fall outside the theoretical framework (Patton 1990, chapter 8).

10.7.4 Do the researchers demonstrate an understanding of the ethical implications of their study?

The indepth, open-ended nature of qualitative methods makes ethical considerations of particular importance (Banister et al. 1994, p. 152). All empirical research should be guided by general ethical principles in recruitment of participants, data collection, analysis, and dissemination of findings. As a general principle, the project should be reviewed and receive guidance from an institutional ethics committee.

Because of the potentially personal nature of information collected and the level of disclosure, researchers should demonstrate care in defining the boundaries of their role, in allowing appropriate debriefing, and in offering referral to professionals where necessary. Anonymity and confidentiality are especially important because of the often smaller number of participants involved in qualitative research. Care should be taken to remove any identifying information from stored data and written reports (Britten et al. 1995, p. 110). Where appropriate, researchers should disclose the source of their funding.

10.7.5 Is the sampling strategy appropriate and will the sample represent the target group?

The researcher should demonstrate how the sampling strategy aligns with the purpose of the study and provide justification for the sample size. As interpretivist and postmodernist perspectives hold that knowledge is produced through the interaction of the researcher and the subjects in an empirical research project, the relationship between the researcher and subjects should be clearly described. The qualitative researcher should specifically define and describe the target group or issue so that the reader can judge whether generalisations to other groups or issues are warranted (Borman et al. 1986).

10.7.6 Do the researchers provide information about data collection procedures and how they were derived?

Researchers should describe the process of collecting their data and the sources used (information derived from literature review, pilot studies, key informants, popular opinion). How structured are the research methods? The rationale for the degree of standardisation (structured versus unstructured interviews) should be explained.

Research methods may change over time or become more structured as research efforts are progressively focused. The rationale behind these changes should be explained in relation to the development of the research questions.

10.7.7 Do the researchers describe the procedures for keeping data organised and retrievable?

Voluminous amounts of data produced by the iterative nature of qualitative research have the potential to leave researchers with 'data overload' (Miles and Huberman 1994, p. 56). Systematic data management is crucial to efficient retrieval and analysis. Researchers should describe the medium through which the data were recorded (audiotape, videotape, researcher notes), the transcribing process, and the method of verifying transcript accuracy (Banister et al. 1994, p. 169). Where computer programs are used to store data and assist with analysis, these should also be described.

10.7.8 What methods of data analysis are used and are they appropriate to address the research question?

In the absence of formal guidelines, reports of data analysis procedures should give enough details for other researchers to follow and assess the quality of analysis. Information about coding systems used and refinements made to them as well as processes of interpretation should be included. Qualitative research is strengthened when more than one person is involved in the data analysis process (see, for example, Miles and Huberman 1994, p. 64), which is an advantage of the TD team approach.

10.7.9 Do the researchers address the threats to reliability and validity (or 'trustworthiness') in data collection, analysis, and interpretation?

Alternate concepts to reliability and validity such as trustworthiness, credibility, transferability, dependability, and confirmability have been proposed as more relevant to qualitative investigations, particularly of the naturalistic or less-structured type (Lincoln and Guba 1985, p. 238). Many qualitative researchers reject the concept of bias as not a useful way of evaluating their work even while they strive to be as rigorous as possible in the processes of data collection, analysis, and interpretation. Ways in which bias can be avoided, or trustworthiness enhanced (depending on the researchers' orientation) are discussed in Miles and Huberman (1994, pp. 262–77).

The researcher's prolonged engagement with the research data can facilitate familiarity with the context and subject of enquiry. The opportunity to consult with other researchers and debrief with peers opens the data and their interpretation to critique and deeper understanding. Each researcher should maintain a diary of their subjective involvement in the research. This record can become the basis of reflexive analysis in which researchers acknowledge and analyse their own roles in the interactions that produce the research data.

Researchers should search for negative cases or disconfirming evidence to extend the interpretation of the data. Member checks or iterative cycling of the data can be undertaken with participants at a number of points in the research project, for example, checking with participants that the information they gave was recorded accurately, or checking that the researcher has accurately summarised and interpreted the data (Miles and Huberman 1994, pp. 275–7). Various types of triangulation (see 10.6.1) could also be considered.

The researcher should undertake to provide an audit trail which can be used to show that all conclusions drawn can be traced to the data which can be traced to the source (Lincoln and Guba 1985, pp. 319–20). Interpretations of the data should be grounded in the data themselves (Stiles 1993, p. 605) and may use *in vivo* codes (taken from the language used by the study subjects) and quotes from the data to aid interpretation (Strauss 1987). Generalisations from the data should be appropriate and related to the study purpose as well as bounded by the scope of the sample used for the study.

10.7.10 Is there a clearly explained relationship between research questions, data, and conclusions?

Strauss and Corbin (1990) argue that a report of qualitative research should contain a strong and clear analytic story throughout the text. Each decision and activity in the project should relate to this analytic logic and be apparent in the description of the process. In research using positivist and postpositivist perspectives, the analytic logic is linear. In interpretive and postmodern studies, the process of relating questions, data, and conclusions may include a non-linear analytic story. For example, conclusions may be multiple and even contradictory where a number of subjective understandings have been incorporated into the research. The ways in which the write-up of the research evokes the emotional quality of subjects' experience may take priority in some studies over a closely argued analytic story. In applied or action research, the relationship between questions, data, and political outcomes may be an important issue.

Table 10.2 Ten key issues in critical appraisal of qualitative research

Key issues in critical appraisal	*Factors to consider in this domain*
1 Is the purpose of the study clearly stated?	• rationale for study explained • research question clearly presented • context in which results will be interpreted
2 Is an appropriate rationale provided for using a qualitative approach?	• maximise strengths of study design to address study purpose
3 Do the researchers clearly outline the conceptual framework of the study?	• use of theory described (that is, descriptive, exploratory only, imposed on or generated from data) • researchers alive to data outside of the theory/framework
4 Do the researchers demonstrate an understanding of the ethical implications of their study?	• appropriate informed consent • opportunity to withdraw • opportunity to retain data • participants given feedback about the study results • appropriate support (that is, debriefing and referral) available to participants • results anonymous/confidential • approval of institutional ethics committee and disclosure of funding source

Table 10.2 (continued)

5 Is the sampling strategy appropriate and will the sample represent the target group?	• sampling strategy explained and related to purpose of study • relationship between researchers and subjects explained • sample size explained • sample specifically defined
6 Do the researchers provide information about data collection procedures and how they were derived?	• relationship of method to research question • description of development of data collection methods (including revisions, changes in structure, reframing of research questions) • theme/concept list for interviews/group discussions • observation schedule for observation
7 Do the researchers describe the procedures for keeping data organised and retrievable?	• recording of data described (for example, audio tape, written notes) • transcriptions checked for accuracy • use of a software program described
8 What methods of data analysis are used and are they appropriate to address the research question?	• detailed outline of procedures • coding systems and interpretation processes clearly described
9 Do the researchers address the threats to reliability and validity (or trustworthiness) in data collection, analysis, and interpretation?	• more than one researcher involved • prolonged engagement and immersion • peer debriefing and consultation • record of reflexive involvement • search for negative cases or disconfirming evidence • member checks and iteration • triangulation • audit trail and grounded interpretation • appropriate generalisation
10 Is there a clearly explained relationship among research questions, data, and conclusions?	• clear analytic logic • incorporation of subjective understandings and emotions • multiple perspectives included • political outcomes

10.8 Levels of TD research

In the preamble to part III, we outlined a framework for thinking about the levels or stages of TD research about health problems. As we saw in chapter 9, the three levels of TD research can be related quite specifically to five basic epidemiological study designs. As we have indicated in this chapter, different qualitative methods in themselves are not seen as distinct research designs. They are more likely to be used as building blocks in research projects that evolve as a result of the iterative nature of qualitative studies. Thus, particular qualitative methods, sampling strategies, or modes of analysis may be useful in more than one level of TD research, depending on the type of research project and stage of the research process in which they are used. While focus groups, for example, are often used for exploratory research before designing a questionnaire (Level I), they may also be used in Level II research. One example would be the focus groups conducted among hospital staff in the Care Aware study after it was discovered that needlestick injuries were not caused by recapping of used needles: these groups were used to assist in identifying the common conceptual framework of mindlessness that became the key to understanding of injuries and intervention to prevent them. In other words, focus groups were a Level II technique in this context.

Some qualitative methods are commonly used in Level I research, to map out or obtain an initial overview of the problem. Counting of recapped needles in disposal bins in the Care Aware study is an example of direct observation used as a Level I technique. Free-listing interview techniques can assist in defining an area of cultural knowledge with which the researcher is unfamiliar. Analysis of similarities and differences in the lists produced by different informants may lead on to Level II research using methods such as semi-structured interviews. Likewise, some health research may begin with unstructured interviews with a maximum variation sample of respondents on a general topic (suburban residents' perceptions of the effects of environmental pollution on health, for example) as a Level I technique. The study could then move on to Level II, incorporating more structured interviews with specified respondents (public health experts, health practitioners, and sufferers of environmentally induced diseases), and documentary analysis of reports and media coverage, in an attempt to discern the elements of influence operating in the problem context. Whittaker's study of perceptions of environment and health in the Australian suburb of Oceanpoint (1998) (see chapter 12) follows the trajectory from Level I to Level II outlined above.

Qualitative approaches such as participant observation that focus on the integration of a large amount of information from diverse sources and methods over a relatively long period of time find their greatest utility in Level III TD research. The complex and evolving research designs that are characteristic of participant observation are likely to provide the strongest evidence for the existence of causal relationships. Participant observation is characterised most strongly by the qualitative research orientation to producing information that is related to particular social contexts. The focus on understanding the subjective point of view of subjects or informants, and the combination of relatively unsystematic exposure to social interaction and the use of more systematic methods such as structured interviews and document analysis, provides a firm empirical ground for understanding the causal web and carrying out interventions.

Qualitative sampling strategies are not as tightly connected to particular methods and designs as are the sampling strategies in epidemiological research.

Nonetheless, particular sampling strategies are typically used at different levels of TD research. For example, maximum variation sampling is a useful strategy in Level I mapping of a problem. Snowball or chain sampling, where the researcher is attempting to learn about the pattern of social networks in a new social environment, is another sampling strategy that can be useful in Level I research. Extreme or deviant case sampling is more likely to be used in Level II research when the researchers already have an overview of the problem but need to find out about the effects of particular variables that have already been hypothesised to be of significance through prior Level I research. Critical case sampling may be particularly useful in Level III research because it is a way of critically evaluating elements of influence that have already been identified at earlier stages of the research. Critical case sampling was used for this purpose in the Care Aware study documented in chapter 7 and in box 10.2.

10.9 Conclusion

Our aim in presenting this broad overview of qualitative methods and approaches is to equip TD researchers to design projects which will combine the most relevant and useful research strategies, whether qualitative, quantitative, or a combination of both. It is possible to carry out TD research using qualitative methods alone, but as noted in the preamble to part III of the book, some of the strongest TD insights come from the combination of qualitative and quantitative approaches to research. This combination is usually achieved through the formation of a TD team with a variety of disciplinary and methodological strengths. The TD team is oriented to maximising the complementarity of these different orientations, as discussed in chapter 4. The following two chapters demonstrate some of the ways in which TD insights can be achieved through hybrid research designs.

Notes

1 Document analysis as discussed later in this chapter is an exception.
2 Other writers, such as Wadsworth, have specified action research as 'research that *recognises explicitly* its action and change-inducing component' (1984, p. 81).
3 A longer list of types of non-probability sampling can be found in Patton (1990, pp. 169–83).
4 Issues of observation reliability are discussed in more detail in 11.2.4.1.
5 'Sub-culture' here refers to an identifiable group within a larger social order, identified by certain cultural traits such as language, dress, and patterns of behaviour.
6 Thanks to J. Porteus for this example.
7 There are other terms encountered in the research literature that refer to much the same concept, for example, *multimethod/multitrait* (Campbell and Fiske 1959), *context sampling* (Stone and Campbell 1984), and *critical multiplism* (Houts et al. 1986).

8 Willms and Johnson also list a fourth type of triangulation: theory triangulation. However, as Lincoln and Guba (1985) point out, there are a number of reasons why this form of triangulation is both 'epistemologically unsound and empirically empty' (p. 307).

9 Like positivism (defined in chapter 2, see endnote 5), postpositivism is a theory of knowledge that holds that reality is knowable by the observer. Postpositivism recognises that our knowledge of reality is mediated by the observer's interaction with the subject studied. The emphasis in the research process is on a critical approach to data collection with strategies that allow the researcher to attain a more comprehensive and thus accurate understanding of a reality which can never be fully apprehended. For further discussion see Guba and Lincoln (1994, pp. 105–17).

10 See 6.1. For explanations of structural and interpretivist perspectives. Postmodernism is an approach to knowledge that, unlike positivism and postpositivism, holds that there is no fixed, immutable reality governed by universal laws. Rather, the nature of reality depends on the position and point of view of the beholder. Reality is necessarily fragmented, non-linear, and multiple. Postmodernism rejects linear narratives of progress, the emphasis on scientific truth, and the value of scientific rationality. All these styles and values are seen as typical of a now superseded modernity. The emphasis in the postmodern research process in the social sciences is on the reflexive position of the observer who is aware of the boundaries of their own knowledge and refuses to speak from a position of expert authority. There is a recognition of the multiple ways in which signs and texts can be interpreted, and an appreciation of the many voices and viewpoints that make up the social world.

11 Strengthening Cross-sectional Studies through Cognitive and Qualitative Methods

NICK HIGGINBOTHAM, KATE D'ESTE, ANN SAUL, AND LINDA CONNOR

11.1 Introduction

Cross-sectional surveys are possibly the most commonly used research method in the social sciences (Babbie 1989, p. 236) and, as we have seen in chapter 9, surveys are also used extensively in epidemiological research. In chapter 9 we introduced cross-sectional surveys as an epidemiological method for finding out the prevalence of a particular health problem or behaviour. This design is central to Level I trans-disciplinary studies in which describing the characteristics of the health issue is the researcher's focus. Our first aim in this chapter is to go into more detail about the nature of cross-sectional surveys in both epidemiology and health social science. We discuss questionnaire aims and administration, sampling bias, types of sampling, sample size, reliability, and validity and measurement error.

Our second aim is to examine how techniques from a range of fields of study are used to improve cross-sectional studies in various ways. As outlined in chapter 4 (see 4.3.2), Step 5 of TD research involves the combination of quantitative and qualitative methods in the implementation of the problem-based enquiry. Where the research method is a cross-sectional survey, for instance, the laboratory skills of cognitive psychologists can identify questions, topics, and questionnaire contexts that are liable to mislead or confuse respondents, leading to errors in the results of large-scale surveys. In a different way, intensive field techniques, as used in anthropology, can help to make survey questions meaningful to people of different backgrounds and to improve the researchers' access to knowledge and practices that are culturally distinct or where the study population is difficult to identify.

11.2 Types and aims of cross-sectional surveys

Survey researchers have a wealth of published expertise to draw upon for advice about designing and administering cross-sectional surveys (for example, Sudman and Bradburn 1982; Cartwright 1983; Babbie 1990; Fowler 1993; Streiner and Norman 1995; Aday 1996). Our aim here is not to summarise this extensive literature. Rather, we provide transdisciplinary insights (combining cognitive psychology and anthropology) for improving the choice of questions, their wording, the social context of questionnaire administration, and choice of respondents. In this section we note the types of questions commonly included in surveys, the importance of specifying the basic aims or purposes of the instrument, and how the nature of the questions themselves influences how they are administered.

A basic technique in cross-sectional surveys is to use standardised measures for the variables we wish to study (that is, exposure or outcome variables). In epidemiology and health social science, these measures are usually standard questions (with pre-coded response options) asking everyone in the sample to indicate their attitudes, beliefs, behaviours, or personal characteristics (for example, satisfaction with clinical services, use of tobacco, marital status, or age). Epidemiological surveys may also consist of some form of health examination or test. When using quantitative methods, standardised measures are very important as they form the basis for future generalisations. If less standardised measures are used, as they may be in qualitative methods, our ability to generalise the study findings may be more limited, although other aspects of the data, such as their richness, may be enhanced.

Survey instruments commonly include one or more *psychometric scales*, that is, a set of items that aim to measure some psychological process such as depression, feelings of social support, perceived well-being, self-efficacy to perform a healthy behaviour, and so forth. To use psychometric scales appropriately (or any of the measures in the survey), it is essential to know something about how reliable and valid these measures are for the group that one is studying (see 11.3.4). However, the methods of assessing reliability and validity will, to some extent, depend on the purpose for which the instrument will be used: prediction, discrimination, or evaluation (Krishner and Guyatt 1985; Phillips et al. 1998).

Predictive instruments aim to predict a future event such as the occurrence of an illness, attempted suicide, or practising safe sex. *Discriminative instruments* aim to separate different respondents according to some theoretical variable (for example, intelligence tests or personality inventories). *Evaluative instruments* aim to sensitively measure how much change has taken place in the individual over a period of time. Such change may include the change in the severity of depression over the course of treatment, or improvement in rational prescribing among hospital interns. Often a single instrument may be used for multiple purposes. For instance, a quality of life scale can be used as a discriminative instrument when comparing different groups of individuals (see, for example, Kaplan 1994) and as an evaluative instrument when assessing changes in individuals over time (see, for example, Byles et al. 1996).

Whether the survey instrument is used for the purpose of prediction, discrimination, or evaluation, the subject matter of the questions posed to the survey respondents will require an appropriate method of administration. Mode of administration is also determined by the characteristics of those to be surveyed. Respondents' feelings of comfort and acceptability will vary depending on whether the task is to answer a self-completion questionnaire, a telephone survey, or a face-to-face interview, and whether closed-ended or open-ended questions are posed (Phillips et al. 1998). In studies of sexual behaviour, sexually transmitted diseases, or activities that are not deemed ethical or legal in that society (for example, pregnancy termination), anonymous self-administered questionnaires may be more acceptable and more honestly answered. On the other hand, when complex concepts such as decision-making about treatment options are to be explored, face-to-face interviews with opportunities for probes and explanations are needed. Similarly, telephone and in-person interviews are most productive with elderly respondents who may have vision difficulties affecting reading skills or for those with low literacy in general. For surveys of marginalised people wary of contact with authorities, such as injecting drug users (for example, heroin users), their cooperation with researchers may be limited to informal conversations and observations of behaviour and context. Finally, there are cost implications for each of these modes of administration; face-to-face interviews are usually the most expensive.

11.3 Fundamentals of cross-sectional surveys: sampling bias, types of sampling, sample size, and measurement error

Cross-sectional surveys are identified with the more positivist and structured types of epidemiological and health social science research. Thus, issues of bias, measurement error, and the distanced neutrality of the observer or researcher are emphasised much more than in the types of qualitative research discussed in chapter 10. Researchers using cross-sectional surveys need to keep in mind two major sources of sampling bias—self-selection of study subjects and people's willingness to act as respondents. As well, the researcher will need to pay particular attention to how the sample was chosen, whether the number of people chosen is enough to answer the research question, and issues of measurement error.

11.3.1 Sampling bias

There are two main forms of bias or error in cross-sectional surveys: sampling and non-sampling. Non-sampling or measurement error is discussed in 11.3.4. One source of sampling error results from the fact that the people who can be included in a cross-sectional study are only those who are actually available. This limitation may lead to *self-selection* or *survivor bias*. For instance:

- If researchers wanted to study the prevalence of sexually transmitted diseases among military personnel, they may miss some subjects who had already left the military due to their symptoms.
- Convulsive disorders were seen more frequently in male children than female children in a district hospital in Indonesia. This may simply reflect the fact that people in the surrounding community seek medical help more readily for boys than for girls.

In reports of surveys the *response rate* must be critically examined. A response rate is the number of people who did respond, expressed as a percentage of those who could have responded. People who did not respond to a survey are usually different from those who did. In a survey of alcohol drinking habits, for instance, the people with highest levels of consumption are those least likely to respond. A response rate in the chosen sample of less than 70 per cent may introduce so much bias in selection of the final study subjects that it will cast doubts on the validity of the study.

11.3.2 Types of sampling in cross-sectional designs

A survey sometimes involves questioning an entire population. For example: What do all children in a high school think about cigarette advertising? What was the number of men in Newcastle who enrolled in the Gut Busters obesity-control program in 1 calendar year? However, if a large population is to be surveyed, a sample must be taken. Information learnt about the sample is then applied (extrapolated) back to the larger population, which is referred to as the *reference population*.

Statistical inference is the term used to describe the process of using a sample to make conclusions about a population. For extrapolation of survey findings to have meaning, the sample needs to be representative of the larger population and to have been taken in an unbiased manner. The degree to which the sample represents a population is known as its *external validity*. The representativeness of the sample should be checked whenever possible. This can be done by reporting a comparison of the sample characteristics with the population characteristics (one way to obtain this information being through census figures). Furthermore, the sampling process should always be described in detail so that others can assess the potential biases in obtaining the sample. If possible, characteristics of responders and non-responders should also be compared.

There are two main types of sampling—probability and non-probability. Non-probability sampling was elaborated in chapter 10 (see 10.3) in connection with qualitative approaches to research. Cross-sectional studies, which typically involve large sample sizes and statistical inference, rarely use non-probability sampling. The role of non-probability sampling for strengthening cross-sectional studies is discussed later in this chapter. Figure 11.1 shows the basic steps to obtaining a

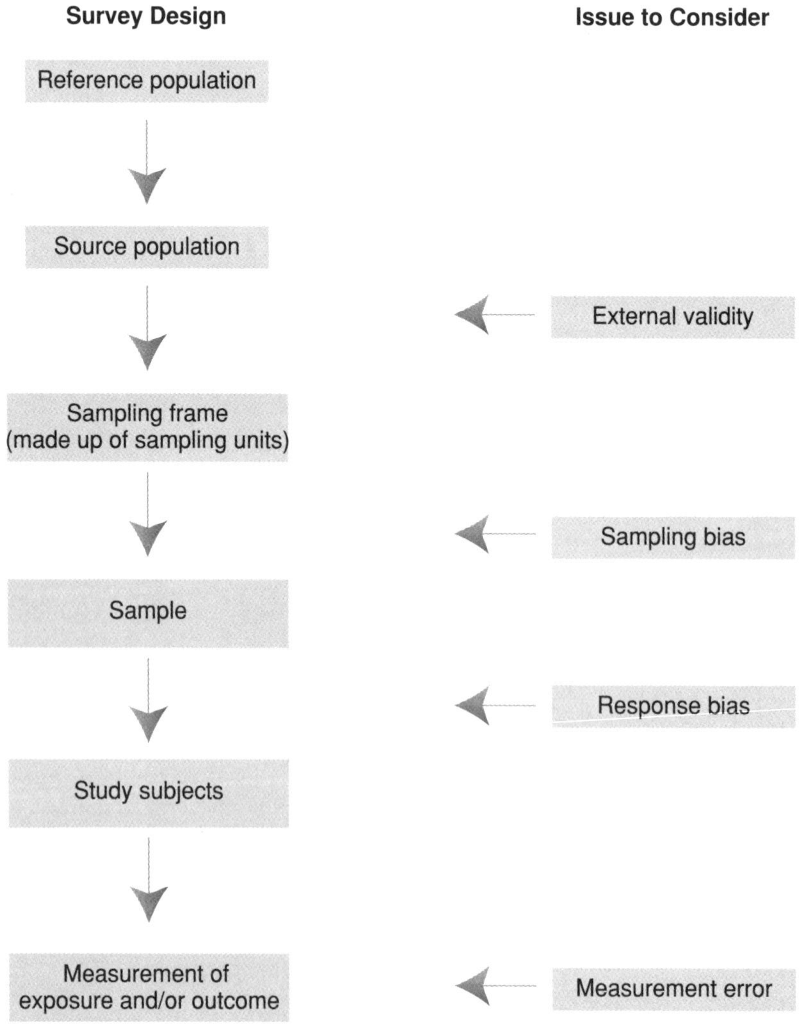

Figure 11.1 Survey design

probability sample and some of the issues to consider at each step. How the investigator can address these issues using qualitative techniques is the focus of this chapter.

11.3.2.1 Probability sampling

In probability sampling, the probability of selection for each person or other unit can be determined. An extensive literature on probability sampling is available, including several excellent textbooks (for example, Kish 1965; Cochran 1977; Moser and Kalton 1979; Schaeffer et al. 1986; Barnett 1991). This section describes the four main types of probability sampling used in cross-sectional studies. Further detail about the calculations which can be performed on each type of sample defined below, and the technical advantages and disadvantages of each, can be obtained from Kelsey et al. (1996).

The *sampling unit* is the unit to be studied and about which generalisations are to be made, for example, a person, household, school, or village. If one wanted to estimate the prevalence of illiteracy in a population, the sampling unit would be people. If one wanted to know the number of households with one or more people who had purchased antibiotics in the past week, the household would be the sampling unit. If one wanted to know the number of villages in a district in which the village leader had endorsed a vaccination program, the village would be the sampling unit. One problem with this method is defining a sampling unit in culturally appropriate terms; this will be discussed a little later.

The *sampling frame* is a list of all the units in the population from which the sample is to be drawn. This could be an alphabetical list of people such as an electoral register or a list of households in the order of their street address. In situations where record keeping is not a priority (for example, rural areas of developing countries), sampling frames have to be compiled by the investigator to ensure reliability (see Naniek Kasniyah's case study, box 11.5). The *sample* is the group of units (people, households, villages) chosen from the sampling frame to be studied.

In order to argue that the sample is representative of the reference population, the aim is to sample in a way that is as random as possible. In other words, to sample so that each unit in the population has a chance of being chosen for the sample that is either equal to every other unit or can be calculated. This can be done in several ways.

Simple random sampling

A simple random sample gives every unit in the population an equal chance of being chosen, using a table of random numbers or a computer-generated selection process. This is simple to understand and carry out. However, it requires advanced knowledge of every unit in the sampling frame. This makes it expensive and difficult in practice for field research.

Systematic sampling

Systematic sampling proceeds by selecting a unit between 1 and k (where k = population size over sample size) and then every kth (for example, second, ninth) unit from a sampling frame. The sampling frame does not need to be known in advance. For instance, the number of patients attending for diabetes education in a year can be estimated and every tenth patient interviewed. It is much more practical for field interviewers to construct the sampling frame as the research proceeds. In a household survey, say, the interviewer might visit every fifth house in the street or examine (audit) every twentieth record in a hospital or health post.

Systematic sampling has several technical advantages. If there is a linear trend in the population (for instance, the houses in the street get progressively more expensive) this method would sample the wealthy, middle-income, and lower-income people. However, if there are peaks and troughs (like the incidence of diarrhoea in the year), choosing every kth month may miss some of the important highs and lows, depending on the starting point chosen.

Stratified sampling

In this method, the population is divided into non-overlapping (that is, mutually exclusive) groups (*strata*) of units that have something in common (for example, age or sex) and a random sample is chosen from each group (*stratum*). Importantly, this method can produce more precise estimates (that is, smaller standard errors) than non-stratified random sampling because the strata consist of units that are similar to each other (homogeneous). The advantage in terms of smaller standard errors occurs if the population is stratified by variables that are associated with the outcome or measurement of interest. Since age and sex are related to most health outcomes, stratification by age and sex is commonly done. Other common stratification variables are location (urban versus rural) or socioeconomic status.

The number of units to be selected from within each stratum can be determined in a number of ways. One method is called *proportional allocation*. In this method the proportions in the sample strata are the same as the proportions in the population strata. For example, assume that we wish to stratify by urban versus rural. If 20 per cent of the population is located in a rural area, then we require 20 per cent of the sample to be from a rural area. If the total sample is 200, we would select forty people from rural areas and 160 from urban areas. However, if we wish to compare rural and urban, then the final number of rural participants may be too small to make meaningful comparisons if we use proportional allocation. In this case we would *oversample* the rural population—that is, have a larger proportion in our sample than is in the population. The follow-on from this is that we then need to weight our analysis so that our final results reflect the population rather than the sample distribution. This is because our sample is not representative of the population as it has a higher proportion of people living in rural areas. There are other methods of selecting numbers within each stratum to minimise the cost in a given situation but they are beyond the scope of this text. Further information can be obtained from Kelsey et al. (1996).

Stratified sampling usually requires advance knowledge of the population and the availability of a sampling frame. It is also possible to use what is termed 'post-stratification' where the final sample (rather than the population or sampling frame) is stratified. The benefits of this are not as good as for stratified sampling, as the original stratification weights need to be estimated.

Cluster sampling

This involves selecting *clusters* or groups of units for study, such as classes in a school or hamlets in a geographical area. Clusters are randomly selected initially, then every member (or sample of members) of the selected class or hamlet is studied. Researchers discussing how to target a skin cancer prevention campaign may want to find the prevalence of hat-wearing among outdoor workers. In a large city, it would be most efficient to select certain workplaces employing outdoor workers (clusters) at random, visit these worksites, and examine all the workers at that site.

Unlike stratified sampling, where the method is deliberately used to obtain more precise estimates or to enable large enough numbers in each strata for comparison, cluster sampling is usually conducted because it is easier administratively or because there is no other way to obtain the sampling units. The important difference between stratified and cluster sampling is that in stratified sampling, units are selected from each stratum or group. In cluster sampling, a random selection of strata, or groups, or clusters is taken. In stratified sampling it is the homogeneity within groups or strata which provides more precise estimates, while in cluster sampling this homogeneity within clusters produces less precise estimates. The amount of homogeneity within clusters can be measured by a parameter or characteristic called the *intraclass correlation coefficient*[1] (if the outcome variable is continuous) or *kappa* (a measure of agreement if the outcome variable is categorical).

The disadvantage of cluster sampling is that special techniques are required for analysis of data. Because of the homogeneity of units within clusters, observations may not be independent, independence being one of the basic requirements for statistical analysis. For example, a dietary survey using a family group as a cluster may find strong similarities in what the adult family members eat. In this case, the units within each cluster are said to be correlated. Adjustments must also be made to the sample size for cluster samples (see section 11.3.3). One method of adjustment for cluster sampling is to calculate what is termed the *design effect*. This is calculated from the formula: $(1 + (m - 1)\rho)$, where m is the average cluster size and ρ is the intraclass correlation coefficient. This factor is also termed the *variance inflation factor* because it is the value that can be used to multiply the variance[2] to adjust for cluster sampling. There are more complex statistical techniques that can be used to adjust for the correlated nature of cluster sampling data (for example, Cochran 1977; Crowder and Hand 1990; Diggle et al.1994).

Stages of cluster sampling

Depending on circumstances, cluster sampling can be performed in one or more stages, described as follows:

- *One stage cluster sampling*: In one stage cluster sampling, all elements of the selected cluster are included in the sample. For example, all students in selected schools would be included in the survey.
- *Two stage cluster sampling*: In two stage cluster sampling, a random sample of clusters is taken and followed by a random sample of units from within the cluster. For example, in each school selected a random sample of students is taken.
- *Multistage cluster sampling*: More complex sampling techniques can also be taken, with several levels of sampling. For example, a random sample of provinces may be taken, followed by a sample of villages and then a sample of households. Finally, combinations of sampling methods can also be used. The initial selection of provinces could be based on a stratified sample, with stratification by rural versus urban, followed by cluster sampling of towns or villages and so forth.

11.3.2.2 Sampling from finite populations

Most of the standard statistical analysis techniques used assume that we have sampled from a large or almost infinite population. Care needs to be taken when sampling from a small or finite population. If the sample size is more than about 5–10 per cent of the population size (*sampling fraction*), then the sample size and variance calculations need to take into account the *finite population correction.*[3] This in effect reduces the variance by an amount equal to the sampling fraction. For example, if we are interested in surveying 200 people to estimate the prevalence of smoking in people over 20 years of age in a particular state or country (with a large population), then the sample is very small relative to the population. The sampling fraction (sample size divided by population size) is a very small value and we can ignore it. If, however, we wish to survey 200 directors of community health centres, from a total of 350 possible community health centres, then the sampling fraction is quite high (200:350). We would then need to use the finite population correction in sample size calculations and analyses. More details can be found in sampling references (for example, Cochran 1977; Barnett 1991).

11.3.3 Sample size

Many different methods and formulae for sample size calculation are possible, depending on what characteristics are being measured or compared in the survey. There are two broad groups of methods of sample size calculation. One is for estimation, the other for hypothesis testing.

If the aim of the survey is to estimate a population parameter (for example, prevalence of smoking), then the estimate should be reported with a confidence interval—usually a 95 per cent confidence interval (CI). A 95 per cent confidence interval is that interval within which you are 95 per cent certain that the true value of the parameter is found. The required sample size will then depend on the expected variance of the parameter estimate and the precision with which you wish to be able to measure it. For example, you may wish to estimate the prevalence of smoking in adolescents, with the 95 per cent confidence interval to be within ± 5 per cent. The confidence interval will then be 10 per cent wide. The sample size formulae for two common parameters—means and proportions—are provided here. Further information can be found in Dobson (1984), Cohen (1988), Pagano and Gauvreau (1993), Rosner (1995), and Daniel (1999), among others.

The sample size required to estimate a mean is:

$$n = \left(z\frac{\sigma}{\Delta}\right)^2$$

Where: n is the required sample size
Z is the value from the standard normal distribution relevant to the confidence interval of interest:
Z = 1.96 for 95% CI
Z = 1.64 for 90% CI
Z = 2.58 for 99% CI
σ is the standard deviation
Δ is the desired precision of the confidence interval.

The sample size to estimate a proportion is:

$$n = \left(\frac{z}{\Delta}\right)^2 p(1-p)$$

Where: n is the required sample size
Z is the value from the standard normal distribution relevant to the confidence interval of interest:
Z = 1.96 for 95% CI
Z = 1.64 for 90% CI

Z = 2.58 for 99% CI
ρ is the expected proportion
Δ is the desired precision of the confidence interval.

For hypothesis testing or comparing groups (for example, quality of life of those with and without asthma), we need to specify the difference to be detected, the variance of the measures, the significance level to be used (usually 5 per cent), and the power required (usually 80–90 per cent). The *significance level* is defined as the probability of rejecting the null hypothesis if the null hypothesis is true (that is, the probability of a false positive). The *power* is the probability of detecting a difference among groups if there really is one (that is, the probability of a true positive). Here we provide the sample size formulae for two common situations. Other sample size or power estimations can be obtained from the references cited above.

Sample size formula for the difference between 2 means (independent groups):

$$n = \frac{2\sigma^2}{\Delta^2}(z_\alpha + z_\beta)^2$$

Where: n is the required sample size *per group*
Z_a is the value from the standard normal distribution relevant to the significance level of interest:
Z = 1.96 for 5% significance level
Z = 1.64 for 10% significance level
Z = 2.58 for 1% significance level
Z_β is the value of the standard normal distribution cutting off probability β (1—power) in the upper (or right hand) tail
$Z_\beta = 0.84$ for 80% power
$Z_\beta = 1.28$ for 90% power
σ is the standard deviation
Δ is the difference to be detected or effect size

Sample size formula for the difference between 2 proportions (independent groups):

$$n = \frac{\rho_1(1-\rho_1) + \rho_2(1-\rho_2)}{(\rho_1 - \rho_2)^2}(Z_\alpha + Z_\beta)^2$$

Where: n is the required sample size per group
Z_α is the value from the standard normal distribution relevant to the significance level of interest:
Z = 1.96 for 5% significance level

$Z = 1.64$ for 10% significance
$Z = 2.58$ for 1% significance level
Z_β is the value of the standard normal distribution cutting off probability β (1—power) in the upper (or right hand) tail
$Z_\beta = 0.84$ for 80% power
$Z_\beta = 1.28$ for 90% power
ρ_1 is the expected proportion in group 1
ρ_2 is the expected proportion in group 2

As a general rule, the sample size will *increase* if:

- the difference to be detected between groups (effect size) *decreases*
- the power *increases*
- the significance level *decreases*.

Two final points can be considered when calculating sample size. The first is that the sample size for hypothesis testing (or comparing two groups) is based on equal numbers in each group. If one group is larger than the other, this needs to be taken into consideration using the formula:

$$N = \frac{1}{4}\left(\frac{1}{Q_1}+\frac{1}{Q_2}\right) N_e$$

Where: N is the total number of subjects adjusted for unequal sized groups
N_e is the total number of units required with equal sized groups
Q_1 is the proportion of units in group 1
Q_2 is the proportion of units in group 2.

The second point is that the sample size calculations assume independent observations, which may not be the case when we have cluster sampling. For cluster sampling, the sample size calculated needs to be multiplied by the design effect (the formula described in the section on cluster sampling). The value of ρ can be obtained from the literature, from previous work, or from a pilot study. In some cases it may be necessary to make an educated guesstimate and calculate sample size for a variety of different circumstances. The most appropriate sample size can then be a compromise between feasibility and having enough numbers to do appropriate analysis and make meaningful conclusions.

Several computer programs (for example, PS, nQuery) are available to calculate sample size and power. (See the review of this software by Thomas and Krebs 1997; also see latest website, http://www.mc.vanderbilt.edu/prevmed/psintro.htm, for PS program.)

11.3.4 Reliability, validity, and measurement error

How do transdisciplinary researchers know that the instrument they plan to use for a cross-sectional survey will work well as a measurement tool? To be working well quantitative measurements must be accurate, precise, reproducible, and self-consistent; only then can one safely compare the scores of different individuals and have confidence about drawing conclusions based on differences between groups. In other words, the scale must have good *reliability*. There are four main types of reliability: test–retest reliability, interobserver reliability, internal consistency, and responsiveness.

The second essential quality of a psychometric scale is *validity*: the extent to which the scale successfully measures the construct (that is, theoretical domain) that it is supposed to measure. A scale with low reliability, in which the scale score includes a lot of measurement error (random or systematic), can never be valid. However, having a highly reliable scale does not ensure validity since it may still not be measuring what is intended. For example, a researcher may believe that diabetic patients' knowledge about good dietary habits reflects actual eating habits. She could develop a highly reliable questionnaire that assesses diabetic respondents' knowledge about the importance of a low-salt diet, but despite the high reliability, the validity of the questionnaire as a measure of eating habits could be poor. As many studies have shown, knowledge about good diet may not reflect actual eating habits. Typically, validity is much harder to assess than reliability. In many published studies, researchers only assess the reliability of the scales they use and make no attempt to establish validity. This is a serious problem that casts doubt on the accuracy and importance of their research results.

11.3.4.1 Reliability and measurement error

Test-retest reliability (sometimes called repeatability) is assessed by administering the instrument to the same group of subjects twice and then comparing the results. A scale has good test–retest reliability if respondents who experience no change in the target condition assessed by the scale have the same results (score) with repeated administrations of the scale. If the survey measure has poor repeatability, one is uncertain whether change scores are due to real change (for example, caused by the impact of an intervention) or simply fluctuation in the measure. The time between the first and second administration of the instrument is typically 1–2 weeks. The time may be shorter if the characteristic assessed changes rapidly (for example, physical fitness of students in an exercise class), or longer if the characteristic is expected to be stable over prolonged periods (for example, diagnosis of a chronic condition). The subjects used to assess the test-retest reliability of the instrument must be similar to those used in the main study. Kappa statistics (Cohen 1960; Chinn and Burney 1987; Donner and Eliasziw 1992; Freedman et al.

1993) are used to estimate test-retest reliability if the outcome is a categorical variable (for example, visit or not visit a healer). Intraclass correlation coefficients (ICC) (Chinn and Burney 1987; Donner and Eliasziw 1987; Rosner 1995) are used if the outcome is a variable measured using a ranking or continuous scale such as the SF-36 Quality of Life Score (McHorney et al. 1993). Although this statistic has the same name, it is calculated differently from ICCs for clustering mentioned in section 11.3.2.1. The sample size required for the test-retest evaluation of an instrument depends on how precise the researcher wishes the estimate of kappa or the ICC to be (see Dobson 1984; Cohen 1988; Pagano and Gauvreau 1993; Rosner 1995; Daniel 1999). Higginbotham, Phillips, and Henderson (1997) have found that thirty to fifty subjects are usually sufficient for acceptable estimates.

Interobserver reliability is only needed if the instrument is completed by external observers (not by the subject him or herself). Interobserver reliability is assessed by looking at the level of agreement between different observers who evaluate the same group of people. Ideally, this should involve completely independent evaluations of the subjects by the different observers, but this is rarely practical, especially when multiple observers are involved in the same session. In most cases two or more observers observe, for example, a series of interviews of behavioural interactions (sometimes on videotape) and then independently code the rating scale based on the interview. The results of the different observers are then compared using kappa or ICC. All the evaluators involved in a study must participate in this reliability check both as interviewers and as coders. Any consistent differences in coding must be discussed and resolved prior to starting the main study. For lengthy studies it is often advisable to reassess the interobserver reliability every 6–9 months during the course of the study and, if necessary, retrain the team of observers to recalibrate their scores (Higginbotham, Phillips and Henderson 1997, p. 7).

Figure 11.2 below summarises our discussion of reliability so far. It shows that the level of agreement between repeated measurements is influenced by variation in the subject (the person may be different at the retest time because of motivation, fatigue, or knowledge) and/or observer variation. *Within* or *intraobserver variation* means random or unpredictable differences in the same interviewer on the two occasions. If the same subject was surveyed by two separate interviewers, disagreement in scores on the same measure may be due to *between* or *interobserver* variation. Systematic differences in the styles of different interviewers can seriously affect the pattern of survey results.[4]

John B. McKinlay (1992, p. 17) comments that survey interviewers affect the quality of results when they conduct interviews that are not carefully standardised (within-observer variability), thus decreasing the extent to which the differences among respondents are detectable in the analysis. He also states that differences between interviewers (interobserver variability) will bias data and reduce validity. In one study, 30 per cent of the variation in key outcome variables (social support

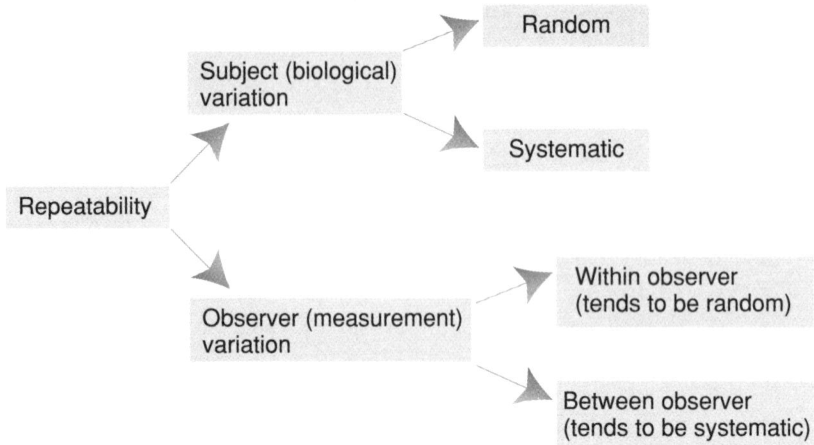

Figure 11.2 Sources of variation in cross-sectional surveys

networks and symptom reporting) was explained by interviewer differences. One internationally respected researcher stated: 'I'd hate to have my data reanalysed controlling for interviewer variability—it could be devastating' (quoted by McKinlay 1992, p. 18).

Internal consistency reliability assesses the extent to which the items in the scale correlate with each other. It shows the extent to which the different scale items all address a common underlying construct (for example, attitude towards hormone replacement therapy). Internal consistency is usually measured by coefficient alpha (Cronbach's alpha). This statistic is an estimate of the proportion of the total variance in the scale scores that is not the result of random errors in measurement. Alpha tells the proportion of total variance due to true score variance between different respondents (see Streiner and Norman 1995).

Responsiveness is the ability of an evaluative instrument to detect change in subjects. Within a clinical population, it is measured by comparing the difference in before versus after scale scores among patients who have improved or deteriorated, to the difference in scale scores of patients who have not shown any clinical change over time. Evaluative instruments that have good responsiveness will be able to detect small but clinically or socially relevant changes in the condition assessed by the instrument. (An excellent evaluation of responsiveness in quality of life measures is found in Buchbinder et al. 1995.)

11.3.4.2 Validity and measurement error

In the health social science literature there is a confusing array of labels for the different types of validity discussed. Moreover, those engaged in the less structured types of qualitative research often reject the notion of validity in favour of the trustworthiness or credibility of qualitative data. These issues are reviewed in chapter 10 (see 10.6 and 10.7). In this section we introduce a few of the more commonly discussed types of validity that are used in quantitative studies as well as in the more structured types of qualitative research.

For predictive scales one is interested in assessing *predictive* or *criterion validity*—the ability of the results of the scale to actually predict what it intends to predict. Does, for instance, the score on a suicide prediction scale actually reflect the likelihood that the respondent will attempt to commit suicide? This type of validity is relatively easy to assess. One could assess the predictive validity of a scale that measures a patient's intention to comply with prescribed medication by conducting a prospective study in which the results of the scale are correlated with a measure of actual medication-taking behaviour assessed at some time after the scale is completed.

For discriminative and evaluative instruments, it is important to assess the content validity and construct validity. *Content validity* is achieved when the scale is made up of a well-balanced sample of items mapping the content domain for the variable. In other words, do the questions that make up the scale give comprehensive coverage of all relevant aspects of the construct the scale is supposed to measure? Judgments of content validity can be made by comparing the range of items in the instrument with information about the content domain gathered through a number of sources, such as the published literature, ethnographic data (for example, domain definition interviews), expert opinion, and/or consensus statements. For example, content validity of a quality of life scale for a particular group may be low if the instrument fails to include social and spiritual dimensions along with conventional measures of physical and emotional functioning.

The most difficult form of validity to establish for a scale is *construct validity*, the ability of the instrument to perform according to theoretical expectations. Do the scores on the scale demonstrate the relationships with other variables that are expected based on the theory about the construct measured by the scale? To test construct validity, one would list some of the interlocking predictions based on the theory (or based on the literature) and see if the data support them (see Streiner and Norman 1995, pp. 150–6). One form of construct validity is *concurrent validity*. The degree of correlation of scale scores with the scores of other, well-validated measures of the same variables (administered at the same time), provides an estimate of concurrent validity. For example, a scale to assess the overall level of health should, theoretically, be inversely related to the number of days taken off work due to illness. If the scores on the scale had a high negative correlation with the days off work, the concurrent validity of the scale would be supported. Similarly, one would expect that knowledge about health-promoting diets and the importance of exercise would be greater among health professionals than the lay public. If the average scores of a scale about level of health awareness were higher in health professionals than in other groups, this would support the concurrent validity of the scale.

In questionnaires that are composed of more than one scale (that is, aim to measure more than one construct), construct validity can also be assessed by confirming, in the matrix of correlations among all items in the questionnaire, the presence of the predicted underlying theoretical variables. This is typically done via *confirmatory factor analysis*. A helpful introduction to this method is provided by Norman and Streiner (1986), while full descriptions of factor analytic methods are found in Tabachnick and Fidell (1996).

Basically, factor analysis determines whether the items that belong to one scale (or subscale in a multiscale instrument) group together (intercorrelate) as expected, or correlate with other items that are not in the same scale. Factor analysis also indicates whether there are more or fewer groupings of items than the researcher predicted. Typically, the expected number of clustered items (factors) is the number of subscales (dimensions) included in the instrument. The number of predicted underlying factors is specified in advance and compared with the number of factors (and their content) produced by the factor analysis (which is derived from the correlation matrix of the item scores). The researcher seeks a high goodness of fit between the observed and predicted factor structures. Generally, an expected factor structure that explains 40–50 per cent of the variance among the items or variables is considered adequate; a scale in which the factor structure explains 60 per cent or more of the variance has good construct validity (Norman and Streiner 1995). For example, when Dupen et al. (1996) developed a new disease-specific Health Locus of Control Scale for asthma, they used confirmatory factor analysis to show that the items written to measure Internal, Powerful Others, and Chance locus of control did group together (formed a common factor) and did not correlate with other subscales.

Epidemiological survey instruments that seek to establish the prevalence of a specific disease (for example, hypertension), other health condition (for example, drug dependency), or health related behaviour (for example, physical exercise) can also be evaluated for their sensitivity and specificity. *Sensitivity* refers to the ability to detect those in the survey who truly have the disease or attribute of interest. A measure lacking sensitivity would miss many cases. *Specificity* refers to the ability to exclude those who do not have the disease. A measure low in specificity would wrongly identify people with the condition (that is, produce a lot of false positives). Unfortunately, it is almost impossible to have a measure that is perfectly sensitive and perfectly specific; there has to be a trade-off between the two. Increased sensitivity will result in a decline in specificity—more people will be picked up who do not really have the disease. In contrast, making a measure more specific may make it less sensitive so that people who have the disease may be left out. Survey designers usually try to find a balance between sensitivity and specificity that is appropriate to the research aims.

Health social science surveys measuring attitudes, knowledge, and behaviours are less concerned with sensitivity and specificity because they do not favour using a dichotomous classification of individuals. Rather, people are seen as having some degree of knowledge, some intensity of attitude, or performing behaviours with some frequency. When measurement is taken using interval scales,[5] more emphasis is placed on determining *concurrent validity* through correlation of the survey scales with similar interval measures of known validity (for example, Dupen et al. 1996).

11.3.4.3 The intersection of quantitative and qualitative concerns

Survey researchers identify validity problems as 'systematic errors', 'artefacts' of the methods used, or 'constructs of *disinterest*' (Judd et al. 1991). Systematic error in survey responses may be due to a number of influences, including recall problems, misunderstanding questions, the cognitive complexity of the task, cultural reinterpretation of sensitive questions, lying, suspicion of authority figures, and courtesy bias or response set (giving responses that one presumes the interviewer wishes to hear).

Survey researchers' concern about systematic errors casting doubt on the validity of their results intersects with the interests of qualitative researchers who have developed methods for overcoming many of these problems. Furthermore, qualitative methods address the ways in which the researcher's (outsider's) perspective articulates with the insider's view (see chapter 10). In the remainder of this chapter, we analyse the sources of invalidity in survey measurement and look at ways in which qualitative techniques, particularly those used in anthropology and psychologists' cognitive laboratory techniques, can assist researchers in anticipating and reducing sources of error when they use surveys. One point to recall from previous chapters is that qualitative techniques (such as indepth interviews and observation) rely on the skill of the fieldworker in gaining detailed accounts of meaning and context. This reduces psychological and cultural misunderstandings and increases the validity or trustworthiness of the findings. However, these techniques do not involve standardised questionnaires—the issues of repeatability and reliability that we have just examined. Designs combining quantitative and qualitative elements aim to improve both validity and reliability. The next section shows some practical approaches that can be used by transdisciplinary researchers to improve cross-sectional designs.

11.4 Cognitive lab techniques for improving surveys

This section introduces qualitative approaches used by psychologists for reducing response bias and measurement error in surveys. The interaction between survey research and cognitive psychology is examined to show both the theoretical rationale and practical procedures that can be used to improve health survey research.

11.4.1 Cognitive lab techniques for improving information retrieval

Cognitive psychologists usually work in laboratories (labs) where subjects, often university students or community volunteers, memorise written materials such as pairs of words that they know they will be asked to recall. In contrast, survey researchers work with large cross-sections of the population and ask people to recall real life events that they did not memorise on purpose. Laboratory studies can measure recall exactly. Survey researchers often have no way to validate what subjects report doing, such as through checking their medical records (Jobe and Mingay 1991, pp. 177–8). Indeed, many surveys, out of necessity, are anonymous. Despite these differences, teams of survey and cognitive laboratory researchers have collaborated to improve questionnaire design with benefits for both disciplines.

11.4.1.1 Cognitive stages in answering questionnaires

When a survey question is asked, the respondent goes through four stages in order to give an answer; problems can arise at any stage of this process (Friedenreich 1994, pp. 1–4; Sudman et al. 1996):

1 understand and interpret the question—*comprehension*
2 search one's long-term memory for relevant information—*retrieval*
3 consider whether the information recalled from memory is relevant and adequate—*estimation and judgment formation*
4 decide what judgments made in step 3 will be disclosed—*editing*.

Our memories about events that take place in time and space are called 'autobiographical' or 'episodic' memories (Sudman et al. 1996). Recall of events from memory is affected by several influences. These include the amount of detail in the survey question, the time period one is asked to recall (some surveys simulate longitudinal studies by asking about past exposures that may have occurred years earlier), how important the experience was to the person (its *salience*), and how often or routine the experience was for the person. Furthermore, survey questions may require information that is *generic* (What usually happens when you go to the doctor?) or *episodic* (How many times did you actually go to the doctor last year? Did she check your blood pressure every time?) (Friedenreich 1994, pp. 1–4).

People suffering chronic illnesses, especially, may have had very many similar episodes of care in the past few years. Large national surveys often ask people about their illness experiences and their visits to health providers, information that is important for understanding health needs and planning services. Validation studies (for instance, checking people's answers against medical records) often show that many chronic conditions are underreported (for example, Means et al. 1989, p. 1). Of equal concern are findings that the use of cancer screening tests such as Pap smears is significantly overreported (Warnecke et al. 1997). Findings such as these can place the validity of survey data in question.

11.4.1.2 Interventions to improve patients' recall

A major source of error is the interviewee's difficulty in accurately recalling specific health events. Based on their study of people's reports of health visits during the 12 months prior to the interview, Barbara Means and colleagues (1989) provided a theoretical explanation for the underreporting of health visits. Subjects convert repeated life events into a generic memory of a 'visit to a doctor' or 'seeing a specialist' rather than using episodic memory, that is, recalling each specific incident. This underreporting of specific events may be complicated by incorrectly *telescoping* events from previous years into the time period covered by the survey. It is useful then to find methods that will improve the accuracy of people's recall of actual events in the reference period (the time period under study). This improves the validity and therefore the usefulness of the survey results.

To achieve this, Means and her colleagues created a two-part intervention to improve the accuracy of subjects' recall. *Decomposition* techniques involve the interviewer prompting for details of travel or waiting times in order to retrieve memories that are specific rather than generic. Construction of a personal time line of significant events, such as illness diagnosis or weddings and birthdays, assists subjects to date their visits more accurately and to distinguish further visits. To see whether their intervention worked, Means and her colleagues compared the recall of experimental subjects who used these techniques with people who answered conventional survey questions. Checked against their actual medical records, the experimental group recalled more actual events and were able to date them accurately to within 15 days. They did not produce false positives or memories of non-existent visits, which may have been created by the intervention method. The researchers concluded that they were using episodic memory to describe actual events.

This intervention demonstrated that a multiple pathways approach can successfully tap into memories of individual events, even when they had been so frequent that the person had constructed a generic memory. This success under laboratory conditions suggests that these procedures are worth considering for large-scale surveys if the increase in accuracy were judged to outweigh the increased cost (Means et al. 1989, pp. 20–1). On the other hand, for very regular behaviour, such as annual health checkups, generic memories may provide better estimates of events than would efforts to remember individual episodes, but could result in overstatements of behaviour when patients forget times when the regular behaviour is interrupted (Warnecke et al. 1997, p. 990).

11.4.2 Cognitive lab techniques for improving questionnaire comprehension

In this section we look at further applications of lab techniques to improve survey question comprehension and assist subjects in retrieving information from memory. Question comprehension can be improved in several ways: by including clear instructions and increasing the length of the question, by simplifying the wording, by asking 'why', 'how', and finally 'when' (as this order fits better with autobiographical memory), and by having a questionnaire administered by an interviewer rather than self-administered (Friedenreich 1994). A vital step in improving questionnaire comprehension has been to test the questionnaire first in a laboratory setting and then undertake pretesting in the field.

The traditional field pretest of questionnaires only detects problems with the flow of questions, the transitions between topics, and the length of the interview. Lab pretests complement these by bringing to light difficulties in the comprehension of questions and the retrieval of information (Royston and Bercini 1987). Cognitive pretests are necessary because the field trials do not detect comprehension problems; questions may be answered quite readily and appear to be satisfactory. The fact that the respondent has misinterpreted an ambiguous phrase or has used a faulty recall strategy will not be obvious and this may cause considerable amounts of response error. Pretests examining the thought processes people use in arriving at an answer will help to improve the questions and reduce the response error (Mingay et al. 1988).

In short, the survey researcher tries to develop an instrument with three essential qualities:

1 The intended meaning of each question is fully understood by the respondent.
2 The retrieval task required of the subject is not strenuous.
3 The response format offers categories that fit easily with the subject's own way of classifying judgments.

The United States National Center for Health Statistics Questionnaire Design Research Laboratory was a pioneer in demonstrating how lab methods can identify poor survey questions and replace them with improved items. The lab's first assignment of this type was to test a knowledge, attitudes, and practice survey of cancer risk factors. In box 11.1 Royston and Bercini (1987) describe how they went about identifying cognitive problems with several of the survey questions and the solutions proposed to clarify the questions.

Box 11.1 Cognitive lab techniques for improving a cancer risk factors survey

At the outset of the interview, respondents were told that the objective was to detect flaws in the questionnaire rather than to collect data on the respondent. They were instructed to comment on any questions that seemed unclear or difficult to answer for any reason. The first round of interviews were conducted in a thinkaloud mode in which respondents were instructed to verbalise their thoughts as they answered questions to shed light on their interpretations of questions and the response strategies used in formulating answers. Because many respondents found it difficult to think aloud as they answered, responses were probed extensively to get at the cognitive aspects of the response process. The following are examples of draft Cancer Research Foundation (CRF) questions and the probes used to get at respondents' thought processes concerning the questions.

- **CRF question: How old were you when you first started smoking cigarettes fairly regularly?**
- Probes: How did you remember how old you were? Are you remembering how old you were when you first smoked or how old you were when you first smoked regularly? What does 'fairly regularly' mean to you?
- **CRF question: Where do you get the most useful information about health care?**
  (Respondent is handed a card with response categories listed.)
- Probes: What does 'most useful' mean to you? (If needed, add:) Does it mean 'believable' or 'information that you would act on'?
- **CRF question: In your opinion, what are the major causes of cancer in this country?**
- Probes: What does 'major cause' mean to you? (If needed, add:) Does it mean 'causes the most cases of cancer', or 'Is most likely to give me cancer', or something else?

These are examples of probes that use follow-up questions to discover people's answering strategies (quoted from Royston and Bercini 1987).

Cognitive interviewing techniques used at the laboratory include focus groups, paraphrasing, confidence ratings, and thinkaloud interviews (Mingay et al. 1988).

Focus group

The lab recruits five to ten volunteers who come in to discuss the subject of a proposed survey or the draft questions. The group may show that a topic is too sensitive to be discussed in a household interview. Some medical terms or concepts may prove to be too technical or difficult to use in a survey.

Paraphrasing

Subjects are asked to put the question in their own words. This shows whether all the terms in the question are understood and, if the person forgets a part of the question, that there may be too many terms for easy recall.

Confidence ratings

Subjects are sometimes asked to say how confident they are in their answers. This indicates whether they found the question difficult to answer and whether or not they were guessing or estimating rather than remembering specific information (Mingay et al. 1988).

Thinkaloud interviews

As indicated in box 11.2, Mingay et al. (1988) record a thinkaloud interview in response to a dietary question. Try and answer this question yourself and compare your own reflections on the process of recall with the example given.

Box 11.2 Thinkaloud interview protocol

Interviewer 'During the past year, how often did you eat turkey meat?'

Respondent: 'Let's see . . . My mother visited me in January . . . she likes turkey so I must have cooked it an extra two times then. I normally make it about once a month, so that would be in January, February, and March [the interview was in early April]. Oh, I nearly forgot—I ate a turkey club sandwich in a restaurant last week so that's twice a month for January to March, an extra couple of times in January and an extra time in March . . . that makes seven times altogether' (Mingay et al. 1988).

This protocol revealed two comprehension problems—'the past year' was meant to be the previous 12 months, but the subject thought it meant this calendar year. She also answered how many times she cooked turkey. She later said that when she cooked a turkey, she would eat it at three meals, not one. Also, in adding up the occasions she had listed, she added up the eating occasions as seven rather than nine. Thinkaloud interviews such as this are now strongly recommended, especially for large surveys, as they can determine what respondents think questions mean, how they retrieve information to form judgments, and pinpoint items that are hard to understand and answer (Sudman et al. 1996).

Mingay and his colleagues conclude that the strengths of the laboratory pretest are that it is economical, detailed, and detects cognitive problems which even very experienced researchers had overlooked. The quiet environment of the laboratory and the skilled interviewer means that problems are really caused by defects in the question, not confusion by an inexperienced interviewer or distractions from household noise or family interruptions. In short, while the field pretest is necessary to obtain frequency distributions (for sample size calculations), and to trial questions on the general population who are less motivated and informed than the laboratory subjects, major cognitive problems can be screened early because *'We can say with considerable confidence . . . that if a question does not work in the lab, it will not work in the field'* (Mingay et al. 1988, pp. 7–8). More recently, these detailed cognitive methods were used to improve wording for sensitive questions in areas such as income, sexual behaviour, and smoking, alcohol, and drug use (Jobe and Mingay 1991, pp. 183–7).

In addition, cognitive lab research suggests several techniques for reducing biases in the final cognitive stage of answering survey questions—the editing stage (Friedenreich 1994, p. 3). Subjects can be motivated to provide honest answers by offering positive feedback about their participation and sufficient time to formulate their responses. Recent experience from HIV/AIDS survey researchers asking sensitive questions about sexual behaviours is also instructive. Subjects are less likely to edit what they say (to make themselves look better) if, after establishing sufficient rapport at the start of the session, the interviewer remains neutral and non-judgmental about the content of his or her replies and uses familiar wording along with open-ended response formats (Catania et al. 1993; see also Boekeloo et al. 1994; Tourangeau and Smith 1996; Turner et al. 1998; Binson and Catania 1998).

11.5 Anthropological techniques for improving surveys

Anthropological fieldwork techniques are ideally suited for improving survey questionnaires. One of the strengths of these techniques is that they were developed for field situations where the investigator works within the social environment of the people concerned. Fieldwork techniques that take account of the complexity of social processes are a way of avoiding the reductionism that we identified in 4.3.1 as a barrier to TD research. Fieldwork techniques (discussed in 10.4.3) provide important contextual information that can be used in various ways to improve cross-sectional survey research.

11.5.1 Qualitative techniques applied to survey development

Typically, anthropological research takes place in the vernacular of the group, where the researcher learns the idioms or local expressions that people use to talk about health issues. Knowledge of local language terms are then fed back into the drafting of survey questions, ensuring that the items are more meaningful for respondents. Using ethnographic research to gain access to local terms is an essential step in developing lists for prevalence surveys of common illness categories that people use to recognise and talk about illness events and seek outside treatment or home remedies (for example, Weller and Romney 1986; Nichter and Nichter 1994).

Chapter 10 presented the main qualitative interview techniques that can be applied to assist the process of survey development. Briefly, *unstructured indepth interviews* and *free listing* allow the survey researcher to become broadly familiar with a new topic. Interviewers can analyse indepth interview data to establish the scope of reactions, the content, the variety and depth of feeling of people's responses in their own words, and how to prioritise material to be included in the questionnaire. After the survey is completed and analysed, *semi-structured interviews* can illuminate relationships between variables, differences between subgroups, and factors that were not measured in the survey. As shown by the cognitive lab examples above, *structured indepth interviews* in the form of probes and thinkalouds can help pretest survey questions.

Bauman and Adair (1992) suggest an important role for focused as well as clinical interviews in survey development. *Focused interviews* use a written or visual (film or video) trigger to start discussion (see, for example, Nichter and Nichter 1994). Four kinds of data are usually collected—the range of responses, their specific content, the depth of reaction, and any personal factors that appear to influence the person's response. This method might be considered when developing recruitment letters, questionnaire instructions, consent forms, new measures, or interview formats (for example, telephone surveys). An understanding of people's reactions to such triggers may improve participation rates in surveys or even recruitment to community interventions or clinical trials. *Clinical interviews* are intended to establish the presence or absence of psychological or physical conditions. As the interviewer generally has a hypothesis in mind, the questions are initially unstructured but they become more focused as the clinician moves towards a diagnosis or conclusion. Survey researchers would use clinical interviews to elicit information about psychological symptoms or to validate standard measures of mental or physical health conditions.

Bauman and Adair (1992) outline a study where *ethnographic interviewing* was used prior to designing a quantitative survey to measure social support among mothers with chronically ill children (see box 11.3). This sequence (qualitative first, quantitative second) appears to conflict with the cognitive lab authors' argument that laboratory testing of items should precede field tests (Mingay et al. 1988). However, we should not confuse field tests of prepared items (following lab work) with field explorations of cognitive domains. Often, ethnographic interviewing or focus group work comes first in order to define the domain of knowledge that potential subjects have, including categories of cultural experience about which questions can be formulated. Once cultural domains are delineated, then items can be written capturing some aspect of such experience.

Box 11.3 Ethnographic interviews used to develop a social support questionnaire

Bauman and Adair (1992) offer an instructive example of the use of ethnographic interviewing to inform questionnaire construction. They designed a questionnaire study to find out the availability, types, sources, and adequacy of social support among African-American and Puerto Rican mothers of children with chronic illnesses. Before designing the questionnaire, though, ten mothers were recruited through doctors and clinics who had experienced caring for a chronically ill child for more than a year.

Women were told that the interviews were designed to find out what the main study should cover. Interviews were between 45 and 90 minutes long. They were taped and transcribed, then analysed separately by two people to identify themes, issues, and word usage. Each interview required 5–6 hours of independent analysis time and 8 hours of joint analysis time. The interviews were designed to alert the researchers to issues that mothers considered important, to give insight into the ways in which social support was planned and accessed, and to help in wording questions for the survey.

Avoiding assumptions
The interviewers had assumed that mothers would find sleep deprivation a problem. Answers to the non-directive question, 'Can you describe what a day is like?' confirmed this, but produced three dimensions—physical exhaustion, mental exhaustion, and broken sleep:

> Sometimes like these two days, I'm being woken up 3 or 4 times during the night. When I cannot go anymore because I'm so tired, then my husband takes her . . . but when he's working, that's another story.

The researchers assumed that the child's illness was a psychological stress, but they had not anticipated that the women's range and depth of involvement with motherhood would lead to role strain in fulfilling their obligations. Strain was particularly felt in meeting the competing demands of other children, in dealing with unpleasant tasks (such as giving injections), and in overload of activities.

> You don't have a life of your own, we live through our children and that's a sad life . . . Atlas couldn't carry what I had to carry the first 3 or 4 years.

Measures of all three types of sleep deprivation and of role strain were included in the questionnaire.

Interview data are descriptive, not analytic
The ethnographic interview produces data on life experiences, thought patterns, metaphors, and structures that people use, without necessarily being aware of it. From descriptions of multiple interactions, it was found that support was rarely asked for; it was exchanged in a reciprocal manner in response to someone's needs.

> Well, just, whenever I have to go out and take care of things . . . we just make arrangements. It's never a matter of asking, we just plan and talk about it ahead of time what she has to do and what I have to do.

It is not likely that people would be able to abstract this idea and report on it intellectually. As a result of the insight into mutual support, the questionnaire did not ask women what people did for them but what people did for each other. They were also asked if these reciprocal arrangements were equal or not.

Language sensitivity

The interviews showed that mothers did not use the word 'problem' about their children; instead they said that things were 'hard'. Problems were practical issues such as picking a child up from daycare or getting away to do the laundry. The impact of the child's illness was difficult or hard.

> It's very difficult, I find it extremely difficult. It's been hard from the beginning and as time goes by it's gotten easier but at the same time it's gotten harder.

The investigators tested this interpretation against the results of previous surveys and it was found that mothers were three or four times more likely to say that parenting was hard than that they had problems.

These results changed the construction of the subsequent questionnaire in several ways. Mothers were conceptualised not as needy dependents but engaged in a web of complex culturally defined obligations. Role strain emerged as an important but unanticipated area. The language of the questionnaire was changed to reflect mothers' idioms—*hardship* rather than *problems*.

11.5.1.1 Better topics

The Bauman and Adair example shows that a key advantage of qualitative research is the way in which it allows themes relevant to the survey to emerge out of the research situation, rather than through the researchers' assumptions prior to using a standardised research instrument. This makes qualitative methods particularly relevant in exploratory research projects. Unforeseen patterns of interrelationship and contrasts between phenomena *from the subjects' point of view* can emerge from unstructured interviews and informal conversations that are conducted in the subjects' social environment and in their own language. Clear examples are Bauman and Adair's identification of the dimensions of fatigue for mothers of ill children and their strong feelings about the nature of motherhood, and the Care Aware team's discovery of automatic pilot as a source of injury among hospital workers (see chapter 7).

The narrative or descriptive way in which subjects are encouraged to talk about their concerns in ethnographic interviews allows certain social processes to be accessed which otherwise the subject may be unable to analyse and report to the researcher. Through anecdotes 'respondents describe multiple instances of the situation under study . . . which together can be examined for patterns' (Bauman and Adair 1992, p. 19). In this case, they are referring to the growth of their understanding that mothers seldom request help as such. Mothers have exchange relationships with members of support networks rather than dependence upon others. Discovery of this pattern using qualitative methods informed the way the topic was conceptualised and questions were constructed in relation to mothers' need for assistance.

11.5.2 Improving cross-cultural sensitivity of survey questions

The survey process is fundamentally a social encounter; in interviewer-administered surveys people are asked questions in a situation akin to ordinary conversation and follow the language and social customs governing conversations (Sudman et al. 1996, p. 245). Therefore, people's understanding of survey questions are affected by personal and interpersonal factors as well as the questionnaire context itself—that is, instructions, order of items, response choices offered, respondent's previous answers, and so forth. The age, sex, education, social status, intelligence, cultural or ethnic identity, and personal experience of health and disease will all make a difference to respondents' comprehension of the researchers' questions and what they feel is an appropriate answer. In every culture, disclosing an answer (editing) can be affected by the sensitivity of the question, whether a particular answer is seen as socially desirable, what the perceived right answer is, and how confident the respondent is about their answer (see, for example, Stone and Campbell 1984; Friedenreich 1994, pp. 1–4).

The survey method was originally designed for respondents in Western industrialised countries where literacy rates are high and participants are familiar with the way in which survey results are applied. Even here there are problems with comprehension and response. This is even more the case when surveys are widely used in health research in developing countries. Various cross-cultural factors can affect the understanding, recall, judgment, and response to survey questions. Kroeger (1983) argues that communication problems make survey research especially problematic in cross-cultural research and that anthropological expertise in cross-cultural communication would improve the validity of the results.

Kroeger (1983) points out that reliable recall can be as little as 2 weeks for structured questions and 3 days for unstructured ones. The recall aids that are used in countries with high rates of literacy, such as health diaries, are of no use where the population cannot read. Standard lists of medical conditions that help people identify illnesses they have experienced are culturally specific and cannot be applied in other contexts unless the local illness categories (idioms of distress) have been thoroughly documented using anthropological methods (Nichter and Nichter 1996).

Illness that does not involve consultation with a doctor or a period in hospital is often underreported. Similarly, some people dislike describing themselves as ill, while others may be more ready to adopt the sick role. Some researchers attempt to minimise these problems by asking people to number the days they did not perform their usual activities. Yet even this measure may pose problems as family, work, or religious demands may lead people to carry on with their activities when they are quite sick.

In cross-cultural situations, the task of completing a survey may be understood differently from what the researchers intend. The assumption that opinions can be sought on all sorts of general issues and the assurance that each individual is kept anonymous and that only collective answers are generated do not necessarily make sense to people who have not encountered them before. Answers to apparently factual questions may be formulated differently in different cultures; guests may count as part of a household, or a new baby may not be seen as a person whose existence should be counted until they are several weeks or months old.

Given the social nature of the survey process, social factors underlie what respondents can express about themselves and why they may resist answering or not be truthful. The presence of other family members or neighbours during the interview may lead to answers that can only be voiced in public. In many societies it is not socially or practically possible to take people away for private interviews, especially women. Giving information may implicate one in political activity. For these and other reasons people are not inclined to answer even factual questions; nor will they acknowledge activities disapproved by the government or religious authorities or even neighbours, including consulting traditional healers or certain forms of family planning.

Proxy reporting, where a mother reports for a child or extended family members report for people outside the household, has been found in industrialised countries to be almost as accurate for attitudes and behaviours as self-reporting (Sudman et al. 1996, chapter 10). However, proxy reporting may not be as useful for estimating disease prevalence rates in a community, as gender taboos and privacy norms may make health events less visible or shared. On the other hand, proxy reporting may yield important information about the family's perception of illness, especially in societies where the family is a dominant social institution.

In short, the social and (often) cross-cultural nature of the survey process benefits greatly from anthropological insights. These insights clarify the domain under investigation, the categories of experience (semantics of illness) and behaviour that are locally meaningful, the appropriate style of conversation, as well as what sorts of people would be suitable informants and appropriate interviewers. Qualitative knowledge of the social context can be combined with quantitative survey principles in order to gain rigour in sampling, measurement, and reliability that allow the results to be both culturally valid and generalisable.

Box 11.4 The use and misuse of surveys in international development: an experiment from Nepal

Large-scale survey research is often relied upon in quantitative research to generate a description of the study problem. However, more valid descriptive data may be obtained using qualitative methods with a smaller sample. For example, Stone and Campbell (1984) highlighted the different results obtained by quantitative and qualitative methods in providing information for fertility and family planning studies in Nepal. An initial study administered a Knowledge, Attitudes, and Practices (KAP) study to over 6000 people. Stone and Campbell then had Nepalese interviewers administer the survey to a purposive sample of Nepalese villagers, comprising people they knew from previous fieldwork. They cross-checked the data derived from the formal surveys with data collected by other methods, including casual conversations or semistructured interviews with their informants, and found a huge difference on many variables. They found a much higher level of awareness for contraceptive methods than did the KAP study. Stone and Campbell comment that money being spent on awareness programs (as a consequence of national KAP studies showing a low degree of awareness) would be better spent on service provision (1984, p. 29).

Stone and Campbell further argued that their small-scale study using qualitative techniques led to a lesser degree of measurement error than large-scale surveys where the anonymity of the investigator and the unsuitability of the questions produced a high proportion of untrue responses. The smaller survey gained greater internal validity. Their review of large-scale national surveys, which used the same basic questionnaire, led them to feel that these problems would not have been reduced by the large sample size due to the high degree of non-sampling error or bias in measurement (Stone and Campbell 1984, p. 29).

11.5.3 Defining the units of analysis

Qualitative methods are sensitive to the wider context in which the phenomena of research interest occur. This can be important for selecting appropriate units of analysis and sampling frames, and in addressing issues of bias, particularly in groups or cultures where the social structure and institutional organisation differs markedly from that of the researchers.

Susan Scrimshaw (1991), an anthropologist interested in the comparative study of household resource allocation, examines the variation in meaning of concepts such as 'household' and 'family' cross-culturally, and how these variations will affect project design. She suggests that quantitative and qualitative methods need to be combined, with what she calls 'exploratory ethnographic work' coming first. Her discussion of definitions of household and family clearly shows the need for culturally informed ethnographic research before surveys are undertaken.

Many surveys are designed using the researcher's definitions of what is to be studied. For instance, researchers who wish to measure a family's material resources and possibly to supplement them in order to improve the children's nutritional status, may run into several problems if they assume that the units of measurement are uncomplicated. Different culture groups make assumptions about what is appropriate for different age or gender groups, so food provided to the family would be divided along these lines. For instance, boys may be given more than girls. A dietary supplementation program may be more successful if people each had access to extra food on a cafeteria system (Scrimshaw 1991, p. 243).

Another common assumption may be that the household is an isolated unit that is easily measured, but this is not necessarily true across cultures. Should close relatives or all members of the common household be counted? Indeed, what does 'household' refer to in different cultures? A couple may receive money from relatives in a distant location or there may be other inputs from the local area that contribute to their level of well-being. 'The family' may be conceptualised as having a 'semi-permeable' boundary; what and how much goes in and out is variable between cultures. These distribution patterns may also be sought in quantitative data (Scrimshaw 1991, p. 244).

It is important to have an understanding of the local or Indigenous meanings of relationships and obligations to obtain valid quantitative data and the anthropologist who knows the community is in the best position to provide them. The anthropologist's position as an insider–outsider may alert survey researchers to other factors that affect resource distribution and nutritional status. These could include privileges given to the children of a first marriage or different amounts of time spent on supervising children's hygiene that the people themselves may not be consciously able to report. Without this culturally sensitive specification of variables, relevant data may be left out of the survey design (Scrimshaw 1991, p. 245).

11.5.4 Identifying the study population

Cross-sectional surveys rely on a valid sampling frame (see 11.3.2.1) for random selection of subjects. In many settings, getting access to such a sampling frame proves exceedingly difficult; incomplete sampling frames result in biased samples of subjects. The researcher may even have to undertake a census of the community in order to enumerate the units of the sampling frame before undertaking random selection. An example of this situation, faced by a medical anthropologist in Indonesia, is shown in box 11.5.

Box 11.5 Ethnographic methods to overcome problems identifying the study population in research on measles vaccination

Naniek Kasniyah, an Indonesian medical anthropologist, planned a survey of Javanese households regarding acceptance of measles vaccine for children under 5 years (referred to as *balita*) using a case-control design. This is her description of the difficulties encountered in identifying the study population before her study could begin (Kasniyah 1992).

The Bayan subdistrict in Central Java was identified as the study location; the next task was to identify the potential subjects. All possible methods for identifying children over 19 months but under 5 years who were not vaccinated for measles (cases) and who were vaccinated (controls) were tried, but all presented problems. For example, the space for immunisation status was never filled out on the child's medical records at the local clinic, and the area vaccinator failed to keep records of those who had never been immunised or the ages of those who had.

Due to the inadequacy of the records held by the medical services and the village government, it was necessary to undertake a household survey in order to establish a reliable sampling frame. Two research assistants carried out the household survey in six villages over a period of 3 months. The village officials suggested that they seek the assistance of hamlet leaders (*Kebayan*), who have an intimate knowledge of the details of the lives of the 175 households in their jurisdiction. The hamlet leaders identified which households contained children under 5 years of age.

The researchers visited each of these households and asked the mother to show them the 'Road to Health' card for each child under 5 years (these cards, issued by the local clinic, show the child's birth date, growth progress, and immunisation status). Nearly all of the women (95 per cent) could produce these cards, so there were no problems unless the card was lost or was a replacement. In some cases, the cards were not accurately filled out and the researchers developed a number of strategies to discover missing birth dates. The immunisation was not recorded for some children although the mothers reported that the child was immunised. Also, cards issued in different years did not use the same method of recording immunisation so the records were not strictly comparable.

To overcome these shortcomings, the mothers were interviewed in order to learn which immunisation the child had received, although often they were not aware of the specific details. In some cases, columns in the immunisation schedule were marked with a tick by the vaccinator because the *balita* had received immunisation elsewhere, but the mothers did not know what the tick meant. The vaccinator himself could not remember in specific cases what the tick signified, so it was difficult to get further information on these cases. Also, *balita* who received measles immunisation during the measles epidemic in 1987 were not recorded, nor were some who had received their injections elsewhere.

From official records then, it was not possible to know the total number of *balita* in the area nor the exact number of known *balita* who had been immunised. In the course of carrying out this survey, the investigators identified problems with all of the data sources that can potentially be used for estimates of prevalence. Using intensive interviewing in the community they arrived at a revised and more accurate estimate of prevalence for measles vaccination in Bayan subdistrict as well as a more valid sampling frame for their case-control study.

11.5.5 Avoiding response bias

Because of the greater familiarity of researchers with subjects in ethnographic research, sources of bias such as courtesy bias can be avoided. Also, errors in recall may be lessened if there are several sessions with the researcher in which the topic can be explored. The immersion of researchers in the social environment of the subjects may alert them to selection bias in cross-sectional surveys that are being carried out or planned.

Helitzer-Allen and Kendall (1992) used ethnographic research done after a knowledge-attitude-practice survey to reveal sources of bias (gaps) in the survey. In their words, 'The KAP–GAP encompasses two sets of behavioural issues: first, the difference between reports of behaviour and actual behaviour, and second, the differences between an intent to act and actual behaviour, (Helitzer-Allen and Kendall 1992, p. 42).

Marilyn Nations criticises epidemiologists for working with models that are too rigid to grasp the complexities of human health behaviour. Nations discusses the contributions that can be made by medical anthropology to the epidemiological task of mortality detection. She points out that in 1970 only 35 per cent of the world's population had reliable mortality statistics available and that this must impact on the planning and evaluation of many health programs (Nations 1986, p. 110). Many studies report serious differences between official figures for deaths, especially for infants, and what can be ascertained locally. In her own study she found that only fourteen out of forty-nine deaths were officially recorded. Such serious discrepancies can bias basic population estimates as well as mislead researchers about sample sizes required for epidemiological studies. Nations suggests that anthropologists' observational methods can remedy this defect (Nations 1986, p. 111).

Accurate information about deaths can be gained from understanding local customs around illness and death and observing the people in the local community who are likely to be involved. For instance, a death may not be announced because of the stigma of illegitimacy or a twin may be buried at home to be near its surviving sibling (Nations 1986, p. 112). In some cultures, newborn infants are not immediately named and given full membership of society—their deaths may go unremarked in formal surveys. An excerpt from Nations's work is given in box 11.6.

Box 11.6 Invisible deaths of 'little angels' in Brazil

In northeastern Brazil, for example, I learned in several instances involving illegitimate births that these newborns were not named, but simply referred to as *angelinhos* (little angels) who, because they had not yet sinned, were expected by parents to fly straight to heaven. *'Little angels'*, I was told, *'were not of this world, but were already in God's keeping.'* Given this belief, it is barely surprising that mothers neglected the secular task of registering their infant's death with the official state registrar or church. Economic sanctions also prevented proper death registration; mothers had to walk to town, pay a registration fee, and risk losing the child's food supplements (her own too, if she was nursing) provided by the state. The deaths of these little angels remained 'hidden' except, of course, to the traditional healer (*rezadeira*) who was treating them, neighbors who lit votive candles as tributes, the local craftsman who built the rustic wooden coffin, the school children who carried the open boxes in processions through the village streets, and the men and cemetery keeper who dug the graves and buried the *angelinhos*. These are not the people who customarily report vital statistics to health bureaucracies (quoted from Nations 1986, p. 114).

11.5.6 Improving the interpretation of survey data

Qualitative methods are not only useful for preparing for survey research. Sometimes survey findings may pose more questions than answers for the researcher, in that the reasons for particular responses may not be evident from the results. In this case, qualitative research may assist in providing an explanatory framework for the outcomes. The *hybrid design* of Helitzer-Allen and Kendall (1992) is a good example of this strategy. Their study included a survey and clinical tests on the topic of malaria infection and use of prophylactic medication, and a subsequent ethnographic study.

Helitzer-Allen and Kendall (1992) began their study because women attending an antenatal clinic in Malawi did not appear to be taking the medicine recommended for malaria prevention (prophylaxis). While 54 per cent of women reported taking chloroquine within the past 7 days, only 29 per cent had blood levels showing that they had taken a large enough dose. To strengthen the research design, this study used multiple methods to find out why women were not taking the recommended drugs. At the clinic, biochemical assays showed whether the women had taken the recommended dose of chloroquine and whether the malaria parasites were present. A questionnaire and collected economic and educational data asked about their knowledge and use of chloroquine, and their malarial history. The researchers then carried out a community ethnography to explore local knowledge and ideas about malaria and pregnancy.

The ethnographic study found that *malungo* (the local word for the aches and pains of malaria) can be caused in adults by many factors, including mosquitoes, wet weather, hard work, witchcraft, airborne pollution, and dirty water and food. Pregnant women were believed to inevitably suffer from those *malungo* that did not require treatment. Small amounts of chloroquine or some paracetamol could be taken for *malungo* from mosquitoes (Helitzer-Allen and Kendall 1992, pp. 48–9).

In some respects the ethnographic results differed from the questionnaire data. Women who had been to school expressed doubts about chloroquine, while those without an education did not. There was a high level of knowledge about the use of chloroquine for cure and prevention—but prevention was thought to be unnecessary, ineffective, and unwise.

The cultural understanding gained from the ethnographic study casts light on the questionnaire findings. It seemed that women reported chloroquine use for prophylaxis out of courtesy to clinic staff. They knew this was the right answer to give staff, but not one that they believed and acted upon, as shown in the biochemical results. In the ethnographic interviews the women were more frank about what they really believed. There was a strong cultural association between bitter, strong medicine and abortion. Chloroquine was a powerful medicine with a bitter taste so women avoided taking it in pregnancy, unless there was strong support from their family. However, they may take it in low doses to relieve symptoms. The ethnography also revealed that some confusing results were due to the way people classified symptoms. Several categories of aches and pains were included with malarial fever; these were believed to be inevitable during pregnancy and so required neither prophylaxis nor cure.

The ethnography cast light on the reasons for low chloroquine use in this community. It confirmed the questionnaire findings that husbands supported their wives in following clinic recommendations, whereas the larger sample in the questionnaire study corrected the impression that more highly educated women were less likely to use chloroquine. Without the multiple methods employed by this study, the problems with malaria prophylaxis would have been overlooked. An intervention based on this improved understanding of cultural commonsense about medicines, *malungo*, and pregnancy successfully increased the uptake of malarial prophylaxis.

11.6 Conclusion

In this chapter we have discussed a variety of strategies that TD researchers can use to combine research approaches and improve the quality of findings of cross-sectional surveys. The basic survey design can be used to establish the prevalence of a problem, to describe its characteristics, or to demonstrate associations among variables. It is thus a key mode of enquiry in Level I TD research of a quantitative nature. We have provided an overview of questionnaire design and administration, sampling methods, size of samples, and problems that can be encountered with sample selection, reliability, and validity.

This chapter has also addressed other issues that may not always appear in standard accounts of survey research. Problems of question comprehension and recall and issues of cross-cultural sensitivity and communication can lower the validity of a conventionally designed survey. We discuss collaborative work that has been done by survey researchers and cognitive psychologists, and by teams that incorporate anthropologists with epidemiologists and health promotion experts. Some examples of these studies have been discussed in detail to demonstrate how such collaborations actually work in practice and to show the impact they have on the design of surveys and the analysis and comprehension of results.

Despite their widespread use, cross-sectional surveys have limitations as a research method. They can only provide information about phenomena from one point in time, although some survey designs have a longitudinal component that relies on recall of previous events. We have shown how cognitive lab techniques can improve this aspect of data quality in cross-sectional studies. Surveys are also a limited tool for explaining complex social processes: the relationships they most readily explicate are of a linear nature. As we have argued in earlier chapters, the relationships between elements in dynamic, complex systems are non-linear. Linear associations among variables revealed by a cross-sectional survey need to be followed up with other methods and research designs in order to identify the elements of influence of a health problem (Level II TD research), and clarify the causal links (Level III TD research). In the next chapter we discuss more hybrid designs—qualitative case-control and contrasting groups framework, and case studies—that are important in Level II and Level III TD research respectively.

Notes

1 A correlation is a measure of how closely related two variables are. Correlation coefficients vary from –1 to +1. A value of –1 or +1 indicates a perfect relationship between the two variables: in graphing the values for the two variables they lie on a straight line. Correlation coefficients close to 0 indicate little or no relationship between the two variables. A positive value indicates that as one variable increases the other also increases, while a negative correlation indicates that one variable decreases as the other increases. The intraclass correlation coefficient (ICC) is a measure of how correlated or homogeneous the units within a cluster are. It is a value between –1 and +1, with values greater than one indicating a positive correlation, and values less than 1 indicating a negative correlation. Values close to 1 indicate very homogeneous units within clusters.

2 The variance is a measure of the variability of the observations and is used in calculation of confidence intervals and hypothesis testing. The main problem with cluster sampling is that the variance is underestimated by standard analysis techniques (that is, smaller than it should be). The variance can be multiplied by the variance inflation factor to obtain a more appropriate (and usually larger) variance.

3 The finite population correction (FPC) is a value which incorporates the sampling fraction of the study. Adjusting by the FPC will reduce the variance.

4 For a highly readable discussion of reliability and validity, see William Trochim's web-based textbook, *Research Methods Knowledge Base*, 2nd edn, http://trochim.human.cornell.edu.

5 Variables can have four levels of measurement. *Nominal* and *ordinal* scales are qualitative in nature, with the former consisting of named categories (for example, men, women, African) and the latter comprising a set of categories that can be ordered on a continuum (for example, thin, normal, fat). *Interval* and *ratio* variables are measured quantities, such as weight, length, or blood pressure. Interval scales achieve equal intervals of measurement in the phenomenon being measured (for example, 5–6 years of age is the same as 10–11 years and so forth). In addition to interval properties, ratio scales have a true 0 point. Hence, scale values represent multipliable quantities (a 3600 g newborn is twice as heavy as an 1800 g neonate) (see Judd et al.1991, chapter 3, for further explanation).

12
Qualitative Case-control and Case-study Designs

JENNY PORTEOUS, NICK HIGGINBOTHAM, SONIA FREEMAN, AND LINDA CONNOR

12.1 Introduction

In this chapter we introduce another two hybrid study designs useful for transdisciplinary research—the qualitative case-control design and its close associate, the contrasting groups framework. These designs are used for Level II transdisciplinary research, where the investigators are seeking to identify the range of causal factors that may underlie a specific health problem. Building upon the framework of the quantitative case-control design, the basic principles of the qualitative case-control design are described. Next we discuss potential problems using this design and some ways to improve the reliability and validity of information gained. The qualitative contrasting groups framework, a type of qualitative case-control design for use with continuous outcome variables, is then introduced. The last sections of the chapter introduce case studies as a flexible design for Level III TD enquiry. Examples of hybrid and qualitative case study designs are discussed.

12.2 The quantitative case-control design

We first described the features of case-control studies in chapter 9 as part of the discussion of epidemiological research designs. In this section, we briefly review the basic principles of case-control design and then go on to discuss in more detail the advantages and problems, as well as ways of avoiding problems, of selection and measurement.

12.2.1 Basic principles of the case-control design

In classic epidemiological research the case-control design, in which subjects are selected on the basis of whether or not they have a particular health outcome of interest, can offer significant advantages over alternative research strategies (Schlesselman 1982). The key distinguishing feature of a case-control study is that it begins with people who are known to have a certain disease (cases) and then compares their exposure to certain factors to people who are known not to have the disease in question (controls). When examining the influence of smoking on lung cancer, for example, subjects would be selected on the basis of whether or not they have lung cancer. We then ask subjects in both groups if they have a past history of smoking (exposure). Relatively simple calculations are then done to determine whether there is any association between the exposure of interest (smoking) and the specified outcome (lung cancer) (figure 12.1).

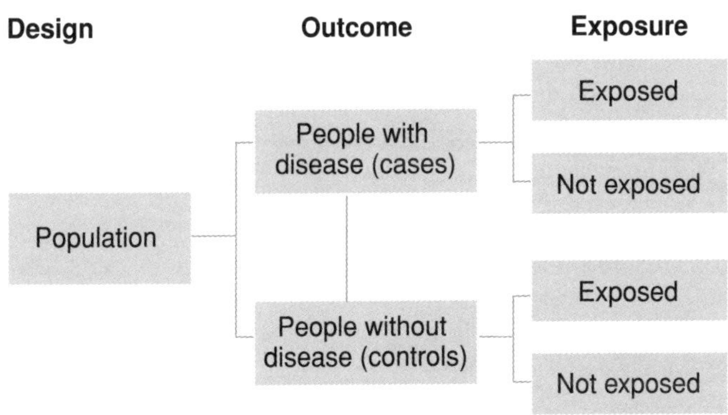

Results

		Outcome	
		Present	Absent
Exposure	Yes	a	b
	No	c	d

Direction of sampling ↓

Figure 12.1 Case-control studies

Let us suppose that in our study of smoking and lung cancer we select 500 cases (people with lung cancer) and 500 controls (people without lung cancer). From subsequent interviews we learn that 350 of the group with lung cancer have a history of smoking, compared to 175 of the group without lung cancer. This is illustrated in table 12.1.

Table 12.1 Case-control study examining the relationship between smoking and lung cancer

	Lung cancer (cases)	*No lung cancer (controls)*
History of smoking	350	175
No history of smoking	150	325
Total	500	500

Using the figures given above, the odds that a subject with lung cancer (case) will have a history of smoking is (350 ÷ 150) = 2.3, while the odds that a subject without lung cancer (control) will have a history of smoking is (175 ÷ 325) = 0.54. In a case-control study the relationship between the exposure (smoking) and outcome of interest (lung cancer) would be expressed in terms of the odds ratio (OR). This is simply the odds that a subject with the outcome of interest (case) has been exposed divided by the odds that a subject without the outcome of interest (control) has been exposed. Using the example given above the odds ratio is (2.3 ÷ 0.54) = 4.3. As this odds ratio is greater than 1.0, it indicates that smoking is indeed associated with lung cancer.[1]

12.2.2 Advantages of the case-control design

The example chosen shows a number of important advantages of the case-control design. Given that we start by selecting people with and without a given disease, we can begin our investigation into the factors which may or may not have influenced the development of that disease immediately. We do not have to follow subjects for years or even decades to see who does and does not develop a disease after a specified exposure. This makes case-control studies very economical in their use of time and money (Beaglehole et al. 1993; Friis and Sellers 1999). Because people are selected into the study on the basis of whether or not they have a disease, they are often the best way of studying a rare disease. Moreover, since the numbers of subjects required for case-control studies tend to be smaller than those required by other research strategies, they have a greater chance of being replicated and their findings confirmed or clarified (Hennekins and Buring 1987; Friis and Sellers 1999).

However, the case-control design is not without its potential disadvantages, and there are particular issues that need to be considered when selecting subjects into the study and when attempting to measure an exposure of interest. These are discussed in detail below.

12.2.3 Potential problems using a case-control design

Despite its apparent simplicity, great care is required when using a quantitative case-control technique. We need to consider three problems:

1. the selection of appropriate subjects for the study (particularly controls)
2. measuring exposure to the risk factor of interest
3. distinguishing between true causal factors and factors that only appear to be associated with the outcome in question (confounding).

A brief outline from the quantitative perspective is given here, before we come back to these issues when considering the *qualitative* case-control design.

12.2.3.1 Selecting cases

When selecting cases for a study, the investigator must first decide what sort of generalisability of study results is most desired. Is the aim to achieve a representative sample of *all* people with lung cancer, or would it be enough to simply include only women, only people above a certain age, or only people of a given ethnic group or social status? Will selection include people with all different types of lung cancer, or one type of cancer only? Will people with all different grades of severity of lung cancer be enrolled, or only a subset of people with either very early or very late disease? Can recruitment draw cancer patients from the general population, or would recruiting cases using hospital admission lists, specialist chest clinics, surgery lists, or cancer support groups offer certain advantages?

It is important to realise that researchers do not always need to have representative samples of the entire population with the outcome of interest, and that important information is gained from looking at only certain groups within the population in greater detail (Beaglehole et al. 1993; Gordis 1996). What is important is to recognise the potential impact of these decisions on the generalisability of the study findings when the results are interpreted.

The other critical issue epidemiologists need to consider when selecting cases (and controls) for a case-control study is that the study subjects are *selected independently of the exposure of interest* (Beaglehole et al. 1993; Friis and Sellers 1999). In other words, using the lung cancer example, a subject's smoking status should not in any way influence their selection into the study. For example, it would not be appropriate to recruit cases or controls from among people enrolled in quit-smoking classes.

12.2.3.2 Selecting controls

Potential problems can also arise when selecting control subjects for a case-control study. It is important that the controls are selected from the *same source population* as the cases. In practical terms this means that control subjects are selected in such a way that they would still have been recruited into the study if they had had the disease in question, but as cases instead of controls (Friis and Sellers 1999). This is so we can be reasonably sure that there are no other factors (age, socioeconomic status, area of residence, health care, dietary habits, and so forth) that may partly account for any observed differences in health outcome between the two groups. Having first ensured that the controls are selected from the same source population as the cases, the investigator needs to consider the representativeness of the control subjects compared to the general population when interpreting the study findings.

As with cases, it is important to select control subjects *independently of the exposure of interest*. In certain situations, this may not be as straightforward as it first appears. For example, when undertaking a hospital-based case-control study examining the link between smoking and lung cancer, researchers may be tempted to recruit both cases and controls from patients attending the hospital's chest clinic. Patients diagnosed with lung cancer would become cases while patients attending the same clinic with other respiratory problems would become controls. The problem with this strategy is that smoking is associated with a wide range of chest problems in addition to lung cancer (for example, bronchitis, emphysema), so that control subjects would be more than likely attending the clinic because they suffer from a smoking-related health problem. In this situation, the selection of control subjects has not been independent of exposure to smoking. It would have been better to select control subjects from patients attending another clinic where the disease was not associated with smoking, or from among patients attending the hospital for elective surgery. This is an important point because the odds ratio derived from the first study would tend to underestimate the true association between smoking and lung cancer (as the control subjects selected in the study would be more likely to be smokers compared to other potential control groups).

12.2.3.3 Measuring exposure

In case-control studies the exposure to a given risk factor for a disease is measured retrospectively. However, accurately measuring an exposure that may have occurred several years in the past is often very difficult. First, recall of certain past events and exposures will vary depending on individual differences and contextual influences as was described in chapter 11 (11.4). Subjects already diagnosed with a disease will have a better recollection of past exposure than subjects who are not, simply because they would have given a lot of thought to what could have contributed to their illness (see, for example, Mackenzie and Lippman 1989). The mother of a baby born with a congenital defect, for example, would be more likely to be able to tell you the number and nature of any headache tablets she took during her pregnancy compared with the mother of a baby born without any congenital problems (Rothman 1986, p. 85). This is known as *recall reporting*, or sometimes *rumination bias* (Hennekens and Buring 1987; Gordis 1996).

The manner in which information about exposure is collected is also important. This information may be collected in a number of different ways:

- by asking study subjects to complete a questionnaire
- by interviewing them
- by asking their relatives or friends about their exposure
- by examining medical or other written records.

What is important is that the information is collected in the same way for both cases and controls. If questionnaires are being used to gather information from cases, they should also be used to gather information from controls. If cases are being interviewed for a study, then controls should be interviewed as well, otherwise differences in exposures between the two groups may appear to be present when in fact they are due to variation in the technique used to collect the data. If more than one interviewer is to be used, there must be strict controls in place to ensure that the interview technique is comparable, otherwise differences in the data may appear because of the differences between the two interviewers. This threat to measurement reliability was defined in chapter 11 as *interobserver variability*. Even if one researcher interviews all the respondents in a study, the same great care must be taken to ensure that the researcher conducts the interview in exactly the same manner for every study subject. Not doing so may produce group differences due to the differences in questioning or other data collection methods used with study subjects. Chapter 11 referred to this reliability problem as *intra-observer variability*.

Problems can also arise in a study if the person collecting the information is aware of either the specific hypothesis being tested or the outcome status of the subject. This is particularly important when the information about a person's exposure is being collected either by interview or by examining medical records. An interviewer, aware of a participant's outcome status, may inadvertently ask a case more detailed questions about exposure. Similarly, the interviewer may be more likely to assume that a control subject has not been exposed to a certain risk factor if written records are inadequate to make a clear-cut decision (Gordis 1996; Friis and Sellers 1999). Subjects who are aware of the study hypothesis being examined, or who have obtained information on possible factors which may have contributed to their illness after being diagnosed with a disease, may also be more likely to report certain exposures than those who are not (Hennekens and Buring 1987).

12.2.3.4 Confounding

Because we are measuring exposure to a risk factor some time after it has occurred, it may be difficult to be sure that exposure to the specific risk factor of interest, and not exposure to something else, led to the outcome. For example, a number of risk factors, including smoking, diet, and exercise, are associated with heart disease.

Research has shown that people who smoke are also more likely to eat high-fat diets (see, for example, Emmons et al. 1994; Tonstad et al. 1999). Investigators examining the relationship between smoking and heart disease who fail to take this fact into account will tend to overestimate the true effect of smoking in their study results. Chapter 9 defined confounding in relation to cohort studies (9.3.1.2). In this case-control example, high-fat diets would be known as a confounder or a confounding variable. Confounding occurs when two factors are associated with each other (for example, people who smoke are also more likely to eat high-fat diets), and the influence on the outcome of one of them is distorted by the effect of the other. It is important to realise that if non-smokers were just as likely to eat high-fat diets as smokers, then there would have been no distortion of the effect of smoking on heart disease and consequently no confounding.

Confounders have three important properties. First, a confounder is a predictor of the outcome of interest (previous research has shown that people who consume high-fat diets are more likely to develop heart disease). Second, confounders are associated with some outcome independently of the actual exposure of interest (high-fat diets have been shown to be associated with heart disease among non-smokers). Third, they are not an intermediate step in the possible causal pathway between the exposure of interest and the outcome (a high-fat diet does not influence the mechanism by which smoking exerts its effect on the heart).

In the example given above, confounding led to an overestimation of the effect of the exposure of interest. However, depending on the factors being studied, it can also lead to an underestimation of the effect of an exposure of interest. To determine whether a potential confounder is present in a study, we need to answer the following two questions:

1 *Is any other factor, apart from the exposure of interest, associated with the outcome?* If the answer is 'Yes',
2 *Is that factor unevenly distributed between the exposed and non-exposed subjects?*

If the answer to the latter question is also 'Yes', then confounding may well be present and we need to work out whether it is likely to lead to an underestimation or overestimation of the true effect of the exposure of interest.

Alternatively, a number of multivariate statistical methods can be applied to examine the effect of the exposure of interest while controlling for the presence of any confounders (see, for example, Rothman 1998).

12.3 Introduction to the qualitative case-control design

Investigators operating at the more structured end of the qualitative research continuum (see chapter 10) aspire to increase the credibility, generalisability, and degree of causal inference associated with findings from qualitative methods. At the same time, TD researchers are able to enhance the validity and understanding of quantitative measures by combining both approaches to examine the same research question. A qualitative case-control study involves integrating the well-defined subject selection criteria of the epidemiological case-control design with qualitative enquiry techniques for illuminating factors influencing the outcome of interest.

12.3.1 Basic principles of the qualitative case-control design

Subjects may be categorised as cases or controls using a range of criteria such as disease status (presence or absence of heart disease), health behaviour (smoking or non-smoking, Pap smear or no Pap smear), or psychological profile (depressed, not depressed). The important thing is that the cases, those having the outcome of interest, can be clearly distinguished from those that do not (controls). A range of qualitative techniques such as structured or unstructured indepth interviews, focus groups, and participant observation are then employed to fully explore the sociocultural, environmental, and other factors relevant to both groups. However, as shown in chapter 10, once a qualitative approach is added, the subjects' interactions with the researcher become part of the evidence. Such data lead to theories not only about whether any observed factors or processes are associated with the outcome of interest, but also to insights into how those factors may operate and interact.

The key distinguishing features between a quantitative and qualitative case-control study lie in the nature of the outcome variable being studied and the methods used to assess exposure. In quantitative case-control studies, the outcome is usually restricted to a disease or other medical condition of interest. In qualitative case-control studies, the outcome can be defined much more broadly and can include classifications based on intentions (subjects who intend to give up smoking, those who do not), behaviours (mothers who have their children immunised, those who do not), or emotional or psychological states (people reporting high or low quality of life). In both quantitative and qualitative case-control studies, however, the outcome is defined as a single dichotomous entity. Furthermore, as noted above, methods used in qualitative case-control studies are usually of the more structured type and rely more on researcher-defined categories of analysis as opposed to purely inductive categories (for example, Pillemer 1985).

In the classic epidemiological approach, we are generally interested in testing a hypothesised causal association between a given exposure and outcome. To achieve this, the exposure is usually quantified in some way, whether it was initially measured by way of questionnaire, review of medical record, or subject interview. In a qualitative case-control study, we are generally more interested in exploring and understanding the interaction between social, psychological, environmental, and personal factors which influence the development of a given outcome. The investigator systematically explores the broad context of the health issue using various means of qualitative enquiry as required. Such a measurement process rarely produces numerical data.

12.3.2 Potential problems using the qualitative case-control design

Investigators wishing to apply the qualitative case-control design need to avoid several problems with its use. Among these are bias in selecting subjects and interviewer sources of error when gathering data. This section also looks at how to combine several types of qualitative measures to improve identification of exposure factors (that is, triangulation of methods).

12.3.2.1 Selecting subjects

The qualitative case-control approach typically uses non-probability sampling of subjects as described in chapter 10 (10.2.3.1). Information-rich examples are deliberately chosen based on previous work in the local area, such as a prevalence survey, which has identified subgroups of cases and controls. As with quantitative research, it is critical that a clear, objective, valid, and reliable measure of outcome is used if the results of the research are to be meaningful.

In qualitative research, cases and controls do not necessarily represent all people with and without the outcome of interest, but are chosen because of the richness of the data they are able to provide (see 10.2.1 and 10.2.2). For example, instead of examining the determinants of smoking behaviour in everyone, investigators may wish to explore the influence of peer pressure among a certain subgroup of women or among adolescent boys. Ideally, subjects should come from the general population, but this is not always possible, especially if the outcome of interest is uncommon. Given the nature of qualitative enquiry, where the emphasis is on the richness of the data that are provided rather than on numbers for statistical analysis, it may still be possible to select cases and controls using predefined criteria from among respondents of a random population survey. If so, then the investigator could approach all, a random subset, or a specified subgroup of interest to participate in further qualitative research (see Kasniyah's sampling strategy, section 12.4). In addition to the potential problems of quantitative case-control studies raised in chapter 9 and section 12.2.3, there are further concerns that need to be considered when undertaking qualitative work using this design. Foremost among these is selection bias. The fieldworker seeking to undertake interviews, focus groups, or observations may only be able to talk with or see a highly selected or somehow unusual group of people. Often those to whom the researcher gains access are the 'articulate, insightful, attractive, and intellectually responsive informants' (Miles and Huberman 1994, p. 264)—in other words, the local élite. Others may never fall within the investigator's gaze because of the type and demands of work they do, their marginal social status, their lack of desire to cooperate, or simply because of an absence of transport by which they can gain access to the places where subjects are being recruited or where the observations are taking place. Physical or intellectual disabilities may also exclude individuals from consideration and introduce systematic bias into a study in the same way.

It is also necessary to think about the time at which the data collection is undertaken. Is it essential to conduct the study within and after normal working hours and on weekends to gain a representative sample of your target population? Or, would targeting a certain day of the week or time of the day be more appropriate? It is vital to recognise the calendar of local events and routine schedules of social life that will influence the people available for interview or observation during the study period. For example, markets may only be held on certain days of the week, more retired people may visit shopping centres the day after they receive their social security (pension) payment than on other days of the week, religious observance at certain times of the year may make it impossible to locate desired respondents (for example, during Christmas or Ramadan).

People with language, speech, or vision difficulties may select themselves out of the study because they feel they have difficulties with participating in an interview. People with low self-esteem, or who are elderly, may decline to participate simply because they feel they would be unable to contribute much and don't want to waste the researcher's time.

12.3.2.2 Measuring exposure

In any case-control study, measuring exposure to a hypothesised causal agent reliably and validly is of the utmost importance. In a qualitative case-control study, the epidemiological concept of exposure is broadened to include sociocultural contexts that may be quite complex. The main objectives are to explore the sociocultural contexts of selected cases and controls in order to first identify potential exposures, and second, to describe the *in situ* processes whereby these variables interact to influence outcomes. In this section we address two key considerations for researchers assessing exposure using a qualitative case-control design:

1 avoiding interviewer sources of error when gathering information from the two groups
2 the value of combining several qualitative methods (that is, *methods triangulation*).

Sources of non-sampling or measurement error in interviews

The investigator undertaking interviews or making observations within the sociocultural context of contrasting informant groups is a potential source of bias in the information gathered. In the more highly structured types of qualitative enquiry, the researcher is seen to act as a filter through which the informant's knowledge and experience is assessed and interpreted (see 10.2.1; see also Borman et al. 1986). The researcher's own personal preconceptions and assumptions about what exposure factors are present and how they operate are seen as a major source of bias (Miller and Crabtree 1994, p. 342). Such preconceptions, whether explicit or not, can influence not only what questions are asked, and hence the information that is elicited (Morse 1994), but also the interpretation of the data once they are collected (Bernard 1994, chapter 10). Reflexive investigators, who continuously examine their relationship with the informant and the emerging material, can achieve greater consistency by documenting preconceptions and assumptions as they become evident during the data collection process (Janesick 1994; Borman et al. 1986). Reason (1994, p. 327) refers to this self-aware and discriminating state of consciousness as *critical subjectivity*: as researchers, we accept that our knowing is from a particular perspective and are able to articulate this in our communications. Added to this is the awareness that our prior expectations of what will occur during data gathering can actually shape the occurrence of those events themselves through subtle interpersonal interactions (Higginbotham et al. 1988, chapter 4).

As with quantitative studies, it is important to use the same basic techniques to collect the information from cases and controls. If interviews or focus groups are being used, the interviewer or group moderator should ensure that the same core sets of issues and topics are discussed in each session. However, new topics that emerge through discussion may be pursued as is customary in qualitative fieldwork. If using a *funnel sequence*, in which the interview starts with a very broad question followed by successively narrower questions, then, as far as possible, the same order of questions should be used. If using filter questions, whereby the next question asked in an interview depends upon the informant's answers to the preceding enquiry, it is important to develop an interview guide so that the general topics discussed in each session are comparable (see Sudman and Bradburn 1982, chapter 8; Bernard 1994, chapter 11; Babbie 1998, chapter 10). What is most important, as Oppenheim (1992, p. 67) points out, is that the data collector finds 'ways of making the questions *mean* the same for each respondent even if this should require greater flexibility in the role of the interviewer'.

Systematic measurement bias can be introduced into the qualitative enquiry if informants' answers to common questions are probed differently (see Bernard 1994, pp. 215–18). A researcher may ask a case either different or more detailed questions concerning exposure than a control. Unless subjects are approached and their knowledge and experiences explored in the same way, any differences that may appear between cases and controls may be the result of the difference in technique being employed rather than any true differences in exposures.

In quantitative case-control studies, measurement bias from *interobserver variation* is introduced when cases and controls are administered the research instruments by different investigators. Such bias can also occur in qualitative case-control designs if the same observers or interviewers do not gather information from both groups evenly. As noted in chapter 10 (see 10.1.3), when gathering qualitative information, the scope and richness of the data collected depend on various characteristics of the researcher. These characteristics range from sex, age, and physical appearance, to skills and experience as an interviewer, self-presentation, ability to establish rapport, body language repertoire, cultural sensitivity, verbal and non-verbal cues, voice tone, and so forth (see, for example, Stone and Campbell 1984; Mechanic 1989; Bernard 1994, chapter 10; Punch 1994; Rice and Ezzy 1999, chapter 3).

Moreover, it is important that the investigator tries to avoid studying all members of one group first (for example, control subjects) before moving on to the other group (for example, cases). If this occurs, it will exaggerate *intra-individual variation* bias. Changes in the investigator, such as increases in knowledge about the topic, language fluency (if the researcher is working outside his or her first language), motivation, fatigue, interview skills, and so forth, will be felt more strongly by the second group. As such, differences in the richness and interpretation of the knowledge gained may be more related to the investigator's development than underlying differences in the two study groups (see Miles and Huberman 1994, pp. 265–9).

The type of relationship that develops between the researcher and informant can also influence the information sought. For example, the interviewer may remind an elderly respondent of her son, daughter, or perhaps even grandchild, so will tend to react to the interviewer accordingly. Similarly, certain respondents may remind the interviewer of their parents or grandparents. The way the interviewer conducts the interview, and the way she interacts with the respondent, may be unknowingly influenced by the relationship she had with her own parents or grandparents. Such dynamics may modify not only what topics are raised for discussion, but also the depth and interpretation of the information gathered during an interview. In order to maintain the integrity of the qualitative data collection technique, it is important for the researchers to critically evaluate whether such factors are introducing potential biases into an interview (critical subjectivity) and adjust their technique accordingly (see Stone and Campbell 1984; Miles and Huberman 1994, pp. 265–6; Morse 1994).

People who have difficulty expressing themselves need to be given as much opportunity as those who confidently put forward their ideas. If not, biases will be introduced related to the informant's education level or degree of self-confidence. In a one-to-one interview this may simply be a process of allowing an individual more time to answer a question, providing encouragement through verbal and non-verbal cues, or using drawings, photos, or even videotapes of familiar situations to stimulate discussion (for example, Nichter and Nichter 1994). In a focus group situation, it may require the use of specific strategies to steer the conversation away from being dominated by one or two people who are highly assertive or like to talk a lot (see Krueger 1988, pp. 84–5; Morgan 1993; Yelland and Gifford 1995).

The information collected may be significantly affected by the presence or absence of other individuals during the course of the qualitative data collection technique. Informants may say different things and behave differently with their spouses or mothers-in-law present than without those individuals (see Stone and Campbell 1984; and 11.5.2). Similarly, the presence of researchers and their indepth questions about meaningful aspects of the informant's life situation may actually change those individuals' views of the world and perceptions of self. While for some researchers (for example, those using interpretivist perspectives) such changes are seen as inevitable during the discovery of human knowledge, for others (for example, those using postpositivist perspectives) this process is considered a source of bias in data collection (see Greene 1994).

Finally, when collecting information from respondents using a qualitative case-control design, cultural norms and expectations may affect the interview context differently for the two groups. For example, among Australian Aborigines, people are generally never referred to by their names after death. A case-control study of Sudden Infant Death Syndrome (SIDS) among Aborigines would need to respect this cultural norm. In other cultures it may be deemed inappropriate to have a male researcher interview a female respondent, or a member of one caste system or religion interview or observe a member of another. Failure to be aware of, and observe, such cultural norms could result in superficial and awkward interviews, with some respondents using deception or even refusing to cooperate at all (see Stone and Campbell 1984, pp. 31–2; Punch 1994).

In review, sociocultural sources of measurement error can occur whenever interviewers gather qualitative information from informants. However, they become more prominent in qualitative case-control fieldwork when the consistency of data collection across all participants is critical for maintaining the integrity of the design, enabling the investigator to maximise the information learned from both groups of informants.

Methods triangulation to strengthen results

A second consideration for assessing exposure is the value of combining multiple measures to identify potentially influential factors. In this context, methods triangulation (see 10.6.1.3) involves using several different qualitative data collection techniques, such as focus group interviews, participant observation, and indepth interviews. The key is to select complementary methods that will provide data that can be integrated to provide a comprehensive, indepth understanding of the situational influences affecting the case and control informants. Importantly, triangulation enables the researcher, 'to regard his or her own material critically, to test it, to identify its weaknesses, to identify where to test further doing something different' (Fielding and Fielding 1986, p. 24).

Although not a qualitative case-control study *per se*, a clear example of qualitative methods triangulation to explore exposure factors is found in Mark and Mimi Nichter's ethnographic study of acute respiratory infection (ARI) in the Oriental Mindoro region of the Philippines (Nichter and Nichter 1994). One facet of their fieldwork was to investigate Filipina mothers' recognition and experience of ARI, their explanations of this disease, care management practices, and health care decision-making. A non-probability sample of lower-class rural carers (mothers and grandmothers) from fishing and agricultural households participated in open-ended and indepth interviews, focus groups, and a mix of structured research exercises. The structured research exercises included a free listing of children's illness categories, a pile-sort exercise, attribute recognition exercises (using illness names and attributes identified from the content analysis of interview data), and projective illness story exercises (vignettes). Focus groups were structured around a series of short video presentations showing the sight and sound of children with ARI. The original aim of all these strategies was to investigate possible differences in health care knowledge and illness classification between carers of different ages and educational levels. By adopting a qualitative case-control approach, the Nichters could have applied their rich combination of methods to examine potential differences between carers who effectively managed ARI in their children compared with those who did not (for example, had children who died or had critical care in hospital).

12.3.3 When to use the qualitative case-control design

As noted in chapter 9, the quantitative case-control design is considered useful when the emphasis is on examining the factors influencing one particular outcome:

- when that outcome itself is fairly uncommon
- when there is a long period of time between exposure and outcome

- when time and cost considerations are paramount when conducting the research
- when it is unethical to either undertake experimental work or passively wait for serious health problems to develop following certain exposures.

The qualitative case-control design has additional advantages. It is useful not only when we wish to validate or enrich the findings of an initial quantitative survey, but also when we wish to understand the process by which sociocultural, environmental, and other factors interact and exert their influence on the outcome of interest. When an apparent inconsistency exists between knowledge or attitude and observed behaviour, defining subjects in terms of those who are and are not consistent and then undertaking indepth qualitative work with them allows you to fully explore the factors that may influence this discrepancy. The strategy may also be used to magnify certain processes that are operating in the community at large. For example, exploring the factors that determine whether or not people who have had heart attacks change their diet (cases) may highlight key issues that are important in understanding factors that influence whether or not members of the community who have not had heart attacks (controls) also change their diet.

12.4 Examples of qualitative case-control studies

Surprisingly, despite its strong popularity among epidemiologists, few published studies have combined qualitative methods with the case-control design. Below are three fieldwork examples showing the depth and versatility of this hybrid design.

12.4.1 Uptake of measles immunisation in Java

Naniek Kasniyah's fieldwork in Java, Indonesia,[2] demonstrates the benefits of using a qualitative case-control design in medical anthropology research. Observing from a prior epidemiological survey that a particular district of Central Java had measles immunisation coverage of only 38 per cent, she undertook a qualitative case-control study to reveal the sociocultural factors influencing participation in the immunisation program. In her investigation, she used the results from a household survey she had completed to identify all mothers in the study area (n = 551) who had children under 5 years of age. Kasniyah then classified them as cases (236 mothers who had not taken their children for measles immunisation) and controls (315 mothers with at least one child who had received measles immunisation). She next took a random sample of thirty mothers from each group and administered a structured indepth interview. These data were supplemented by participant observation that proceeded in the study area over a period of 5 months.

Kasniyah's enquiry found that most rural Javanese still adhere to many traditional beliefs about illness and use local healers and therapies. These combine elements of a personalistic system of health beliefs, in which illness is thought to be caused by sentient beings such as spirits, deities, and ancestors—a cure is effected by ritual exorcism or by placation of the responsible supernatural being—with a 'naturalistic system' (Foster and Anderson 1978). In naturalistic systems, bodily imbalances are identified as contributing to illness, for example an imbalance in the humours of the body. Imbalances are attributed to a variety of circumstances such as weather, diet, and strong emotions; a cure requires that the balance of bodily elements be restored.

Javanese villagers also use biomedical treatments. Most people, in fact, have a pluralistic orientation to health care in which they may utilise a variety of health care resources in the course of an illness. Health workers in the area need to acquaint themselves with local knowledge and practices because they have an effect on the acceptance of new health programs, such as childhood vaccinations. Indeed, health workers themselves could be said to share the pluralistic orientation of Javanese to health care.

The findings of the qualitative case-control study indicated that while all mothers believed measles to be a common disease of childhood (77 per cent of cases and 83 per cent controls), mothers of non-immunised children were less likely to believe that it was a dangerous illness compared to mothers whose children were immunised (17 per cent versus 40 per cent). Measles was considered serious only when complications developed. For example, the women knew that children could become blind if 'the spots came out in the eyes', and believed that the disease could be fatal 'if the spots do not come out' and the fever became very high.

The qualitative work further showed that mothers frequently believed it was in the child's best interest to be exposed to and infected with measles, because only then could the child be considered safe. One grandmother recounted to the researchers: 'When I was small, my elder sibling had measles. She tried to make me catch it. Finally I did get it, and I thought this was the right thing.'

By using a qualitative case-control design, Kasniyah showed that for future measles immunisation programs to be effective in the area, health teams first had to address the mothers' perception that measles was not a dangerous disease for their children, and other community members' deep-seated belief that children were not safe from the disease until they had suffered its effects.

12.4.2 Exposure to HIV among injecting drug users in Canada

Harvey and colleagues (1998) and Pillemer (1985) have also applied the qualitative case-control design to health problems, although neither describes their research using these terms. As a first step in a quantitative case-control investigation for identifying risk factors for HIV seroconversion among injecting drug users (IDUs) in Vancouver, Harvey et al. (1998) selected sixteen subjects for indepth interviews. Eight participants had two documented HIV-negative tests and the other eight had received a recent positive test with a known negative test in the previous 18 months. Open-ended questions covered perceptions of risk, choice, and decision-making related to needle use practices and safe sex. Using a grounded theory approach (see chapter 10), dominant themes that emerged from the interviews concerned addiction, prevention, and the social determinants of one's actions, such as past abuse, homelessness, racism, and squalid living conditions. Commonality between the HIV-positive and -negative participants was strong for themes dealing with addiction and the social determinants of risk behaviour. However, group differences were found for ideas about prevention. HIV-positive participants reported needle sharing despite seroconversion status. This happened, they felt, because at the critical moment the drug injector does not care about the risk of infection; the HIV-positive person may not want to let others know about the presence of disease or may purposely want to expose others (Harvey et al. 1998, p. 316). In contrast, some HIV-negative participants spoke of feeling invincible to the disease because they had continuously avoided seroconversion despite engaging in high-risk behaviour.

12.4.3 Physical abuse of the elderly in the USA

Pillemer (1985) combined qualitative and quantitative data collection with a case-control design to examine the influence of dependency on elder abuse among Americans living on the east coast of the USA. Forty-two physically abused elders (over 65 years) and forty-two controls (individually matched on sex and living conditions) were recruited from a social agency and participated in a 60–90 minute interview. Standardised scales (physical health, functional impairment, and dependency) and open-ended questions about the nature of the elder's relationship with the person who abused them, were both used. Pillemer worked his qualitative material into case descriptions that gave a picture of the way dependency relationships are played out in families where an elderly person is physically abused. He found a strong correspondence between the questionnaire data and the case material. Strikingly, the abusers appear as people with few resources who are unable to meet their own basic needs. Indeed, they are heavily dependent on those they abuse—sometimes children unable to separate from their parents, sometimes disabled or demented spouses. Rather than having power in the relationship, as some researchers had hypothesised, they are relatively powerless (Pillemer 1985, p. 154).

12.5 Qualitative contrasting groups framework: a qualitative case-control design for use with continuous variables

In the qualitative case-control design about measles immunisation in Java described above, the outcome was defined using a dichotomous variable such as immunised child versus non-immunised. In this instance, case definition is relatively clear, and assignment of subjects to case and control groups routinely follows agreed criteria. However, some outcomes, such as child nutrition score (weight-for-age), grams of alcohol consumed weekly, frequency of unprotected sex, and so forth, are measured with some form of continuous score (11.3.4.1).

In the contrasting groups design, subjects in a survey are first assigned a score according to some agreed performance criteria and then rank ordered according to that score, from greatest to least. The researcher then selects subjects from the top and bottom of the rankings. In so doing, two contrasting groups are created that will become the focus for intensive qualitative follow up. The criteria on which subjects are ranked can be derived from previous work in the area or *de novo* by the researcher. There are no strict rules for how to define the contrasting groups, although it seems reasonable to consider that subjects in the top and bottom quartiles—or perhaps top and bottom quintiles or deciles—would provide sufficient heterogeneity to generate hypotheses. Depending upon the number of potential subjects within each group and the resources available for indepth work, either the whole of the group, or some random selection from it, can be invited to participate in further qualitative work.

An obvious problem with the contrasting group framework approach lies in setting the cut-off point for cases and controls if conventions have not been established. As a general rule, the greater the disparity between the top and bottom groups, the better the chances of identifying underlying themes that may help explain the discrepancy. While it is true that this approach ignores potentially valuable information that may be learned from the middle groups, it is believed to be an acceptable trade-off for clarity of interpretation and qualitative analyses. If time and resources permit, a third group, selected from among subjects with middle scores, can be used to both test the theory that has emerged from the earlier data and to explore any relationship between the exposure and outcome that might exist for the middle group.

12.6 Examples of qualitative contrasting groups design

Three examples of a contrasting groups framework are provided below. The first focuses on determinants of child health in Yemen, while the second illustrates the design's value for exploring the interaction between social support and perceptions of health and well-being among the elderly in Australia. The third example highlights problems involved in identifying contrasting groups of physicians in Thailand, when criteria of 'good' prescribing practices are highly complex.

12.6.1 Social determinants of child health in Yemen

Using demographic and nutritional data collected from a systematic survey of 50 per cent of village households in South Yemen, anthropologist Cynthia Myntti (1993) constructed a 'child health score' that she used to rank order thirty-seven mothers with children under 5 years of age. She then focused on the eight mothers who ranked lowest and the eight mothers who ranked highest on the child health score and asked them to complete an interviewer-administered knowledge, attitudes, and practice survey. She also undertook unstructured interviews and participant observation with a total of ten women, five from each extreme of the child health score.

No differences between the high and low child health score groups were found using the demographic data, socioeconomic status, or responses to the interviewer-administered knowledge, attitudes, and practice questionnaire. However, the unstructured interview, coupled with the participant observation, revealed that women who ranked well on the child health score had regular sufficient income, even if it was rather low, and that they controlled the allocation of at least part of that income themselves. These women were socially integrated, with networks of friends or kin to whom they could turn for help. While they viewed life as 'hard work' and were either content or angry about their conditions, they were not passive in their response to it. Women who ranked poorly on the child health score, on the other hand, suffered insecurity due to illness or periods of unemployment. Even if their household income was large, these women did not necessarily have access to or control of it. Money tended to be spent on expensive habits of the husband, such as attending *qat* parties (social occasions where men chew the leaves of a local shrub for its mildly euphoric effect) to make business contacts. These women were socially isolated, with no supportive friends or family to turn to. They tended to blame fate for their ill fortune and were bitter or helpless, sometimes depressed.

Myntti's analysis confirms the links between poverty and ill health but also shows the importance of examining the allocation of resources within households when understanding the interplay of factors influencing the distribution of child mortality. The insights gained were facilitated using the contrasting groups technique.

12.6.2 Social support and perceptions of health and well-being among the elderly in Australia

Brendan Goodger (2000) used a contrasting groups design with elderly Australians to explore how varying levels of social support (high versus low) affect people's attitudes about growing older and their perceptions of health and well-being. He began by administering the eleven-item Duke Social Support Index (DSSI) to 301 people aged 70 years and over randomly selected from the electoral roll in Newcastle, Australia. The DSSI measures people's evaluation of the adequacy of support they receive from members of their social network as well the number of social interactions they had over the last week. Goodger then ranked subjects according to their scores on the DSSI and identified subjects in the top and bottom 20 per cent. He then randomly selected ten people from within each extreme group and asked them to participate in indepth interviews in which a number of topics, including social support, perceptions of the ageing process, physical and emotional health, social ties, and social activities were discussed.

Subjects recording high levels of social support reported having a personal sense of accomplishment and self-direction in their life, even if that life had presented them with a few hard knocks. In contrast, subjects recording low levels of social support felt strongly an unfolding sense of destiny. They felt like passive recipients of life events over which they had little control. Two quotes reflect these differences:

> I still think you've got your place in the world in your life. I think it's up to you to make the most of what you've got, whether you're 18 or 78, you make the most of what was given to you (Ron, high social support group).

> I have just gone along with the tide . . . I'm a great believer in what's to be will be. What's the use of worrying? It's going to happen, isn't it? I always maintain our life is mapped out for us from the day we are born and I don't think anyone is going to change it much (Jane, low social support group).

Overall, the contrasting groups design, with indepth interviews, led to a number of insights about how the ageing process affected the use, maintenance, and dismantling of social support networks among elderly people in this Australian community. It also showed how people could mobilise their social networks to continue enjoying activities thoroughly as long as they lived.

12.6.3 Doctors' prescribing patterns for children with diarrhoea in rural Thailand

An observational study carried out in rural Thailand to investigate the factors influencing doctors' prescribing habits for diarrhoea shows the difficulty in identifying contrasting groups. Nopporn Howteerakul (1997) first observed the case management of 424 childhood diarrhoea cases treated by thirty-eight doctors to see how closely they followed the treatment guidelines recommended by WHO and the Thai Control of Diarrhoeal Disease Program. Next, he attempted to rank order the physicians according to their level of compliance with the formal guidelines so that contrasting groups could be followed up with indepth interviews.

However, compliance with guidelines turned out to be a complex, multidimensional outcome variable, with at least six major indicators (using oral rehydration solution for all cases, not giving antidiarrhoeal preparations [absorbents], using antibiotics only for bloody diarrhoea, etc.). This made it hard to rank doctors on a single scale in order to identify extreme cases. One issue was that the mix of different types of childhood diarrhoea cases was not standard. Each doctor saw a different combination of conditions in terms of diagnosis, severity, complications, and age. Second, Howteerakul was uncertain if each of the six criteria should be given equal weight when it is clear that some prescribing practices, such as overuse of broad spectrum antibiotics, are more harmful than others, such as giving absorbent medication.

Third, Howteerakul found that most doctors did not follow the guideline about restricting use of antibiotics to cases of bloody diarrhoea. Therefore, physicians who happened to have more of these cases got higher compliance scores. In brief, it seemed that no consistent pattern emerged of adherence or non-adherence to the guidelines. Each doctor showed an idiosyncratic mixture of prescribing practices that they explained as the 'therapeutic art' as opposed to scientific side of medicine. Nevertheless, taking these complexities into account, Howteerakul was able to identify eight doctors who appeared to be most consistent adherents to the national guidelines and who, along with eight physicians who followed the guidelines less consistently, were recruited for indepth interviews.

In the next section, we direct our attention to another hybrid design valuable to TD researchers—case studies.

12.7 Case-study designs

In epidemiological research, a 'case' refers to an individual known to have a certain disease of relevance to the research. In the field of health social science and social science more generally, a 'case study' is a term used to describe a type of research design that is focused on the intensive empirical study of an issue or problem. Often, but not always, this is done by integrating a range of methods. The case may be an individual or a more complex unit of analysis such as a town or suburb (Whittaker 1998), or a category of people such as 'mothers of chronically ill children' (Bauman and Adair 1992). Case-study designs are eclectic designs in that the researcher can draw on any methods that are useful in illuminating the research problem. Nonetheless, there are principles for case-study design that ensure the research is rigorous and trustworthy or valid. Case studies are a useful design for TD researchers because multiple methods and perspectives may be integrated in the quest to gain an understanding of often complex empirical phenomena.

In a well-known book on case study research, Robert Yin has defined a case study as:

> An empirical inquiry that investigates a contemporary phenomenon within its real-life context, especially when the boundaries between phenomenon and context are not clearly evident (1994, p. 13).

Yin is here emphasising the contemporary nature of phenomena chosen for case study, because thorough empirical research is usually undertaken as part of the case-study design. However, historical events or processes where no empirical research is possible can also be the subject of case studies. Yin also emphasises the real-life character of case study phenomena. In other words, the researchers are not trying to control or limit the variables under study, as would be done in a controlled experiment, but are attempting to incorporate more naturalistic methods of enquiry. Finally, Yin points to the broad scope and complexity of research questions that may be addressed through case studies. Case-study designs similar to the qualitative research discussed in chapter 10, stress the importance of understanding a problem in relation to a broader context. Case-study designs that do not prematurely separate the phenomenon of concern and its context can be powerful means for TD researchers to investigate the way in which different levels of the health hierarchy (see chapter 2) are implicated in a particular problem. For example, in a case study with a research question focused on the development of resistant antibiotics in the treatment of tuberculosis, it would be difficult at the outset of the study to exclude any level of the health hierarchy from consideration as not being part of the causal phenomena, as the examples in chapter 6 (6.9) show.

While case-study designs may incorporate a range of different methods, this does not imply that these methods are used in an unconsidered or random way. Like the less structured types of qualitative methods discussed in chapter 10, the sequence of the methods used can evolve as the research proceeds in response to new opportunities and new insights on the part of the researchers. However, each method must be justified in terms of the research question(s) guiding the study and in terms of the information about the problem that the researchers have already produced. Information obtained from different methods and sources must be rigorously compared and weighted by the researchers, in accordance with the principles for assessing research quality (including triangulation) discussed in chapter 10 (see 10.7). Case-study research often incorporates qualitative and quantitative methods. However, one type of method, or just one method (such as an illness narrative or life history interview) may produce the data for the case study. There are no hard and fast rules about the number or type of methods that should be used in a case study.

12.7.1 Types of case studies

Willms and Johnson (1996) have discussed the ways in which case studies may be generated from a larger existing body of data, particularly ethnographic data. For example, in an ethnographic study of health in a community, preliminary analysis of data may reveal that certain themes emerge repeatedly. In this situation, the researcher may extract case studies from the larger body of data that highlight these salient themes. A case study drawn from the larger body of information will be analysed and written up not just for its intrinsic value, that is, because 'one wants better understanding of this particular case' (Stake 1994, p. 237), but also because it gives a theoretical insight or is generalisable to a larger collection of cases. These last two purposes of case studies are referred to by Stake as *instrumental* and *collective* respectively (1994, p. 237).

Yin has provided a formalised typology of case studies, based not on purpose but on design. He distinguishes four basic types of designs, depending on whether single or multiple cases are used and whether there is only a single unit of analysis (such as a person) or whether there are multiple or *embedded* units of analysis (1994, p. 39). Yin makes the important point that multiple case studies use a replication, not a sampling logic, whereby the results of each case (similar or contrasting) are predicted using theoretical propositions.

For example, the case study of chronic illness discussed in 12.7.3 is one of a series of multiple case studies that were generated as part of a larger ethnographic study. These case studies were used to test some of the theoretical propositions about chronic illness that other researchers had developed (including the problematic search for a diagnosis, the role of stress, and changes in social roles and relationships). The larger research project of which the case studies of chronic illness formed a part was not in itself designed as a case study but rather as an ethnography of health and illness in an Australian suburb. The Coalfields heart disease example discussed in chapter 5, by contrast, was designed as a case study and conforms to Yin's Type 2 design: a single case study with multiple units of analysis.

12.7.2 A TD case study design of heart disease in the Coalfields

The TD team at the University of Newcastle included epidemiologists, a cardiologist, biostatisticians, social scientists, nutritionists, nurses, health promoters, and

	Sing e-case designs	Mu tip e-case designs
Holistic (single unit of analysis)	Type 1	Type 3
Embedded multiple units of analysis)	Type 2	Type 4

Source: Adapted from Yin (1994, p. 39)

Figure 12.2 Basic types of designs for case studies

others who cooperated for 10 years on a project focused on finding an explanation of the epidemic of heart disease in the Australian Coalfields. The primary research question—evaluation of a community development strategy for preventing heart disease in this community—required that the problem be investigated using many research methods. The case—the geographically, socially, and occupationally defined area known as the Coalfields—incorporated many units of analysis, including individuals (CHD sufferers and their family members), health services, statistical data sets, and voluntary organisations. The team, membership of which changed over time, focused on many different data sources that were hypothesised to be relevant to the understanding of CHD.

As the understanding of the problem increased, the units of analysis broadened from analyses of traditional risk factors (for example, smoking rates, diet practices, obesity) to aspects of social life such as recreational pursuits, gender relations, and the political history of the area. Information from different fields of study, different methods, and different data sources was constantly compared and discussed; contradictory findings raised new questions that spurred further data gathering and analysis. In other words, the process of triangulation took place. For example, survey data from mailed questionnaires indicated that the heart disease epidemic was a low priority, although historical evidence showed tremendous community interest in building up clinical services and emergency care. Subsequent ethnographic probes looked at the cultural communitarian spirit that could account for both findings (Higginbotham et al. 1999, p. 691). Theoretical propositions were tested and rejected (such as the hypothesis that the socioeconomic indicators of the Coalfields could account for the higher rates of CHD; see 5.3.3.1 and Dobson et al. 1991). The long timeframe of the case study and the range of disciplines and methods involved allowed the development of a new theory of CHD (the 'larrikin heart'), which is outlined in chapter 5. Researchers with expertise in different fields of study followed the recognised procedures to ensure quality data collection in their own fields, and these procedures included both quantitative and qualitative methods. However, the overall design of the project did not follow any predefined pattern. As Yin points out, for case studies:

> the data collection procedures are not routinized. In laboratory experiments or in surveys, for instance, the data collection phase of a research project can be largely, if not wholly, conducted by a research assistant. The assistant is to carry out the data collection activities with a minimum of discretionary behavior, and in this sense the activity is routinized—and boring. There is no such parallel in conducting case studies (1994, p. 55).

The multiple publications and reports of this complex case study provide the 'chain of evidence' (Yin 1994, pp. 98–9) that establishes the reliability of the findings and allows outsiders to follow the development of the theories. Importantly, the Coalfields case study showed how the lived experiences of a community are tightly connected to both its industrial history and evolving biology.

12.7.3 A case study of chronic illness

In 1994–96, a team of researchers (primary care physicians and anthropologists) undertook an ethnographic study of health and illness in an Australian suburb from the point of view of residents of the suburb rather than of patients or medical practitioners. The researchers were interested in the spectrum of health resources utilised by residents of the small beachside community, as well as their understandings of health and illness. Interviews, focus groups, health diaries, and analyses of secondary data such as census figures and health statistics, were the primary methods used in this ethnographic study of the meanings and practices that constituted health-related actions of residents of the suburb. The primary researcher lived in the suburb as a participant-observer for the 18 months that the research was carried out (Whittaker et al. 1996).

During the course of long semistructured interviews (see 10.4.1), a number of respondents recounted narratives of chronic illness. These narratives became a subject of particular interest to the research team, because of both the rich information they contained about the meanings attributed to illness and the range of health resources used by some residents, and because they were amenable to comparative analysis with other health social scientists' work on chronic illness. In other words, the illness narratives provided important information for the primary aims of the study as well as being an interesting data set in themselves. In Yin's terms, the collection of illness narratives led to a multiple case design with single units of analysis (the sufferers and their relatives who were interviewed).

Other researchers have reported on the common themes that occur in sufferers' narratives of chronic illness. These themes can be regarded as a set of propositions about the experience and effects of chronic illness that can be tested with further case study research. Two studies of illness narratives, concerning multiple sclerosis (Robinson 1990), and problems with the temporomandibular joint (TMJ) (Garro 1994), reported the following recurring themes.[3]

12.7.3.1 Problematic search for diagnosis

Garro's study of people eventually diagnosed as suffering problems with the temporomandibular joint of their jaw revealed a common pattern of a 'protracted and taxing search for diagnosis . . . with conflicting interpretations for their illness' (Garro 1994, p. 776). Robinson (1990, p. 1184) also found that a common experience of sufferers of multiple sclerosis was a 'problematic initial search for a diagnosis through the formal health system'.

12.7.3.2 Body–mind duality

Garro states that narrative representations often depict the body as a biomedical machine. This metaphor was commonly encountered among residents of Oceanpoint (see Whittaker and Connor 1998) and is based on a cultural schema which separates mind and body, although interaction may occur. A recurrent concern of chronic sufferers in Garro's study was whether their pain and dysfunction were attributable to the body or the mind. This question emerged either implicitly or explicitly in their interactions with others, particularly the medical profession. Doubt about whether an illness is of the body or of the mind generally arises when symptoms diverge from the usual expectations of what happens when a patient is ill. Attributing the problem to a malfunctioning mind rather than the body implies that it is the sufferer who is to blame, both for the symptoms and for the failure of the practitioner to achieve a diagnosis or cure. According to Garro, this is a widely accepted cultural schema, evident in the discourse of health professionals and laypeople (1994, pp. 779-80).

12.7.3.3 Legitimation of complaints

Chronic illness narratives often express the struggle to resolve the patients' concern that they be judged as having a legitimate complaint (Garro 1994, p. 779). Biomedical legitimacy may rest on the patient being able to fit into a preconceived pattern of disease. Legitimacy is best exemplified by a diagnosis based on classic symptoms or a description of a disease as a classic case.

Chronic sufferers must also deal with the implications of community judgments about the legitimacy of certain illnesses. Relatively new diseases, about which little is known and which are difficult to diagnose and/or treat, such as chronic fatigue syndrome (CFC) and repetitive strain injury (RSI), may be less well accepted as the basis for adopting the sick role. Sometimes the stigma attached to a certain disease label is such that an alternative, more acceptable, label is preferred either by the patient or the doctor.

12.7.3.4 The changing significance of psychogenic explanations

Garro notes that stress has become a popular explanation for illness in North America (Garro 1994, p. 779). The Oceanpoint study revealed that this was also the case in this Australian suburb (Whittaker and Connor 1998). Other authors have noted that the cultural schema that defines stress as a cause of ill-health may be accepted both by doctors and the lay public (Lock 1982; Fitzpatrick 1984; Helman 1985). Explanations of the workings of stress are interlinked with cultural schemata concerning the separation of the mind and the body. Garro's study revealed that patients suffering from TMJ were prepared to consider explanations based on stress in the initial stages when efforts at diagnosis or treatment were unsuccessful. When the problem persisted and patients became less receptive to purely psychological explanations, health care workers were more likely to offer psychogenic interpretations and to view their patients as 'problem patients' (Garro 1994, p. 780).

12.7.3.5 Life changes

Fitzpatrick has stated that the importance of understanding personal narratives of chronic illness is that for sufferers, 'making sense of illness, and understanding the meaning of sickness and disease' involve 'ordering and sequencing a myriad range of phenomena in everyday life which may or may not be perceived as related to health and illness' (quoted in Robinson 1990, p. 1185). The degree to which chronic illness affects the quality of life varies between individuals. However, the search for some control over their illness, in terms of knowledge about the cause of their ailment, the relief of symptoms, or mastery of disabilities, was a constant theme in personal illness narratives of sufferers of TMJ dysfunction (Garro 1994, p. 783).

12.7.3.6 Social relations

Garro (1994, p. 775) suggests that illness narratives may serve the purpose of upholding or reinforcing appropriate social roles. In some cases, they may serve as a *moral commentary* by contrasting appropriate and inappropriate responses to illness. In chronic illness narratives, stressing one's ability to continue to play a useful part in society, either as a paid or unpaid worker, is often an important consideration.

Because of the prolonged nature of chronic disease, economic changes are often at the forefront of illness narratives. Economic difficulties may interact with and compound the suffering of the ill person as well as those around them. In addition to coping with the breakdown of their health, chronic sufferers may also be faced with the disintegration of their marriage and other social relationships. These concerns are interwoven into the illness narratives of chronic sufferers. The illness narrative therefore bears witness to the interdependence of the biomedical realities of chronic ill health with other levels of the health hierarchy.

12.7.4 Case study of Graham from the Oceanpoint study

This case study, one of several CFS sufferers in Oceanpoint, echoes many of the themes highlighted by Robinson (1990) and Garro (1994), suggesting that their findings may have generalisability to a broader universe of phenomena. Like Garro's narrative (1994, pp. 775–7), Graham's narrative was derived using the method of a long, semistructured interview. Robinson analysed undirected written personal narratives or autobiographies of multiple sclerosis sufferers (1990, pp. 1175–8). The mode of analysis used in the case study of Graham is one that Yin (1994, pp. 106–8) refers to as *pattern-matching*: the Garro and Robinson studies provide the predicted pattern of experience of chronic illness (the six emergent themes summarised above), and the case of Graham provides the empirical test of their propositions.

Graham is a 41-year-old railway worker. His wife, Kylie, is a 32-year-old registered nurse. At the time of interview, in which both Graham and Kylie participated, Graham had been sick for 3 years. Graham has struggled to make some sense of the sequence of events that unfolded over the long period during which his symptoms remained undiagnosed. He explained that he was originally treated for stress and anxiety:

> Stress and anxiety led to an over-active thyroid. An over-active thyroid . . . mind you this took over 14 months to get solved. Anyway that led to a tumour on my pituitary gland.

Kylie explained that initial treatment for stress and anxiety and the subsequent inability to adequately diagnose puzzling physical symptoms led doctors to conjecture that all Graham's problems were due to psychological causes. She interjected at one point:

> Hang on, you forgot the trip to the psychiatrist in the middle of all that because you weren't really sick and there was nothing really wrong with you. And they didn't see any symptoms so of course you must have a screw loose, so we will send you to the psychiatrist.

Graham first noticed symptoms while doing some work-related training:

> I went through the second day of the course into a so-called stress symptom. That was all right . . . I just couldn't handle the exam. It was like I was under a lot of pressure. Like a person with stress.

Graham's symptoms included anxiety, headaches, and an inability to cope; he was 'really upset' and suffered sleeplessness. According to Kylie, the general practitioner (GP) treated Graham for 'stress and anxiety and having depression and the whole bit'. One of the reasons for this course of action was that the GP thought that Graham was depressed because of the death of a friend:

> because previously to him getting sick in the July of 1992, his best mate had committed suicide in the May. And it was about 6 weeks from the time he committed suicide to the time Graham took crook. And so they put it down to the fact that he wasn't coping very well with the situation. And it was just a total build up of that. So from the July to the October they treated him primarily for stress and anxiety and depression (Kylie).

Four months later, Graham was not getting better and was beginning to doubt the diagnosis of stress. His mother suggested a thyroid test.

As Garro notes, chronic sufferers sometimes 'seesaw between different interpretations', especially when their illness is not responding to treatment (Garro 1994, p. 780). Graham initially accepted the diagnosis of stress on the advice of doctors but came to doubt this diagnosis based on his own embodied knowledge of his symptoms and also on the advice of relatives. Thus, the subjective understanding and the professional definition of the symptoms, while initially convergent, began to diverge with the passage of time. However, convergence was again achieved when a psychiatric evaluation carried out in December 1992 ruled out psychiatric causes for Graham's problems:

> And he [the psychiatrist] said to him [Graham], 'Look, you certainly don't have a psychological problem. You have a definite physical problem, and your physical problem is causing your mental problem.' Those were his words (Kylie).

A respiratory test carried out in January 1993 showed that Graham had an overactive thyroid. His doctors explained that they had been initially reluctant to diagnose an overactive thyroid on the basis of Graham's description of his symptoms because he 'didn't have all the classic symptoms that present with an overactive thyroid and that is why they said that is why we don't believe him. But this test proved he did (Kylie)'.

For both patients and doctors the term 'classic symptoms' has a very important legitimating function. In Graham's case legitimation was dependent on scientific tests showing that his symptoms were characteristic of a narrowly defined disease category.

By February 1993 Graham was experiencing severe symptoms and both he and his family were suffering greatly. Graham had not worked since July 1992:

> I spent a lot of time on the lounge. I was always tired . . . I could sleep through the day and through the night. I was worn out (Graham).

> And that's true. He slept for 14 months. He slept, he ate. He didn't do anything, he didn't move off that lounge. He didn't go anywhere, he didn't see anybody, he didn't talk to anybody unless they came here to see him. And that was the end of it. There was nothing. He couldn't look sideways at his kids. The children couldn't sit at the table to eat their tea. If they sat down and put a cup on a plate, it was 'Don't do that!' and it was like World War III (Kylie).

These problems were threatening to break up what had previously been a very strong marriage:

> That's how he was and I said to all of the specialists, 'I don't give a shit what you do, but pull your finger out and sort something out with him because,' I said, 'we have been married for 12 years', it was 10 years then, and I said to them, 'We aren't going to make another year, because I don't have to put up with this and neither do my children.' And it's killing us and the relatives and the neighbours wondered how long it was before I was going to pack up my bags and leave.

Shortly after, an endocrinologist diagnosed that Graham's symptoms were the result of a pituitary tumour. However, following an operation to remove the tumour and beginning thyroid hormone replacement therapy, Graham continued to experience tiredness and lethargy. At this stage, having exhausted the limits of his expertise, the endocrinologist stated that there was nothing more he could do and referred Graham to an immunologist. Tests by the immunologist revealed 'glandular fever plus he had the Epstein Barr virus'. As was the case with his pituitary tumour, Graham's complaints were again outside the range of classic symptoms. According to Kylie, the professor of immunology stated:

> 'You can't have both. You are not supposed to have glandular fever *and* Epstein Barr virus at the same time. Because one is a marker or a titre that shows up if you have had the glandular fever.' Anyway Graham has both (Kylie).

Despite being an unusual case, having his illness legitimated by scientific tests was reassuring. One of the most positive aspects of the diagnosis and subsequent encounters with the immunologist was being taken seriously:

> And he [the immunologist] believed him straight up when Graham said to him, 'I can't mow the lawn. If . . . I try to mow the lawn in one day flat, I can't do anything for three or four days.' And he said to Graham, 'Yes, and I quite believe you, because these results tell me exactly that.' And that was just wonderful after all the other crap that we had from all the other hierarchy (Kylie).

Even though Graham's symptoms were finally diagnosed, the specialist explained that there was no specific treatment. Since biomedicine was not able to answer all Graham's questions about his illnesses, he began delving into his family history to see if his complaints may be hereditary:

> OK. Looking back to when I took the Aurorix for stress and anxiety. Talking to the GP she said if it runs in the family it can come up. I have just been looking at the family tree at the moment and it looks a bit shaky. My mother is a manic depressive and looking back to my father's mother . . . see my mum and dad are first cousins, so it makes it all a bit too close to home.

Graham is very bitter that it took so long for doctors to find what was wrong with him. He is particularly upset that he was unable to work for so long, even though the sick leave provisions of the government authority that employs him are more generous than he would have encountered in a private sector job:

> They should have turned around and done it better and done it properly. The trouble is this, I got in with a bunch of donkeys in there, I feel dirty about it. It cost me 5 months of my sick pay, out of work for no reason at all.

The economic implications of being out of work for so long were discussed by Kylie, who struggled to meet the family's financial commitments and keep up the payments on private health insurance to avoid long waiting lists in the public health system.

Graham feels that he has been in the sick role for longer than necessary because of the delays and inefficiencies of diagnosis and treatment. He has had to cope with living with an illness about which little is known and which is not well recognised or accepted in the community. This was implied by the specialist who chose an alternative disease label when diagnosing Graham.

> Now Professor C says he doesn't like to call it chronic fatigue syndrome because too many people have such an emotional response to it. So he prefers to speak about it as Epstein Barr virus (Kylie).

Overall, Graham's case reveals how the meaning of the illness experience is shaped by everyday interactions with the medical profession, friends, family, and the community generally. At the structural level, personal illness experience is also affected by political and economic forces relating to the health system within which the drama is played out. All the themes that emerged in the Robinson and Garro studies also emerged in this case study from Oceanpoint, strengthening the explanation of the process of chronic illness that the original two authors had proposed.

12.7.5 Understanding case studies of chronic illness using TD frameworks

Case studies of chronic sufferers' illness narratives provide a means of situating the lay perspective within a TD framework. This lay perspective complements the specialist knowledge of professionals who are not personally experiencing an illness. Robinson and Hawpe have differentiated between narrative and scientific thinking:

> Both are attempts to organise and give meaning to human experience, to explain and guide problem solving. But the products of these two modes of thought, story, and principle respectively are quite distinct. The product of scientific thinking is a principle or law . . . testable only by further formal scientific activity. The product of narrative thought is context-bound, concrete, and testable through ordinary interpersonal checking (1986, p. 114).

In chapter 4, we discussed how researchers can synthesise findings from different fields of knowledge and ways of knowing to construct TD frameworks. We outlined the processes by which a single researcher draws together threads from single, interdisciplinary, and multidisciplinary insights into a TD framework to analyse a complex health problem. In some cases the TD thinker utilises one or more dynamic principles to provide a coherent meaning to the diverse strands, as Stephen Kunitz demonstrated by his explanation of population declines among Indigenous peoples. This integrative way of thinking may also be undertaken by lay people endeavouring to come to terms with their illness. This is particularly the case with chronic sufferers who, like professional TD researchers, also draw together inputs from many different strands of knowledge. For example, during a prolonged search for the meaning of signs and symptoms of illness the chronic patient must integrate information about the condition from a primary care physician who usually then refers the patient to a specialist. Each specialist brings their own expertise to bear in an attempt to diagnose and treat the symptoms. When the limits of knowledge are reached, the specialist may refer the patient to another specialist or health professional, all of whom have different, sometimes contradictory, insights into the patient's condition. In addition, sufferers must come to terms with the way family, friends, and the wider society interpret their illness. On occasions, alternative explanations and therapies are also sought.

The chronic sufferer is pulled in different directions by the structural imperatives of the health system that provides care, as well as by the need to restore personal biological, psychological, and social integrity. In Australia, as in many Western countries, the formal health system encourages chronic patients to fragment their experience in terms of the different inputs from different specialist groups. However, this goes against a more compelling process, which is to integrate their whole experience in a framework that merges individual bodily and lifestyle experiences with wider cultural understandings. The sufferer has various ways of knowing in the form of biomedical diagnoses, alternative therapy explanations, advice from friends and relatives, knowledge gained from the printed media or through the internet, and forced changes in life circumstances. As Graham's case shows, there is an ongoing attempt to integrate this knowledge into a coherent framework. This

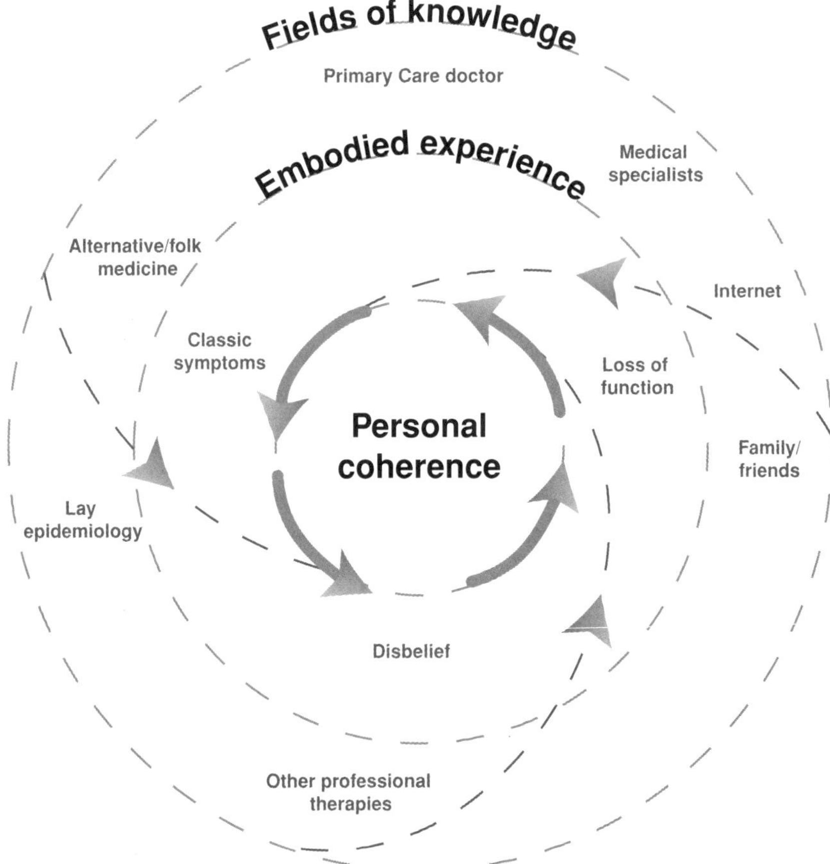

Figure 12.3 The chronic illness sufferer as a TD thinker

process, shown in figure 12.3, parallels the way that TD researchers synthesise information from many different perspectives and disciplines.

12.8 Conclusion: levels of TD enquiry and the case-control and case study designs

We classify qualitative case-control and contrasting groups designs as hybrid study designs that take advantage of the strengths of both quantitative and qualitative methods to identify potential causal factors influencing a specific health problem (table III.1, preamble to part III). These designs are of particular value in Level II transdisciplinary research when the investigators move beyond a description of the problem to specification of elements of influence. Many of the biases that distort the findings of quantitative case-control studies in relation to selecting subjects (cases and controls) and measuring exposure, must also be overcome when using the qualitative case-control design. Structured qualitative methods are used in these designs in order to maximise the consistency of findings and minimise the measurement error that may occur in the situation of researcher as instrument. In other words, efforts are made to take into account the influence of subjectivity while minimising its effects (Rice and Ezzy 1999, p. 32). In particular, researchers need to avoid:

- interobserver variation that may occur when cases and controls are interviewed by different researchers
- intra-observer variation arising when the same investigator interviews one group first, followed by the second.

Methods triangulation, the selective combination of complementary qualitative methods, improves the researcher's depth and breadth of understanding of the health problem context. In so doing, meaningful differences between the groups, in their characteristics or situation (exposures), are likely to come into focus.

From the perspective of complexity theory, the qualitative case control design is a vehicle for exploring non-linear relationships. It is a tool for illuminating and understanding complex relationships among elements within a dynamic system. When methods triangulation is applied, the key is to uncover patterns that may exist amid a seemingly disparate and chaotic range of information produced using multiple qualitative methods (observations, focus groups, depth interviews). In general terms, the qualitative case-control method, as with other non-linear approaches, helps us analyse self-organising systems in order to understand patterns of dynamic behaviour that are naturally present in such systems (Barton 1994, p. 12). An intriguing notion of self-organising in complexity theory is that such patterns will emerge from qualitative data even in the presence of bias, distortion, and discrepancy of interpretation that may characterise the study findings.

On the other hand, our review of case study designs showed that they are used at different levels of TD research. They are frequently used to generate a rich problem description (Level I). However, the main strength of case study designs is their capacity to clarify causal links (Level III TD research). The examples of heart disease in the Coalfields and the narratives of chronic illness both show how case studies can assist in the clarification of causal relationships. This is particularly true where participants' subjective understandings are important to the theoretical propositions that emerge. The case study that incorporates long interviews and/or participant observation is a powerful means of capturing the way in which subjects themselves construct the meaning of their situation, and how this in turn affects their interactions with other individuals and systems.

Case studies often collect data longitudinally, and are focused on processes rather than events. Thus the case study allows the researcher to understand the way phenomena change over time. Theoretical propositions that relate to causal links over time, particularly where subjective interpretations are crucial to the processes that occur, can be investigated more readily using case studies than almost any other method. The open-ended nature of many case-study designs, where new methods and approaches may be incorporated as desired, allows a greater opportunity to understand the broadest context in which the problem of interest is located. It also helps avoid premature judgments about the relationship between problem and context, or between causes and effects. This strength can also be a disadvantage if the boundaries of the case become so difficult to define that explanation is inhibited.

In the preamble to part III we also classified the case study as a hybrid research design. This is in recognition of the range of methods that may be used in case studies, especially those with multiple units of analysis such as the Coalfields heart disease study. However, some case studies, such as the narratives of chronic illness sufferers, rely only on a single method, usually from the less-structured end of the qualitative research spectrum. In addition, it is important to recognise that case studies lend themselves to constructing images of health problems as part of a complex, dynamic system. For example, we can infer from the Oceanpoint case study that the dynamic underlying the chronic sufferer's quest for coherence within himself and his family was an attempt to end uncertainty and restore self-regulation. If illness is viewed as a far-from-equilibrium system, then chronic patients' attempts to organise experiences and meanings associated with their illness are examples of the tendency towards self-organisation in new and unpredictable ways. Similarly, at varying times and in response to varying circumstances, the chronic patient may be drawn to differing attractors by accepting or rejecting opposing or contradictory bodies of knowledge. The acceptance of various perspectives (for example, bio-medical diagnoses, alternative therapists' explanations, internet advice, or the opinions of friends or relatives) could be seen as the tendency to be drawn to a particular attractor. In attempting to reconcile or synthesise the varying views, chronic patients, like other dynamic systems at the edge of chaos, are attempting to gain control over their state.

Notes

1 An odds ratio less than 1.0 would suggest that subjects exposed to the risk factor of interest have less risk of developing the outcome of interest. However, an odds ratio of 1.0 indicates that there is no association between the exposure of interest and the outcome being examined.

2 This fieldwork was carried out in 1992 as research for a Master of Medical Science Degree at the University of Newcastle.

3 This represents a sample of common themes in these studies. Not all the themes appear in both the studies.

Conclusion: The Future and Health Social Science

NICK HIGGINBOTHAM, GLENN ALBRECHT, AND LINDA CONNOR

The future health environment

We can consider the future of health social science by imagining an array of health priorities that will challenge health social scientists as the twenty-first century unfolds. Any predictions we may make now about the central health issues that will dominate the twenty-first century are clearly speculative. Yet, looking at contemporary interacting systems that produce health and illness and operate across different levels in the health hierarchy, we can imagine a number of events taking place.

First, the disease profiles of newly industrialised nations, such as those in Southeast Asia, will show a dramatic rise in chronic diseases (cardiovascular diseases, cancer, and especially diabetes) while retaining a high infectious disease burden. Western postindustrial countries will suffer the re-emergence of infectious diseases (hepatitis, TB, whooping cough), while increasing their chronic disease profiles as an even greater proportion of the population reaches old age, supported by ever-increasing and costly levels of medical intervention. In both contexts, the changing disease profiles and new biomedical technology available will challenge the adequacy of existing health care systems and require new initiatives in preventative health and clinical medicine.

Second, we will see an explosion of concern globally about multiple-drug resistant organisms (parasites, bacteria, and viruses, including HIV) causing disease in humans and livestock and the emergence of new infectious diseases. The pharmaceutical and biotechnology industries will have trouble staying ahead of these challenges and the expense of developing and applying new treatments will mean a dramatic sharpening in barriers of access to therapeutics among the poor.

Third, wealth (class) differentials in health status, longevity, and quality of life will increase based on one's ability to consume biotechnology innovations, such as regenerative organs, transplants, and bionic parts that prolong and improve life.

Fourth, massive geographic movements of populations will take place both within nation states and across borders. Some will be refugees from conflict and repressive governments. Some migrants will be giving up degraded and unproductive environments or fleeing the areas made inhospitable by global warming and ozone depletion. Others will be economic refugees—victims of trade globalisation—seeking places where jobs and a higher standard of living are available. Irrespective of cause, the health consequences of such population displacement and migrations are predictable: spread of pathogens into new environments (including harmful soil and plant materials), pressures on ecosystems, burden on health systems, undermining the foundations of health in new sites, and worsening of conditions for those left behind.

Fifth, a greater burden of disease may emerge from conditions that have long incubation periods. Absence of accurate knowledge about numbers exposed and length of incubation makes effective health planning impossible until the disease outbreak. For example, the upper estimate for the expression of new variant Creutzfeldt-Jacob Disease (nvCJD) (see chapter 3) in the population within the next 20 years is 500 000 cases (von Radowitz 2000). Such projections are based on nvCJD deaths in recent years in relation to the amount of infected beef that entered the food chain from the early 1980s to 1996, when all contaminated beef was removed. Should the incubation period be longer than 20 years, however, the total number of infected people could rise into the millions worldwide. Similarly, an epidemic time bomb of malignant cancer caused by exposure to asbestos fibres (mesothelioma) may be ticking away. Given that asbestos has been used worldwide in common materials such as automobile brake linings and is still found in many building structures, it is not surprising that we are already seeing an upward trend in the annual number of cases of malignant mesothelioma in the industrialised world (American Cancer Society 1999).

The future of health social science

Faced with these scenarios of diminishing human health, what does the transdisciplinary perspective developed in this book offer health social scientists? TD thinking enriches health social scientists' action in the future through four principles:

- inclusiveness
- reflexivity
- openness to change
- the response to complexity.

First, TD thinking is inclusive in important ways. By making the explanation of the health problem the central focus of TD teamwork, it is capable of synthesising insights and enquiry approaches across the health hierarchy. Such inclusivity links behavioural and social science perspectives on health to those of the physical, biological, and medical sciences, as well as the knowledge of both professional researchers and laypeople. Significantly, the TD research framework incorporates multiple research strategies (quantitative and qualitative) and hybrid study designs, as required to provide enlightenment on a particular health problem. By being inclusive, TD thinking ensures that the fullest range of ideas and methods—and the expertise required to apply them—can be brought to bear on priority health problems that crystallise at any moment in time.

Second, TD thinking is reflexive in that it encourages health social scientists to question the accepted ways of conceptualising issues and doing research. Reflexivity into the motives, strategies, and perceptions of the researchers and a willingness to incorporate new and sometimes controversial insights and methods as a result of that reflection ensures that the TD process achieves evolutionary synthesis of knowledge and, at times, completely novel understandings of health problems. The notion of transdisciplinary space, the domain beyond disciplinary reach wherein problem explanations lie, is central to reflexive TD thought. Reflexive awareness enables TD thinkers to process and use new information associated with novel aspects of emerging health problems and to adjust, discard, or create new strategies as required.

Third, TD thinking anticipates, as the hallmark of the twenty-first century, accelerated change at all levels of the health hierarchy. TD reasoning and teamwork interactions provide the means for accommodating these rapid changes and generating new modes of understanding and knowledge about them. Another reason the TD approach is receptive to change is because it is open *a priori* to all theories of knowledge, not only those traditionally associated with health research. As the twenty-first century progresses, predicting and directing change will be central features of TD conceptual frameworks.

The fourth principle of transdisciplinary thinking that enables health social scientists to deal with future health scenarios is the response to complexity. We have used complexity theory as a particularly powerful TD framework showing how all health problems evolve as properties of open, dynamic systems incorporating many levels of the health hierarchy. TD offers strategies for setting health policies and creating interventions depending on the nature of the system involved. Systems, as has been observed, can range from far-from-equilibrium, creative, and ordered to near-equilibrium and disordered. Complexity theory has offered the important insight that even systems at the edge of chaos can be understood through the concepts of attractors, basin of attraction, and point of balance between creative activity (chaos) and higher level organisation. The evolution of more highly ordered systems is explained through concepts such as dissipative structures, self-regulation, and adaptive features (see chapters 3 and 6). In essence, the transforming vision of complexity theory is both evolutionary and revolutionary. Evolutionary in that it is 'part of a slow, gradual change of vision that is accruing as we develop new tools, new abilities and more subtle understandings of how things work' (Goerner 1994, p. 7) and revolutionary in that complexity theory has become a key to the 'physical understanding of how order arises' (Goerner 1994, p. 7).

In this text we have advanced transdisciplinary thinking as a much-needed bridge between the sciences, and between approaches to knowledge that emphasise the organic and the mechanical. Systematic use of transdisciplinary thinking makes comprehensible a range of seemingly opposite concepts, including holism/reductionism, chaos/order, subjective/objective, organic/mechanical, mind/body, and physical/spiritual. A dialectical understanding of the continuity and tensions between these concepts is an integral part of what we describe as an organically unified vision of reality—the basis of transdisciplinary thinking.

Transdisciplinary thinking ideally prepares health social scientists to address contemporary and future problems facing human populations. While health social science has a legitimate focus on cultural, political, psychological, and economic dimensions of health, we have seen in this text that such a focus cannot ultimately be seen in isolation from the other levels within the health hierarchy. The transdisciplinary theorist and researcher, no matter what specialty, has an obligation to go further and use tools and methods, such as those presented in this book, to more fully connect their expertise with those of others (professionals and other, nonprofessional, community members) in the pursuit of solutions to the health problems of the twenty-first century.

References

Aday, L.A. 1996, *Designing and Conducting Health Surveys: A Comprehensive Guide* (2nd edn), Jossey-Bass Publishers (Wiley), San Francisco.

Adler, N.E. et al. 1994, 'Socioeconomic Status and Health: The Challenge of the Gradient', *American Psychologist*, vol. 49, pp. 15–24.

Adler, P.A. and Adler, P. 1994, 'Observational Techniques', in N.K. Denzin and Y.S. Lincoln (eds), *Handbook of Qualitative Research*, Sage Publications, Thousand Oaks, California.

Albrecht, G. 1990, 'Philosophical Thoughts on a Transdisciplinary Model of Human Health', in N. Higginbotham and G. Albrecht (eds), *Sociocultural Studies 1, Module 2: Transdisciplinary Thinking in Health Social Science Research: Definition, Rationale and Procedures*, Centre for Clinical Epidemiology and Biostatistics, University of Newcastle, Newcastle, Australia.

—— and Higginbotham, N. (eds), 1992, *Sociocultural Studies 1, Module 2: Transdisciplinary Thinking in Health Social Science Research: Definition, Rationale and Procedures*, Centre for Clinical Epidemiology and Biostatistics, University of Newcastle, Newcastle, Australia.

——, Freeman, S. and Higginbotham, N. 1998, 'Complexity and Human Health: The Case for a Transdisciplinary Paradigm', *Culture Medicine and Psychiatry*, vol. 2, pp. 55–92.

Alland, A. 1970, *Adaptation in Cultural Evolution: An Approach to Medical Anthropology*, Columbia University Press, New York.

American Cancer Society 1999, 'Malignant Mesothelioma', <www2:cancer.org/CID/171.00/index.html>, accessed 2 December 1999.

Anderson, R. 1996, *Magic, Science, and Health: The Aims and Achievements of Medical Anthropology*, Harcourt Brace College Publishers, Fort Worth.

Angulo, F. 1998, 'Antimicrobial-Resistant Salmonella Infections in Humans', *The C.A. USE,* (Careful Antibiotic Use to Prevent Resistance) Winter Quarter, vol. 2, January. www.cdc.gov/ncidod/dbmd/cause/jan98.htm.

Arora, N.K. et al. 1999, *Aims-INDIACLEN National Pulse Polio Immunisation Program Evaluation 1997–98,* Clinical Epidemiology Unit, All India Institute of Medical Sciences, Delhi.

Ashton, J. 1986, *Healthy Cities: Action Strategies for Health Promotion: Attachment 3,* University of Liverpool, Liverpool.

—— 1992, *Healthy Cities,* Open University Press, Philadelphia.

Australian Bureau of Statistics 1988, 'Profile of Local Government Areas—Usual Resident Counts, New South Wales', *ABS Census of Population and Housing,* 30 June 1986, cat. no. 2470.0., ABS, Canberra.

Australian Institute of Health 1996, *The Fifth Biennial Report of the Australian Institute of Health: Australia's Health,* Australian Government Publishing Service, Canberra.

Babbie, E.R. 1990, *Survey Research Methods* (2nd edn), Wadsworth Publishing, Belmont, California.

—— 1998, *The Practice of Social Research* (8th edn), Wadsworth Publishing, Belmont, California.

Baer, H. 1996, 'Toward a Political Ecology of Health in Medical Anthropology', *Medical Anthropology Quarterly,* vol. 10, no. 4, pp. 451–4.

Bak, P. and Chen, K. 1991, 'Self-organised Criticality', *Scientific American,* vol. 264, pp. 6–33.

Banister, P. et al. 1994, *Qualitative Methods in Psychology: A Research Guide,* Open University Press, Buckingham.

Barker, D.J.P. (ed.) 1992, 'Foetal and Infant Origins of Adult Disease', Papers written by the Medical Research Council Environmental Epidemiology Unit, University of South Hampton, *British Medical Journal,* London.

—— et al. 1989, 'Weight in Infancy and Death from Ischaemic Heart Disease, *Lancet,* vol. 9, pp. 577–80.

Barnett, V. 1991, *Sample Survey Principles and Methods,* Edward Arnold, London.

Barrett-Connor, E.L. 1985, 'Obesity, Atherosclerosis and Coronary Artery Disease', *Annals of Internal Medicine,* vol. 103, pp. 1009–10.

Barton, S. 1994, 'Chaos, Self-organisation and Psychology', *American Psychologist,* vol. 49, pp. 5–14.

Bauman, L.J. and Adair, E.G. 1992, 'The Use of Interviewing to Inform Questionnaire Design', *Health Education Quarterly,* vol. 19, no. 1, pp. 9–23.

Beaglehole, R., Bonita, R. and Kjellstrom, T. 1993, *Basic Epidemiology,* World Health Organization, Geneva.

Becker, Howard 1953, 'Becoming a Marihuana User', *American Journal of Sociology,* vol. 59, pp. 235–42.

Beekmann, S.E. et al. 1990, 'Risky Business: Using Necessarily Imprecise Casualty Counts to Estimate Occupational Risks for HIV-1 Infection', *Infection Control and Hospital Epidemiology*, vol. 11, pp. 371–9.

Begg, C. et al. 1996, 'Improving the Quality of Reporting of Randomized Controlled Trials', *Journal of the American Medical Association*, vol. 276, no. 8, pp. 637–9.

Bellini, J. 1986, *High Tech Holocaust*, Greenhouse Publications, Richmond.

Berg, K. 1983, 'Genetics of Coronary Heart Disease', *Progress in Medical Genetics*, vol. 5, pp. 35–90.

Berlin, J.A. and Colditz, G.A. 1990, 'A Meta-Analysis of Physical Activity in the Prevention of Coronary Heart Disease', *American Journal of Epidemiology*, vol. 132, pp. 612–28.

Bernard, H.R. 1994, *Research Methods in Anthropology: Qualitative and Quantitative Approaches*, Sage Publications, Thousand Oaks, California.

Bierlich, B. 1999, 'Sacrifice, Plants, and Western Pharmaceuticals: Money and Health Care in Northern Ghana', *Medical Anthropology Quarterly*, vol. 13, no. 3, pp. 316–37.

Bijnen, F., Caspersen, C. and Mosterd, W.L. 1994, 'Physical Inactivity as a Risk Factor for Coronary Heart Disease: A WHO and International Society and Federation of Cardiology Position Statement', *Bulletin of the World Health Organization*, vol. 72, pp. 1–4.

Binson, D. and Catania, J.A. 1998, 'Respondents' Understanding of the Words Used in Sexual Behavior Questions', *Public Opinion Quarterly*, vol. 62, pp. 190–208.

Blois, M.S. 1988, 'Medicine and the Nature of Vertical Reasoning', *New England Journal of Medicine*, vol. 318, pp. 847–51.

Bloom, B.L. 1988, *A Psychosocial Perspective*, Prentice Hall, New Jersey.

Bodenheimer, T.S. 1984, 'The Transnational Pharmaceutical Industry and the Health of the World's People', in J.B. McKinlay (ed.), *Issues in the Political Economy of Health Care*, Tavistock, London and New York.

Boekeloo, B.O. et al. 1994, 'Self Reports of HIV Risk Factors by Patients at a Sexually Transmitted Disease Clinic: Audio vs Written Questionnaires', *American Journal of Public Health*, vol. 84, no. 5, pp. 754–60.

Boodman, S. 1997, 'Hospitals Promote Hand-washing to Reduce Spread of Infection', *Detroit News*, 6 November, http://detnews.com/1997/accent/9711/06/11060029.htm, accessed 15 January 2000.

Booth-Kewley, S. and Friedman, H.S. 1987, 'Psychological Predictors of Heart Disease: A Quantitative Review', *Psychological Bulletin*, vol. 101, pp. 343–62.

Borman, K.M., LeCompte, M.D. and Goetz, J.P. 1986, 'Ethnographic and Qualitative Research Design and Why it Doesn't Work', *American Behavioral Scientist*, vol. 30, no. 1, pp. 42–57.

Bradshaw, J. 1981, 'A Taxonomy of Social Need', in P. Henderson and D. N. Thomas (eds), *Readings in Community Work*, George Allen and Unwin, London.

Britten, N., Jones, R., Murphy, E. and Stacy, R. 1995, 'Qualitative Research Methods in General Practice and Primary Care', *Family Practice*, vol. 12, no. 1, pp. 104–14.

Brown, L.R. and Halweil, B. 1999, 'HIV Epidemic Slowing Population Growth', *A Worldwatch News Release on HIV*, http://www.worldwatch.org/alerts/990928.html, accessed 29 October 1999.

Brown, P.J., Inhorn, M. and Smith, D.J. 1996, 'Disease, Ecology and Human Behavior', in C.F. Sargent and T.M. Johnson (eds), *Medical Anthropology: Contemporary Theory and Method*, Praeger, London.

Brown, Peter 1998, 'Understanding Medical Anthropology: Biocultural and Cultural Approaches', in P. J. Brown (compiler), *Understanding and Applying Medical Anthropology*, Mayfield Publishing, California.

Brown, V. 1994, 'Health and Environment: A Common Framework and a Common Practice', in C. Chu and R. Simpson (eds), *Ecological Public Health: From Vision to Practice*, Institute of Applied Environmental Research, Griffith University, Queensland.

Buchbinder, R., Bombadier, M.Y. and Tugwell, P. 1995, 'Which Outcome Measures Should be Used in Rheumatoid Arthritis Clinical Trials?', *Arthritis and Rheumatism*, vol. 38, no. 11, pp. 1568–80.

Byles, J., Harris, M., Nair, B. and Butler, J. 1996, 'Preventive Health Programs for Older Australians', *Health Promotion Journal of Australia*, vol. 6, no. 2, pp. 37–43.

Byles, J., Feldman, S. and Mishra, G. 1999, 'For Richer, for Poorer, in Sickness and in Health', *Women and Health*, vol. 29, no. 1, pp. 15–30.

Byrne, D. 1998, *Complexity Theory and the Social Sciences: An Introduction*, Routledge, London.

Caldwell, J.C. 1992, 'Old and New Factors in Health Transitions', *Health Transition Review*, vol. 2, Supplementary issue, pp. 205–16.

—— 1994, 'New Challenges for Demography', *Journal of the Australian Population Association*, vol. 11, no. 2, pp. 9–19.

—— and Santow, G. 1989, 'Introduction', in J.C. Caldwell and G. Santow (eds), *Selected Readings in the Cultural, Social and Behavioural Determinants of Health*, Health Transition Centre, Australia National University, Canberra.

—— et al. (eds) 1990, *What We Know about the Health Transition: The Cultural, Social and Behavioural Determinants of Health*, Health Transition Centre, Australian National University, Canberra.

—— and Caldwell, P. 1995, 'Synthesis: Where Are We Now?', *Health Transition Review*, vol. 5, no. 2, p. 255.

Caldwell, P. et al. (eds) 1999, *Resistance to Behavioural Change to Reduce HIV/AIDS Infection in Predominantly Heterosexual Epidemics in Third World Countries*, Health Transition Centre, National Centre for Epidemiology and Population Health, Australian National University, Canberra.

Calnan, M. 1990, 'Food and Health: A Comparison of Beliefs and Practices in Middle-Class and Working-Class Households', in S. Cunningham-Burley and N. McKeganey (eds), *Readings in Medical Sociology*, Tavistock, London.

Campbell, D.T. and Fiske, D.W. 1959, 'Convergent and Discriminant Validation by the Multitrait-Multimethod Matrix', *Psychological Bulletin*, vol. 56, pp. 81–105.

Carswell, J.W., Lloyd, G. and Howells, J. 1989, 'Short Communication: Prevalence of HIV in East African Lorry Drivers', *AIDS*, vol. 3, no. 11, pp. 759–61.

Cartwright, A. 1983, *Health Surveys in Practice and in Potential: A Critical Review of Their Scope and Methods*, King Edward's Hospital Fund for London, London.

Casey, A. 1993, 'The Power Behind Your Doctor', *Green Left*, 7 April, pp. 14–15.

Catania, J.A. et al. 1993, 'Response Bias in Surveys of AIDS-Related Sexual Behavior', in D.G. Ostrow and R.C. Kessler (eds), *Methodological Issues in AIDS Behavioural Research*, Plenum Press, New York.

Centers for Disease Control (CDC) 1987, 'Recommendations for Prevention of HIV Transmission in Health-Care Settings', *Morbidity and Mortality Weekly Report*, vol. 36, pp. 3s–18s.

Centers for Disease Control and Prevention 1992, 'Surveillance for Occupationally Acquired HIV Infection—United States, 1981–1992', *Journal of the American Medical Association*, vol. 268, p. 3294.

—— 1993, 'Update: Hantavirus Disease—Southwestern United States', *Morbidity and Mortality Weekly Report*, 30 July, pp. 570–2.

—— October 1998, *Antimicrobial Resistance: A Growing Threat to Public Health*, Hospitals Infection Program, www.cdc.gov/ncidod/hip/Areist/am_res.htm, accessed 15 January 2000.

Chetley, A. 1990, *A Healthy Business? World Health and the Pharmaceutical Industry*, Zed Books, London.

—— 1993, 'The Future of the Bangladesh National Drug Policy', *Essential Drugs Monitor*, no. 15, pp. 10–11.

Chinn, A. and Burney, P.G.J. 1987, 'On Measuring Repeatability of Data from Self-Administered Questionnaires', *International Journal of Epidemiology*, vol. 16, pp. 121–7.

Chowdhury, Z. 1995, *The Politics of Essential Drugs: The Makings of a Successful Health Strategy: Lessons from Bangladesh*, Zed Books, London.

Chu, C. 1994a, 'Healthy Cities Update', in C. Chu and R. Simpson (eds), *Ecological Public Health: From Vision to Practice*, Institute of Applied Environmental Research, Griffith University, Queensland.

—— 1994b, 'Integrating Health and Environment: The Key to an Ecological Health', in C. Chu and R. Simpson (eds), *Ecological Public Health: From Vision to Practice*, Institute of Applied Environmental Research, Griffith University, Queensland.

—— and Simpson, R. (eds) 1994, *Ecological Public Health: From Vision to Practice*, Institute of Applied Environmental Research, Queensland.

—— and Rickson, D. 1994, 'Social Impact Assessment and the Ecological Public Health', in C. Chu and R. Simpson (eds), *Ecological Public Health: From Vision to Practice*, Institute of Applied Environmental Research, Griffith University, Queensland.

Cleland, J. and Hill, A. 1991, 'Studying the Health Transition: An Overview', in J. Cleland and A. Hill (eds), *The Health Transition: Methods and Measures*, Health Transition Centre, Australian National University, Canberra.

Cobb, A.K. and Hagemaster, J.N. 1987, 'Ten Criteria for Evaluating Qualitative Research Proposals', *Journal of Nursing Education*, vol. 26, no. 4, pp. 138–43.

Cochran, W. 1977, *Sampling Techniques* (3rd edn), John Wiley & Sons, New York.

Cohen, J. 1988, *Statistical Power Analysis for the Behavioural Sciences* (2nd edn), Lawrence Erlbaum, New Jersey.

Cohen, J.A. 1960, 'A Coefficient of Agreement for Nominal Scales', *Educational Psychological Measurement*, vol. 20, pp. 37–46.

Colborn, T., Dumonoski, K. and Myers, J.P. 1996, *Our Stolen Future: Are We Threatening Our Fertility, Intelligence, and Survival? A Scientific Detective Story*, Abacus, London.

Collignon, P. 1999, 'Vancomycin-Resistant Enterococci and the Use of Avoparcin in Animal Feed: Is There a Link?', *Medical Journal of Australia*, vol. 171, pp. 144–6.

Colwell, R.R. and Patz, J.A. 1997, *Climate, Infectious Disease and Health: An Interdisciplinary Perspective*, American Academy of Microbiology, Washington DC.

Commonwealth of Australia 1994, *National Goals, Targets and Strategies for Improving Cardiovascular Health. Report of the National Health Goals and Targets Implementation Working Group on Cardiovascular Disease*, Australian Government Publishing Service, Canberra.

Cooke, J. 1998, *Cannibals, Cows and the CJD Catastrophe*, Random House, Sydney.

Cosminsky, S. 1994, 'All Roads Lead to the Pharmacy: Use of Pharmaceuticals on a Guatemalan Plantation', in N.L. Etkin and M.L. Tan (eds), *Medicines: Meanings and Contexts*, Health Action Information Network, Quezon City, Philippines.

Courington, K.R., Patterson, S.L. and Howard, R.J. 1991, 'Universal Precautions Are Not Universally Followed', *Archives of Surgery*, vol. 126, pp. 93–6.

Creswell, J.W. 1998, *Qualitative Inquiry and Research Design: Choosing Among Five Traditions*, Sage Publications, Thousand Oaks, California.

Crowder, M.J. and Hand, D.J. 1990, *Analysis of Repeated Measures*, Chapman and Hall, London and New York.

Cuff, E. and Payne, G. 1984, *Perspectives in Sociology* (2nd edn), George Allen and Unwin, Sydney.

Daniel, W. 1999, *Biostatistics: A Foundation for Analysis in the Health Sciences*, (7th edn), John Wiley & Sons, New York.

Danzon, Patricia Munch 1998, *Pharmaceutical Price Regulation: National Politics Versus Global Interests*, AEI Press, Washington DC.

Darzins, P.J., Smith, B.J. and Heller, R.F. 1992, 'How to Read a Journal Article', *Medical Journal of Australia*, vol. 157, no. 6, pp. 389–94.

Davies, B. et al. 1995, 'Challenges of Conducting Research in Palliative Care', *Omega*, vol. 31, no. 4, pp. 263–73.

Davies, P. 1989, *The Cosmic Blueprint*, Unwin Hyman, London.

Davison, C., Frankel, S. and Smith, G. 1992, 'The Limits of Lifestyle: Re-assessing "Fatalism" in the Popular Culture of Illness Prevention', *Social Science and Medicine*, vol. 34, no. 6, pp. 675–85.

de Bono, E. 1992, *Teach Your Child How to Think*, Penguin, London.

Dean, A. 1997, *Chaos and Intoxication: Complexity and Adaptation in the Structure of Human Nature*, Routledge, London.

Deitz, B. 1992, *Network for Healthy School Communities—Case Studies*, Network of Healthy School Communities, Canberra.

Denzin, N.K. 1978, *The Research Act* (2nd edn), McGraw-Hill, New York.

—— 1989, *The Research Act* (3rd edn), Prentice Hall, New Jersey.

—— and Lincoln, Y.S. 1994, *Handbook of Qualitative Research*, Sage Publications, Thousand Oaks, California.

Derrickson-Kossmann, D. and Drinkard, L. 1997, 'Dissociative Disorders in Chaos and Complexity', in F. Masterpasquia and P.A. Perna (eds), *The Psychological Meaning of Chaos*, American Psychological Association, Washington DC.

Desowitz, R.S. 1981, *New Guinea Tapeworms and Jewish Grandmothers: Tales of Parasites and People*, W.W. Norton, New York.

DeWalt, B.R. and Pelto, P.J. 1985, 'Microlevel/Macrolevel Linkages: An Introduction to the Issues and a Framework for Analysis', in B.R. DeWalt and P.J. Pelto (eds), *Micro and Macro Levels of Analysis in Anthropology: Issues in Theory and Research*, Westview Press, London.

Dey, I. 1993, *Qualitative Data Analysis: A User-Friendly Guide for Social Scientists*, Routledge, London.

Diggle, P., Liang, K.L. and Zeger, S. 1994, *Analysis of Longitudinal Data*, Oxford Science Publications, New York.

Dobson, A.J. 1984, 'Calculating Sample Size', *Transactions of the Menzies Foundation*, vol. 7, pp. 75–9.

—— 1987, 'Trends in Cardiovascular Risk Factors in Australia, 1966–1983: Evidence from Prevalence Surveys', *Community Health Studies,* vol. 11, pp. 2–14.

——, Halpin, S. and Alexander, H. 1991, 'Does the Occupational Structure of the Hunter Region Explain the High Rates of Ischaemic Heart Disease Among its Men?', *Australian Journal of Public Health,* vol. 15, no. 3, pp. 172–6.

Doll, R. and Peto, R. 1981, *The Causes of Cancer,* Oxford University Press, Oxford.

Donner, A. and Eliasziw, M. 1987, 'Sample Size Requirements for Reliability Studies', *Statistics in Medicine,* vol. 6, pp. 441–8.

—— 1992, 'A Goodness-of-Fit Approach to Inference Procedures for the Kappa Statistic: Confidence Interval Construction, Significance Testing and Sample Size Estimation', *Statistics in Medicine,* vol. 11, pp. 1511–19.

Dressler, W.W. 1990, 'Education, Lifestyle and Arterial Blood Pressure', *Journal of Psychosomatic Research,* vol. 34, no. 5, pp. 515–23.

Dupen, F. et al. 1996, 'Validation of a New Multidimensional Health Locus of Control Scale (Form C) in Asthma Research', *Psychology and Health: The International Review of Health Psychology,* vol. 11, pp. 493–504.

Dyke, C. 1988, 'Cities as Dissipative Structures', in B.H. Weber, D.J. Depew and J.D. Smith (eds), *Entropy, Information, and Evolution: New Perspectives on Physical and Biological Evolution,* MIT Press, Cambridge, Massachusetts.

Elliott, S.J. 1995, 'Psychosocial Stress, Women and Heart Health: A Critical Review', *Social Science and Medicine,* vol. 40, pp. 105–15.

Elmendorf, M. and Isely, R. 1983, 'Public and Private Roles of Women in Water Supply and Sanitation Programs', *Human Organisation,* vol. 42, no. 3, pp. 195–204.

Emmons, K.M. et al. 1994, 'Mechanisms in Multiple Risk Factor Interventions: Smoking, Physical Activity, and Dietary Fat Intake Among Manufacturing Workers, Working Well Research Group', *Preventive Medicine,* July, vol. 23, no. 4, pp. 481–9.

Engel, G.L. 1977, 'The Need for a New Medical Model: A Challenge for Biomedicine', *Science,* vol. 196, pp. 129–36.

—— 1980, 'The Clinical Application of the Biopsychosocial Model', *American Journal of Psychiatry,* vol. 137, pp. 535–44.

—— 1982, 'The Biopsychosocial Model and Medical Education', *New England Journal of Medicine,* vol. 306, no. 13, 1 April, pp. 802–5.

Essential Drugs Monitor, <http://www.who.org/programmes/dap/edm.html>.

Etkin, N.L. and Tan, M.L (eds) 1994, *Medicines: Meanings and Contexts,* Health Action Information Network, Quezon City, Philippines.

Fielding, N.G. and Fielding, J.L. 1986, 'Linking Data', *Qualitative Research Methods,* Series 4, pp. 23–35.

Firth, W.J. 1991, 'Chaos—Predicting the Unpredictable', *British Medical Journal*, vol. 303, pp. 1565–8.

Fischer, F. 1998, 'Beyond Empiricism: Policy Inquiry in Postpositivist Perspective. (The Evidentiary Basis of Policy Analysis: Empiricist vs Postpositivist Positions)', *Policy Studies Journal*, vol. 26, no. 1, pp. 1–13.

Fiske, S.T. and Neuberg, S.L. 1990, 'A Continuum of Impression Formation, from Category-based to Individuating Processes: Influences of Information and Motivation of Attention and Interpretation', *Advances in Experimental Social Psychology*, vol. 23, pp. 1–74.

Fitzpatrick, R. 1984, 'Lay Concepts of Illness', in R. Fitzpatrick, J. Hinton, G. Scrambler and J. Thompson (eds), *The Experience of Illness*, Tavistock, London.

Fontana, Andrea and Frey, James H. 1994, 'Interviewing: The Art of Science', in N.K. Denzin and Y.S. Lincoln (eds), *Handbook of Qualitative Research*, Sage Publications, Thousand Oaks, California.

Foster, G.M. and Anderson, B.G. 1978, *Medical Anthropology*, John Wiley & Sons, New York.

Fowler, F.J., Jr 1993, *Survey Research Methods* (2nd edn), Sage Publications, Newbury Park, California.

Freedman, L., Parmar, M. and Baker, S. 1993, 'The Design of Observer Agreement Studies with Binary Assessments', *Statistics in Medicine*, vol. 12, pp. 165–79.

Freeman, W. et al. 1990, 'Association Between Risk Factors for Coronary Heart Disease in Schoolboys and Adult Mortality Rates in the Same Localities', *Archives of Disease in Childhood*, vol. 65, pp. 78–83.

Fridkin, S.K. and Gaynes, R.P. 1999, 'Antimicrobial Resistance in Intensive Care Units', *Clinics in Chest Medicine*, vol. 20, no. 2, p. 303.

Fridkin, S.K. et al. 1996, 'The Role of Understaffing in Central Venous Catheter-Associated Bloodstream Infections', *Infection Control and Hospital Epidemiology*, vol. 17, no. 3, pp. xx–xx.

Friedenreich, C.M. 1994, 'Improving Long-Term Recall in Epidemiologic Studies', *Epidemiology*, vol. 5, no. 1, pp. 1–3.

Friedman, H.S. and DiMatteo, M.R. 1989, *Health Psychology*, Prentice Hall, New Jersey.

Friis, R.H. and Sellers, T.A. 1999, *Epidemiology for Public Health Practice* (2nd edn), Aspen Publishers, Geneva.

Garrett, L. 1994, *The Coming Plague: Newly Emerging Diseases in a World Out of Order*, Virago Press, London.

Garro, L.C. 1994, 'Narrative Representations of Chronic Illness Experience: Cultural Models of Illness, Mind, and Body in Stories Concerning the Temporomandibular Joint (TMJ)', *Social Science and Medicine*, vol. 38, no. 6, pp. 775–88.

Glaser, B. and Strauss, A. 1967, *Discovery of Grounded Theory: Strategies for Qualitative Research*, Aldine de Gruyter, Chicago.

Glover, J. and Woolacott, T. 1992, *A Social Atlas of Australia*, vol.2, cat. no. 4385.0., Australian Bureau of Statistics, Canberra.

Goerner, S.J. 1994, *Chaos and the Evolving Ecological Universe*, Gordon and Breach, South Australia.

Goffman, E. 1961, *Asylums: Essays on the Social Situation of Mental Patients and Other Inmates*, Doubleday, New York.

Goldberg, R.J. 1992, 'Coronary Heart Disease: Epidemiology and Risk Factors', in I.S. Ockene and J.K. Ockene (eds), *Prevention of Coronary Heart Disease*, Little, Brown and Company, Boston.

Goodger, B. 2000, An Examination of Social Support Amongst Older Australians, Unpublished PhD thesis, University of Newcastle, Newcastle, Australia.

Goodwin, B. 1995, *How the Leopard Changed its Spots: The Evolution of Complexity*, Phoenix Giants, London.

Gordis, L. 1996, *Epidemiology*, W.B. Saunders, Philadelphia.

Gotto, A.M. et al. 1990, 'The Cholesterol Facts. A Summary of Evidence Relating Dietary Fats, Serum Cholesterol, and Coronary Heart Disease', *Circulation*, vol. 81, pp. 1721–33.

Greater Irvine Health Promotion Center 1993, *Greater Irvine Health Promotion Center Report*, University of California, Irvine, March, pp. 4–5.

Greene, J.C. 1994, 'Qualitative Program Evaluation: Practice and Promise', in N.K. Denzin and Y.S. Lincoln (eds), *Handbook of Qualitative Research*, Sage Publications, Thousand Oaks, California.

—— 2000, 'Understanding Social Progress Through Evaluation', in N.K. Denzin and Y.S. Lincoln (eds), *Handbook of Qualitative Research* (2nd edn), Sage Publications, Thousand Oaks, California.

Guastello, S.J. 1995, *Chaos, Catastrophe, and Human Affairs: Applications of Nonlinear Dynamics to Work, Organizations, and Social Evolution*, Lawrence Erlbaum, New Jersey.

Guba, E.G. and Lincoln, Y.S. 1989, *Fourth Generation Evaluation*, Sage Publications, Newbury Park, California.

—— 1994, 'Competing Paradigms in Qualitative Research', in N.K. Denzin and Y.S. Lincoln (eds), *Handbook of Qualitative Research*, Sage Publications, Thousand Oaks, California.

Hadley, W.K. 1989, 'Infection of the Health Care Worker by HIV and Other Blood-Borne Viruses: Risks, Protection, and Education', *American Journal of Hospital Pharmacy*, vol. 46, pp. s4–s7.

Halstead, S.B., Tugwell, P. and Bennett, K. 1991, 'The International Clinical

Epidemiology Network (INCLEN): A Progress Report', *Journal of Clinical Epidemiology*, vol. 44, p. 579–89.

Hancock, T. 1992, 'Promoting Health Environmentally', in K. Dean and T. Hancock, *Supportive Environments for Health*, WHO, Copenhagen.

—— 1994, 'Sustainability, Equity, Peace and the (Green) Politics of Health', in C. Chu and R. Simpson (eds), *Ecological Public Health: From Vision to Practice*, Institute of Applied Environmental Research, Griffith University, Queensland.

Hardon, A. 1992, 'Consumers Versus Producers: Power Play Behind the Scenes', in N. Kanji et al. (eds), *Drugs Policy in Developing Countries*, Zed Books, London.

Harvey, E. et al. 1998, 'A Qualitative Investigation into an HIV Outbreak Among Injection Drug Users in Vancouver, British Columbia', *AIDS Care*, vol. 10, no. 3, pp. 313–21.

Hayles, K.N. 1991, *Chaos and Order: Complex Dynamics in Literature and Science*, University of Chicago Press, Chicago.

Heading, G. 1996, Missing Bodies: Exclusionary Health Discourses and Participatory Heart Disease Programmes, PhD thesis, University of Newcastle, Australia.

Heart Foundation, n.d., *Promoting Heart Health: An Educational Resource Manual for Rural and Remote Health Workers*, Heart Foundation, Queensland.

Hegel, G.W.F. 1976, *The Philosophy of Right*, translated by T. M. Knox, Oxford University Press, Oxford.

Helitzer-Allen, D. and Kendall, C. 1992, 'Explaining Differences Between Qualitative and Quantitative Data: A Study of Chemoprophylaxis During Pregnancy', *Health Education Quarterly*, vol. 19, no. 1, pp. 41–54.

Helman, C.G. 1985, 'Communication in Primary Care: The Role of Patient and Practitioner Explanatory Models', *Social Science and Medicine*, vol. 20, pp. 923–31.

Henderson, D.K. et al. 1990, 'Risk for Occupational Transmission of Human Immunodeficiency Virus Type 1 (HIV-1) Associated with Clinical Exposures: A Prospective Evaluation', *Annals of Internal Medicine*, vol. 113, pp. 740–6.

Henderson, G.E. and Fischer, W.A. 1999, The Cephalosporin Wars in China: Competing in the Chinese Antibiotic Market (unpublished draft), Department of Social Medicine, University of North Carolina School of Medicine, Chapel Hill, North Carolina, pp. 1–25.

Hennekens, C.H. and Buring, J.E. 1987, *Epidemiology in Medicine*, Little, Brown and Company, Boston.

Hetzel, B. and McMichael, A. 1987, 'Diet and Coronary Heart Disease: Insights into a Modern Epidemic', in *The Lifestyle Factor*, Penguin, New York.

Higginbotham, N. 1984, *Third World Challenge to Psychiatry: Culture Accommodation and Mental Health Care*, University of Hawaii Press, Honolulu.

—— 1992, 'Developing Partnerships for Health and Social Science Research: The International Clinical Epidemiology Network (INCLEN) Social Science Component', *Social Science and Medicine*, vol. 35, pp. 1325–7.

—— 1994, 'Capacity Building for Health Social Science: The International Clinical Epidemiology Network (INCLEN) Social Science Program and the International Forum for Social Science in Health', *Acta Tropica*, vol. 57, pp. 123–38.

—— 1998, 'Methodological Issues in Developing Transdisciplinary Health Social Science', *Proceedings of the Asia Pacific Social Science and Medicine Conference*, Yogyakarta, Indonesia, 7–12 December, Gadjah Mada University Press, Yogyakarta.

—— and Albrecht, G. 1988, *Health Social Science, Module 1: Social, Cultural and Psychological Determinants of Disease*, Centre for Clinical Epidemiology and Biostatistics, University of Newcastle, Newcastle, Australia.

——, West, S.G. and Forsyth, D.R. 1988, *Psychotherapy and Behaviour Change: Social, Cultural and Methodological Perspectives*, Pergamon Press, New York.

—— and Streiner, D.L. 1991, 'The Social Science Contribution to Pharmaco-epidemiology', *Journal of Clinical Epidemiology*, vol. 44, Supplement II, pp. 73s–82s.

—— and Titheridge, C. 1993, Coalfields Healthy Heartbeat Program: A Case Study in Community Development, Unpublished paper presented at the Public Health Association Meeting, University of New South Wales, Sydney, 30 September.

—— et al. 1993, 'Community Worry About Heart Disease: A Needs Survey in the Coalfields and Newcastle Area of the Hunter Region', *Australian Journal of Public Health*, vol. 17, pp. 314–21.

——, Albrecht, G. and Freeman, S. 1997, 'The Case for a Transdisciplinary Paradigm', in L. Hunt (ed.), *Proceedings of the Third Asia and Pacific Conference on the Social Sciences and Medicine*, Faculty of Health Sciences, Edith Cowan University, Perth.

——, Phillips, M. and Henderson, G. 1997, 'Developing Reliable and Valid Measures to Assess the Outcomes of Intervention Trials or to Determine the Level of Exposure in Studies about Etiology', *Clinically Applied Health Social Science: Module 7*, Centre for Clinical Epidemiology and Biostatistics, University of Newcastle, Newcastle.

—— et al. 1999, 'Reducing Coronary Heart Disease in the Australian Coalfields: Evaluation of a Ten-Years Community Intervention', *Social Science and Medicine*, vol. 48, pp. 683–92.

Hill, A.B. 1965, 'The Environment and Disease: Association or Causation', *Proceedings of the Royal Society of Medicine*, vol. 58, pp. 295–300.

Hocking, B., Gordon, I., Grain, H. and Hatfield, G. 1996, 'Cancer Incidence and Mortality and Proximity to TV Towers', *Medical Journal of Australia*, vol. 165, pp. 601–5.

Houts, A.C., Cook, T.D. and Shadish, W.R. 1986, 'The Person–Situation Debate: A Critical Multiplist Perspective', *Journal of Personality*, vol. 30, pp. 147–60.

Howteerakul, N. 1997', Prescribing Patterns and Quality of Care for Children under Five Years of Age with Diarrhoea in Thailand, PhD thesis, Centre for Clinical Epidemiology and Biostatistics, University of Newcastle, Newcastle, Australia.

Hussain, S.P. and Harris, C.C. 1998, 'Molecular Epidemiology of Human Cancer', *Recent Results in Cancer Research*, vol. 154, pp. 22–36.

Inhorn, M. and Brown, P. 1990, 'The Anthropology of Infectious Disease', *Annual Review of Anthropology*, vol. 19, pp. 89–117.

Institute of Food Science and Technology (UK) (IFST) 1996, Bovine Spongiform Encephalopathy: Part 1/3, *IFST: Current Hot Topics*, <http://www.easynet.co.uk/ifst/hottop5.htm>, accessed 18 July 1999.

—— 1999, Bovine Spongiform Encephalopathy (BSE): Part1/3, *IFST: Current Hot Topics*, <http://www.easynet.co.uk/ifst/hottop5.htm>, accessed 7 June 1999.

International Forum for Social Science in Health (IFSSH) 1993, *An Introduction to the International Forum for Social Science in Health*, Mahidol University, Faculty of Social Sciences and Humanities, Nakornpathom, Thailand.

Jagger, J. and Pearson, R.D. 1991, 'Universal Precautions: Still Missing the Point on Needlesticks', *Infection Control and Hospital Epidemiology*, vol. 12, pp. 211–13.

Janes, C. 1995, 'The Transformations of Tibetan Medicine', *Medical Anthropology Quarterly*, vol. 9, no. 1, pp. 6–39.

Janesick, V.J. 1994, 'The Dance of Qualitative Research Design: Metaphor, Methodolatry and Meaning', in N.K. Denzin and Y.S. Lincoln (eds), *Handbook of Qualitative Research*, Sage Publications, Thousand Oaks, California.

Jantsch, E. 1972, *Technological Planning and Social Futures*, Cassell, London.

Javholm, B., Englund, A. and Albin, M. 1999, 'Pleural Mesothelioma in Sweden: An Analysis of the Incidence According to the Use of Asbestos', *Occupational and Environmental Medicine*, vol. 56, no. 2 , pp. 110–13.

Jick, T.D. 1983, 'Mixing Qualitative and Quantitative Methods: Triangulation in Action', in J. Van Maanen (ed.), *Qualitative Methodology*, Sage Publications, London.

Jobe, J.B. and Mingay, D.J. 1991, 'Cognition and Survey Measurement: History and Overview', *Applied Cognitive Psychology*, vol. 5, pp. 175–92.

Johansson, S.R. 1995, 'Health Transition Research, Health Policy and Human Welfare', *Health Transition Review*, vol. 5, pp. 227–30.

Johnson, A. 1977, 'Sex Differentials in Coronary Heart Disease: The Explanatory Role of Primary Risk Factors', *Journal of Health and Social Behaviour*, vol. 18, pp. 46–54.

Johnson, E. 1994, 'Strength of Kurri People', letter to the editor, *Newcastle Herald*, 28 November, p. 6.

Judd, C.M., Smith, E.R. and Kidder, L.H. 1991, 'Measurement: from Abstract Concepts to Concrete Representations', *Research Methods in Social Relations* (6th edn), Holt, Rinehart and Winston, Fort Worth.

Kamat, V.R. and Nichter, M. 1998, 'Pharmacies, Self-medication and Pharmaceutical Marketing in Bombay, India', *Social Science and Medicine*, vol. 47, pp. 779–94.

Kanji, N. 1992, 'Action at Country Level: The International and National Influences', in N. Kanji et al., *Drugs Policy in Developing Countries*, Zed Books, London.

Kannell, W.B. 1983, 'An Overview of the Risk Factors for Cardiovascular Disease', in N.M. Kaplan and J. Stamle (eds), *Prevention of Coronary Heart Disease*, W.B. Saunders, Philadelphia.

Kaplan, R.M. 1994, 'Using Quality of Life Information to Set Priorities in Health Policy', *Social Indicators Research*, vol. 33, nos 1–3, pp. 121–63.

——, Sallis, J. and Patterson, T.L. 1993, *Health and Human Behavior*, McGraw-Hill, New York.

Kasniyah, N. 1992, Social Psychological Determinants of Javanese Mothers' Failure to Immunize Their Children Against Measles, Masters thesis, Centre for Clinical Epidemiology and Biostatistics, University of Newcastle, Newcastle, Australia.

Kauffman, S.A. 1993, *The Origins of Order: Self-Organisation and Selection in Evolution*, Oxford University Press, New York.

Kelsey, J.L., Thompson, W.D. and Evans, A.S. 1986, *Methods in Observational Epidemiology*, Oxford University Press, New York.

—— 1996, *Methods in Observational Epidemiology* (2nd edn), Oxford University Press, New York.

Kemmis, S. and McTaggart, R. 1988, *The Action Research Planner* (3rd edn), Deakin University Press, Geelong.

Khachatourians, G. 1998, 'Agricultural Use of Antibiotics and the Evolution and Transfer of Antibiotic-Resistant Bacteria', *Canadian Medical Association Journal*, no. 3, pp. 1129–36.

Kirkwood, I. 1996, 'Cessnock Coalmine Could Close', *Newcastle Herald*, 7 August, p. 1.

Kirschner, B. and Guyatt, G. 1985, 'A Methodological Framework for Assessing Health Indices', *Journal of Chronic Disorders*, vol. 38, no. 1, pp. 27–36.

Kish, L. 1965, *Survey Sampling,* John Wiley & Sons, New York.

Kleinman, A.M. 1973, 'Medicine's Symbolic Reality: On a Central Problem in the Philosophy of Medicine', *Inquiry,* vol. 16, pp. 206–13.

Kleinman, J.C. et al. 1988, 'Mortality Among Diabetics in a National Sample', *American Journal of Epidemiology,* vol. 128, pp. 389–401.

Knafl, K.A. and Howard, M.J. 1984, 'Interpreting and Reporting Qualitative Research', *Nursing and Health,* vol. 7, pp. 17–24.

Knutsson, A. et al. 1986, 'Increased Risk of Ischaemic Heart Disease in Shift Workers', *Lancet,* vol. 2, pp. 89–92.

Kotler, P. and Roberto, E.L. 1989, *Social Marketing: Strategies for Changing Public Behaviour,* The Free Press, London.

Kresh, J. Yasha and Izrailtyan, I. 2000, 'The Heart as a Complex Adaptive System', in Y. Bar-Yam (ed.), *Unifying Themes in Complex Systems,* Perseus Books, New York.

Kresh, J. et al. 2000, 'Phase-Plane (Poincaré Plots) of Heart-Beat Interval from a Healthy Individual', *Journal of Thoracic and Cardiovascular Surgery,* in press.

Kroeger, A. 1983, 'Health Interview Surveys in Developing Countries: A Review of the Methods and Results', *International Journal of Epidemiology,* vol. 12, no. 4, pp. 465–81.

Krueger, R.A. 1988, *Focus Groups: A Practical Guide for Applied Research,* Sage Publications, Thousand Oaks, California.

Kuhn, Thomas S. 1970, *The Structure of Scientific Revolutions* (2nd edn), University of Chicago Press, Chicago.

Kunitz, S.J. 1997, 'Disease and the Destruction of Indigenous Populations', in T. Ingold (ed.), *Companion Encyclopedia of Anthropology: Humanity, Culture and Social Life,* Routledge, London.

Kunstadter, P. 1990, 'Methods in the Study of Human Biological Responses to Cultural and Environmental Change', *Medical Anthropology Quarterly,* vol. 4, no. 3, pp. 348–53.

Labonte, R. 1994, 'Econology: Health and Sustainable Development', in C. Chu and R. Simpson (eds), *Ecological Public Health: From Vision to Practice,* Institute of Applied Environmental Research, Griffith University, Queensland.

Lacy, R. 1996, 'How Now Mad Cow?, *Viva Guides,* p. 3, <http://www.veg.org/veg/Orgs/Viva/Guides/madcow.html>.

Lancet 1984, 'Needlestick Transmission of HTLV-III from a Patient Infected in Africa', vol. 2, pp. 1376–7.

Langer, E.J. 1989, *Mindfulness,* Addison-Wesley, Massachusetts.

—— and Piper, A.I. 1987, 'The Prevention of Mindlessness', *Journal of Personality and Social Psychology,* vol. 53, pp. 280–7.

Lannin, D.R. et al. 1998, 'Influence of Socioeconomic and Cultural Factors on

Racial Differences in Late-Stage Presentation of Breast Cancer', *Journal of the American Medical Association*, vol. 279, no. 22, pp. 1801–7.

Last, J.M. 1995, *A Dictionary of Epidemiology* (3rd edn), Oxford University Press, New York.

Le Guenno, B. 1995, 'Emerging Viruses', *Scientific American*, October, pp. 30–7.

Leatherman, T.L. 1996, 'A Biocultural Perspective on Health and Household Economy in Southern Peru', *Medical Anthropology Quarterly*, vol. 10, no. 4, pp. 476–95.

Lee, P.R. et al. 1991, 'Drug Promotion and Labeling in Developing Countries: An Update', *Journal of Clinical Epidemiology*, vol. 44, Supplement II, pp. 495–555.

Leeder, S. et al. 1983, 'Attack and Case Fatality Rates for Acute Myocardial Infarction in the Hunter Region of NSW, Australia, in 1979', *American Journal of Epidemiology*, vol. 118, pp. 42–51.

Leigh, J. et al. 1991, 'The Incidence of Malignant Mesothelioma in Australia, 1982–1988', *American Journal of Industrial Medicine*, vol. 20, no. 5, pp. 643–55.

Levins, R.T. 1994, 'Introduction: Basic Elements in a Conceptual Framework for New and Resurgent Disease', in M.E. Wilson, R. Levins and A. Spielman (eds), *Disease in Evolution: Global Changes and Emergence of Infectious Diseases*, Academy of Sciences, New York.

—— et al. 1994, 'The Emergence of New Diseases', *American Scientist*, vol. 82, pp. 52–60.

Levy, S.B. 1991, 'Antibiotic Availability and Use', *Journal of Clinical Epidemiology*, vol. 44, Supplement II, pp. 83s–7s.

—— 1998, 'The Challenge of Antibiotic Resistance', *Scientific American*, vol. 278, no. 3, pp. 32–9.

Lewin, R. 1993, *Complexity: Life on the Edge of Chaos*, Phoenix, London.

Lincoln, Y.S. and Guba, E. 1985, 'Designing a Naturalistic Inquiry', *Naturalistic Inquiry*, Sage Publications, Newbury Park, California.

Lincoln, Y.S. and Denzin, N.K. 1994, 'The Fifth Moment', in N.K. Denzin and Y.S. Lincoln (eds), *Handbook of Qualitative Research*, Sage Publications, Thousand Oaks, California.

Linn, L.C. 1968, 'The Mental Hospital from the Patient Perspective', *Psychiatry*, vol. 31, pp. 213–23.

Litva, A. and Eyles, J. 1995, 'Coming Out: Exposing Social Theory in Medical Geography', *Health and Place*, vol. 1, no. 1, pp. 5–14.

Lock, M. 1982, 'Models and Practice in Medicine as Syndrome or Life Transition?', *Culture, Medicine and Psychiatry*, vol. 6, pp. 261–80.

Lomas, J. 1993, 'Retailing Research: Increasing the Role of Evidence in Clinical Services after Childbirth', *Milbank Quarterly*, vol. 71, no. 3, pp. 439–73.

Lupton, D. 1995, *The Imperative of Health and the Regulated Body*, Sage Publications, London.

McAuliffe, K. 1990, 'The Killing Fields: Latter-day Plagues', *Omni*, May, pp. 52–4, 94–6, 98.

McCormick, R.D. et al. 1991, 'Epidemiology of Hospital Sharps Injuries: A 14-Year Prospective Study in the Pre-AIDS and AIDS Eras', *American Journal of Medicine*, vol. 91, pp. 301s–7s.

McElroy, A. 1990a, 'Biocultural Models in Studies of Human Health and Adaptation', *Medical Anthropology Quarterly*, vol. 4, no. 3, pp. 243–65.

—— 1990b, 'Rejoinder', *Medical Anthropology Quarterly*, vol. 4, no. 3, pp. 379–87.

—— and Townsend, P. 1999, *Medical Anthropology in Ecological Perspective* (3rd edn), Macmillan Education Australia, Melbourne.

McHorney, C., Ware, J.E. and Raczek, A.E. 1993, 'The MOS 36-Item Short-Form Health Survey (SF-36): 11. Psychometric and Clinical Tests of Validity in Measuring Physical and Mental Health Constructs', *Medical Care*, vol. 13, no. 3, pp. 247–63.

Mackenzie, S.G. and Lippman, A. 1989, 'An Investigation of Report Bias in a Case-Control Study of Pregnancy Outcome', *American Journal of Epidemiology*, vol. 129, no. 1, pp. 65–75.

McKinlay, J.B. 1992, 'Health Promotion through Health Public Policy: The Contribution of Complementary Research Methods', *Canadian Journal of Public Health, Special Supplement on Health Promotion Methods*, March, pp. 11–19.

McMichael, A.J. 1993, *Planetary Overload: Global Environmental Change and the Health of the Human Species*, Cambridge University Press, Cambridge, Mass.

Maddow, R. 2000, *New Drugs Have Cut US AIDS Death Rates in Half—What About Prisoners?*, http://users.javanet.com/~maddow/MDR-HIV.html, accessed 15 January 2000.

Malcolm, J. 1993, Social Factors in Outcomes after Acute Myocardial Infarction, PhD thesis, University of Newcastle, Newcastle, Australia.

Mamdani, M. and Walker, G. 1986, 'Essential Drugs in the Developing World', *Health Policy and Planning*, vol. 1, no. 3, pp. 187–201.

Manderson, L. and Aaby, P. 1992, 'Can Rapid Anthropological Procedures be Applied to Tropical Disease?', *Health Policy and Planning*, vol. 7, no. 1, pp. 46–55.

Manson, J.E. et al. 1992, 'The Primary Prevention of Myocardial Infarction', *New England Journal of Medicine*, vol. 326, pp. 1406–16.

Maslow, A. 1968, *Toward a Psychology of Being*, Van Nostrand Reinhold, New York.

Masterpasquia, F. and Perna, P.A. (eds) 1997, *The Psychological Meaning of Chaos*, American Psychological Association, Washington DC.

Means, D., Nigam, A. and Zarrow, M. 1989, 'Autobiographical Memory for Health-Related Events', *Vital and Health Statistics*, National Center for Health Statistics, Hyattsville, Maryland, Series 6, no. 2, pp. 1–6, 20–21.

Mechanic, D. 1989, 'Medical Sociology: Some Tensions among Theory, Method and Substance', *Journal of Health and Social Behaviour*, vol. 30, pp. 147–60.

Metcalfe, A. 1988, *For Freedom and Dignity: Historical Agency and Class in the Coalfields of NSW*, Allen &Unwin, Sydney.

—— 1993, 'Living in a Clinic: The Power of Public Health Promotions', *Australian Journal of Anthropology*, vol. 4, pp. 31–44.

Miles, M.B. and Huberman, M. 1994, *Qualitative Data Analysis: An Expanded Sourcebook* (2nd edn), Sage Publications, Thousand Oaks, California.

Millard, A.V. 1994, 'A Causal Model of High Rates of Child Mortality', *Social Science and Medicine*, vol. 38, no. 2, pp. 253–68.

Miller, G. T. 1995, *Environmental Science*, Wadsworth, California.

Miller, K. 1994, 'Students Letters from "Poisoned" Young Minds', *Newcastle Herald*, 3 November, p. 1.

Miller, William L. and Crabtree, Benjamin F. 1994, 'Clinical Research', in N.K. Denzin and Y.S. Lincoln (eds), *Handbook of Qualitative Research*, Sage Publications, Thousand Oaks, California.

—— et al. 1998, 'Understanding Change in Primary Care Practice Using Complexity Theory', *Journal of Family Practice*, vol. 46, no. 5, pp. 369–76.

Mingay, D. et al. 1988, *A Cognitive Approach to Questionnaire Design*, Paper presented at the American Association of Public Opinion Research Annual Convention, National Centre for Health Statistics, Toronto, Canada, May 1988, pp. 1–9.

Morgan, D.L. (ed.) 1993, *Successful Focus Groups: Advancing the State of the Art*, Sage Publications, Newbury Park, California.

Morgan, Lynn M. 1987, 'Dependency Theory in the Political Economy of Health: An Anthropological Critique', *Medical Anthropology Quarterly*, vol. 1, no. 2, June, pp. 131–54.

Morse, J.M. 1994, 'Designing Funded Qualitative Research', in N.K. Denzin and Y.S. Lincoln (eds), *Handbook of Qualitative Research*, Sage Publications, Thousand Oaks, California.

Morsy, S. 1990, 'Political Economy in Medical Anthropology', in T.M. Johnson and C.F. Sargent (eds), *Medical Anthropology: Contemporary Theory and Method*, Praeger, New York.

—— 1996, 'Political Economy in Medical Anthropology', in C.F. Sargent and T.M. Johnson (eds), *Medical Anthropology: Contemporary Theory and Method* (revised edn), Praeger, Westport, Connecticut.

Mosely, W.H. and Chen, L.C. 1984, 'Child Survival: Strategies for Research', *Population and Development Review,* vol. 10S, pp. 25–45.

Moser, C. and Kalton, G. 1979, *Survey Methods in Social Investigation* (2nd edn), Gower, Aldershot.

Munishi, G. 1991, 'The Development of the Essential Drugs Program and Implications for Self-Reliance in Tanzania', *Journal of Clinical Epidemiology,* vol. 4, Supplement II, pp. 75–145.

Murray, C.J.L. and Lopez, A.D. (eds) 1996, *The Global Burden of Disease,* Harvard University Press, Boston.

—— 1997, 'Global Mortality, Disability and the Contribution of Risk Factors', *Lancet,* vol. 349, 17 May, pp. 1436–42.

Murray, D.M. 1998, *Design and Analysis of Group-Randomised Trials,* Oxford University Press, Oxford.

Myntti, C. 1993, 'Social Determinants of Child Health in Yemen', *Social Science and Medicine,* vol. 37, no. 2, pp. 233–40.

Nations, M. 1986, 'Epidemiological Research on Infectious Disease: Quantitative Rigor or Rigormortis? Insights from Ethnomedicine', in C.R. Janes, R. Stall and S.M. Gifford (eds), *Anthropology and Epidemiology,* D. Reidel Publishing, Boston.

Newcastle Herald 1986, 'Cessnock Runs Last in Unfit Hunter', 8 January, p. 3.

—— 1986, 'Cessnock Slams "Fatties" Label', 9 January, p. 1.

—— 1986, 'Health Study Not Intended to Wound', 10 January, p. 3.

—— 1994, 'Angry Kurri Sends Dross Plan Back to Council', 13 October, p. 3.

—— 1996, 'Editorial: Dross Recycling Argument', 3 April, p. 16.

Newcombe, P.A. and Carbonne, P.P. 1992, 'The Health Consequences of Smoking: Cancer', *Medical Clinics of North America,* vol. 76, no. 2, pp. 305–31.

Nichter, M. and Nichter, M. 1994, 'Acute Respiratory Illness: Popular Health Culture and Mothers' Knowledge in the Philippines', *Medical Anthropology,* vol. 15, pp. 353–75.

—— (eds) 1996, *Anthropology and International Health: Asian Case Studies* (2nd edn), Gordon and Breach, Reading.

Nichter, M. and Vuckovik, N. 1994, 'Understanding Medication in the Context of Social Transformation', in N.L. Etkin and M.L. Tan (eds), *Medicines: Meanings and Contexts,* Health Action Information Network, Quezon City, Philippines.

Nickson, P. 1993, 'Community-determined Health Development in Zaire', in J. Rohde, M. Chatterjee and D. Morley (eds), *Reaching Health for All,* Oxford University Press, Bombay.

Nicolescu, Basarab 1998, 'A New Vision of the World: Transdisciplinarity', extract from *Transdisciplinarity—A Manifesto* (in press), Watersign Press, http://www://perso.club-internet.fr/nicol/ciret/english/visionen.htm, accessed 1 August 1999.

Norman, D.A. 1981, 'Categorization of Action Slips', *Psychological Review,* vol. 88, pp. 1–15.

Norman, G.R. and Streiner, D.L. 1986, *PDQ Statistic,* B.C. Decker, Toronto.

Ntozi, J.P.M. et al. (eds) 1997, 'Vulnerability to HIV Infection and Effects of AIDS in Africa and Asia/India', *Health Transition Review*, Supplement to vol. 17.

Oakley, A. 1992, *Social Support in Motherhood: The Natural History of a Research Project*, Blackwell, London.

Oppenheim, A.N. 1992, *Questionnaire Design, Interviewing and Attitude Measurement*, St Martin's Press, London.

Ormerod, P. 1998, *Butterfly Economics*, Faber and Faber, London.

Pagano, M. and Gauvreau, K. 1993, *Principles of Biostatistics,* Wadsworth, California.

Page, T., Lam, P. and Gibberd, R.W. 1990, *Mortality in the Hunter Region of New South Wales, 1984–1988,* Hunter Health Statistics Unit, Newcastle, September.

Pais, A. 1991, 'Niels Bohr's Times', in A. Pais, *Physics, Philosophy and Polity,* Clarendon Press, Oxford.

Pappas, G. 1990, 'Some Implications for the Study of the Doctor–Patient Interaction: Power, Structure and Agency in the Works of Howard Waitzkin and Arthur Kleinman', *Social Science and Medicine,* vol. 30, no. 2, pp. 190–204.

Patton, M.Q. 1980, *Qualitative Evaluation Methods*, Sage Publications, Beverley Hills, California.

—— 1987, *How to Use Qualitative Methods in Evaluation*, Sage Publications, Newbury Park, California.

—— 1990, *Qualitative Evaluation and Research Methods,* Sage Publications, Newbury Park, California.

Pelletier, A. 1997, 'Deaths Among Trespassers. The Role of Alcohol in Fatal Injuries', *Journal of the American Medical Association*, vol. 277, no. 13, pp. 1064–6.

Percy-Smith, J. 1996, 'Assessing Community Needs', in J. Percy-Smith (ed.), *Needs Assessments in Public Policy,* Open University Press, Philadelphia.

Peto, J. et al. 1999, 'The European Mesothelioma Epidemic', *British Journal of Cancer,* vol. 79, nos 3–4, pp. 666–72.

Peto, R. 1994, 'Smoking and Death: The Past 40 years and the Next 40', *British Medical Journal,* 8 October, vol. 309, pp. 937–9.

Peyser, P.A. 1997, 'Genetic Epidemiology of Coronary Artery Disease', *Epidemiology Review,* vol. 19, no. 1, pp. 80–9.

Pfaffenberger, B. 1988, *Microcomputer Applications in Qualitative Research, Qualitative Research Methods,* vol.14, Sage Publications, Newbury Park, California.

Phillips, M., Higginbotham, N. and Henderson, G. 1998, *Integrating Health Social Science in the Design and Assessment of Health Research Protocols, Module 7: The Development and Assessment of Questionnaires and Surveys (Part 1)*, Department of Clinical Epidemiology, Beijing Hui Long Guan Hospital and Department of Social Medicine, Harvard Medical School, Massachusetts.

Pillemer, K. 1985, 'The Dangers of Dependency: New Findings on Domestic Violence Against the Elderly', *Social Problems*, vol. 33, no. 2, pp. 146–58.

Plotnikoff, R. 1994, An Application of Protection Motivation Theory to Coronary Heart Disease Risk Factor Behaviour in Three Australian Samples: Community Adults, Cardiac Patients and Schoolchildren, PhD thesis, University of Newcastle, Newcastle, Australia.

Pont, J. 1990, 'Heart Attack . . . We Believe It Will Never Happen to Us', *Cessnock Advertiser*, 24 October, p. 44.

Porteous, D. 1996, 'Methodologies for Needs Assessment', in J. Percy-Smith (ed.), *Needs Assessments in Public Policy*, Open University Press, Philadelphia.

Price, B. 1997, 'Analysis of Current Trends in United States Mesothelioma', *American Journal of Epidemiology*, vol. 145, no. 3, pp. 211–18.

Prigogine, I. and Stengers, I. 1984, *Order Out of Chaos: Man's New Dialogue with Nature*, Bantam, New York.

Prusiner, S.B. 1995, 'The Prion Diseases', *Scientific American*, January, vol. 30, p. 37.

Punch, M. 1994, 'Politics and Ethics in Qualitative Research', in N.K. Denzin and Y.S. Lincoln (eds), *Handbook of Qualitative Research*, Sage Publications, Thousand Oaks, California.

Rabkin, J.G. and Chesney, M.A. 2000, 'Adherence to HIV Medications: The Achilles Heel of the New Therapies', in D.G. Ostrow and S.C. Kalichman (eds), *Psychological and Public Health Impacts of New HIV Therapies*, Plenum Press, New York.

Reason, J. 1979, 'Actions not as Planned: The Price of Automatization', in G. Underwood and R. Stevens (eds), *Aspects of Consciousness: Psychological Issues*, vol. 7, Academic Press, London

—— 1984, 'Absent-Mindedness and Cognitive Control', in J.E. Harris and P.E. Morris (eds), *Everyday Memory, Actions and Absent-Mindedness*, Academic Press, London.

Reason, P. 1994, 'Three Approaches to Participative Inquiry', in N.K. Denzin and Y.S. Lincoln (eds), *Handbook of Qualitative Research*, Sage Publications, Thousand Oaks, California.

Reddy, P.H. 1995, 'Health Transition Research in India can Improve Health', *Health Transition Review*, vol. 5, pp. 248–53.

Reice, S. 1994, 'Nonequilibrium Determinants of Biological Community Structure', *American Scientist*, September–October, vol. 82, p. 434.

Reich, M. 1994, 'Bangladesh Pharmaceutical Policy and Politics', *Health Policy and Planning*; vol. 9, no. 2, pp. 130–43.

Rice, P.L. and Ezzy, D. 1999, 'In-Depth Interviews', *Qualitative Research Methods: A Health Focus*, Oxford University Press, Melbourne.

Rizzo, T.A. and Corsaro, W.A. 1995, 'Toward a Potential Integration of Interpretive and Quantitative Research in Psychology: A Reply to Shadish and Rosenblatt and Howes', *American Journal of Community Psychology*, vol. 23, no. 3, pp. 435–45.

Robinson, I. 1990, 'Personal Narratives, Social Careers and Medical Courses: Analysing Life Trajectories in Autobiographies of People with Multiple Sclerosis', *Social Science and Medicine*, vol. 30, no. 11, pp. 1173–86.

Robinson, J.A. and Hawpe, L. 1986, 'Narrative Thinking as a Heuristic Process', in T.R. Sarbin (ed.), *Narrative Psychology*, Praeger, New York.

Romney, A.K. et al. 1986, 'Culture as Consensus: A Theory of Culture and Informant Accuracy', *American Anthropologist*, vol. 88, pp. 313–38.

Rondinelli, D. 1991, 'Decentralizing Water Supply Services in Developing Countries: Factors Affecting the Success of Community Management', *Public Administration and Development*, vol. 11, no. 5, pp. 415–30.

Rosenberg, E. 1999, 'US Frees Up AIDS Drugs for Africans', *Sydney Morning Herald*, 24 July, p. 29.

Rosenfield, P. 1992, 'The Potential of Transdisciplinary Research for Sustaining and Extending Linkages between the Health and Social Sciences', *Social Science and Medicine*, vol. 11, pp. 1343–57.

Rosenman, R.H. et al. 1975, 'Coronary Heart Disease in the Western Collaborative Heart Study: Final Follow-up Experience of 8½ years', *Journal of the American Medical Association*, vol. 233, pp. 872–7.

Rosner, B. 1995, *Fundamentals of Biostatistics* (4th edn), Duxbury Press, Pacific Grove, California.

Rothman, K.J. 1986, *Modern Epidemiology*, Little, Brown and Company, Boston.

—— and Greenland, S. 1998, *Modern Epidemiology* (2nd edn), Lippincott-Raven Publishers, Philadelphia.

Royston, P. and Bercini, D. 1987, *Questionnaire Design in a Laboratory Setting: Results of Testing Cancer Risk Factor Questions*, Paper presented at the American Statistical Association Convention, Survey Methods Section, August.

Sackett, D. et al. 1996, *Clinical Epidemiology: A Basic Science for Clinical Medicine*, (2nd edn), Little, Brown and Company, Boston.

Sallis, J.F. and Owen, N. 1998, *Physical Activity and Behavioral Medicine*, Sage Publications, Thousand Oaks, California.

Sandar, Z. and Abrams, I. 1999, *Introducing Chaos*, Allen & Unwin, Sydney.

Saradamma, R.D., Higginbotham, N. and Nichter, M. 2000, 'Social Factors

Influencing the Acquisition of Antibiotics without Prescription in Kerala State, South India', *Social Science and Medicine*, vol. 50, pp. 891–903.

Scheaffer, R.L., Mendenhall, W. and Ott, L. 1986, *Elementary Survey Sampling* (3rd edn), Duxbury Press, Boston.

Schlesselman, J.J. 1982, *Case-control Studies: Design, Conduct and Analysis*, Oxford University Press, New York.

Schneider, E.D. and Kay, J.J. 1995, 'Order from Disorder: The Thermodynamics of Complexity in Biology', in M.P. Murphy and L.A.J. O'Neill (eds), *What is Life? The Next Fifty Years*, Cambridge University Press, Cambridge.

Schwartz, M.N. 1997, 'The Use of Antimicrobial Agents and Drug Resistance', *New England Journal of Medicine*, vol. 337, no. 7, pp. 491–2.

Schwartz, S. 1994, 'The Fallacy of the Ecological Fallacy: The Potential Misuse of a Concept and its Consequences', *American Journal of Public Health*, vol. 84, no. 5, pp. 819–24.

Scrimshaw, N.S. 1991, 'Combining Quantitative and Qualitative Methods in the Study of Intra-Household Resource Allocation', in J. Cleland and G. Hill (eds), *The Health Transition: Methods and Measures*, Health Transition Centre, Australian National University, Canberra, pp. 243–5.

—— and Gleason, G.R. (eds) 1992, *RAP. Rapid Assessment Procedures: Qualitative Methodologies for Planning and Evaluation of Health Related Programs*, International Nutrition Foundation for Developing Countries (INFDC), Boston.

Seidman, E. 1994, 'Ecological Theory and Research: Dilemmas for Action Scientists', *Community Psychologist*, vol. 28, no. 1, pp. 3–34.

Sellick, J.A., Hazamy, P.A. and Mylotte, J.M. 1991, 'Influence of an Educational Program and Mechanical Opening Needle Disposal Boxes on Occupational Needlestick Injuries', *Infection Control and Hospital Epidemiology*, vol. 12, pp. 725–31.

Sewankambo, N.K., Spittal, P.A. and Willms, D.G. (in press), 'Representing HIV/AIDS Concerns in Uganda: The Genogram as a Visual Complement to Ethnographic and Epidemiological Evidence', in N. Higginbotham, R. Briceño-Leon and N. Johnson (eds), *Applying Health Social Science: Case Studies from the Developing World*, Zed Books, Ottawa.

Sewell, W.H. 1989, 'Some Reflections on the Golden Age of Interdisciplinary Social Psychology', *Annual Review of Sociology*, vol. 15, pp. 1–16.

Shadish, W.R. 1995, 'The Logic of Generalization: Five Principles Common to Experiments and Ethnographies', *American Journal of Community Psychology*, vol. 23, no. 3, pp. 419–28.

Short, L.J. et al. 1991, 'Economic Implications of Accidental Needle-Stick Injuries (NSI) at a Large Urban Hospital', *CDC AIDS Weekly*, 25 November, p. 21.

Siegrist, J. et al. 1990, 'Low Status Control, High Effort at Work and Ischaemic Heart Disease: Prospective Evidence from Blue-Collar Men', *Social Science and Medicine*, vol. 31, pp. 1127–34.

Silverman, D. 1985, *Qualitative Methodology and Sociology: Describing the Social World*, Gower, Brookfield, Vermont.

Silverman, M., Lydecker, M. and Lee, P.R. 1992, *Bad Medicine: The Prescription Drug Industry in the Third World*, Stanford University Press, California.

Singer, M. 1995, 'Beyond the Ivory Tower: Critical Praxis in Medical Anthropology', *Medical Anthropology Quarterly*, vol. 9, pp. 80–106.

Sorenson, T. 1994a, 'Dross Focus Switches to Alcan Smelter', *Newcastle Herald*, 11 November, p. 1.

—— 1994b, 'Dross "Death" Threats', *Newcastle Herald*, 17 November, p. 1.

Soumerai, S.B., McLaughlin, T.J. and Avorn, J. 1989, 'Improving Drug Prescribing in Primary Care: A Critical Analysis of the Experimental Literature', *Milbank Quarterly*, vol. 67, pp. 268–317.

Soumerai, S.B. and Avorn, J. 1990, 'Principles of Educational Outreach ("Academic Detailing") to Improve Clinical Decision Making', *Journal of the American Medical Association*, vol. 263, pp. 549–56.

Spicer, J. and Chamberlain, K. 1996, 'Developing Psychosocial Theory in Health Psychology: Problems and Perspectives', *Journal of Health Psychology*, vol. 12, pp. 161–71.

Spittal, P. et al. 1997, ' "We are dying. It is finished!": Linking an Ethnographic Research Design to an HIV/AIDS Participatory Approach in Uganda', in S.E. Smith, D.G. Willms and N.A. Johnson (eds), *Nurtured by Knowledge: Learning to do Participatory Action-Research*, Apex Press, New York.

Spradley, J.P. 1979, *The Ethnographic Interview*, Holt, Rinehart and Winston, New York.

Stake, R.E. 1994, 'Case Studies', in N.K. Denzin and Y.S. Lincoln (eds), *Handbook of Qualitative Research*, Sage, Thousand Oaks, California.

Steele, P. and McElduff, P. 1995, *Hunter Region Heart Disease Prevention Programme: Newcastle MONICA Date Book—Coronary Events 1984–94*, Centre for Clinical Epidemiology and Biostatistics, University of Newcastle, Newcastle, Australia.

Stiles, W.B. 1993, 'Quality Control in Qualitative Research', *Clinical Psychology Review*, vol. 13, no. 6, pp. 593–618.

Stock, R. 1985, 'Drugs and Underdevelopment: A Case Study of Kano State, Nigeria', *Studies in Third World Societies*, December, no. 34, pp. 115–39.

Stokols, D. 1988, 'Transformational Processes in People–Environment Relations', in Joseph McGrath (ed.), *The Social Psychology of Time: New Perspectives*, Sage Publications, Newbury Park, California.

—— 1992, 'Establishing and Maintaining Healthy Environments: Towards a Social Ecology of Health Promotion', *American Psychologist*, January, pp. 6–23.

Stone, L. and Campbell, J. 1984, 'The Use and Misuse of Surveys in International Development: An Experiment from Nepal', *Human Organisation*, vol. 43, no. 1, pp. 27–37.

Strauss, A.L. 1987, *Qualitative Analysis for Social Scientists*, Cambridge University Press, Cambridge, UK.

Strauss, A. and Corbin, J. 1990, *Basics of Qualitative Research: Grounded Theory Procedures and Techniques*, Sage Publications, Newbury Park, California.

—— 1994, 'Grounded Theory Methodology: An Overview', in N.K. Denzin and Y.S. Lincoln (eds), *Handbook of Qualitative Research*, Sage Publications, Thousand Oaks, California.

Streiner, D.L., Norman, G. and Blum, H. 1989, 'Epidemiologic Research Strategies', *Epidemiology*, B.C. Decker, Toronto.

Streiner, D.L. and Norman 1995, *Health Measurement Scales: A Practical Guide to their Development and Use* (2nd edn), Oxford University Press, Oxford.

—— 1996, *Epidemiology* (2nd edn), Mosby, St Louis.

Sudman, S. and Bradburn, N.M. 1982, *Asking Questions: A Practical Guide to Questionnaire Design*, Jossey-Bass Publishers, San Francisco.

—— 1996, *Thinking About Answers: The Application of Cognitive Processes to Survey Methodology*, Jossey-Bass Publishers, San Francisco.

Susser, M. 1994, 'The Logic in Ecological: I. The Logic of Analysis', *American Journal of Health*, vol. 84, no. 5, pp. 825–9.

Swan, N. 1993, 'Return of the Deadly Diseases', *Sunday Telegraph*, Sydney, 9 May, p. 122.

Sydney Morning Herald 2000, 'Nine Patients Face Threat of Brain Disease', *Sydney Morning Herald*, 4 May, p. 3.

Tabachnick, B.G. and Fidell, L.S. 1996, *Using Multivariate Statistics* (3rd edn), Harper Collins College, New York.

Tandberg, D., Stewart, K.K. and Doezema, D. 1991, 'Under-Reporting of Contaminated Needlestick Injuries in Emergency Health Care Workers', *Annals of Emergency Medicine*, vol. 20, pp. 66–70.

Taylor, D. 1986, 'The Pharmaceutical Industry and Health in the Third World', *Social Science and Medicine*, vol. 22, no. 11, pp. 1141–9.

Taylor, S.E. 1999, *Health Psychology*, (4th edn), McGraw-Hill, New York.

Tench, Watkin 1996, 'Transactions of the Colony in April and May 1789', in T. Flannery (ed.), *Watkin Tench 1788*, The Text Publishing Company, Melbourne, pp. 102–10.

Tesch, S.A. 1988, 'Multicausal Solution', *Hidden Arguments: Political Ideology and Disease Prevention Policy*, Rutgers University Press, New Jersey.

Theorell, T. and Karasek, R.A. 1996, 'Current Issues Relating to Psychological Job Strain and Cardiovascular Research', *Journal of Occupational Health Psychology*, vol. 1, no. 1, pp. 9–26.

Thomas, L. and Krebs, C. 1997, 'A Review of Statistical Power Analysis Software', *Bulletin of the Ecological Society of America*, vol. 78, no. 2, pp. 126–39.

Timmermans, K. 1996, 'DAP Support: Making a Difference in Guinea', *Essential Drugs Monitor*, no. 22, pp. 7–8, http://www.who.int/dap/edm.html.

Tonstad, S. et al. 1999, 'Under-Reporting of Dietary Intake by Smoking and Non-Smoking Subjects Counseled for Hypercholesterolaemia', *Journal of Internal Medicine*, April, vol. 245, no. 4, pp. 337–44.

Tourangeau, R. and Smith, T.W. 1996, 'Asking Sensitive Questions: The Impact of Data Collection, Question Format, and Question Context', *Public Opinion Quarterly*, vol. 60, pp. 275–304.

Townsend, P.K. and McElroy, A. 1992, 'Toward an Ecology of Women's Reproductive Health', *Medical Anthropology*, vol. 14, pp. 9–14.

Treloar, C.J. 1994, Details of Social Marketing Materials from Concept to Product to Actual Use: The Care Aware Programme, Unpublished paper, Centre for Clinical Epidemiology, University of Newcastle, Newcastle, Australia.

—— 1997, 'Developing a Multilevel Understanding of Heart Disease: An Interview Study of MONICA Participants in an Australian Centre', *Qualitative Health Research*, vol. 7, no. 4, pp. 468–86.

—— et al. 1995, 'The Personal Experience of Australian Health Care Workers Accidentally Exposed to Risk of HIV Infection', *AIDS*, vol. 9, no. 12, pp. 1385–6 (letter).

—— et al. 1996, 'An Academic Detailing Education Program Aimed at Decreasing Exposure to HIV Infection among Health Care Workers', *Journal of Health Psychology*, vol. 1, no. 40, pp. 455–68.

—— et al. 2000, 'A Critical Appraisal Checklist for Qualitative Research Studies within Clinical Epidemiology', *Indian Journal of Pediatrics*, vol. 67, no. 4, pp. 22–7.

Trochim, W. 1999, *Research Methods Knowledge Base* (2nd edn), http:// trochim.human.cornell.edu, accessed 2 September 1999.

Turner, I. 1974, '1914–19', in F. Crowley (ed.), *A New History of Australia*, Heinemann, Melbourne.

—— 1979, *Industrial Labor and Politics*, Hale and Iremonger, Sydney.

—— 1983, *In Union is Strength: A History of the Trade Unions in Australia, 1788–1939* (3rd edn), Thomas Nelson, Melbourne.

—— et al. 1998, 'Adolescent Sexual Behavior, Drug Use, and Violence: Increased Reporting with Computer Survey Technology', *Science*, vol. 280, pp. 867–73.

United Nations Development Program 1997, *Human Development Report 1997*, Oxford University Press, New York.

University of California 1992, *The School of Social Ecology: A Bold Venture*, University of California, Irvine, August, pp. 1–7.

Van der Geest, S. 1985, 'Unequal Access to Pharmaceuticals in Southern Cameroon: The Context of a Problem', *Studies in Third World Societies*, December, no. 34, pp. 141–66.

—— 1988, 'Pharmaceutical Anthropology: Perspectives for Research and Application', in S. Van der Geest and S.R. Whyte (eds), *The Context of Medicines in Developing Countries*, Kluwer Academic, Boston.

—— and Whyte, S.R. (eds) 1988, *The Context of Medicines in Developing Countries*, Kluwer Academic, Boston.

——, Hardon, A. and Whyte, S.R. 1990, 'Essential Drugs: Are We Missing the Cultural Dimension?', *Health Policy and Planning*, vol. 5, no. 2, pp. 182–5.

Velasquez, G. and Boulet, P. 1999, 'Essential Drugs in the New International Economic Environment', *Bulletin of the World Health Organization*, vol. 77, no. 3, pp. 288–92.

Verrusio, A.C. 1989, 'Risk of Transmission of the Human Immunodeficiency Virus to Health Care Workers Exposed to HIV-Infected Patients: A Review', *Journal of the American Dental Association*, vol. 118, pp. 339–42.

von Radowitz, J. 2000, 'Mad Cow Death Fears Allayed', *Sydney Morning Herald*, 21 January, p. 10.

Wadsworth, Y. 1984, *Do It Yourself Social Research*, Victorian Council of Social Service, Melbourne Family Care Organisation in association with Allen & Unwin, Melbourne.

—— 1993, *How Can Professionals Help . . . Groups Do Their Own Participatory Action Research?*, ARIA, Melbourne.

Waldrop, M.M. 1994, *Complexity: The Emerging Science at the Edge of Order and Chaos*, Penguin Books, London.

Warnecke, R.B. et al. 1997, 'Cognitive Aspects of Recalling and Reporting Health-Related Events: Papanicolaou Smears, Clinical Breast Examinations, and Mammograms', *American Journal of Epidemiology*, vol. 146, no. 11, pp. 982–91.

Wass, A. 1994, *Promoting Health: The Primary Health Care Approach*, Harcourt Brace, Sydney.

Weber, B.H., Depew, D. and Smith, J. (eds) 1988, *Entropy, Information, and Evolution: New Perspectives on Physical and Biological Evolution*, MIT Press, Cambridge, Massachusetts.

Weber, M. 1968, *Economy and Society: An Outline of Interpretive Sociology*, G. Roth and C. Wittich (eds), 1978, University of California Press, Berkeley.

Weerasuriya, K. and Brudon, P. 1998, 'Essential Drugs Concept Needs Better Implementation', *Essential Drugs Monitor*, nos 25–6, pp. 32–3.

Weinstein, Raymond 1979, 'Patient Attitudes Toward Mental Hospitalization: A Review of Quantitative Research', *Journal of Health and Social Behaviour*, vol. 24, pp. 237–58.

—— 1983, 'Labeling Theory and the Attitudes of Mental Patients', *Journal of Health and Social Behaviour*, vol. 24, pp. 70–84.

Weller, S.C. and Romney, A.K. 1986, 'Systematic Data Collection', *Qualitative Research Methods*, vol. 10, Sage Publications, Newbury Park, California.

Weller, S.C., Romney, A.K. and Orb, D.P. 1987, 'The Myth of a Sub-Culture of Corporal Punishment', *Human Organization*, vol. 16, no. 1, pp. 39–47.

Whitby, M., Stead, P. and Najman, J.M. 1991, 'Needlestick Injury: Impact of a Recapping Device and an Associated Education Program', *Infection Control and Hospital Epidemiology*, vol. 12, pp. 220–5.

White, K.L. 1991, *Healing the Schism: Epidemiology, Medicine, and the Public's Health*, Springer-Verlag, New York.

Whittaker, A. 1998, 'Talk About Cancer: Environment and Health in Oceanpoint', *Health and Place*, vol. 4, no. 4, pp. 313–25.

—— et al. 1996, *The Oceanpoint Study: 'General Practice in its Community Context'*, University of Newcastle, Newcastle, Australia (available at the Auchmuty Library, University of Newcastle).

—— and Connor, L. 1998, 'Engendering Stress in Australia: The Embodiment of Social Relationships', *Women and Health*, vol. 28, no. 1, pp. 97–115.

WHO 1976, 'Methodology of Nutritional Surveillance: Report of a Joint FAO/UNICEF/WHO Expert Committee', *WHO Technical Report Series*, no. 593, WHO, Geneva.

—— 1993, 'Results of Drug Use Survey in Bangladesh', *Essential Drugs Monitor*, Geneva, no. 16, p. 20.

—— 1998, 'Antimicrobial Resistance', *Fact Sheet No.194*, www.who.int/inf-fs/en/fact194.html.

Whyte, W.F. 1955, *Street Corner Society: The Social Structure of an Italian Slum* (2nd edn), University of Chicago Press, Chicago.

Wilkinson, S. 1998, 'Focus Groups in Health Research: Exploring the Meanings of Health and Illness', *Journal of Health Psychology*, vol. 3, no. 3, pp. 329–48.

Williams, P. and Plotnikoff, R. 1995, 'The Kurri Kurri Public School Healthy Heartbeat Project', *Health Promotion Journal of Australia*, vol. 5, no. 1, pp. 35–9.

Willms D.G., Chingono, A. and Wellington, M. 1996, *AIDS Prevention in the 'Matare' and the Community: A Training Strategy for Traditional Healers in Zimbabwe*, Department of Anthropology, McMaster University, Ontario.

Willms, D.G. and Johnson, N. 1996, *Essentials in Qualitative Research: A Notebook for the Field*, McMaster University, Ontario.

Willms, D.G. and Sewankambo, N. 1994, An Intervention Discourse: Emerging Questions, Evolving Research Designs, and Epistemological Relevances Encountered in the Dialogue Between Epidemiology and Anthropology, Unpublished paper presented at the XII Annual INCLEN Meeting, Chiangmai, Thailand, 28 January, pp. 3–18.

Willms, D.G. et al. in press, 'AIDS Prevention in the *Matare* and the Community: A Training Strategy for Traditional Healers in Zimbabwe', in N. Higginbotham, R. Briceño-Leon and N. Johnson (eds), *Applying Health Social Science: Case Studies from the Developing World*, Zed Books, London.

Winett, R.A., King, A. and Altman, D. 1989, *Health Psychology and Public Health: An Integrative Approach*, Pergamon, New York.

Wingate, P. and Wingate, R. 1988, *The Penguin Medical Encyclopedia* (3rd edn), Penguin Books, London.

Wolinsky, H. 1979, 'Atherosclerosis', in P. Beeson, W. McDermott and J.B. Wyndarden (eds), *Textbook of Medicine*, W.B. Saunders, Philadelphia.

Wright, J. 1994, 'Phone Your Say', *Newcastle Herald*, 27 October, p. 7.

Yelland, J. and Gifford, S. 1995, 'Problems of Focus Group Methods in Cross-Cultural Research: A Case Study of Beliefs about Sudden Infant Death Syndrome', *Australian Journal of Public Health*, vol. 19, no. 3, pp. 257–63.

Yin, R.K. 1994, *Case Study Research: Design and Methods* (2nd edn), *Applied Social Research Methods Series*, vol. 5, Sage Publications, Thousand Oaks, California.

Young, J.C. 1981, *Medical Choice in a Mexican Village*, Rutgers University Press, New Jersey.

Index

Bold indicates major entries.

ACUTE MEDICINE 2015

DECLAN O'KANE, MD, FRCP

Consultant Physician
Northampton General Hospital

Scion

First published 2015

A CIP catalogue record for this book is available from the British Library.
ISBN 978 1 907904 25 7

Scion Publishing Limited
The Old Hayloft, Vantage Business Park, Bloxham Road, Banbury OX16 9UX, UK
www.scionpublishing.com

Important Note from the Publisher

Typeset by Phoenix Photosetting, Chatham, Kent, UK
Printed in the UK

Contents

Preface

This is the book that I want to have in my back pocket whilst dealing with the acute take. It is a quick reference of 'what and why' that covers common and not so common emergencies. I am very aware of the frailties of human memory and decision-making and a simple checklist at hand can hopefully enhance safety and clinical acumen. Included at the back is a quick emergency drug reference where drug information is consolidated to avoid repetition. This does not replace the BNF for drugs with which you are unfamiliar. To some the information will be new and to others it is simply a reminder. It needs to be compact and concise so let us not waste further words or space.

Declan O'Kane, August 2014

Acknowledgements

I'd like to thank my wife and my two girls for their love, patience and forbearance when I disappear to my office.

This book is dedicated to the memory of my good friend, Jeremy Sherman FRCS.

In my training I was fortunate to work for many wonderful hard-working clinicians. I am particularly indebted to Professor Jennifer Adgey CBE and the late Dr James I. Coyle.

I'd like to thank those who have read the manuscript and made helpful suggestions and additions, including Dr Jacob F. de Wolff, Dr Andrew Solomon, Dr Pad Boovalingam, Dr Omar Kirresh, Dr Peter Rhead and Dr Christopher Miller. Any remaining errors are mine. If you have any comments, questions or suggestions, please write to me at drokane@gmail.com. Errata will be available on my website at www.dok.org.uk.

Disclaimer

Every effort has been made in preparing this publication to provide accurate and up to date information in accord with accepted standards and practice at the time of publication. The author can make no warranties that the information contained herein is totally free from error, not least because clinical standards are constantly changing. The author therefore disclaims all liability for direct or consequential damages resulting from the use of material within this publication. Readers are recommended to check all drugs doses, indications and C/I and interactions used with the *British National Formulary* or drug data-sheet prior to use. If a reader is unsure what to do then they should seek support from their senior medical adviser. Patients should seek help from their own doctor/healthcare provider.

Decision making for the medical registrar

The first medical registrar year is tough and stressful, but with the years it gets easier and more enjoyable: you recognise the same patterns and problems and the solutions become easier to resolve in seconds, and it becomes more enjoyable because you can solve other people's puzzles for them. Sometimes, however, a problem is completely new so you need to sit down and work it out from first principles and/or ask for help from someone who may have encountered the situation before. Referrals will come thick and fast – regard these as compliments to your skills in problem solving. Get help once you have thought (time allowing) it through yourself and presented your plan. If you are unhappy or concerned call for advice. Share diagnostic dilemmas and don't sit on them. Don't go home without resolving your concerns. As consultants we constantly discuss interesting and difficult cases. Good medical practice is about reflective practice and seeking feedback. Good luck.

Abbreviations

5-ASA	5-amino salicylic acid
AAA	abdominal aortic aneurysm
ABC	airway, breathing and circulation
ABG	arterial blood gas
ABU	asymptomatic bacteriuria
ACA	anterior cerebral artery
ACE	angiotensin converting enzyme
ACS	acute coronary syndrome
ACTH	adrenocorticotrophic hormone
ADA	adenosine deaminase
AED	automated external defibrillators
AF	atrial fibrillation
aHUS	atypical haemolytic uremic syndrome
AICD	automated implantable cardioverter-defibrillator
AIDP	acute inflammatory demyelinating polyneuropathy
AIDS	acquired immunodeficiency syndrome
AKI	acute kidney injury
ALF	acute liver failure
ALI	acute lung injury
ALP	alkaline phosphatase
ALT	alanine aminotransferase
AMAN	acute motor axonal neuropathy
AMTS	abbreviated mental test score
ANA	antinuclear antibody
ANCA	antineutrophil cytoplasmic antibody
APKD	adult polycystic kidney disease
APS	antiphospholipid syndrome
APTT	activated thromboplastin time
AR	aortic regurgitation
ARDS	acute/adult respiratory distress syndrome
AS	aortic stenosis
ASD	atrial septal defect
ATN	acute tubular necrosis
AV	arteriovenous or atrioventricular
AVM	arteriovenous malformation
AVNRT	atrioventricular nodal re-entrant tachycardia
AVPU	awake, voice, pain, unresponsive
AVRT	atrioventricular re-entrant tachycardia
BBB	bundle branch block
BD/bd	twice daily
BE	base excess
BHL	bihilar lymphadenopathy
BiPAP	bilevel positive airway pressure
BJP	Bence-Jones protein
BMS	bare metal stents
BP	blood pressure
CABG	coronary artery bypass grafting
CAD	coronary artery disease
CBG	capillary blood glucose
CCB	calcium channel blocker
CCF	congestive cardiac failure
CEA	carcinoembryonic antigen
CHB	complete heart block
CI-AKI	contrast-induced acute kidney injury
CIDP	chronic inflammatory demyelinating polyneuropathy
CK	creatine kinase
CKD	chronic kidney disease
CLO test	*Campylobacter*-like organism test (rapid urease test)
CMP	cardiomyopathy
CMV	cytomegalovirus
CO	cardiac output
CP	chest pain
CPAP	continuous positive airways pressure
CPR	cardiopulmonary resuscitation
CRP	C reactive protein
CSF	cerebrospinal fluid
CSM	carotid sinus massage
CTG	cardiotocogram
CTPA	computed tomography pulmonary angiogram
CVA	cerebrovascular accident (stroke)
CVP	central venous pressure

CVVH	continuous veno-venous haemofiltration
DCM	dilated cardiomyopathy
DES	drug-eluting stents
DI	diabetes insipidus
DIC	disseminated intravascular coagulation
DKA	diabetic ketoacidosis
DM	diabetes mellitus
DNAR	do not attempt resuscitation
DOB	date of birth
DSA	digital subtraction angiography
DWI	diffusion weighted imaging
EBV	Epstein–Barr virus
ECG	electrocardiogram
EEG	electroencephalogram
EF	ejection fraction
ELISA	enzyme-linked immunosorbent assay
EPO	erythropoietin
EPS	electrophysiological study
ERCP	endoscopic retrograde cholangiopancreatography
ESR	erythrocyte sedimentation rate
EVD	external ventricular drainage
FBC	full blood count
FEV	forced expiratory volume
FFP	fresh frozen plasma
FMF	familial Mediterranean fever
FVC	forced vital capacity
GBS	Guillain–Barré syndrome
GCA	giant cell arteritis
GFR	glomerular filtration rate
GGT	gamma-glutamyl transpeptidase
GH	growth hormone
GHB	gamma-hydroxybutyric acid
GORD	gastro-oesophageal reflux disease
GTCS	generalised tonic clonic seizure
GTT	glucose tolerance test
HAART	highly active antiretroviral therapy
HBV	hepatitis B virus
HCM	hypertrophic cardiomyopathy
HCV	hepatitis C virus
HELLP	syndrome of haemolysis, elevated LFTs, low platelets
HHS	hyperglycaemic hyperosmolar state
HIAA	5-hydroxyindoleacetic acid
HIT(T)	heparin-induced thrombocytopenia +/– thrombosis
HIV	human immunodeficiency syndrome
HONK	hyperosmolar non-ketotic state
HR	heart rate (ventricular rate)
HRCT	high resolution CT
HRS	hepatorenal syndrome
HRT	hormone replacement therapy
HSV	*Herpes simplex* virus
HTLV	human T cell lymphotropic virus
HUS	haemolytic uraemic syndrome
IABP	intra-aortic balloon pump
IAH	impaired awareness of hypoglycaemia
ICA	internal carotid artery
ICD	*see* AICD
ICH	intracerebral haemorrhage
ICP	intracranial pressure
ICS	intercostal space
IDDM	insulin dependent diabetes mellitus
IGF-1	insulin-like growth factor 1
IHD	ischaemic heart disease
IM	intramuscular route
INR	international normalized ratio
ITP	immune (idiopathic) thrombocytopenic purpura
IVC	inferior vena cava
IVDU	IV drug user
IVIG	intravenous immunoglobulin
IVU	intravenous urogram
JVP	jugular venous pressure
KUB	kidneys, ureter, bladder
LAD	left axis deviation
LBBB	left bundle branch block
LCA	left coronary artery
LCHAD	long-chain 3-hydroxyacyl-coA dehydrogenase
LDH	lactate dehydrogenase
LFT	liver function test
LMN	lower motor neuron

LMWH	low molecular weight heparin
LOC	loss of consciousness
LP	lumbar puncture
LSE	left sternal edge
LV	left ventricle
LVH	left ventricular hypertrophy
LVAD	LV assist device
LVEDP	LV end diastolic pressure
LVF	left ventricular failure
LVH	left ventricular hypertrophy
MAOI	monoamine oxidase inhibitor
MAT	microscopic agglutination test
MCA	middle cerebral artery
MDAC	multidose activated charcoal
MG	myasthenia gravis
MGUS	monoclonal gammopathy of undetermined significance
MH	malignant hyperpyrexia
MI	myocardial infarction
MIC	minimum inhibitory concentration
MRSA	meticillin-resistant *Staphylococcus aureus*
MR	mitral regurgitation
MS	multiple sclerosis/mitral stenosis
MSH	melanocyte-stimulating hormone
MST	morphine sulphate
MTS	mental test score
MVP	mitral valve prolapse
NAC	*N*-acetyl cysteine
NBM	nil by mouth
NCSA	non-convulsive status epilepticus
NEWS	national early warning score
NG	nasogastric
NHL	non-Hodgkin lymphoma
NIDDM	non-insulin dependent diabetes mellitus
NIPPV	non-invasive positive pressure ventilation
NIV	non-invasive ventilation
NMS	neuroleptic malignant syndrome
NOAC	new oral anticoagulant
NOS	nitric oxide synthase
NS	normal saline
NSAID	non-steroidal anti-inflammatory drug
NSTEMI	non-ST elevation MI
OCP	oral contraceptive pill
OGD	oesophagogastroduodenoscopy
OPs	organophosphates
PA	pernicious anaemia
PAF	paroxysmal atrial fibrillation
PAN	polyarteritis nodosa
PAWP	pulmonary artery wedge pressure
PBG	porphobilinogen
PCA	posterior cerebral artery
PCC	prothrombin complex concentrates
PCI	percutaneous coronary Intervention
PCP	*Pneumocystis carinii* pneumonia
PE	pulmonary embolism
PEEP	positive end-expiratory pressure
PEFR	peak expiratory flow rate
PEG	percutaneous endoscopic gastrostomy
PEJ	percutaneous endoscopic jejeunostomy
PEP	post-exposure prophylaxis
PET	pre-eclamptic toxaemia
PFO	patent foramen ovale
PICC	peripheral inserted central catheter
PMC	pseudomembranous colitis
PMR	polymyalgia rheumatica
PND	paroxysmal nocturnal dyspnoea
PNH	paroxysmal nocturnal haemoglobinuria
POTS	postural tachycardia syndrome
PPCI	primary percutaneous coronary intervention
PPD	purified protein derivative
PUD	peptic ulcer disease
PPE	plasma protein electrophoresis
PPI	proton pump inhibitor
PPM	permanent pacemaker
PRES	posterior reversible encephalopathy syndrome
PRL	prolactin level

PSA prostate specific antigen
PSM pansystolic murmur
PT prothrombin time
PTH parathyroid hormone
PTX pneumothorax
PVD peripheral vascular disease
PVE prosthetic valve endocarditis
PVO pyrexia of unknown origin
RA rheumatoid arthritis
RAA renin angiotensin aldosterone
RAD right axis deviation
RAS renal artery stenosis
RBBB right bundle branch block
RBC red blood cell
RCA right coronary artery
RF respiratory failure
RIF right iliac fossa
RMZ right mid-zone
ROSC return of spontaneous circulation
RSV respiratory syncytial virus
RTA renal tubular acidosis
rt-PA recombinant tissue plasminogen activator
RVH right ventricular hypertrophy
RVOT RV outflow tract
SAH subarachnoid haemorrhage
SARS severe acute respiratory syndrome
SBE subacute bacterial endocarditis
SBP systolic blood pressure, spontaneous bacterial peritonitis
SC subcutaneous route
SDH sub-dural haematoma
SE status epilepticus
SIADH syndrome of inappropiate ADH secretion
SJS Stevens Johnson syndrome
SLE systemic lupus erythematosus
SOL space-occupying lesion
SR sinus rhythm
STEMI ST elevation MI
SUDEP sudden unexpected death in epilepsy
SUND sudden unexpected nocturnal death
SVC superior vena cava
SVR systemic vascular resistance
SVT supraventricular tachycardia
TAB temporal artery biopsy
TACI total anterior circulation infarct
TB tuberculosis
TCA tricyclic antidepressant
TdP Torsades de pointes
TDS three times a day
TEN toxic epidermal necrolysis
TF typhoid fever
TIA transient ischaemic attack
TIMI thrombolysis in MI
TIPS transjugular intrahepatic portosystemic shunt
TNF tumour necrosis factor
TOE transoesophageal echocardiogram
TPA tissue plasminogen activator
TPN total parenteral nutrition
TPR temperature, pulse, respirations
TRALI transfusion associated lung injury
TSH thyroid stimulating hormone
TTE transthoracic echocardiogram
TTP thrombotic thrombocytopenic purpura
TVR target vessel revascularisation
U&E urea/creatinine and electrolytes
UFH unfractionated heparin
UMN upper motor neuron
URT upper respiratory tract
USS ultrasound scan
UTI urinary tract infection
V/Q scan ventilation / perfusion scan
VATS video-assisted thoracoscopic surgery
VF ventricular fibrillation
VKA vitamin K antagonist
VRIII variable rate intravenous insulin infusion
VSD ventricular septal defect
VT ventricular tachycardia
VTE venous thromboembolism
VZV varicella zoster virus
WPW Wolff–Parkinson–White syndrome
ZIG zoster immune globulin

01 Adult Resuscitation

1.1 Introduction

- Ensure you are up to date with BLS and ALS courses. Be familiar with the excellent American Heart Association basic and advanced cardiovascular life support (ACLS) guidelines and European guidelines, which are freely accessible on the internet in pdf format.
- There is much in common in guidelines. The things that differ are due to a lack of evidence and so either way is defensible. It is difficult to perform trials on resuscitation and much is extrapolated from basic theory as well as laboratory and animal experiments.
- Guidelines are just that and experienced clinicians who know and understand the evidence or lack of evidence can deviate to a degree.

1.2 Running a cardiac arrest

- Resuscitating an unresponsive pulseless apnoeic patient can be stressful and it is never as simple as a basic algorithm suggests. It is not uncommon to find yourself trying to cope with a collapsed patient wedged in a toilet cubicle. All you can do is your best. Such a patient is certifiable as dead and you cannot make that situation any worse. In a small number of cases you can make a significant difference.
- Are you unsure of the rhythm – could it be VF? If so, do not hesitate to defibrillate. If there is **any** delay in defibrillation then get good quality CPR going at least using chest compressions. *Survival depends on the immediate initiation of chest compressions and early defibrillation if there is a shockable rhythm.*
- As soon as you arrive use the ABCs to quickly determine the basics – check the airway is not obstructed, look for breathing, palpate a major pulse, and commence chest compressions as quickly as possible; hopefully someone else will already have done so.
- Your concern is whether unresponsiveness is due to circulatory collapse or not. If unsure start CPR. It is probably less harmful to CPR a patient who turns out to have a pulse than to delay CPR in a pulseless patient. If possible let someone else do CPR as you take stock and look at the bigger picture. This is a very useful reason for the ABCs – to buy you some thinking and information-gathering time.
- Once you have the defibrillator leads on look at the rhythm and assess if it is shockable. If shockable then shock and treat for VT/VF. Go through the standard list of treatable causes ensuring effective CPR continues.

1.3 Is resuscitation appropriate?

- Always consider if resuscitation is appropriate. Is there a 'do not resuscitate' form in the notes? Is there an advance directive or community DNAR order? What was the patient's expressed wish?
- Is this VF due to a small inferior STEMI which is shockable, giving the patient many good years ahead, or an elderly patient with co-morbidities dying a

'natural death' from severe pneumonia and a large stroke, where the chances of a successful outcome are very poor?

- The aim is, fundamentally, to prolong life and not to prolong death/dying and to do what the patient would want us to do. If you can't be sure then continue. Reassess and take senior advice especially in a young patient/hypothermia/ overdose. Stop when continuing is considered futile.

1.4 General advice

- Emphasis should be on cardiac arrest prevention and so care should be instigated pre-arrest when reversible factors can be dealt with. If a patient is *in extremis* and pre-arrest, then call the arrest team.
- The ABC assessment allows you a moment to figure out what is going on and determine what you plan to do next. Let someone else manage these whilst you think.
- Delegate roles. If you are leading the arrest then ask others to get venous/ intraosseous access and obtain notes. Determine the ceiling of care. Contact your senior if unsure or unclear.
- Send away extra staff if there are demands elsewhere. Hospital business goes on and extra hands might be more productive seeing other sick patients and preventing cardiac arrests elsewhere.
- Stop once you all feel that continuing is futile. Thank the team. Complete audit sheets and record all in the patient notes. Arrange to talk with family. Do a self-debrief: anything you would do differently or better? Seek feedback and add to personal development plan.
- Favourable outcome likely from BLS/ALS: witnessed arrest; in-hospital; early effective CPR; shockable rhythm; early defibrillation; hypothermia (e.g. submerged in icy water).

1.5 Basic life support

Signs of impending or established cardiac arrest include unresponsiveness, irregular or absent breathing, impalpable pulse (can be difficult to palpate).

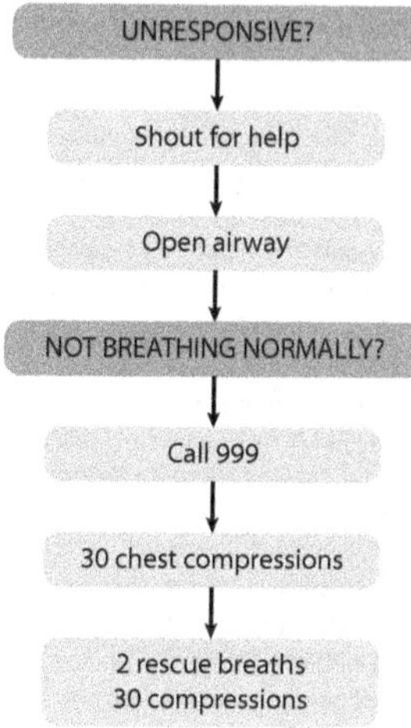

Basic life support algorithm.
Reproduced with permission from the Resuscitation Council (UK).

- **Assessment of a collapsed person:** ensure safe to approach. Check for local hazards; particularly relevant outside hospital when there may be traffic, water, electrical or chemical hazards. Check if patient is unresponsive: shake patient by the shoulders and ask loudly "Are you all right". If patient responds then leave them in the same position unless in danger and assess further to determine what is wrong (consider ABCDE/oxygen/IV access). Get help if needed. Reassess regularly. If the patient **does NOT respond** then shout for help and turn the patient on their back and open the airway using head tilt (if neck is okay) and chin lift. Head tilt involves placing hand on forehead and tilting head back gently. Chin lift is done by using fingertip under the chin and lifting to open the airway. If there are concerns over neck injury use jaw thrust, where fingers at the angle of the jaw lift the mandible forwards whilst keeping the neck immobile.
- **Airway and breathing assessment:** now keep the airway open and look for signs of breathing and for chest movements. Feel for air on your cheek. Difficult, noisy, irregular gasping breathing is seen with cardiac arrest and is not normal. Assess for a maximum of 10 s. If the person is breathing normally then place in recovery position and summon help – 999/911 or send a bystander or go yourself if no other choice. Contine to assess and be prepared to start CPR if deteriorates. If the person is **not breathing normally** then start CPR.
- **Start 30 chest compressions at 100/min:** kneel by the side of the patient, place the heel of one hand in the centre of the chest (which is the lower half of the breastbone (sternum)) and place the heel of your other hand on top of the first

hand. Interlock the fingers of your hands and ensure that pressure is not applied over the ribs. Keep your arms straight. Do not apply any pressure over the upper abdomen or the bottom end of the sternum. Position yourself vertically above the patient's chest and press down on the sternum at least 5 cm (but not exceeding 6 cm). After each compression, release all the pressure on the chest without losing contact between your hands and the sternum; repeat at a rate of at least 100/min (but not exceeding 120/min). Compression and release should take equal amounts of time.

- **Now give two rescue breaths:** open the airway again using head tilt and chin lift. Pinch the soft part of the nose closed, using the index finger and thumb of your hand on the forehead. Allow the mouth to open, but maintain chin lift. Take a normal breath and place your lips around his mouth, making sure that you have a good seal. Blow steadily into the mouth while watching for the chest to rise, taking about 1 s as in normal breathing; this is an effective rescue breath. Mouth to nose breathing can also be considered where mouth to mouth not possible. Maintaining head tilt and chin lift, take your mouth away from the patient and watch for the chest to fall as air comes out. Take another normal breath and blow into the patient's mouth once more to achieve a total of two effective rescue breaths. The two breaths should not take more than 5 s in all. If you are unable to give rescue breaths then continue chest compressions uninterrupted. Where available bag–mask ventilation may be used.
- **Continue with 30 chest compressions at 100/min:** then return your hands without delay to the correct position on the sternum and give a further 30 chest compressions. Continue with chest compressions and rescue breaths in a ratio of 30:2. Stop to recheck the patient only if he starts to wake up, to move, to open eyes and to breathe normally. Otherwise, do not interrupt resuscitation.
- **Now give two rescue breaths: as detailed above.** Continue this cycle until ALS started or BLS is continued. If you are unable to give rescue breaths then continue chest compressions uninterrupted.
- **Additional notes**: if your initial rescue breath does not make the chest rise normally then before your next attempt: look into the patient's mouth and remove any obstruction; recheck that there is adequate head tilt and chin lift; do not attempt more than two breaths each time before returning to chest compressions. If there is more than one doctor present, another doctor should take over delivering CPR every 2 min to prevent fatigue. Ensure that interruption of chest compressions is minimal during the changeover of doctors.
- **Chest-compression-only CPR may be used as follows**: if you are not trained, or are unwilling to give rescue breaths, give chest compressions only; if only chest compressions are given, these should be continuous, at a rate of at least 100/min (but not exceeding 120/min).
- **Do not interrupt resuscitation:** until professional help arrives and takes over, or the patient starts to wake up (to move, to open eyes and to breathe normally), or you become exhausted.
- **Recovery position:** the RC(UK) recommends the following sequence of actions to place a patient in the recovery position. Remove the patient's glasses, if present. Kneel beside the patient and make sure that both his legs are straight. Place the arm nearest to you out at right angles to his body, elbow bent with the hand palm-up. Bring the far arm across the chest, and hold the back of the hand against the patient's cheek nearest to you. With your other hand, grasp the far leg just above the knee and pull it up, keeping the foot on the ground. Keeping

his hand pressed against his cheek, pull on the far leg to roll the victim towards you on to his side. Adjust the upper leg so that both the hip and knee are bent at right angles. Tilt the head back to make sure that the airway remains open. If necessary, adjust the hand under the cheek to keep the head tilted and facing downwards to allow liquid material to drain from the mouth. Check breathing regularly. If the victim has to be kept in the recovery position for more than 30 min turn him to the opposite side to relieve the pressure on the lower arm.

1.6 Adult choking algorithm

Usually occurs when eating and patient clutches neck/chest and may be unable to speak. Can be wheezing and stridor. May become unconscious.

If conscious with airways obstruction give five back blows then five abdominal thrusts

- If the patient shows signs of mild airway obstruction then encourage coughing, but do nothing else. But if patient shows signs of severe airway obstruction and is conscious then give up to five back blows. Stand to the side and slightly behind the patient. Support the chest with one hand and lean the victim well forwards so that when the obstructing object is dislodged it comes out of the mouth rather than goes further down the airway. Give up to five sharp blows between the shoulder blades with the heel of your other hand. Check to see if each back blow has relieved the airway obstruction.
- If this fails then give up to five abdominal thrusts. Stand behind the patient and put both arms round the upper part of his abdomen. Lean the victim forwards. Clench your fist and place it between the umbilicus (navel) and the bottom end of the sternum (breastbone). Grasp this hand with your other hand and pull sharply inwards and upwards. Repeat up to five times. If the obstruction is still not relieved, continue alternating five back blows with five abdominal thrusts.

If unconscious start CPR

- Help the patient carefully to the ground. Call an ambulance immediately. Begin CPR. Healthcare providers who are trained and experienced in feeling for a carotid pulse should initiate chest compressions even if a pulse is present in the unconscious choking victim.
- Following successful treatment for choking, foreign material may nevertheless remain in the upper or lower respiratory tract and cause complications later. Patients with a persistent cough, difficulty swallowing, or with the sensation of an object being still stuck in the throat should therefore be referred for an immediate medical opinion.

1.7 Advanced life support

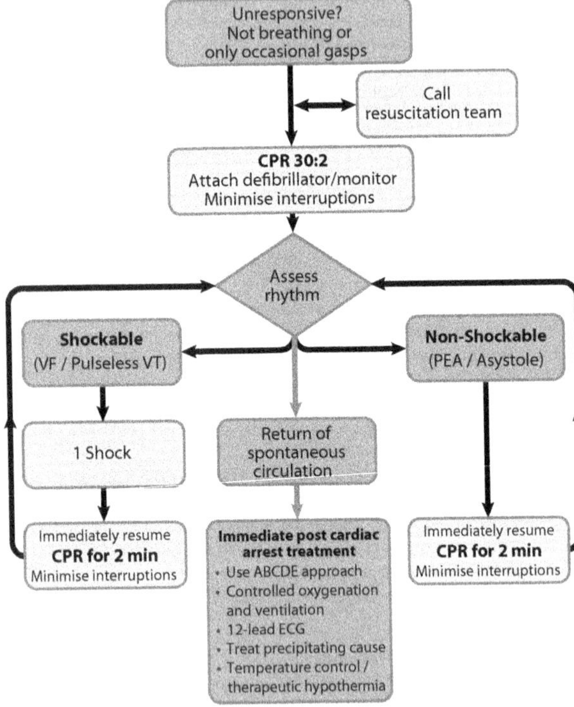

During CPR

- Ensure high-quality CPR: rate, depth, recoil
- Plan actions before interrupting CPR
- Give oxygen
- Consider advanced airway and capnography
- Continuous chest compressions when advanced airway in place
- Vascular access (intravenous, intraosseous)
- Give adrenaline every 3–5 min
- Correct reversible causes

Reversible Causes

- Hypoxia
- Hypovolaemia
- Hypo- /hyperkalaemia/metabolic
- Hypothermia
- Thrombosis – coronary or pulmonary
- Tamponade – cardiac
- Toxins
- Tension pneumothorax

Advanced life support algorithm.
Reproduced with permission from the Resuscitation Council (UK) 2010.

The ALS algorithm

- **Confirm cardiac arrest:** unresponsiveness and absent or gasping breaths. Carotid pulsation can be unreliable and difficult to palpate which delays CPR. Start good quality CPR: even chest-compression-only CPR. Give high quality compressions to a 5 cm depth with full chest recoil. Early defibrillation is key with uninterrupted

CPR unless there is clear ROSC. Continued CPR may augment return of circulation. Good CPR gives about 20% of normal cardiac output. There is a progressive metabolic acidosis. Survival after 30 min is uncommon; exceptions are hypothermia/drug overdoses. Patient should be placed on a hard surface or a board placed behind the patient. Once intubated or other ventilatory device then continue compressions at 100/min and ventilate the lungs at a rate of about 10 breaths/min.

- **Continue CPR:** perform uninterrupted chest compressions while applying self-adhesive defibrillation/monitoring pads – one below the right clavicle and the other in the V6 position in the mid-axillary line. Shave hair if need. Antero-posterior electrode placement is also satisfactory to avoid pacemakers and ICDs and preferred for AF DC cardioversion. Plan actions before pausing CPR for rhythm analysis and communicate these to the team. Stop chest compressions; assess rhythm.

SHOCKABLE RHYTHM

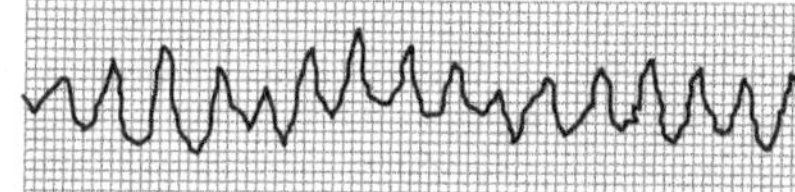

Ventricular fibrillation.

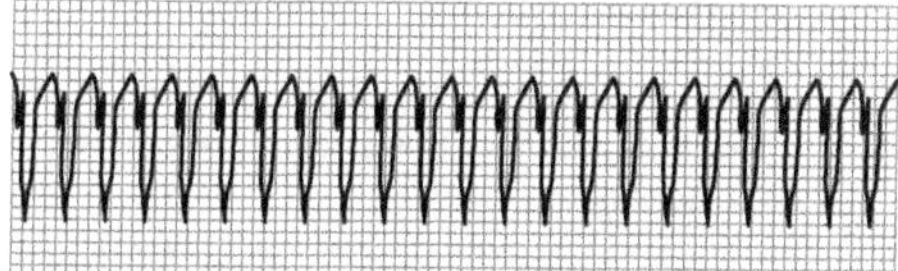

Pulseless VT.

- Confirm VF (or VT) from the ECG. Resume chest compressions immediately; simultaneously, the designated person selects the appropriate energy on the defibrillator (150–200 J biphasic for the first shock and 150–360 J biphasic for subsequent shocks) and presses the charge button.
- While the defibrillator is charging, warn all rescuers other than the individual performing the chest compressions to "stand clear" and remove any oxygen delivery device as appropriate. Ensure that the rescuer giving the compressions is the only person touching the patient.
- When clear, give the shock. Restart CPR without reassessing the rhythm or feeling for a pulse using a ratio of 30:2, starting with 30 chest compressions. Continue CPR for 2 min; the team leader prepares the team for the next pause in CPR.
- Resume chest compressions immediately and then give **ADRENALINE 1 mg IV and AMIODARONE 300 mg IV** while performing a further 2 min CPR. Repeat this 2 min CPR – rhythm/pulse check – defibrillation sequence if VF/VT persists. Give further **ADRENALINE 1 mg IV** after alternate shocks (i.e. approximately every 3–5 min). **Precordial thump**: only for witnessed arrest and where unable to immediately defibrillate.

NON-SHOCKABLE RHYTHM

- Determine if PEA (pulseless electrical activity) or asystole. Continue CPR. Note that atropine is no longer recommended for PEA/asystole.
- **Pulseless electrical activity**: start CPR 30:2. Give **ADRENALINE 1 mg IV** as soon as intravascular access is achieved. Continue CPR 30:2 until the airway is secured, then continue chest compressions without pausing during ventilation. Consider possible reversible causes of PEA. Recheck the patient after 2 min: if there is still no pulse and no change in the ECG appearance: continue CPR. Recheck the patient after 2 min and proceed accordingly. Give further **ADRENALINE 1 mg IV** every 3–5 min (alternate loops). If VF/VT, change to the shockable rhythm algorithm. If a pulse is present, start post-resuscitation care.
- **ASYSTOLE**: start CPR 30:2. Without stopping CPR, check that the leads are attached correctly. Give **ADRENALINE 1 mg IV** as soon as intravascular access is achieved. Continue CPR 30:2 until the airway is secured, then continue chest compression without pausing during ventilation. Consider possible reversible causes of PEA and correct any that are identified. Recheck the rhythm after 2 min and proceed accordingly. If VF/VT, change to the shockable rhythm algorithm. Give **ADRENALINE 1 mg IV** every 3–5 min (alternate loops). Whenever a diagnosis of asystole is made, check the ECG carefully for the presence of P waves because the patient may respond to cardiac pacing when there is ventricular standstill with continuing P waves. There is no value in attempting to pace true asystole.
- Consider early intubation and IV access but ensure chest compressions uninterrupted. Work throxugh the 6 'H' and 4 'T's (see below).

Cause	Action – work through list of 10 (the 6 'H's and 4 'T's)
Hypoxia	Check pre-arrest history and observations and causes. Give O_2 and assess cause. May need intubation and ventilation.
Hypovolaemia	If suspected start IV NS fluid challenge. Give blood if severe haemorrhage: consider O-negative. See *Massive transfusion* protocol (*Section 4.1*).
Hypokalaemia	If suspected start potassium infusion.
Hyperkalaemia	If suspected give CALCIUM CHLORIDE IV which is cardioprotective, then give insulin/dextrose.
Hypoglycaemia	Give 50 ml of 50% dextrose IV or consider IM GLUCAGON.
Hypothermia	Low core temperature: rectal thermometer. Rewarm cautiously. Hypothermia is neuroprotective. Do not stop until patient rewarmed or resuscitation fails.
Thrombosis (PE)	For an acute PE an echo may show RV dysfunction and dilatation. ABG: hypoxia, CPR may dislodge clot. Consider immediate thrombolysis with ALTEPLASE. Surgical embolectomy or mechanical thrombectomy where available immediately. CPR is not a contraindication to thrombolysis with potentially fatal PE. CPR should be continued to allow time to act, e.g. 60–90 min. Give IV fluids to ensure adequate filling pressures.
Thrombosis (MI)	Coronary thrombosis – ECG will show STEMI or new LBBB once defibrillated. Consider primary PCI.
Tamponade	Faint heart sounds, falling BP, raised JVP. ECG may have shown low voltage. Large heart on CXR, bedside echo may be diagnostic. Was there chest trauma, bleed on anticoagulants, recent cardiac surgery? Recent cardiac intervention, e.g. ablation, needs immediate pericardiocentesis.
Toxins	Need drug overdose history – see *Toxicology* section (*Chapter 20*).

Cause	Action – work through list of 10 (the 6 'H's and 4 'T's)
Tension PTX	Moribund cyanosed patient dying. Insert needle in 2nd interspace on affected resonant side (trachea deviated away). Diagnostic 'hiss' hopefully as decompresses. BP should improve. Do not wait for CXR. Insert chest drain. Suspect in ventilated patient who deteriorates.

- **Definition**: pulseless electrical activity (PEA)/electromechanical dissociation = absence of detectable cardiac output in the presence of a coordinated electrical rhythm.
- **Focused echo**: increasing availability of small cheap portable echo machines may be used in the arrest situation without disturbing CPR. Sub-xiphoid views can help exclude pericardial tamponade and other causes of hypotension or PEA.

KEY POINTS

- **Prevention**: emphasis is on prevention and early detection of problems and intervention before cardiac arrest. Implement systems to detect at-risk patients – early warning systems: track and trigger. These should be implemented and the involvement of critical care outreach should help flag up high risk patients before they arrest.
- **If ROSC** does not occur quickly then ensure rapid IV access and intubation with minimal interruption to chest compressions. **Continuous quantitative waveform capnography** for monitoring of ET tube placement is a useful marker that identifies ROSC.
- **ADENOSINE IV/IO**: safe/effective in undifferentiated regular monomorphic wide complex tachycardia (US) and may be diagnostic of terminating SVT with aberrant conduction.
- **Oxygen: 100% O_2 or 15 L/min** with a non rebreather mask gives an FiO_2 of about 85% and is recommended in cardiac arrest and shock, but should be reduced post-arrest to avoid O_2 toxicity. Follow BTS guidance. Watch oxygen saturation. Watch for CO_2 retention which can only be diagnosed by ABG.

When to stop resuscitation

- After 30 min the probability of a successful outcome is very low. There are exceptions and they include patients who are hypothermic (they should be returned to normal core temperature before stopping), near drowning and tricyclic antidepressant overdose. If unsure take senior advice. In reality, futile continuation is usually clear. In younger patients (under 40) try to seek senior advice before stopping CPR unless it is clearly futile.
- Clinical context matters – if in the setting of a massive intracerebral haemorrhage then cardiac arrest is a terminal event and CPR was likely futile all along. If in the setting of VF with a small inferior MI then would continue for longer. If there is VF/VT then shocks and antiarrhythmics should be tried.
- Current guidance is that resuscitation may be discontinued if all of the following apply: 15 min or more has passed since the onset of collapse; no bystander CPR was given before arrival of the ambulance; there is no suspicion of drowning, hypothermia, poisoning/overdose, or pregnancy; asystole is present for more than 30 s on the ECG monitor screen.

Intraosseous infusion

- IO infusion is an alternative option to IV access (tracheal drugs no longer recommended). It allows the injection of fluids and drugs directly into the marrow-filled area of the bone and provides a non-collapsible entry point into the systemic venous system unaffected by vasoconstriction and is useful in emergencies to provide fluids and medication when IV access not available or not feasible.

- A needle is injected through the bone's hard cortex and into the soft marrow interior. An infusion can be used when traditional methods of vascular access are difficult or impossible.
- Typical sites include antero-medial aspect of the tibia, anterior aspect of the femur, the superior iliac crest and the head of the humerus. Often used in paediatrics. Main issue is physical retention. Newer devices such as EZ-IO use specially designed cutting IO needle and are easier to retain.

Cardiac arrest: reasons to consider IV calcium are hyperkalaemia, severe hypocalcaemia, magnesium toxicity, calcium channel blocker toxicity.

1.8 Special cases in resuscitation

Cause	Advice
Patient Has ICD	These patients are at high risk of cardiac arrest. If AICD senses a shockable rhythm it will fire a 40 J shock internally which may cause pectoral muscle contraction. Shocks to rescuers doing CPR are minimal especially if wearing gloves. Generally produces a maximum of 8 possible discharges. Place shock pads away from AICD, e.g. antero-posterior: left precordium to below left scapula. A magnet placed over the AICD will disable any of its activity.
Post-cardiac surgery cardiac catheterization	Cardiac arrest where chests compressions difficult. Give 3 quick consecutive 'stacked' shocks before starting chest compressions. Consider re-sternotomy (reopening the sternal wound) to exclude tamponade. Internal defibrillation with paddles. Direct cardiac compression can be given to the heart. Use 20 J in cardiac arrest but only 5 J if supported on cardiopulmonary bypass.
Post drowning	Immediately start CPR and 15 L/min O_2; ROSC prior to hospital suggests better prognosis. Look for and treat hyperkalaemia with fresh water drowning. Look for and manage compounding issues, e.g. associated hypothermia/exposure, drug overdose or suicide attempt. Duration of hypoxia is the most critical survival factor.
Post electrocution	Extensive burns can affect face and neck and airway. CPR because patient may be in VF or asystole with early intubation if possible. Asystole is seen after DC shock and VF after AC shock (mains supply). Check for secondary spinal injury or other trauma. Muscle paralysis can cause respiratory failure (reduced FVC <1.5 L). Fluid resuscitation as tissue/muscle damage. Ensure good diuresis, watch for AKI and check CK and K^+.
Cardiac arrest in pregnancy	Caesarean section within 5 min of the cardiac arrest can save mother and baby. Call maternal cardiac arrest team and obstetrician immediately and note time. After 20 weeks aortocaval compression so left lateral tilt (right side high and left side low). Use a fixed wedge or a large gravid uterus can be

Cause	Advice
	manually displaced to the left. Optimal chest compressions in higher position on sternum. Ventilate: bag mask 100% O_2 and monitor capnography. Optimal airway control. Follow ALS algorithm using same drugs. Place IV access above diaphragm (not femoral) and give IV fluids as needed. Defibrillation is regarded as safe throughout pregnancy. Remove fetal monitors during defibrillation. If suspect magnesium toxicity stop it and give antidote IV calcium chloride/ gluconate. If no ROSC within 4 min then emergency caesarean section and aim to deliver within 5 min of resuscitation commencing. Delivery can be life saving for mother and fetus and may improve a desperate situation. **Possible causes:** bleeding coagulopathy, DIC, sepsis, acute MI, concealed haemorrhage – placental abruption, ectopic pregnancy, rupture or dissection of aneurysms, pulmonary embolus (thrombolysis if life-threatening PE), amniotic fluid embolism (immediate caesarean), anaesthetic complication, known or new cardiac disease, HTN, pre-eclampsia/eclampsia, placenta abruptio/placenta praevia. Discuss an urgent management plan for these if ROSC – most are obstetric.

1.9 Return of spontaneous circulation

- **ROSC:** palpable central pulse or sudden increase in end-tidal CO_2 trace. If signs of ROSC then complete assessment: ABC. O_2/ventilation. You bring the patient back from death so the immediate questions are why the cardiac arrest and anticipate possible complications. Get an ECG, ABG, U&E, troponin.
- Key considerations: is it STEMI needing primary PCI, acute PE needing thrombolysis, hyperkalaemia needing calcium and insulin/dextrose?
- **ABC: high FiO_2** can now be reduced to give O_2 as per BTS guidance. Check FBC, U&E, ABG, CXR, 12-lead ECG, Mg, Ca, troponin, lactate. Of these the ECG is the most useful as a large MI should be evident. If STEMI then PPCI is the next approach if stable.
- **AIRWAY**: maintain patency of airway: ensure no obstruction. Place patient onto back and listen for snoring or stridor which all may suggest some degree of obstruction. If no suspected cervical spinal injury then open airway by tilting the head back (hand on forehead to tilt head back) and chin lift (fingertips under the point of the chin). If neck injury suspected then use jaw thrust to lift the mandible and tongue keeping C-spine immobile. Inspect the oropharynx and remove any foreign bodies with a finger sweep and extract any obstructed material with forceps and suction. Consider oropharyngeal or nasopharyngeal airway if additional airway protection needed. Advanced airway support will involve bag–valve mask delivering O_2 with a good seal. Ensure adequate preparation and pre-oxygenation with 100%. Pre-ventilate with high flow O_2 prior to intubation to ensure full oxygenation.
- **BREATHING**: open airway and look, listen and feel for normal breathing. Assess for a maximum of 10 s and if breathing place in recovery position. If not breathing or agonal breaths then immediately commence CPR. Hypoventilation alone may need ventilatory support – bag and mask, intubation or NIPPV.

- **CIRCULATION**: if AED not instantly available then start CPR with 30 compressions with open airway. Pinch nose. Give 2 rescue breaths. Kneel by side, place heel of hand on the lower sternum. Press down firmly 4–5 cm allow recoil, 100/min. Recommence 30 chest compressions with ratio of 30: 2. CPR is performed at 100/minute in 2 minute episodes followed by reassessment. Do not interrupt unless definite signs of recovery. Plan for any pauses to be as short as possible. Compression-only CPR where unable/unwilling to give rescue breaths. Continue until help comes, exhaustion or patient improves and recovers. Bag–mask ventilation if available or consider intubation.
- **DISABILITY**: look for CNS injury. Assess level of consciousness. This can be with the GCS or the **AVPU score** – are they **A**lert, respond only to **V**erbal stimulus or does it require a **P**ainful stimulus or are they **U**nconscious with no response at all. General neurological assessment is dealt with below. Check pupils especially in the comatose patient where they can signify serious brain injury, coning and stroke. Check neurology, e.g. seizure, hemiparesis, sensory level and paraparesis. Cardiac arrest may be due to massive brain injury/stroke or other pathology.
- **EXPOSURE:** expose, with modesty in mind, the patient and do a full top to toe evaluation if the diagnosis is not obvious. If spine safe roll over and check the back and spine. Check orifices, eyes, etc. Palpate abdomen, feel the back of head and scalp for bumps and evidence of trauma.
- **Induced hypothermia** may be neuroprotective. Indicated in those comatose following ROSC due to VF arrest. Involves cooling to 32–34°C for 12–24 h or longer post-ROSC. Evidence in non-VF arrest lacking but is used in comatose patients after either form of arrest. Methods include cooling blankets and ice bags as well as ice-cold isotonic infusion. Up to 3 L has been given in some trials.
- **Glycaemic control**: aim for glucose control of 6–10 mmol/L. Avoid hypoglycaemia which can cause or exacerbate brain injury.
- **Coagulopathy**: watch for signs and check APTT, FBC, PT, platelets, fibrinogen if any doubt.
- **Hypotension:** treat (SBP <90 mmHg) by addressing cause with a choice of vasopressor, e.g. ADRENALINE, DOPAMINE or NORADRENALINE. Fluids: 1–2 L of IV NS or Ringer's lactate. Chilled to 4°C for induced hypothermia. Other vasopressors are listed later.
- **Post-arrest myocardial dysfunction:** may be related to an underlying STEMI but a period of hypoperfusion can result in temporarily impaired pump function for up to 72 h which can be bridged with inotropes and IABP if required. In some cases hypotension and shock may be partly driven by a SIRS type mechanism with a drop in systemic vascular resistance and in these cases noradrenaline may be useful – take expert advice. This is best delivered within an ITU setting with access to invasive monitoring.
- **Arrhythmias:** see below for management of tachy/bradyarrhythmias
- **Seizures and myoclonic jerks**: can be seen post-ROSC in up to 10% of patients. These can be managed conservatively but if significant and frequent then may consider anticonvulsants. Clonazepam can be used for myoclonus as well as valproate and some of the newer agents. Consider neurology input.

Bradycardia management

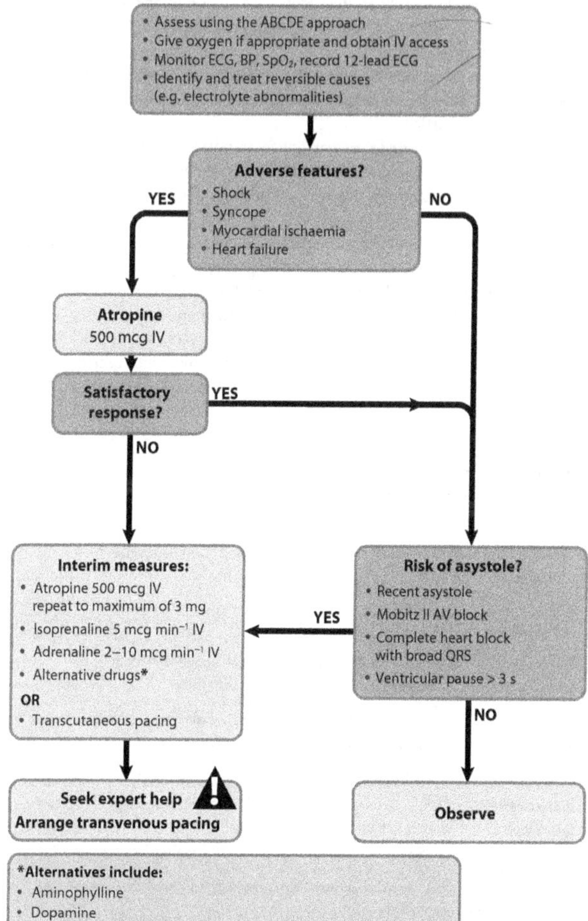

Adult bradycardia algorithm.
Reproduced with permission from the Resuscitation Council (UK) 2010.

Assess

- Give O_2 if appropriate as per BTS and obtain IV access. Monitor ECG, BP, SpO_2, record 12-lead ECG. Identify and treat reversible causes (e.g. electrolyte abnormalities). *If there is evidence of shock, syncope, myocardial ischaemia, or heart failure, then treat as below otherwise observe.*

- **Give ATROPINE 500 mcg IV** and observe and if no improvement or risk of asystole (e.g. risk of asystole – recent asystole, Möbitz II AV block, complete heart block with broad QRS, ventricular pause >3 s) then give additional **ATROPINE 500 mcg IV** up to a maximum of 3 mg.
- Failure to respond consider **ISOPRENALINE IV OR ADRENALINE IV** or **AMINOPHYLLINE, DOPAMINE, GLUCAGON** (if beta-blocker or CCB overdose). Glycopyrrolate can be used instead of atropine.
- Set up **transcutaneous pacing** as preparation for transvenous pacing. Initiate transcutaneous pacing immediately if there is no response to atropine, or if atropine is unlikely to be effective. It can be painful and so use analgesia and sedation.
- If atropine is ineffective and transcutaneous pacing is not immediately available, **fist pacing** can be attempted while waiting for pacing equipment. Give serial rhythmic blows with the closed fist over the left lower edge of the sternum to pace the heart at a physiological rate of 50–70 beats/min.
- **Emergency transvenous pacing** is the treatment of any severe bradycardia with significant haemodynamic compromise. Temporary transvenous pacing should be considered if there is a history of recent asystole, Möbitz type II AV block, complete heart block (especially with broad QRS or initial heart rate <40 beats/min), or evidence of ventricular standstill of more than 3 s.

Tachycardia management

Based on Adult tachycardia algorithm (Resuscitation Council (UK) 2010).

Assess

- ABCDE approach. Give oxygen if appropriate and obtain IV access.
- Monitor ECG, BP, SpO_2, record 12-lead ECG. Troponin.

Clinical and ECG	Advice
Stable **Unstable**	Absence of shock, syncope, myocardial ischaemia, heart failure Shock, syncope, myocardial ischaemia, heart failure
Unstable + HR >150	Usually ventricular rate >150/min then 3 synchronized shocks and if this fails then **AMIODARONE IV as below**
Stable and regular narrow QRS complex	Try vagal maneouvre and consider repeated adenosine. (1) sinus tachycardia; (2) AV nodal re-entry tachycardia (AVNRT, the commonest type of SVT); (3) AV re-entry tachycardia (AVRT), which is associated with Wolff–Parkinson–White (WPW) syndrome; (4) atrial flutter with regular AV conduction (usually 2:1).
Stable and irregular narrow QRS complex	Probable fast AF. Try beta-blocker or diltiazem or amiodarone or digoxin (not with WPW). Digoxin or IV amiodarone preferred if in failure. Avoid Digoxin or verapamil if WPW.
Stable and broad complex QRS irregular	(1) **AF with BBB** treat as for narrow complex. (2) **Pre-excited AF** consider amiodarone (not digoxin or verapamil). (3) **Polymorphic VT,** e.g. TdP – give **MAGNESIUM 2 g IV over 10 min.** Consider overdrive pacing. Take advice. Check U&E, Mg, Ca. Causes of long QTc.
Stable and broad QRS complex regular	Assume VT and give **AMIODARONE IV as below. Consider ADENOSINE IV (as above)** if unsure of rhythm, e.g. SVT + BBB try **ADENOSINE** IV to terminate.

Clinical and ECG	Advice
AMIODARONE: 300 mg IV over 10–20 min if unstable or 20–60 mins if stable and a further shock and a further 900 mg IV infusion over 24 hours. Infusion through central line. **ADENOSINE: 6 mg fast IV into large vein** with immediate saline flush and look for termination of arrhythmia. If no success repeat with 12 mg and then a further 12 mg.	

Implantable cardioverter defibrillator (ICD)

Looks like and can function as a pacemaker; however, it can also deliver low-energy synchronized cardioversion and high-energy defibrillation shocks that successfully terminate 99% of ventricular fibrillation attacks

Indications for an implantable cardioverter defibrillator (EPS = electrophysiological study)
• Cardiac arrest due to VF or VT not due to a transient or reversible cause • Spontaneous sustained VT in association with structural heart disease • Syncope of undetermined origin with clinically relevant, haemodynamically significant sustained VT or VF induced at EPS when drug therapy is ineffective, not tolerated, or not preferred • Non-sustained VT in patients with coronary disease, prior myocardial infarction, LV dysfunction, and inducible VF or sustained VT at EPS that is not suppressible by a class I antiarrhythmic drug • Spontaneous sustained VT in patients without structural heart disease not amenable to other treatments

Emergency DC cardioversion

- **Indication:** DC cardioversion (only if we treat VF is it called defibrillation) should be considered in all fast and unstable tachyarrhymias. Usually the ventricular rate is >150/min. If there is chest pain, breathlessness due to pulmonary oedema, or hypotension due to the arrhythmia, then arrange urgent DC shock.
- **Contraindications:** digitalis toxicity as danger of ventricular arrhythmias – usually 1 or 2 doses omitted if elective. Not for sinus tachycardia or multifocal atrial tachycardia as futile. Concerns about unanticoagulated AF of duration >48 h and embolic/stroke risk needs to be weighed against the need for improving haemodynamics. Ideally they should have a TOE to identify left atrial appendage thrombus, but in reality this is not practical or feasible or available in the emergency situation. Take expert advice. In these cases some form of rate control rather than rhythm control may be tried, but DC cardioversion is quick and often effective.
- **Sedation:** enlist help of anaesthetist to protect airway. Needs sedation, e.g. **MIDAZOLAM IV** is the sedation of choice and provides amnesia and sedation. Maximum total of 7.5 ml (1 mg/ml) can be given. Annexate should be available for oversedation. Written consent if possible, however, patient may be too unwell for this. Use pulse oximetry and continuous monitoring which can be done via the pads. Remove nitrate patches. Ensure good IV access.
- **DC cardioversion:** place pads on the chest (anterior posterior may be preferred for AF). Use a biphasic shock of 120–150 J or monophasic 200 J; for atrial flutter or SVT, a lower shock strength can be considered. Ensure that the defibrillator is 'synced' with the R wave of the QRS complexes. There is a sync button which does this and a bright dot appears on the R wave – this avoids shocking on a T wave and inducing VF. Give 3 successive shocks if there is no immediate cardioversion,

giving up to full energy available. Ensure you warn all before giving the shock. If no success, consider repeating after **AMIODARONE 150–300 mg IV** over 20 min.

- Elective cardioversion for AF: those on warfarin should have evidence of levels of INR within the therapeutic window for the past 4 weeks prior to the procedure. Evidently in the emergency situation this is waived, but therapeutic LMWH should be given if not anticoagulated and continued for 4 weeks.
- **Complications:** skin soreness like a sunburn over the pads, arrhythmias, stroke (DC cardioversion may precipitate systemic emboli from intracardiac thrombus) especially in AF which is not anticoagulated, failure is seen in many with AF but more successful in VT and atrial flutter and SVT, mild troponin rises.

Emergency pericardiocentesis

- Relative contraindications are uncorrected bleeding disorders, e.g. low platelets, raised INR. A long needle is passed using a sub xiphoid approach under strict asepsis and local anaesthesia, with echo/ultrasound control, aspirating with needle at 30° to skin with the patient sitting up at 45° angle, aiming for tip of the left shoulder.
- Connect a 20 or 50 ml syringe to the spinal needle, and aspirate 5 ml of NS into the syringe. While advancing the needle, the occasional injection of up to 1 ml of NS helps to keep the needle lumen patent. Seldinger technique is used and a wire is passed; once the pericardial space is entered then a floppy soft-tipped guide-wire is passed into the space and around the heart.
- A pig tailed or soft straight multiperforated sterile drainage catheter is inserted over the wire and the wire removed. This allows rapid drainage and improved BP. Take senior advice if available and transfer patient to cardiology centre as soon as possible. Drainage of large effusions, especially if chronic ones, must be evacuated very slowly; otherwise, there may be acute ventricular dilation or pulmonary oedema.
- **Complications:** PTX, damage to myocardium, coronary vessels, arrhythmias, pulmonary oedema.

02 Early Management of Acutely Ill Patients

2.1 Levels of care

Clinicians need to classify patients according to their needs to enable best possible care in the most appropriate part of the hospital. These have been designated as differing levels and you should know the terminology.

Level	Details
Level 0	Patients whose needs can be met through normal ward care in an acute hospital, e.g. intravenous therapy. Observations required less frequently than every 4 h.
Level 1	Patients at risk of their condition deteriorating, or those recently relocated from higher levels of care, whose needs can be met on an acute ward with additional advice and support from the critical care team, e.g. patients requiring observations more than every 4 h, tracheostomy, CVP line, chest drain, continuous infusion of insulin, PCA, post-op.
Level 2	Patients requiring more detailed observation or intervention including support for a single failing organ system or post-op care and those 'stepping down' from higher levels of care. Needing hourly monitoring, needing >50% O_2 delivered by face mask.
Level 3	Patients requiring advanced respiratory support alone or basic respiratory support together with support of at least two organ systems. This level includes all complex patients requiring support for multi-organ failure.

The care delivered depends on several factors. These include the skills of the nurses predominantly and the skill mix, i.e. appropriately trained nurses, their seniority and the number of healthcare assistants available. The ratio of skilled staff to patients is fundamental in allowing time for the correct level of care and observation. When a patient is sick there is a need to move the patient to a level of care that is appropriate, which may mean moving them to the medical assessment unit (MAU), or to an HDU or ITU bed. For the latter two groups of patients it is good to involve critical care outreach as early as possible.

Advice before you call a senior doctor

- Seeking help from seniors, peers or other disciplines is a key skill at all levels. Organisation is crucial. It depends on what time available. If *in extremis* get the notes, observations and call quickly whilst others continue to manage the patient. If more time get the notes and make a quick summary list of clinical details. Get lab results, imaging and pathology and make a summary note. Check notes, drug chart, fluid balance and observations charts and bring all of this to the phone with you.
- Know FiO_2, IV drugs and infusions. What was premorbid state and the patient's wishes? If the patient had stated they didn't want intubation and ventilation for a chronic worsening lung condition then best to confirm this before calling ITU (ring the family if needed for baseline and other such information if you think it will alter the escalation decision).
- State up front (**S**ituation) why you are ringing, e.g. "I need a CT or ITU bed" or just advice. Now give **B**ackground (SBAR, see below) remembering that it is not a case presentation. Give vital findings quickly. If it's a complex clinical question by all

means suggest the plan you thought you might follow and then seek approval – the senior doctor might agree or change your plans, but either way it will be a good learning experience.

SBAR

Heading	Discussion
Situation	Identify yourself and the ward and speciality. Identify the name, age and sex of patient. What is the immediate concern to resolve?
Background	Explain clinical context. What has happened? Reason admitted. Main past medical history. Relevant medications, procedures, resus status, other input already taken. Relevant lab results.
Assessment	Latest observations and NEWS. Bring the notes and observations charts and lab results to the phone with you.
Recommendation	For nursing staff explain what you need – if you feel patient needs to be seen now, or can it be dealt with in 20 min, or an hour. If it is an SHO/Registrar/ST calling a consultant follow the above advice.

2.2 ABCDE quick check

Focus	Assess	Warning signs	Actions
Airway	Normal speech and no added airways noises	Reduced GCS especially <9, paradoxical chest movements, snoring, drooling, grunting, stridor	Chin lift, jaw thrust, removal of foreign bodies, oropharyngeal airway, suction secretions, recovery position, intubation, treat any suspected anaphylaxis
Breathing	Talking full sentences, comfortable, RR 12–20. O_2 sats >96%	Too breathless to talk, RR <8 or >20. Wheeze, reduced chest expansion one side, silent chest, accessory muscles, cyanosis, tracheal deviation	High concentration O_2 via reservoir mask 15 L/min. CPAP, NIV, cough assist device, ventilation, IV antibiotics
Circulation	Cap refill <2 sec. HR 50–90 bpm. SBP 120–140 mmHg. Urine output 40 ml/h	Cold, shut down, peripheral cyanosis, SBP <90 mmHg or >220 mmHg. Raised JVP. Urine output <40 ml/h.	Repeated 250 ml fluid bolus. IV antibiotics. Coronary revascularization, thrombolysis (ACS/PE), LMWH (PE), inotropes, balloon pump
Disability	Normal GCS orientated	Low GCS, confused, comatose, pupil signs, Cheyne–Stokes. Assess using **A**lert, **V**oice, **P**ain, **U**nresponsive	Check ABC. Look for hypoglycaemia or opiates. Give glucose, naloxone, treat sepsis or encephalitis or stroke

Focus	Assess	Warning signs	Actions
Exposure	Full examination	Meningism, peritonitis, hypothermia, fractures, spinal injury	Cautious rewarming, watch observations, bloods
DEFGH	**D**on't **E**ver **F**orget **G**lucose or **H**eroin (opiates)		

Important signs of impending demise: hypotension, cold peripheries, oliguria or anuria, fall in GCS (coma) or new confusion, developing cyanosis, tachy/bradycardia, tachy/bradypnoea.

There has been much work done to help spot sick patients early on to allow early intervention. Early warning scores provide a 'track-and-trigger' system to efficiently identify and respond to patients who present with or develop acute illness. The RCP has developed National Early Warning Scores (NEWS). There is also a recommendation that escalation communication uses the SBAR protocol. NEWS should be an aid and not a substitute for competent experienced clinical judgement.

2.3 National Early Warning Scores

Parameter	0	+1	+2	+3
Respiratory rate (breaths/min)	12–20	9–11	21–44	≥ 25 or ≤8
SpO_2* (%)	≥96	94–95	92–93	≤91
Temp (°C)	36.1–38.0	35.1–36.0 or 38.1–39.0	≥39.1	≤ 35
Systolic BP (mmHg)	111–219	101–110	91–100	≤ 90 or >220
Pulse rate (bpm)	51–90	41–50 or 91–110	111–130	≥ 131 or ≤40
Conscious	A	A	A	VPU
Supplemental O_2	No		Yes	

*For patients with known Type 2 respiratory failure due to COPD, recommended BTS target saturations of 88–92% should be used. These patients will still 'score' if their oxygen saturations are below 92% unless the score is 'reset' by a competent clinical decision-maker and patient-specific target oxygen saturations are prescribed and documented on the chart and in the clinical notes.

Clinical Risk and Response

Score	Notes
Low risk (0–4)	Should prompt assessment by a trained nurse who decides if a change to frequency of clinical monitoring or an escalation of clinical care is required.
Medium risk (5–6 or a RED score)	Needs an urgent review by a clinician competent to assess acute illness – ward-based doctor or acute team nurse, who can escalate to a team with critical care skills as required.

Score	Notes
High risk (≥7)	Prompts emergency assessment by a clinical team/critical care outreach team with critical care competencies and there is usually transfer of the patient to a higher dependency care area.
Exceptions	Extreme values in one physiological parameter (e.g. heart rate <40 bpm, or a respiratory rate of <8 per minute or a temperature of <35°C) should not be ignored and on its own requires urgent clinical evaluation.

Reference: Royal College of Physicians (2012) National Early Warning Score (NEWS): standardising the assessment of acute-illness severity in the NHS. Report of a working party. London: RCP.

2.4 Assessment of hydration

- This is a key clinical skill which needs care and attention. Gather evidence from patient, from fluid balance, clinical context, blood results, urine output and weight. Rarely a need for a central line to tell if patient under/overloaded. Fluid challenge is a useful dynamic and potentially therapeutic assessment.
- **Hypovolaemia:** check for signs of thirst, low BP, tachycardia, reduced skin turgor, dry tongue and mucous membranes, oliguria, capillary return, cold nose and fingers and toes. JVP not visible. Thready pulse. Postural drop even lying to sitting. Reduced GCS. Confusion. Improvement of parameters with 250–500 ml of N-Saline (NS) or Hartmann's solution (or more depending on context), fluid challenges to improve BP, reduce HR, improve urine output.
- **Hypervolaemia:** oedema, normal or high BP, tachycardia if in LVF, raised JVP, good pulse possibly. No postural drop. Normal urine output. Ascites, heart failure. Fails to respond or worsens with fluid challenge.

2.5 Basis of cardiovascular support

- The heart is a four chamber muscular pump forcing blood around in parallel pulmonary and systemic circulations. The direction of flow between the atria and ventricles and the ventricles and aortic and pulmonary arteries is controlled by valves which allow only one-way flow.
- The heart is about the size of a clenched fist. It is enveloped in a layer of fibrous pericardium within the pericardial sac. It is suspended by the major vessels. It lies between the lungs and behind the sternum. Inferiorly the surface is formed by the right ventricle and left ventricle and part of the right atrium posteriorly. The inferior surface is in contact with the diaphragm. Posteriorly lies the base of the heart formed by the left atrium in close contact with the descending aorta and oesophagus.
- The two atria act as storage vessels for blood returning to the heart. The two ventricles act as pumps. On the left side the left atrium receives oxygenated blood from the lungs from the four pulmonary veins. The left atrium and left ventricle are separated by the semilunar mitral valve. The mitral valve has anterior and posterior leaflets. The left ventricle pumps blood into the systemic circulation and has a thick muscular wall
- On the right side the right atrium receives deoxygenated blood from the systemic circulation from the inferior and superior vena cava. The right atrium and

ventricle are separated by the tricuspid valve which has three leaflets. Blood is ejected with systole across the pulmonary valve into the pulmonary artery. Right-sided pressures are low and the RV is thin walled compared with the left.

- The right border of the heart is formed almost entirely by the right atrium. The left border of the heart is formed almost entirely by the left ventricle with the left atrial appendage superiorly. The base or posterior surface is formed almost entirely by the left atrium which is closely opposed to the oesophagus (important for transoesophageal echo). Inferior or diaphragmatic surface of the heart is made up by the right and left atrium

Coronary arteries

- **Left coronary artery**: arises from the left aortic sinus. It forms the left main stem and branches almost immediately into the left anterior descending (LAD) artery which travels between right and left ventricles towards the apex and the circumflex.
- **Left anterior descending (LAD) (anterior intraventricular)**: the LAD gives off the diagonal branches (D1), diagonal branches (D2)and septal branches. Supplies anterior 2/3rd of IV septum and a major portion of left ventricular walls.
- **Circumflex artery** (CX) which lies in the left AV groove between the left atrium and left ventricle and supplies the vessels of the lateral wall of the left ventricle. CX gives off the posterior descending artery (PDA) (10% of patients have a left dominant circulation in which the CX also supplies) and the obtuse marginal branches.
- **Right coronary artery** is the first branch of the aorta and arises from the anterior aortic sinus and runs in the AV grove between right atrium and ventricle. It gives off the acute marginal branch which runs along the margin of the right ventricle above the diaphragm, Sinus node branch in 60% (otherwise supplied by the CX) and atrioventricular node branch and continues as the posterior descending artery (RCA dominant) in over 65% which supplies the inferior wall of the left ventricle and inferior part of the septum.
- **Blood flow in coronary arteries** is usually maximal during diastole when the ventricle relaxes and oxygen extraction is near maximal so increased demand requires increased flow so any significantly partially obstructive lesion (>70%) will cause ischaemia. Slowing the heart lengthens diastole which aids coronary perfusion. Devices such as intra-aortic balloon pumps improve coronary perfusion.
- **Cardiac output (CO)** is about 5 L/min. CO = stroke volume × heart rate. In the normal heart ventricular performance measured as CO depends on adequate stretching of the myocytes and appropriate LV filling. In heart failure excess filling cannot be accommodated. Contractility of the heart measured as that fraction ejected from LV per systole and and is normally >60%. The ability to move blood also depends on afterload made up of systemic vascular resistance (SVR).
- **Blood pressure (BP)** = CO × SVR. SVR is maintained by vasoconstrictors, e.g. angiotensin II and aldosterone. Mean arterial BP = (SBP−DBP)/3 + DBP.

2.6 Basis of neurological management

Anatomy and physiology: the brain is 1% of body weight but gets over 10% of cardiac output for its high metabolic demand. It is sensitive to embolism and ischaemia and any reduction in global cerebral perfusion for more than a few seconds causes collapse. The brain is irrigated by four arteries. Two internal carotid arteries anteriorly (anterior circulation) and the two vertebrals posteriorly (posterior circulation).

Vertebrals arise from ipsilateral subclavians. The branches of these arteries meet again with the circle of Willis with posterior communicating artery connecting ICA to PCA and the anterior communicating between R and L anterior cerebral arteries.

The brain is contained within a bony box and so as pressure increases the only exit is the foramen magnum. Skull contains, by volume, 80% brain, 10% blood, 10% CSF. Within the skull there are further compartments due to the falx and tentorium. These limit the scope of expansion such that any increase in intracranial volume will cause a gradual and ultimately exponential rise in ICP which leads to brainstem compression and death. Raised ICP will also reduce cerebral perfusion pressure, which is mean systemic arterial pressure (MAP) minus ICP. Normal 'opening' pressure is 10–25 cm CSF. Always measure opening pressure at LP. Rising ICP can result in focal signs and herniation syndromes.

Wakefulness is controlled by the reticular activating system, which is a fine network of nerves within the brainstem ascending as far as the thalamus and hypothalamus bilaterally. Compression, stroke, tumours and any other pathology can cause disruption with coma. Progressive rises in ICP compresses the medulla and eventually respiratory centres in the brainstem and medulla are compromised and respiration ceases. It is important to understand the different forms of cerebral oedema which are detailed below.

Glasgow Coma Scale

Communicate what patients can do rather than just the absolute score. Describe score as X out of 15 to ensure no misunderstanding. Changes may be more important than actual values. Difficult to deal with aphasic patients who get a reduced score. Possibly ignore speech and mark best eye and best motor out of 10. No best approach.

Score	Best eye response (E4)	Best verbal response (V5)	Best motor response (M6)
1	No eye opening	None	No motor response
2	Eye opening to pain (supraorbital and sternal pressure/rub)	Incomprehensible sounds (moaning but no words)	Arm extends to pain (decerebrate response, adduction, internal rotation of shoulder, pronation of forearm)
3	Eye opens to speech (wake patient if asleep)	Inappropriate words (random or exclamatory articulated speech, but no conversational exchange)	Arm flexes to pain (decorticate response)
4	Eye opens spontaneously	Confused (patient responds but some disorientation and confusion)	Arm withdraws from pain (pulls part of body away when pinched; flexion ok)
5		Normal (patient responds coherently and appropriately to questions – month, age)	Hand localises to pain (e.g. gets above chin when supra-orbital pressure applied)

Score	Best eye response (E4)	Best verbal response (V5)	Best motor response (M6)
6			Obeys commands (patient follows simple commands)

Herniation syndromes

Herniation syndrome	Pathogenesis and symptoms
Sub-falcine herniation	Unilateral pressure from above and laterally pushing down and medially pushes the cingulate gyrus under the falx and can nip the anterior cerebral artery and cause infarction. Usually a superior cortical space occupying lesion or SDH/EDH. Coma usually, leg weakness, abulia.
Trans-tentorial herniation	Compresses IIIrd nerve (ipsilateral), stretching VIth nerve. Posterior cerebral artery (C/L hemianopia), cerebral peduncle (C/L hemiparesis); posterior midbrain: bilateral ptosis, upward gaze; reticular activating system: coma, medulla: HTN and bradycardia.
Uncal herniation	Uncal herniation occurs when the uncus is displaced medially and inferiorly over the free edge of the tentorium cerebelli. This type of herniation is usually secondary to a mass located inferiorly in the cerebral hemisphere in the temporal lobe. Indentation of the contralateral cerebral peduncle, known as Kernohan's notch, causes ipsilateral hemiparesis, which falsely localizes the symptoms to the other side. Clinical: coma, ipsilateral IIIrd nerve palsy, ipsilateral hemiparesis.
Tonsillar herniation	Compression of the medulla (apnoea and death), compressed PICA (lateral medullary syndrome).

Cerebral oedema

Types	Notes	
Vasogenic 'vascular permeability of blood–brain barrier , e.g. tumour (steroids potentially useful)	Increased permeability of brain capillary endothelial cells, tumour, abscess, around a haemorrhage, contusion, meningitis. The neurons and glia are relatively normal in appearance.	This form of oedema may respond to therapies intended to reduce it, e.g. steroids. On CT the grey–white matter differentiation is maintained and the oedema involves white matter, extending in finger-like fashion.
Cytotoxic 'cell death', e.g. ischaemic stroke	Failure of the normal homeostatic mechanisms that maintain cell size: neurons, glia, and endothelial cells swell. Due to cellular energy (ATP) failure	Hypoxic ischaemic/infarction, osmolar injury, some toxins; part of the secondary injury sequence following head trauma. Does not respond to steroids. BBB remains intact.
Interstitial or transependymal	Characterised by an increase in the water content of the periventricular white matter.	Due to obstruction of CSF flow, e.g. hydrocephalus.

03 Ventilation of acutely ill patients

3.1 Basis of respiratory support

- Normal ventilation is driven by external intercostals and diaphragm creating a negative airways pressure. Active process vulnerable to fatigue and neuromuscular weakness. 21% oxygen at atmospheric pressure (760 mmHg or 101.3 kPa) reaches the alveoli.
- In a perfect system arterial PO_2 = alveolar PO_2 but due to AV shunting in lungs and cardiac venous drainage into pulmonary veins there is a normal 2.5 kPa (20 mmHg) difference. In some pathological states this is increased. Moist atmospheric air at 37°C has a PO_2 of 20 kPa (150 mmHg) and there is an increased A–a gradient. This is seen with impaired diffusion across the alveolar capillary membrane or V/Q shunting. Hypoventilation and Type 2 RF has a normal A–a gradient.
- PCO_2 is a useful guide of alveolar ventilation and rises with any hypoventilatory state. The alveolar–arterial difference in PCO_2 is only 1 mmHg.
- Blood transports oxygen bound to haemoglobin. O_2 carriage is not directly proportional to partial pressure of O_2. The relationship is sigmoidal (see figure below) due to cooperative sequential binding of four oxygen molecules with haemoglobin. This enables it to load well when O_2 is plentiful and unload well when O_2 is scarce, giving it some advantage over the relationship being completely linear.
- The flat upper portion is alveoli and shows that the Hb is over 90% saturated even with reduced PO_2 down to 60 mmHg (8 kPa). Giving additional O_2 above 100 mmHg (13 kPa) adds little to oxygen carrying capacity. Where the graph is steepest this reflects the tissues with a PO_2 of 40 mmHg (5 kPa) and shows that increased metabolic demand is met with offloading of oxygen within a very small range of PO_2. It also shows that in giving appropriate oxygen even small increases can improves blood oxygen carriage markedly.
- Metabolic by-products, e.g. DPG, acidosis and raised PCO_2 or temperature move the curve towards the right, which makes Hb release oxygen more readily.
- This only works if there is accurate real-time monitoring of oxygen sats using pulse oximetry +/– ABG. Hypercarbia can only be detected by ABG.

A–a (O_2) = (FiO_2%/100) * (P_{atm} – 47 mmHg (6.2 kPa) – ($PaCO_2$/0.8) – PaO_2)

Hypoxia +	**Causes**
Normal A–a Gradient	1. Hypoventilation (decreased respiratory drive or neuromuscular disease) 2. Low FiO_2 especially <21% oxygen, e.g. at altitude
Increased A–a Gradient	1. Diffusion defect 2. V/Q mismatch 3. Shunting

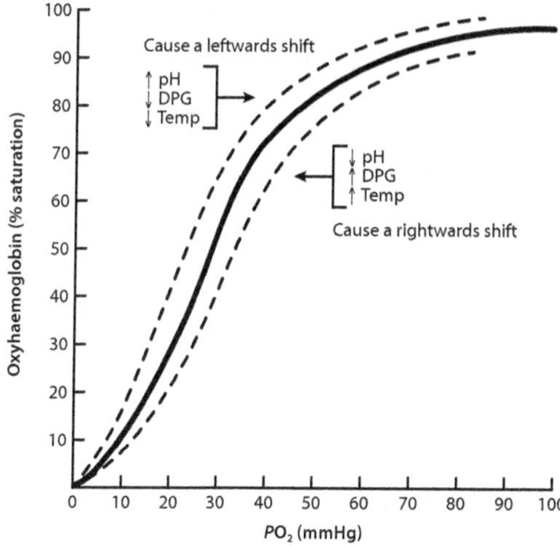

Oxygen dissociation curve.

Reproduced from http://openi.nlm.nih.gov under a Creative Commons License.

3.2 Oxygen therapy

All acute physicians should be familiar with the BTS guidance on oxygen therapy which depends upon prescribing a target SpO_2 of 94–98% and of 88–92% in those with severe COPD.

- The naïve may simply prescribe 100% O_2 in all acutely ill patients. However, excessive O_2 may lead to formation of oxygen free radicals and cause absorption atelectasis and V/Q mismatch. It may also hide significant deteriorations. Prescribe enough oxygen to achieve an O_2 saturation of 94–98% except in those patients with severe COPD where a target of 88–92% would be more appropriate and the ward staff should adjust FiO_2 to get to that level.
- **Simply giving all acutely ill patients a high FiO_2 over what is needed can hide significant deteriorations.** A patient with pneumonia may be saturating at 98% on 2 L O_2 via nasal route but begins to desaturate to 90%, but her saturation improves to 98% when increased to FiO_2 of 0.4. This suggests a clinical worsening, which would have been hidden if she was on a non-rebreather at 15 L/min from the outset. In this situation a CXR showed a small PTX that would have been missed.
- **Prescribe the desired saturation and not the delivery rate or flow or mask** which should be left to ward level policy. Desaturations and increases in FiO_2 to respond to falling desaturations should be escalated to medical staff and acted upon as needed.
- Where **COPD-related CO_2 retention** is likely it is recommended that treatment should be commenced using a 28% Venturi mask at 4 L/min in prehospital care or a 24% Venturi mask at 2–4 L/min in hospital settings, with an initial target saturation of 88–92% pending urgent blood gas results. This is seen mostly in those with severe COPD, morbid obesity, chest wall deformities or neuromuscular disorders.

Blood gas monitoring needed because oxygen saturations give no guide to CO_2 retention.

- **Precautions: monitor with O_2 saturation probe** – therapy may in some cases depress ventilation in those with chronic hypercapnia (CO_2 retainers) where the main drive to breathe is hypoxia. Often the true reasons are mixed and involve shunting and hypoventilation.
- **If in peri arrest and unable to maintain saturations**: bag–valve mask ventilation with 100% O_2 and urgently fast bleep anaesthetists or arrest team and consider intubation and ventilation. Consider humidified oxygen for patients who require high-flow oxygen for more than 24 h or in those who report upper airway discomfort due to dryness.
- **Hyperbaric oxygen therapy**: occasionally 100% O_2 is required at greater than atmospheric pressure. There are still concerns that increased oxygen can lead to oxygen toxicity and this must be borne in mind. Indications for hyperbaric oxygen: CO poisoning, decompression sickness, air embolism, cyanide poisoning, gas gangrene, to improve wound healing (decubitus ulcers), refractory osteomyelitis, thermal burns, improves skin grafting success.

Step	Using a Venturi mask	Using nasal specs
1	24% (2–4 L/min)	1 L/min
2	28% (4–6 L/min)	2 L/min
3	35% (8–10 L/min)	4 L/min
4	40% (10–12 L/min)	Simple face mask 5–6 L/min
5	60% (12–14 L/min)	Simple face mask 7–10 L/min
6	Reservoir mask at 15 L/min O_2	

Oxygen delivery devices

Method	Notes
Room air: FiO_2 21%:	Room air is 21% oxygen and 78% nitrogen. Small increases in inspired O_2 can produce larger improvements in tissue oxygenation.
Nasal cannula: FiO_2 24–44% at 1–6 L/min	A nasal cannula (NC) is a thin tube with two small nozzles to go into the patient's nostrils. Provides O_2 at low flow rates, e.g. 1–6 L/min, and provides FiO_2 24–44%. Well tolerated – some find this preferable to a facemask. No dead space. High flow rates (>6 L/min) cause nasal mucosal drying and nose bleeds.
Simple facemask: FiO_2 40–60% at 5–8 L/min	Fits over a patient's nose and mouth. Delivers O_2 as the patient breathes via nose or mouth. Open side ports allow room air to enter and dilute the O_2 and allow exhaled CO_2 to leave. Connected to oxygen source by a narrow plastic tube. Mask held in place by an adjustable elastic band. Can deliver moderate to high concentrations of O_2 from FiO_2 40% to 60% at 5–8 L/min.

Method	Notes
Non-rebreather with reservoir bag: FiO_2 up to 85–90% at 15 L/min	Similar to face mask but has 3 one-way valves with the 2 side ports. This prevents room air from entering the mask but allows exhaled air to leave the mask. It has a reservoir bag like a partial rebreather mask. Reservoir bag has a one-way valve preventing exhaled air from entering the reservoir. Allows larger concentrations of O_2 to collect in the reservoir bag for the patient to inhale. High flow delivery systems giving high FiO_2. Flow rate of 15 L/min supplies up to 90% FiO_2, but requires tight fitting mask. Use when very high FiO_2 required and in critically ill patients.
Venturi mask [max = 50% FiO_2]	Variable fixed amounts. High flow delivery system with flow rate between 4 and 12 L/min, FiO_2 can be set specifically with different flow rate and air ports. FiO_2 can be 24%, 28%, 31%, 35%, 40% and 50%. External ports must remain open to entrain room air. Can be used in COPD CO_2 retainers who require a fixed O_2 level. Start at 28% mask and adjusting depending on ABG.
Bag–valve mask with intubation or nasopharyngeal or oropharyngeal airways	Used for basic emergency ventilation until expected recovery or intubation attempted. Bag–valve mask ventilation requires a good seal and a patent airway with usual airway opening techniques. It is used with high flow O_2 to an O_2 reservoir and the operator. The O_2 flow rate equals the minute volume of the patient so 100% O_2 is delivered. The bag–valve mask can deliver O_2 to a spontaneously breathing patient. Can also be used to manually ventilate a patient via a mask or tube, or with an oral or nasopharyngeal airway.

3.3 Advanced airways management

Method	Notes
Endotracheal intubation	A bridging measure to allow treatment/recovery. Not indicated in those with little expectation of recovery. Inappropriate in terminal disease or other end-state cardiac or respiratory disease. Planned elective intubation is much safer than emergency intubation. Ensure adequate preparation. Ensure pre-oxygenated with 100% O_2 before commencing. Intubation must only be by appropriately trained personnel.
Tracheostomy	Preferred in those needing on-going airways protection. Better tolerated and more comfortable than endotracheal tube. Less sedation is required. Less dead space to ventilate and airways resistance is reduced. It avoids many of the upper airways complications of an ET tube. Those with tracheostomies are sometimes managed in step-down units outside an HTU/ITU facility. Ensure nursing and medical staff are trained in their use.
Oropharyngeal airway	The Guedel is J shaped and is passed between teeth into oropharynx. Usually rotated from pointing up to pointing down during insertion over tongue. Often used when bag–valve mask ventilation being used. In a semi-comatose patient a nasopharyngeal airway is better tolerated.

Method	Notes
Nasopharyngeal airway	Used in semi-comatose patient who is making satisfactory attempts at breathing. Can place patient in the recovery position with O_2 and a nasopharyngeal airway and monitor closely. The main contraindication is basal skull fracture (major trauma, CSF, coma, should be seen on CT). General advice to choose the size of nasopharyngeal airway to match the width of the patient's little finger or nares. Average height females require a size 6 Portex and males a size 7. Lubricate the end with KY jelly. They go straight back into the nasal cavity and turn downward towards the posterior pharynx. Insert into largest nares. Usual practice is to attach a safety pin at the nose end to prevent further tube movement into airway.

Non-invasive ventilation (NIV/NIPPV)

Method	Notes
Positive pressure	Normal physiology involves using intercostal muscles and diaphragm to create a negative airways pressure relative to atmospheric pressure, sucking air in to reach the alveoli. Pushing air in which is the most practical way to oxygenate lungs therapeutically alters normal physiology. This can be done invasively by full endotracheal intubation and ventilation, or non-invasively using face masks or hoods and a ventilator device that provides positive pressure. Positive airway pressure can then be given continuously (CPAP) throughout the respiratory cycle or varied with the cycle (e.g. BiPAP). The main reasons to use NIV instead of invasive ventilation in acute care are to avoid complications of intubation and invasive ventilation, to improve outcomes (e.g. reduce mortality rates, decrease hospital length of stay), and to decrease the cost of care. It is mainly used in those with type II RF. The machine can automatically detect episodes of inspiration and expiration. NIV is usually used to improve oxygenation and increase minute volume, thus reducing $PaCO_2$
Continuous positive airways pressure (CPAP)	CPAP is the application of continuous positive pressure whilst the patient continues to initiate and generate breaths. Prevents collapse of airways, recruiting more alveoli for gas exchange. The positive pressures are maintained even on expiration. Work of breathing is reduced. Can be accompanied by high FiO_2. Pressures used are 5–20 cmH_2O. Adjust FiO_2. Main use is cardiogenic pulmonary oedema at typical pressures of 2.5–12.5 cmH_2O. Primarily helps hypoxaemia rather than CO_2 retention and can help avoid intubation. Patient wears a tight-fitting mask which is essential to maintain the positive pressure. Outside of the acute setting it is useful for those with obstructive sleep apnoea in keeping the airways open.
Bi-level positive airways pressure (BiPAP)	BiPAP usually refers to the application of positive pressure ventilation similar to CPAP except that pressures are changed for inspiration and expiration. Needs a tight fitting face mask and a ventilator that is capable of delivering two levels of pressure: inspiratory (high pressure, e.g. 8 cmH_2O) and expiratory (lower pressure, e.g. 4 cmH_2O).

Advantages

- NIV reduces intubation and mortality in those with decompensated respiratory acidosis. It is non-invasive (lower risk of infection) and requires a shorter hospital stay (it can be used at home depending on indication). Mortality rates are lower.

- NIV and COPD related Type 2 RF: non-invasive ventilation (NIV) in the ICU and the ward environment, has been shown in randomised controlled trials (RCTs) and systematic reviews to reduce intubation rate and mortality in COPD patients with decompensated respiratory acidosis (pH <7.35 and $PaCO_2$ >6 kPa) following immediate medical therapy.
- NIV should therefore be considered within the first 60 minutes of hospital arrival in all patients with an acute exacerbation of COPD in whom a respiratory acidosis persists despite maximum standard medical treatment.

Application

- NIV can be used in both type I and II RF. Indications include exacerbations of COPD and cardiogenic pulmonary oedema. An effective seal is necessary and the patient needs to be able to tolerate the mask as well as the feeling of breathing out against resistance. Intolerable for some.
- Positive pressure aids the inspiratory phase of breathing, which is active. Reduces respiratory muscle work, maintains alveoli patency during expiration which improves the ventilatory process. Increased alveolar recruitment and so air comes into more contact with pulmonary blood flow, which reduces V/Q mismatches and blood traversing the lung alveoli which is never in contact with oxygenated air as alveoli are closed off (shunting – which obviously does not respond to increased FiO_2 since it never gets there).
- NIV is described as trying to breathe with your head out of the window of a speeding car. The flow rate of O_2 is prescribed and administered via the port on the mask or, if available, into the disposable filter attached to the generator. Start at oxygen 2–4 L/min depending on the FiO_2 needed. Humidified O_2 is usually given. NIV may be trialled in some conditions, e.g. asthma and pneumonia, but only if the patient is in ITU and can be intubated immediately. **It is not for hypoxic asthmatics or those with reversible pathology who are tiring and decompensating. They need immediate access to invasive ventilation.**
- NIV is not indicated in: impaired consciousness, severe hypoxaemia or patients with copious respiratory secretions

Indications for using NIV	Contraindications to NIV
• COPD with a respiratory acidosis pH 7.25–7.35 (H^+ 45–56 nmol/L) • Hypercapnic respiratory failure secondary to chest wall deformity (scoliosis, thoracoplasty) or neuromuscular diseases • Cardiogenic pulmonary oedema unresponsive to CPAP • Weaning from tracheal intubation	• Exacerbations of COPD with a pH <7.25 (assess for ITU, intubation and ventilation) • Cardiac or respiratory arrest, haemodynamic instability, moribund, untreated PTX • Delirium, agitation, GCS <10 • Vomiting, upper GI bleeding, bowel obstruction • Facial trauma, upper airway obstruction • Unable to clear sputum, high risk of aspiration

NIV protocol and settings

- See machine's instruction manual. In Spontaneous/Time (S/T) mode, the ventilator delivers pressure support breaths with PEEP. Patient's spontaneous inspiratory effort triggers the ventilator to deliver inspiratory positive airway pressure (IPAP)

- It cycles to expiratory positive airway pressure (EPAP) during expiration. If the patient's breathing rate is lower than a prescribed rate, the ventilator triggers a pressure-controlled breath according to the IPAP prescribed. The breath is ventilator-triggered, pressure-limited and time-cycled. The actual level of pressure support is equal to the difference between IPAP and EPAP.
- The monitor of the ventilator can display expired tidal volume, minute ventilation, peak inspiratory pressure, inspiratory time/total cycle time, and patient peak flow and % patient triggered breaths.

Suggested protocol for NIV

- Sit patient up in a position of comfort, explain NIV and what to expect.
- Chose smallest mask providing a proper fit and place over the patient's face.
- Start with IPAP of +10 cmH_2O and EPAP of +5 cmH_2O.
- Gradually increase IPAP as tolerated by patient up to 40 cmH_2O.
- Observe respiratory rate and tidal volume (target 5–7 ml/kg).
- Set back-up breath rate of 10–15 breaths per minute.
- Monitor for any distress, coma, vomiting, and secretions ++.
- Adjust FiO_2 to maintain SpO_2 >90%. Repeat ABG at 2 h.
- EPAP may be increased in acute pulmonary oedema.
- Apply strapping to the mask once patient used to NIPPV.
- Straps: tight enough to prevent leaks, but allow entry of 1 or 2 fingers.
- Dressing on nasal bridge can help avoid pressure sores.

Parameters you need to prescribe

- Broadly, IPAP helps lower PCO_2 and EPAP improves PO_2.
- IPAP ranges from 4 to 40 cmH_2O (usual max 25) with increments of 2 cm.
- EPAP ranges from 4 to 20 cmH_2O (usual max 15) with increment of 2 cm.
- Rate ranges from 4 to 40 breaths per minute.
- Timed inspiration ranges from 0.5 to 3 s with increment of 0.1 s.
- IPAP rise time: 0.05, 0.1, 0.2, 0.4 s, and FiO_2 ranges from 21 to 100%.
- Back-up respiratory rate: 12–16 breaths/minute.
- The FiO_2 can be adjusted according to the ABG and SpO_2.

For cardiogenic pulmonary oedema without hypercapnia: CPAP 8–15 cmH_2O via face mask, normal I:E ratio is 1:2 (inspiration:expiration).

Measure success: reduction in $PaCO_2$ or improved pH by + 0.06 and/or correction of respiratory acidosis associated with a clinical improvement.

- **Failure**: signs of failing NIV and need for escalation include: worsening acidosis or hypercapnia and/or falling GCS, especially if < 9. Determine ceiling of therapy so that escalation if appropriate is rapid.
- **Difficulties**: include copious respiratory secretion with difficulty in clearance may be the issue. Intubation and mechanical ventilation may be necessary depending on the ceiling of therapy which should have been ascertained.

Invasive ventilation

- Involves similar concepts to NIV but requires intubation and ventilation and oxygenation by placing of an endotracheal tube, laryngeal mask or tracheostomy. It can require a mixture of sedation and neuromuscular blockade. The settings usually allow timing to the patient's inspiratory effort. Air is pushed in and increases intra-alveolar pressure or lung tidal volume until a point where the lungs are allowed to deflate passively. Pressures generated can cause a PTX or reduce venous return or cause lung injury. Ventilators can be set basically using either volumes (tidal volume is preset and fixed and pressures vary) or pressure settings. Benefits should be improved gas exchange and a decreased work of breathing.

- **Complications of mechanical ventilation:** lung injury, difficulties in intubation, laryngeal injury, PTX, tension pneumothorax, pneumo-mediastinum, airway injury, alveolar damage, ventilator-associated pneumonia, weakness and atrophy of the diaphragm, reduced cardiac output, oxygen toxicity, acute lung injury (ALI) and acute respiratory distress syndrome (ARDS).
- **Monitoring the effectiveness of mechanical ventilation:** use pulse oximetry, ABG, effort of breathing, tidal volume, respiratory rate, HR and BP, mortality, CXR findings.

Indications for endotracheal intubation and ventilation

- Protection of the airway and/or need to remove secretions.
- GCS <9, airway obstruction, severe respiratory fatigue or drowsiness.
- Apnoea with cardiac/respiratory arrest.
- Hypoxaemia (PO_2 <8 kPa) despite high FiO_2 +/– NIV.
- SaO_2 <90% despite CPAP with FiO_2 >0.6.
- Control CO_2 (hyperventilate to lower PCO_2 for raised ICP).
- Control O_2/CO_2 (type II RF with acidosis).
- Respiratory rate >35/min or <10/min.
- FVC <15 ml/kg or 1 L or <30% predicted.
- Tidal volume <5 ml/kg or inadequate inspiratory force <25 cmH_2O.
- Surgery to head and neck or involving muscular paralysis.

References:

British Thoracic Society Standards of Care Committee (2002) Non-invasive ventilation in acute respiratory failure. *Thorax*, 2002; 57:192.

O'Driscoll *et al.* (2008) BTS guideline for emergency oxygen use in adult patients. *Thorax*, 63 (Suppl 6):1.

Royal College of Physicians (2008) Non-invasive ventilation in chronic obstructive pulmonary disease: management of acute type 2 respiratory failure. London: RCP.

Capnography

Capnography is the measurement of exhaled CO_2. The return of spontaneous circulation is sometimes difficult to assess with other methods, but it is clearly demonstrated on capnography measurements by an abrupt increase in the $PEtCO_2$ (end-tidal PCO_2) value. If $PEtCO_2$ abruptly increases to a normal value (35–40 mmHg), it is reasonable to consider that this is an indicator of ROSC. Continuous end-tidal CO_2 monitoring can confirm a tracheal intubation. A good wave form indicating the presence of CO_2 ensures the ET tube is in the trachea.

04 Shock

Introduction and definition

- Shock is a clinical syndrome where there is generalized tissue hypoxia due to reduced oxygen delivery or increased O_2 extraction. It may be worsened by anaemia, reduced cardiac output, pyrexia, hypoxaemia.

Clinical syndrome

- Pale, sweating, cold, clammy, confused, obtunded, tachycardic, SBP <90 mmHg.
- Tachypnoeic, oliguric, raised JVP may suggest cardiogenic or PE or tamponade.
- Warm peripheries, bounding pulse, hypo- or hyperthermia, sepsis, rash, erythema.

Clinical severity assessment score	
Class 1	10–15% blood volume loss. Physiological compensation and no clinical changes appear.
Class 2	15–30% blood volume loss. Partial compensation. Postural hypotension, generalized vasoconstriction, urine output 20–30 ml/h. Identify and treat to prevent progression.
Class 3	30–40% blood volume loss. Decompensating shock with hypotension. HR >120, tachypnoea, oliguria <20 ml/h, confused.
Class 4	40% blood volume loss. Marked hypotension, tachycardia and tachypnoea. Anuric, comatose. Irreversible shock heading to multi-organ failure. Rapid intervention for any recovery.

Pathophysiology

- O_2 extraction increases, but anaerobic lactic acidosis can occur.
- Sepsis causes release of bacteria and other molecules with vasodilatation.
- Increased cardiac output, capillary permeability and hypovolaemia.
- Reduced oxidative phosphorylation, ATP and cell pump dysfunction.
- Progressive downward spiral of multi-organ failure and death.

Findings

- **Mean arterial pressure:** <60 mmHg and systolic BP <90 mmHg.
- **Lactate: >4 mmol/L** (value correlates with mortality).
- **Cardiac output:** <2.2 L/min/m^2 (except sepsis).
- **Urinary catheter**: oliguric unless polyuric state, e.g. HHS/ DKA.

Investigations

- **FBC:** Hb normal or low if bleeding, raised if fluid loss alone. Raised WCC.
- **U&E**: raised urea/creatinine, e.g. AKI, dehydration, consider prerenal, renal, postrenal.
- **Others:** raised troponin, dimer (DIC/PE), lactate (can guide severity).
- **Echocardiogram:** assess LV, valves, exclude pericardial fluid/blood collection or vegetations.
- **CXR** for suspected chest disease – heart, lungs, mediastinum, perforation.
- **CTPA or V/Q scan**: PE and CT may show lung and aortic pathology.
- **Sepsis screen:** blood cultures, urinalysis, sputum, USS for fluid collection/liver abscess.

- **12-lead ECG**: arrhythmias, ischaemia, infarction, electrolyte changes, cardiomyopathy.
- **Arterial blood gases**: metabolic or respiratory acidosis, or both.
- **AXR:** if bowel obstruction or perforation suspected.
- **CT abdomen:** if suspected AAA, pancreatitis or suspected retroperitoneal bleeding or fluid collection or bowel obstruction or ischaemia.
- **Abdominal–pelvic USS:** renal obstruction, cholecystitis, jaundice, liver abscess or pelvic collection.
- **Coagulation screen**: DIC: low fibrinogen, platelets and raised APTT and PT.
- **Invasive monitoring** such as CVP and pulmonary artery (capillary) wedge pressure (PAWP) can be useful when the type of shock is not clear, e.g. PE where PAWP is normal and CVP raised, LVF where PAWP raised and CVP normal or elevated and cardiac tamponade where PCWP and CVP raised.
- **Urgent endoscopy:** for diagnosis and therapy of suspected upper GI bleed.

Types	Causes	Clinical	Key considerations
Cardiogenic (bedside echo is very useful)	'Pump failure', ACS, myocarditis, CMP, drug toxicity (Ca-blocker overdose), VT, CHB, tachy/bradyarrhythmia, valve failure: acute MR, AR, MS, AS	Obtunded, cold peripheries oliguria, postural hypotension, dizziness, presyncope, drowsiness, confusion, tachycardia, rapid breathing (acidotic). CRT (press over nailbed for 5 s) abnormal if >2 s for pink colour to return	Cautious fluid challenge CXR to confirm pulmonary oedema ECG – STEMI needs urgent PCI/thrombolysis Consider inotropes Consider IABP Can BP tolerate nitrates/ loop diuretics? Can I get an echo?
Obstructive	Pulmonary embolism, cardiac tamponade, tension PTX	As above + raised JVP. Muffled heart sounds with tamponade, hyper-resonant hemithorax and deviated trachea with tension PTX. Obvious DVT with PE	Needle 2nd ICS for tension PTX Thrombolysis for PE Pericardiocentesis for CT
Hypovolaemic: non-haemorrhagic	Fluid loss, e.g. cholera, DKA, HHS, pancreatitis	Fluid loss – severe urine or GI fluid loss (diarrhoea, vomiting), polyuria	Treat DKA/HHS Hypercalcaemia Treat diabetes insipidus Oral/IV rehydration therapy for cholera or GI loss

Types	Causes	Clinical	Key considerations
Hypovolaemic: haemorrhagic	Haemorrhage – think AAA, GI bleed, retroperitoneal, obvious traumatic lesion	As above + sign of bleeding (internal/external), e.g. pulsatile bleeding, AAA, melena, Grey Turner, Cullen signs, thigh haematoma, psoas haematoma, ectopic pregnancy	Transfuse blood. O negative if critical. Reverse coagulopathy – Beriplex/Octaplex for warfarin Fluid resus with NS. Leaking AAA: vascular urgent surgical consult for repair Upper GI bleed: endoscopic therapy or laparotomy Beta-hCG if ectopic suspected and laparotomy
Distributive	Septicaemic shock, anaphylaxis, neurogenic, Addisonian crisis	Warm vasodilated peripheries, hypotension, oliguria, tachycardia, confusion, rapid breathing (acidotic). DBP drops more quickly than SBP. Anaphylaxis (drug, transfusion, sting, nut allergy): flushed, wheeze, urticaria Sepsis: meningococcal sepsis with purpura, retained tampon	IV fluids: NS Sepsis: IV antibiotics + NS Adrenal: IV hydrocortisone + NS Anaphylaxis: IM adrenaline + IV fluids + nebs.

Immediate actions

- Get good IV access, e.g. x2 antecubital fossa green/brown/grey venflons, good access to monitoring, e.g. intra-arterial lines on HDU, O_2 to give sats 94–98%. Get ECG, CXR, send FBC/U&E/LFT/lactate and cultures and consider troponin and dimer. Cross match if haemorrhage.
- Get help if patient expiring before you even summon arrest team. If no bleeding, inpatient, no MI on ECG then think PE or sepsis. But keep reviewing. You may rationally treat multiple aetiologies, e.g. sepsis and PE until the diagnosis is confirmed.

Choosing an inotrope (also see Drug formulary)

- Patients presenting with cardiogenic and distributive and septic shock are managed with vasoactive drugs and inotropes. Inotropes are usually sympathomimetic agents that can affect heart rate (chronotropic), and heart contractile function (inotropic). They may also affect vascular resistance and flow to various vascular beds (vasopressor). Vasoactive agents and inotropes can improve physiological measurements, but there is no evidence that they improve outcome.

- Vasopressors only affect vascular tone alone and can change the systemic and pulmonary vascular resistance. This can alter flow to skin, muscles and other organ groups. In shock the emphasis is to maintain cerebral, coronary and renal perfusion, often at the cost of flow to skin and other less vital areas. Effects depend on the production of intracellular secondary messengers. Adrenergic receptors act through G proteins. It is suggested that multiple agents at low dose preferable in cardiac disease. Vasopressin in low or moderate doses can spare catecholamines and inotropes are not generally indicated in end-stage heart failure.
- Other physical methods to help flow include **intra-aortic balloon pump**. These may be used in cardiogenic shock. Anti-shock suits are sometimes used pre-hospital in hypovolaemia. Usage of these IV inotropic and chronotropic agents is usually restricted to the ITU, CCU or HDU because these drugs need close and careful monitoring and adjusting, usually on the basis of invasive monitoring.

Indication	Recommended inotropes
Initiate diuresis	**DOPAMINE** at 1–2 mcg/kg/min dilates renal, mesenteric and cerebral vessels and may improve renal perfusion.
Cardiogenic shock	**NORADRENALINE**: BP <70 mmHg especially if low peripheral vascular resistance. Vasoconstrictor, increasing PVR and also cardiac output (*Circulation*, 2008;118:1047).
Cardiogenic shock (mean BP <70–100 mmHg)	**DOBUTAMINE** at 2–20 mcg/kg/min is a positive inotrope but does not vasoconstrict and is also considered first line. **DOPAMINE** (inotropic) at 2–10 mcg/kg/min increases HR and is a positive inotrope but may increase O_2 demand. **DOPAMINE** (vasopressor) produces some vasoconstriction especially at higher doses, such as 10–20 mcg/kg/min.
Septicaemic shock	**NORADRENALINE** (0.2–1.0 mcg/kg/min) **or DOPAMINE** to maintain MAP≥65 mm Hg. Dobutamine inotropic therapy when cardiac output remains low despite fluid resuscitation and combined inotropic/vasopressor therapy (*Crit Care Med*, 2008;36:296).

4.1 Haemorrhagic shock

Acute traumatic blood loss: aim for an SBP of 80 mmHg or palpable radial pulse or cerebration. Use small boluses of 250 ml of fluid crystalloid and tranexamic acid.

Introduction

- Trauma is the commonest cause of young deaths worldwide after HIV/AIDs. Death is usually due to brain injury or exsanguination. The current strategy is that of damage control resuscitation (DCR) with concepts such as permissive hypovolaemia. Reduced administration of crystalloid has seen a reduction in mortality.
- Crystalloids and colloids increase BP, dilute clotting factors, destabilize formed clots and lead to further bleeding. They have no significant O_2 carrying capacity. In reducing initial fluid challenge there is a balance in allowing on-going tissue hypoperfusion but maintaining haemostasis and clot control.

- **Major haemorrhage is defined as loss requiring a >2–4 unit transfusion.** Young patients can often cope with loss with physiological reserve and can look better than expected. They can then suddenly decompensate. These patients must be identified early so that appropriate fluid strategies are applied.
- BP is usually the physiological parameter that defines shock, but cardiac output is also important and determines tissue O_2 delivery. A normal BP may simply be a product of raised peripheral resistance with a low CO (remember BP = CO × PR). A bleeding patient with signs of shock already has a significant blood loss. **Cryptic shock** is found in those with normal BP and pulse despite significant blood loss. Blood pressure is also directly related to blood loss.
- Where there is brain injury a higher SBP >90 mmHg is advocated. Avoid a coagulopathy and ensure haemostasis maintained using a ratio of 1 FFP to 1–2 units packed cells from the start. Platelets also given. Consider giving fibrinogen. There is no resolution to the crystalloid vs. colloid debate and either is acceptable with the above provisos.
- **Tranexamic acid**, which reduces clot breakdown, may be given and has been shown to reduce mortality if commenced within 3 h of injury.

Reference: Harris T, *et al*. (2012) Early fluid resuscitation in severe trauma. *BMJ*, 345:e5752.

Look for a cause of bleeding

- **Trauma:** needs trauma management and direct compression and control of bleeding points. Further explanation beyond the scope of this text.
- **Ruptured spleen:** usually with abdominal trauma. Increased risk with splenomegaly or glandular fever. Requires urgent laparotomy. Urgent USS or CT abdomen.
- **Abdominal aortic aneurysm**: pulsatile expansile mass + abdominal or back pain. Needs urgent vascular referral and laparotomy. If clinical suspicion high then surgery may proceed on clinical suspicion alone. Otherwise urgent USS or CT abdomen.
- **Upper gastrointestinal bleed**: see separate topic (*Section 14.3*). Is it variceal or non-variceal bleeding? If patient is moribund then it becomes a surgical issue and laparotomy is needed to arrest bleeding.
- **Ectopic pregnancy**: fertile female, abdominal pain, missed period, positive beta-hCG. Needs urgent surgery and urgent USS abdomen.
- **Retroperitoneal bleeding**: palpable mass in abdomen, pelvis, bruising round umbilicus or flanks. Can be seen especially if anticoagulated. Urgent USS or CT abdomen. Reverse anticoagulation.

In a bleeding patient check FBC and clotting profile and treat any coagulopathy/give platelets if platelet function or numbers are impaired. The immediate risks of bleeding in a shocked patient override thrombotic risks even in those with prosthetic metal heart valves or previous PE. Take haematological advice if needed.

Massive transfusion protocol

- Massive haemorrhage and resuscitation can result in a refractory coagulopathy. Trauma patients do better if given blood components and transfused early. Give red cells, FFP, cryoprecipitate and platelets as Trauma or Shock Packs in those with massive bleeding, such as those with surgical or medical life-threatening haemorrhage needing over 10–20 units of RBCs in 24 h.

- Surgical control of haemorrhage with volume resuscitation using fluids and blood components is needed. Once bleeding controlled, a restrictive approach to blood product transfusion is preferred because of the risks and negative outcomes of transfusion such as multiple organ failure, systemic inflammatory response syndrome, TRALI, increased infection, and increased mortality.
- Increased ratios of plasma and platelets to RBCs and their timely administration are thought to improve outcome in trauma, decrease coagulopathy and transfusion requirements based on retrospective data.
- Large volumes of plasma are required to correct coagulopathy, so early administration is best and may limit consumptive coagulopathy and thrombocytopenia, and the need for blood and blood products. Limiting the use of isotonic crystalloid will avoid a dilutional coagulopathy. Limiting the use of NS may prevent further acidosis.
- Evidence is growing for use of point of care coagulation testing to guide haemostatic therapy. Standard coagulation tests such as PT, APTT, INR, platelet count, and fibrinogen usually require 30–60 min for results to be available. For massive transfusion patients requiring acute interventions, results of standard coagulation tests may not be an accurate reflection of coagulation function. Measurement of platelet count and fibrinogen only provides absolute amounts, not functional activity and may overestimate the levels.

Resuscitation targets

- Hypotensive resuscitation (SBP 80–100 mmHg) until haemorrhage is controlled is generally recommended, unless there is concern for traumatic brain injury when higher BP acceptable.
- Monitor base deficit and lactate levels to assess adequacy of resuscitation.
- Correct electrolyte abnormalities, e.g. hyperkalaemia from large volume of banked RBCs, hypocalcaemia from citrated anticoagulants, and Na and Cl abnormalities from crystalloid resuscitation.
- Aim for Hb 7–9 g/dL, PT and APTT within normal range (APTT/INR >1.5 give 4 FFP). Aim for platelet count $>80\times10^9$/L (<30 give 2 units platelets, <80 give 1 unit platelets). Aim for fibrinogen level >1 g/L (<1 g/L then 2 cryoprecipitate).
- Give 5 ml 10% calcium gluconate by slow IV injection if ionised calcium level low.

Additional notes

- Maintain/achieve normothermia. Avoid/correct acidaemia. Avoid/treat hypocalcaemia. In obstetric haemorrhage FFP use may be delayed because patients are hypercoagulable.
- Use forced air warmers and rapid infusion devices where indicated
- Warfarin reversal: give **VITAMIN K** slow IV and **OCTAPLEX/BERIPLEX**.
- Low platelets or dysfunction (clopidogrel/aspirin). Give additional platelets – take haematology advice.
- Heparin has short half-life and protamine causes significant hypotension. Consider protamine with care and reluctance – it may have some effect with LMWH. Give **PROTAMINE IV** slowly.

New oral anticoagulants: Factor Xa inhibitors (e.g. rivaroxaban, apixaban) not easily reversed. Thrombin inhibitors (e.g. dabigatran) not easily reversed. Seek advice from haematologist. May need dialysis.

Bleeding and prosthetic heart valves

- Worst case scenario is a metal mitral ball and cage valve (aortic and newer tilting-disc valves lower risk) which has an annual risk of thromboembolism of 30% if anticoagulation is stopped. Other valves have a much lower incidence, possibly 12% per annum, of thromboembolism.
- The weekly risk of thromboembolism for the worse case is still less than 1%, so in patients with potentially life threatening acute bleeds, anticoagulation must be stopped temporarily/completely reversed as the risk of death by exsanguination will be significantly higher.
- In ischaemic stroke the advice from national guidelines for patients with metal valves is to switch to aspirin for a week and then restart anticoagulation. For those with haemorrhagic stroke the risks need to be finely balanced but again anticoagulation should be reversed completely acutely for at least 1–2 weeks.

Example of a Massive Transfusion PROTOCOL (follow local guidance)

- Establish good IV access × 2. Give blood products through warmer. ABC. High flow O_2, IV NS 1 L initially over 10–20 min unless pulmonary oedema. Send cross-match and bloods.
- Constantly reassess fluid balance and status. Repeat bloods (FBC, PT, APTT, fibrinogen, U&E, calcium) every 30 min.
- **Consider if immediate surgery indicated to stop bleeding.** Try to focus management on assessment and cause as well as replacement. Liaise with laboratory to ensure packs arrive as needed.
- **Contact blood bank** with patient name, gender, DOB or approximate age and hospital number if known, location. Give brief clinical details, on warfarin, NOAC, pregnant or not.
- **Tranexamic acid** 1 g IV over 10 min + infusion 1 g over 8 h.
- Vitamin K + Octaplex or Beriplex if on warfarin
- Blood bank should send: **Shock pack 1**: (4 U uncrossmatched O RhD negative red cells). **Shock pack 2**: (6 U red cells, 4 FFP, 1–2 platelets + 1 cryoprecipitate). Send bloods. **Shock pack 3** (6 U red cells, 2 FFP, 1–2 platelets + 1 cryoprecipitate). Send bloods.
- Discuss with haematology about recombinant Factor VIIa/fibrinogen concentrate.
- **Continue as clinically indicated.** Reassess situation constantly and if MTP ceases at any time then tell switchboard to stand down. Continue with further shock packs until stand down. Identify specific cause of shock and determine any specific remedies.

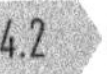

4.2 Hypovolaemic shock

About

- Primary water/salt loss. For blood loss alone see *Section 4.1*.

Causes

- Severe gastroenteritis, HHS, DKA, cholera, burns, overdiuresis.
- Diabetes insipidus: cranial or nephrogenic, hypercalcaemia, heat stroke.
- Surgical drains and stomas losing excessive fluids which are unreplaced.
- Addison's disease, major burns, erythroderma.

Clinical

- Assess state of hydration. Reduced skin turgor, cold, clammy, cold peripheries.
- Tachycardia, postural hypotension, obtunded, reduced capillary return.
- Oliguria, progressive confusion and coma.

Investigations

- **ABG**: hypoxia PO_2 <8 kPa, low HCO_3, **lactate** >4.0 mmol/L.
- **FBC**: Hb initially normal and may fall. **APTT/PT**: look for coagulopathy.
- **U&E**: raised urea (GI bleed or AKI/CKD), raised creatinine (AKI/CKD), raised K^+ if AKI or haemolysis.
- **Others:** calcium, cortisol and SynACTHen test.

Management

- IV access (2 grey venflons antecubital fossa), baseline bloods, urinary catheter, physiological monitoring. Manage cause. Watch for AKI. Consider central venous line and HDU with monitoring.
- Volume replacement: 1 L NS over 30 min, then 1 L over 1 h and replace in response to clinical change. If there is concern over volume overload then consider 200 ml NS fluid challenges and reassessment. Replace electrolytes as needed. Manage Na^+ and K^+ levels. Body weight can help manage fluid status.
- Determine if there is any steroid deficiency, e.g. Addison's disease, and give **IV HYDROCORTISONE 100 mg IV** and then via IM 6 hourly if suspected as longer effect for steroid replacement.
- If there is diabetes insipidus investigate if either cranial or nephrogenic. Consider giving ADH if cranial.

4.3 Acute heart failure/cardiogenic shock

About

- Perilous peri-arrest state needing rapid action and senior help. Mortality is high (70%).
- A bedside echocardiogram confirms the diagnosis and possible aetiology.
- Acute heart failure and cardiogenic shock differ by degrees of cardiac damage.

Aetiology

- Failure of the LV leads to forward failure and failure to perfuse organs. Backward failure due to rise in LA pressure, pulmonary artery pressure, and then venous pressure. Increased pressure moves fluid into the interstitium and alveoli.
- There is perfusion without oxygenation (VQ mismatch) and so hypoxia.
- Mitral stenosis causes pulmonary oedema but LV function is normal.
- Chronic mitral regurgitation better tolerated as left atrium has dilated so lower LVEDP.

Diagnosis

- Severely impaired tissue perfusion and PCWP >18 mmHg.
- Cardiogenic shock when MAP <60 mmHg or SBP <90 mmHg.

Causes

- **Acute coronary syndromes:** usually STEMI and left coronary artery disease. Check 12-lead ECG. If acute escalate for PPCI/thrombolysis. Check troponin.
- **Pre-existing cardiac disease:** with new or fast AF, ischaemia or infarction, fluid overload, new medications (negative inotropes, NSAIDs).

- **Precipitants:** missed medications, e.g. diuretics, co-morbidities, pneumonia, excess alcohol, fluid overload, arrhythmias, ischaemia.
- **Cardiomyopathy or myocarditis:** possible potential recovery with supportive management.
- **Valve failure:** aortic stenosis, mitral stenosis, severe aortic regurgitation, severe mitral regurgitation (papillary muscle infarction or endocarditis; endocarditis can often destroy valves with massive regurgitation).
- **Arrhythmias:** fast AF, VT, CHB reducing cardiac output.
- **Cardiac tamponade:** impaired diastolic filling reduces output. Needs echo and pericardiocentesis.
- **Hypertensive crisis:** rare but consider renal artery stenosis or phaeochromocytoma.
- **Neurogenic**: SAH.

Clinical

- BP usually normal or low <90/60 mmHg. Can be high – hypertensive crisis.
- Severe dyspnoea, cyanosed, agitated, low volume pulse with cold peripheries.
- Pink frothy sputum and haemoptysis, and dyspnoea, oliguria.
- Triple rhythm S3, pulsus alternans, tachycardia, AF.
- Right heart failure: raised JVP, dependent oedema, ascites, hepatomegaly.
- High output cardiac failure – AV fistula, Paget's disease.

NYHA grading of breathlessness related to heart failure

I. No symptoms
II. Symptoms with moderate exercise
III. Symptoms with minimal exercise
IV. Symptoms at rest

Investigations

- **FBC/U&E:** detect anaemia AKI/CKD. Raised LFTs and PT with severe liver congestion.
- **ABG**: type 1 RF, lactate: >2.0 mmol/L.
- **Troponin or CKMB:** raised with NSTEMI/STEMI or myocarditis.
- **ECG**: arrhythmia, low voltage, ST elevation (STEMI consider PCI). New LBBB, true posterior MI.
- **Urgent echocardiogram:** LV or RV dysfunction, assess valve integrity and exclude tamponade or VSD.
- **BNP:** echo is always preferred but in patient where the aetiology of dyspnoea is unclear brain natriuretic peptide (BNP) levels correlates with impairment of left ventricular function.
- **CXR:** pulmonary oedema, cardiomegaly and increased upper lobe venous markings, bat wing oedema, Kerley B lines, bilateral pleural effusion.
- **Swan–Ganz:** invasive monitoring may be attempted if diagnosis or management uncertain.
- **Cardiac catheterisation**: image coronary vessels looking for occluded vessel, culprit lesion, poor LV, severe AR, dilated root. Can perform angioplasty, stenting.

General management

- **Sit patient up. ABC O_2** if needed as per BTS guidance. Opiate: **DIAMORPHINE** 2.5–5 mg or **MORPHINE** 5–10 mg IV + **METOCLOPRAMIDE** 10 mg IV antiemetic can relieve chest pain/dyspnoea.
- **Treat any cause,** e.g. cardiovert patient in sustained VT, or PCI the STEMI, or cardiac surgery for the valve disease.

- **IV diuretics:** large dose **FUROSEMIDE 50–100 mg IV** when SBP >120 mmHg. More modest doses of **IV FUROSEMIDE 20–40 mg** venodilate and cause diuresis without further reducing the BP.
- **Nitrates**: (do not use if hypotension) **give sublingual GTN (150–300 mcg) 2 sprays/pills** and consider **IV GTN** if SBP >100 mmHg. Titrate to pain, breathlessness and BP.
- **Admit to HDU/CCU/ITU** with cardiac monitoring, physiological monitoring, urinary catheter. Venous/arterial line. Give O_2 as per BTS guidelines and reassess after ABG. May be a role for CVP line.
- **Acute coronary syndrome**: see *Section 11.2*. If STEMI then PCI with angioplasty/stenting of culprit vessel recommended or urgent thrombolysis if PCI not possible.
- **SALBUTAMOL 2.5–5.0 mg** nebuliser QDS and PRN if any bronchospasm. Can worsen tachycardia.
- **IV AMINOPHYLLINE** has been used. However, concerns over arrhythmias. Consider only if significant element of bronchospasm.
- **Arrhythmias**: if not already on **DIGOXIN** then load with **DIGOXIN** or consider **IV AMIODARONE** via a large or central cannula which can treat VT with SBP >90 mmHg, otherwise DC shock for any tachyarrhythmia and hypotension.
- **Anticoagulate** with LMWH if patient in AF or LV thrombus.
- **Inotropes:** those in shock – low 'renal' dose **DOPAMINE** is usually first line. **DOBUTAMINE** infusion is also indicated.

Specific additional issues

- **Severe hypertension**: manage with IV nitrates/IV diuretics.
- **Ultrafiltration:** venovenous isolated ultrafiltration can remove fluid in patients, although is usually reserved for those unresponsive or resistant to diuretics or in severe renal failure
- **Cardiac tamponade**: globular heart on CXR. Urgent bedside echo if available. Consider needle pericardiocentesis.
- **Hypovolaemia or RV failure or PE:** a fluid challenge may help with CVP monitoring if possible. Patients often feel better lying flat. Give IV plasma expander (100–200 ml aliquots given over 10–15 min) or NS and reassess.
- **CPAP:** where available it can improve oxygenation. Start at 5 and increase as needed to 10–12 cmH_2O. Check ABG 30 min and 1 h post-CPAP. When changing pressure turn flow up in 2 cmH_2O steps at 2–3 min intervals over the first 10–15 min. CPAP can improve oxygenation but may compromise venous return.
- **Intubation and ventilation**: will reduce work of breathing and O_2 demand so mechanical ventilation should be considered.
- **Intra-aortic balloon pump** (IABP): is a 25–50 ml elongated helium-filled balloon inserted via the femoral artery and placed distal to the left subclavian artery, but proximal to the renal arteries. Balloon inflates with diastole and deflates with systole. Improves cerebral and coronary perfusion in cardiogenic shock and acute LVF, refractory unstable angina and ischaemic ventricular arrhythmias. Most coronary perfusion is in diastole. C/I: significant aortic regurgitation, aortic arch aneurysm. Patients should be anticoagulated with heparin.
- **Ventricular assist devices:** provide bridging cardiac support. Requires cardiopulmonary bypass. Various different types. Bridge to transplant or recovery or revascularisation.
- **VTE prophylaxis:** advocated because high risk of PE.

Avoid drugs which can worsen heart failure, e.g. calcium channel blockers such as verapamil, antiarrhythmics, NSAIDs, COX-2 inhibitors, steroids.

In stabilised heart failure consider:

- **ACE inhibitors,** e.g. RAMIPRIL low dose and titrate gradually up to full dose over several weeks + beta-blockers (once stable), e.g. carvedilol. In those with EF <40%, reduces the risk of hospitalisation and the risk of premature death. If ACE inhibitors not tolerated, usually due to cough, consider angiotensin II receptor blockers, e.g. Candesartan. Monitor U&E for renal dysfunction and hyperkalaemia. Contraindicated in pregnancy and renal artery stenosis.
- **Diuretics:** oral FUROSEMIDE or BUMETANIDE (hypokalaemia), often combined with aldosterone antagonists, should be considered in those who are breathless with minimal exertion and worse. Watch for hyperkalaemia and AKI. METOLAZONE is a particularly potent diuretic which is sometimes used with intractable volume overload.

The emphasis should be on maximising vasodilator therapy (ACE inhibitor/ARB) before diuretic therapy.

- **Angiotensin receptor antagonists:** usually for those who cannot tolerate ACE inhibitor. Consider titrating up the dose of CANDESARTAN. Can cause hyperkalaemia. Monitor U&E.
- **Aldosterone antagonists: Spironolactone**/Eplerenone: in NYHA III/IV failure (symptoms at rest or minimal exercise). Can be added to conventional treatment including an ACE inhibitor/ARB (87%) and a beta-blocker (75%). Spironolactone can cause hyperkalaemia and worsening renal function. Eplerenone is a similar drug with proven benefits post-MI and in heart failure but with less gynaecomastia.
- **Beta-blockers:** e.g. CARVEDILOL, BISOPROLOL or METOPROLOL have shown benefit in clinical trials. Start low dose slowly titrated up. These should not be started until patient stable otherwise they can lead to worsening of condition. Nebivolol is recommended for stable mild–moderate heart failure in patients over 70 years old.
- **Ivabradine:** should be considered to reduce the risk of hospitalization in patients in sinus rhythm with an EF <35%, a heart rate remaining >70/min, and persisting symptoms despite maximal standard treatment.
- **Hydralazine and oral nitrates** for those who do not tolerate ACE inhibitor/ARB.
- **Digoxin:** for those with heart failure and AF. Evidence that it reduces hospitalisations.
- **Non pharmacological:** exercise rehabilitation programmes have been shown to improve functional capacity. Combine with salt restriction and weight loss and smoking cessation.
- **Revascularisation:** consider angiogram and revascularisation by PCI or CABG.
- **Implantable cardioverter–defibrillator** if at high risk for lethal arrhythmias.
- **Warfarin/new oral anticoagulant** if in AF or LV thrombus. Start LMWH and warfarinise. Role in dilated cardiomyopathy is debatable. Consider new oral anticoagulants for non-valvular AF. Heart failure increases risk of stroke with AF.
- **Biventricular pacing** if LVEF <35% and QRS >120 ms NYHA III/IV failure (symptoms at rest or minimal exercise).
- **Surgery:** CABG where appropriate, valve surgery (mitral valve repair or replacement) where appropriate, repair of LV aneurysms, ventricular assist

devices mentioned above, transplantation is considered in end-stage cardiac failure in those suitable.

Reference: European Society of Cardiology (2012) *ESC guidelines for the diagnosis and treatment of acute and chronic heart failure.*

4.4 Anaphylactic/anaphylactoid shock

About

- A severe and potentially life threatening systemic reaction.
- Can occur in an acute and unexpected manner and can recur, so on-going monitoring for 6–12 h needed.

Aetiology

- Antigen exposure causes IgE antibody generation. Later re-exposure produces mast cell degranulation due to antigen cross-linking IgE-releasing histamine. Histamine activates receptors with massive release of cytokines and chemokines. Increases postcapillary venule permeability and fluid loss into interstitium. Oedema and hypotension exacerbated by vascular smooth muscle relaxation.
- Release of vasoactive mediators cause laryngeal/pharyngeal/bronchial oedema or bronchospasm and/or hypotension. Anaphylactoid reactions are identical but not immune generated.

Causative agents

- Drugs (e.g. penicillin), radiological contrast media, insect bites/stings, eggs, fish, peanuts.
- Latex allergy (e.g. gloves, tourniquets, and sphygmomanometer cuffs). Consider if allergic reaction occurs during a medical or dental procedure.
- Blood products. IV immunoglobulin to those with selective IgA deficiency.
- NSAIDs, ACE inhibitor and Alteplase can cause angioedema/angioneurotic oedema.
- Aspiration of a hydatid cyst.

Clinical

- Comes on over minutes with hypotension, flushing, itching, and urticaria.
- Chest pain, tachycardia, bradycardia, hypotension, incontinence.
- Laryngeal oedema causing stridor and hoarseness, staccato cough.
- Wheeze and bronchoconstriction. Periorbital itching. Skin flushing, erythema.
- Urticaria (not seen with C1 esterase deficiency) or oedema.
- Abdominal pain, colic, diarrhoea and vomiting, angioedema.
- Facial swelling, lips, nasal itching, sneezing. Metallic taste in mouth, confusion.

Investigations

- **FBC:** increased WCC. Increased CRP if sepsis/malignancy/inflammatory cause considered.
- **Mast cell tryptase:** initial, after 1–2 h and 24 h/follow up.
- **ECG**: SR, tachycardia, ST/T wave changes, new AF.
- **Infection screen**: blood/urine cultures.
- **C1 esterase inhibitor:** deficiency is a rare cause of angioedema without urticaria. Check C4 and C1 inhibitor levels because treatment for this condition is different.
- **Allergy testing**: allergen skin testing; RAST identifies specific IgE.

Differential

- Vasovagal syncope, sepsis, scombroidosis (histamine release), systemic mastocytosis.
- Panic attack, causes of syncope/presyncope, causes of breathlessness.

Management

Anaphylactic shock : lie flat, airway, oxygen, good IV access, crystalloid fluids, **ADRENALINE** 0.5 ml (0.5 mg) of 1 in 1000 IM and 200 mg **HYDROCORTISONE** IM and 10 mg **CHORPHENAMINE** IM/IV.

- **Lay person flat**: if hypotensive or faint then lay patient supine and raise legs to increase venous return.
- **Remove causes:** stop drug infusion, blood or blood product, remove bee sting.
- ABC: high (15 L/min) O_2 if shocked and then give O_2 as per BTS guidelines and reassess after ABG. Physiological monitoring BP, HR, SaO_2 and ECG.
- Call anaesthetics for help if any concerns of airway obstruction and oedema or any stridor, severe bronchospasm or respiratory compromise. Get IV access and start 1 L NS over 20 min.
- **ADRENALINE IM: if there is wheeze, stridor, respiratory distress, or shock then give ADRENALINE 0.5 ml of 1/1000 (0.5 mg) IM.** Adrenaline reduces histamine release and causes cutaneous vasoconstriction (which can reduce absorption of the bee sting or other allergen). Repeat dose after 5–10 min if poor response. Give into anterolateral aspect of muscle bulk of the middle third of the thigh using a green needle in adults. Do not give adrenaline subcutaneously. IM route post-thrombolysis is safer than IV and a muscle haematoma is unlikely to be significant with such a small volume. Apply pressure over the injection site to help haemostasis. Benefits may be lifesaving.
- **HYDROCORTISONE** 200 mg IV should be given.
- **SALBUTAMOL 2.5–5.0 mg** for bronchoconstriction which may be repeated.
- **AMINOPHYLLINE** IV if SOB + wheeze in cases usually where patient is asthmatic and symptoms persist.
- **CHLORPHENAMINE** 10 mg slow IV/IM (H_1 blocker).
- **GLUCAGON 1–2 mg IV** (doses up to 5 mg given) is rarely needed and is only considered if there is persisting hypotension and the patient is on beta-blockers. It bypasses the β-adrenergic receptor and directly activates adenylyl cyclase.
- **VASOPRESSIN** has been used when hypotension has not been responsive to ADRENALINE.
- **INOTROPES:** e.g. dopamine infusion may be considered.
- If still no improvement with airway oedema or bronchospasm and symptoms worsening consider anaesthetic review for intubation and mechanical ventilation, invasive monitoring and inotropes.

Discharge and follow up

- Patients need monitoring for 6–12 h post full recovery to ensure no late biphasic reactions. Continue **PREDNISOLONE** 40 mg PO OD for 3 days along with an antihistamine.
- Discharge with **2 EPIPENS** each containing **0.3 mg ADRENALINE for IM usage** with instructions on how to self-administer a dose. The second Epipen is in case one injector fails or patient needs a second dose. Teach to only use Epipen if anaphylaxis occurs with difficulty breathing or becoming faint. Give self-injection in the lateral thigh. It may be given through clothing, avoiding seams and

pockets. Hold needle in place for 10 s to ensure the adrenaline dose has been delivered completely. Check the patient's injection technique regularly to ensure doing it correctly (there are self-teach videos on youtube.com).

- Long term patient should wear a medic-alert bracelet.
- All need referral to specialist for allergy clinic/immunology opinion and identification of cause and antigen avoidance.

4.5 Toxic shock syndrome

Otherwise healthy patients with rapid onset fever, rash, hypotension, erythema, diarrhoea due to toxins from *Staphylococcus aureus* or *Streptococcus pyogenes*.

About

- Toxic shock syndrome (TSS) is potentially fatal. Early signs may be subtle.
- Septic focus may be a minor skin trauma, post-surgical wound, or tampon.
- Beware low BP, rash, erythema, fever and diarrhoea. Spot it and act quickly.

Aetiology

- **Toxic shock syndrome**: Staphylococcal: exotoxin from *Staph. aureus* (called toxic shock syndrome toxin 1 (TSST-1)) acts as a super antigen and causes release of cytokines (TNF, interleukin-1, M protein and gamma interferon). Induces a huge immune response and overstimulation of Th cells. Seen initially with tampons.
- **Toxic shock-like syndrome**: Streptococcal: usually group A beta-haemolytic streptococci. Mortality higher with this form. Due to *Strep. pyogenes* exotoxin A and B (SPEA/SPEB). Seen in healthy adults. There may be evidence of soft tissue infection and necrosis.

Clinical

- Signs are subtle and initially easily missed; then inexorable decline in otherwise healthy person.
- SBP <90 mmHg and increased HR and warm peripheries possibly.
- Erythematous rash, pyrexia, agitation, delirium, diarrhoea.
- Vaginal examination for retained tampon or a simple infected wound.
- Later: desquamation of the palms and soles.

Investigations

- **FBC**: increased neutrophil, WCC and thrombocytopenia.
- **U&E:** increased urea/creatinine (AKI), lactate, CRP, CK, AST.
- **Clotting:** increased APTT but PT and fibrinogen normal unless patient develops DIC.
- **Blood/urine/sputum** dipstick and cultures. **CXR:** look for infection.

Complications

- AKI, rhabdomyolysis, acute liver failure, circulatory collapse. DIC mortality is 5%.

Management

- **ABC: high FiO_2** initially then give O_2 as per BTS guidelines and reassess after ABG.
- **Urgent often aggressive fluid resuscitation (5–10 L per day)** is required with IV crystalloids and colloids due to the extreme hypotension and diffuse capillary leak.
- **Eliminate source:** wound cleaning and debridement if there is one. **Pelvic examination** to remove any retained tampons. Look for any source of sepsis. Abscess drainage. Topical antibiotics.

- **Inotropes**: may be needed but give volume support first. Monitor ABG.
- **Critical care**: patients need critical care as multi-organ failure can occur.
- **IV FLUCLOXACILLIN +/− IV CLINDAMYCIN** for streptococcal antigens reduces toxin production and **VANCOMYCIN IV** for staphylococci.
- **High dose IV immunoglobulin** has been suggested as a potential adjunctive therapy for streptococcal TSS to neutralize a wide variety of superantigens and to facilitate opsonization of streptococci. There is no evidence for steroid usage.

4.6 Septicaemic shock

Systemic Inflammatory Response Syndrome (SIRS) ▶Sepsis ▶Severe sepsis ▶Death. This can happen over anything from hours to days.

Systemic inflammatory response syndrome (SIRS)

- A generic systemic immunological response to infective, traumatic, malignant or inflammatory insults. Severe infections can manifest as a systemic inflammatory response.
- Causes include microbial invasion of normally sterile blood and tissue, acute pancreatitis, severe trauma, ischaemic insult and so on. Insults may be multiple, e.g. cholangitis + acute pancreatitis.

Definitions

SIRS	Sepsis	Severe sepsis
SIRS needs 2 or more of the following • **WCC <4 × 10^9/L or** • **WCC >12 × 10^9/L or** • **WCC >10% immature neutrophils** • **Core temp <36°C or >38°C** • **RR >20/min** • ***Pa*CO_2 <4.3 kPa** • **HR >90 bpm**	**SIRS with a presumed or confirmed infectious process**	**SIRS + evidence of organ dysfunction as shown by one or more of these** • Unexplained/lactic acidosis • CNS: obtunded, coma • Renal failure: creatinine >177 µmol/L • Urine output <0.5 ml/kg/h • Liver failure: bilirubin >34 µmol/L • Plt <100 × 10^9/L, INR >1.5 • Respiratory: hypoxia, SpO_2 <90% • CVS: cardiac failure, arrhythmias

Septic shock = severe sepsis + refractory SBP <90 mmHg despite fluid resuscitation and/or inotropes.

Pathophysiology

- Infected causes induced by endo/exotoxins. Release of cytokines (TNF, IL-1, IL-6) and inducible NOS relaxes vascular smooth muscle and bradykinin.
- This is opposed by IL-4 and IL-10 which reduce TNF-alpha, IL-1, IL-6, and IL-8. Result is hypoxaemia, hypovolaemia, vasodilation and capillary leak.
- There is a fall in SVR with increased CO and SBP <90 mmHg and a fall in DBP and warm extremities with a good capillary refill. Non-vital organs are hypoperfused at the expense of heart, kidneys, liver, and brain.
- With a severe insult the actual systemic inflammatory response may lead to severe hypotension and end-organ damage, a pro-coagulant state and eventually **multiple organ dysfunction syndrome** (MODS).

- Therapeutic regimens try to reverse this. Compounded by subcellular mitochondrial level dysfunction with reduced O_2 extraction, despite adequate supply, exacerbating tissue acidosis and production of lactate.
- Critically low perfusion of the gut is also key in the further downward spiral leading to multi-organ failure. Loss of integrity of the gut leads to the release of further cytokines and the entry of more organisms.

> Clinical presentation may be masked in those who are on steroids or immunosuppressives. They may be more ill than they appear and this must be borne in mind in terms of escalating therapy for sepsis.

Clinical assessment for symptoms and signs of septic sources

- Have a logical system and work top to toe in symptoms and signs.
- General: malaise, fever, night sweats, weight loss give idea of onset.
- **Respiratory:** chest signs for cough, fever, pneumonia, empyema, TB.
- **Urinary**: renal angle tenderness, urinary symptoms. Urinalysis.
- **Hepatobiliary:** RUQ pain, jaundice, pale stools, positive Murphy's sign.
- **Peritonism**: appendicitis, paralytic ileus, abdominal distension, previous appendectomy.
- **Endocarditis**: new murmurs, stigmata, recent cardiac operations/interventions.
- **Dermatology**: abscesses, boils – check perineum, cellulitis, and burns.
- **Gynaecology**: pelvic pain, STI, retained tampons.
- **Foreign bodies**: new heart valves, catheter, central line, hip replacement.
- **Immunosuppression**: neutropenia, myelodysplasia, haematological malignancy, HIV.
- **Sore throat**: tonsillitis, peri-tonsillar abscess, Lemierre's syndrome, glandular fever.
- **Foreign travel:** viral illness (dengue, VHF), malaria, HIV conversion.
- **CNS infection**: headache, seizure, encephalopathy, focal signs, cold sores.
- **Joint pain/back/bone pain**: septic joint, prosthesis, osteomyelitis, brucellosis.

Non-infectious causes of SIRS

- Pancreatitis, liver failure and cirrhosis, bowel ischaemia, infarction or perforation.
- Any major surgery (general or obstetric), trauma and tissue damage, malignancy.
- Transfusion reaction, GI bleed / haemorrhagic shock, drug reaction.
- Systemic vasculitis, myocardial infarction, skin reactions (TEN, SJS), seizures.

Potential complications of SIRS

- DIC (low fibrinogen, raised clotting times, low platelets).
- Respiratory failure/ acute respiratory distress syndrome.
- Acute kidney injury, multi-organ failure.
- Gastrointestinal bleeding/stress ulcer, anaemia, coagulopathy.
- DVT and VTE, hyperglycaemia, electrolyte disturbances.

> There is a combination of reduced intravascular volume with vasodilatation producing hypotension.

Clinical

- Classically warm but may have cool peripheries, delirium, and be obtunded and agitated.
- Deterioration can be rapid with rigors, fever or hypothermia.
- Vomiting, diarrhoea. Fall in BP <90/60 mmHg, low volume central pulse.
- Purpura (meningococcal), macular rash (toxic shock syndrome).

Investigations

- **FBC**: anaemia, WCC and platelets up or down with sepsis. Raised CRP/ESR.
- **Infection screen: blood cultures**: aerobic/anaerobic. **Urine:** urinalysis and culture.
- **CSF**: consider LP if meningitis/abscess considered and no contraindication.
- **Skin: take scrapings if any haemorrhagic lesions.** Swab any infected sites or infected lines or pressure sores or wounds.
- **Faeces**: send for culture if diarrhoea.
- **Effusions:** tap any pleural or ascitic fluid.
- **Abdominal/pelvic USS/CT** can show infected fluid collections, liver abscesses.
- **CXR**: pneumonia may show consolidation/effusion/empyema.
- **ABG:** metabolic acidosis +/− respiratory failure.
- **Lactate** >4 mmol/L with sepsis. **Thick/thin blood films** if malaria suspected.

Management actions in the first 6 h	Physiological targets in the first 6 h
• Check if serum lactate >4 mmol/L and administer high flow oxygen. • Give IV fluid challenges, e.g. IV 20 ml/kg crystalloid (NS) and measure hourly urine output. • Take at least 2 good quality blood cultures (not from the venflon insertion) using strict asepsis within 45 min (aerobic and anaerobic bottles) before antimicrobial therapy. • Give broad spectrum antibiotics, e.g. **TAZOCIN IV** within 1 h.	• Arterial O_2 saturation >93%. • Mixed/central venous O_2 sat >70% and haematocrit >30%. • CVP 8–12 mmHg (12–15 mmHg if ventilated). • Urine output ≥0.5 ml/kg/h and normalize lactate. • Apply vasopressors if not responding to initial fluid resuscitation to get a MAP ≥65 mmHg.

Management

- **ABC: give high FiO_2** if shocked, otherwise O_2 as per BTS guidelines. Consider ITU/HDU admission if severe sepsis, i.e. before patient is shocked. Involve clinical outreach. Severity: lactate >4 mmol/L and base deficit of −5 to −10 being moderately severe and −10 or worse suggests severely ill.
- **Circulation:** establish IV access. CVP line if needed (concerns over overfilling/cardiac failure). HDU intra-arterial BP monitoring if possible. Watch FBC, U&E, lactate and ABG. Transfusion to get Hct >30%.
- **Monitor:** urine output (catheterization also excludes post-renal obstruction if AKI).
- **Treat hypotension and/or a lactate >4 mmol/L** with IV fluids with 30 ml/kg (approximately 2 L in a 70 kg adult) of crystalloid (NS or Hartmann's solution). Repeated 250 ml saline boluses titrated to response. The typical patient may need 4–6 L of fluid in total.
- **Intubation and ventilation**: reduces work of breathing and helps oxygenation.
- **Blood cultures**: take before antibiotics with strict asepsis. Avoid taking as part of cannula insertion which is notoriously unreliable with false positives.
- **Broad spectrum IV antimicrobial (follow local guidance where possible)**: administer antibiotics within 1 h of arrival. If no allergy and renal function normal then consider **TAZOCIN IV +/− GENTAMICIN IV OD** if hospital-acquired. If penicillin allergic then give **MEROPENEM IV TDS**. Consider **VANCOMYCIN IV BD for MRSA**. Consider **CEFTRIAXONE IV BD** for suspected meningococcal infection. If MRSA considered then IV Vancomycin. Delayed administration increases mortality. Haematological malignancies: consider IV antifungal agents.

- **Surgical consult and management**: if abscesses or pus collections or necrotizing fasciitis or acute abdomen or suspected perforation or intra-abdominal sepsis. Consider **TAZOCIN.**
- **Inotropes/vasopressors:** use vasopressors for hypotension not responding to fluid resuscitation to aim for a mean arterial pressure >65 mmHg. Aim for a CVP >8 mmHg and central venous O_2 saturation (SvO_2) >70%, or mixed venous O_2 saturation (SvO_2) >65%. Consider **NORADRENALINE** and **ADRENALINE**. Give **DOBUTAMINE** if myocardial depression.
- **Non-infective SIRS:** usually the cause is apparent and therapy should be directed at that. Fluid replacement, oxygenation, critical care monitoring and focused therapies and interventions are key.
- **Corticosteroids,** e.g. consider **HYDROCORTISONE 50 mg IV followed by HYDROCORTISONE 50 mg IM qds** when BP is vasopressor-dependent and response to fluid has been poor. Monitor blood glucose.
- **Blood glucose**: maintain blood glucose level 4.0–8.2 mmol/L. Consider a variable rate insulin infusion if hyperglycaemia. Avoid hypoglycaemia.
- **Human activated C protein** was previously advocated in selected severe sepsis cases in ITU. *In vivo* activated protein C (APC) has antithrombotic, antifibrinolytic and anti-inflammatory properties, and its use has been discontinued.
- **Other considerations: in all patients ensure**: Analgesia, Nutrition (oral or NG preferable), Pressure care. **VTE prophylaxis:** is important. **Stress ulcer prophylaxis**: with PPI or Ranitidine.
- **Transfusion:** consider blood transfusion if Hb less than 7 g/dL or actively bleeding. Transfusion at a higher Hb if there are other co-morbidities. Target 7.0 to 9.0 g/dL.
- **Final thoughts:** ask about foreign travel. Malaria, dengue or viral haemorrhagic fever?

Multiorgan dysfunction syndrome

A complication of severe sepsis

- **Pulmonary**: acute lung injury and acute respiratory distress syndrome.
- **Cardiac**: myocardial dysfunction but vasodilation; drop in SVR causes increased cardiac output.
- **Gastrointestinal tract**: breakdown in normal mucosal integrity. The large surface area for nutritional uptake becomes a large area for entry of bacteria from the gut lumen. The liver is overwhelmed and is also dysfunctional. Systemic entry of toxins and bacteria to the pulmonary and systemic circulations. Develop ileus, pancreatitis, ischaemic colitis and acalculous pancreatitis and GI haemorrhage.
- Progressive kidney and liver failure.
- **Neurological**: progressive coma.

References:

Identifying Sepsis Early: www.scottishintensivecare.org.uk/education/ise.pdf.
Surviving Sepsis Campaign Guidelines 2012: www.survivingsepsis.org/

05 Acute breathlessness

The breathless patient may not be hypoxic and the patient with severe hypoxia may not appear to be breathless. Check O_2 saturation and ABG.

5.1 Assessment

- When asked to see a patient with breathlessness there are a range of possible diagnoses. Look for clues in the patient's current and past medical history and whether it came on a background of dyspnoea or not.
- What are observations: RR, BP and HR, are they hypoxic? Why are they in hospital? Ask about any other symptoms such as chest pain. Have a low threshold for suspecting PE in any inpatient.
- If the patient is hypoxic or respiratory rate is fast or slow, or nurse is concerned, see immediately. Mildly breathless or *in extremis*? If *in extremis* hurry because it could be pre-arrest.
- Start O_2 aiming for sats of 94–98% unless there is chronic COPD (28% O_2). Get ECG, especially if chest pain, looking for VT/fast AF/sinus tachycardia or ST changes. Ischaemic ECG and chest pain or suspected pulmonary oedema then give some sublingual GTN if systolic BP >110 mmHg.
- If wheeze or known COPD/asthma advise to start a **SALBUTAMOL 2.5 mg** nebulizer.
- Sudden unexpected breathlessness, especially if hypoxic or hypotensive in hospital, consider as PE if there is no obvious better alternative diagnosis.

Diagnostic clues

- **Sudden onset**: pulmonary oedema, pulmonary embolism, acute anaphylaxis and airway oedema, acute PTX, aspiration pneumonia, hyperventilation syndrome, inhaled foreign body.
- **Gradual onset:** pulmonary oedema, non-cardiogenic pulmonary oedema (ARDS), COPD/bronchiectasis, acute asthma, pneumonia, small PTX, lymphangitis carcinomatosis.
- **Exacerbation of known cause**: exacerbation of COPD, bronchiectasis, asthma, CCF, pulmonary fibrosis, cystic fibrosis.
- **Breathlessness with normal CXR**: PE, early pneumonia, PCP pneumonia, hyperventilation, COPD, small PTX (easily missed), metabolic acidosis with Kussmaul's breathing.

Clinical findings

- O_2 sats, RR and temperature. Wheeze, pursed lips, prolonged expiration, tripod position of COPD. Is there wheeze (PEFR)? Check HR: tachycardia, fast AF, VT. BP: hypotension or JVP elevated (pulmonary oedema, PE, tamponade, SVC obstruction).
- Auscultation – murmurs, S3, S4, triple rhythm, systolic murmurs. Chest – dull at bases, stony dull effusion. Air entry and breath sounds – is much air moving? Always get patient to breathe through mouth and listen to chest. Chest pain: ACS, PE, dissection, pericarditis. Legs: pedal oedema or ?DVT.

Differentials and management for acute breathlessness

Differential	Information and notes
Acute severe asthma	Usually a known asthmatic with increased breathlessness, wheeze, cough, reduced PEFR. May also be infection or other triggers. May be a history of previous episodes needing A&E attendance, hospitalization and even ITU. Difficult socioeconomic circumstances, alcohol and drug issues are all associated with poor outcomes.
Upper airway obstruction	Distress, breathless with stridor. Causes include laryngeal oedema, angioedema, inhaled foreign body, chemical burns, physical burns; inspect and remove if possible and consider Heimlich procedure if foreign body suspected. If intubation impossible then a cricothyrotomy may be needed - call ENT and anaesthetic fast bleep. Anaphylaxis or angio-neurotic oedema of laryngeal mucosa: stridor or hoarseness may suggest histamine release, oedema and anaphylaxis. See *Section 4.4.*
Pneumothorax	Breathless +/− pain. Look for underlying lung disease or chest trauma. If chest examination shows reduced air entry, hyper-resonant quiet side may be a PTX – CXR diagnostic. Follow PTX pathway (see *Section 12.4*). Those with underlying lung disease are at higher risk and may need aspiration and a chest drain. 100% O_2 helps resorption but caution if COPD.
Tension pneumothorax	Breathless and BP drops as RA filling compromised and signs and situation suggest tension PTX (ventilated patient or chest trauma). Immediate needle aspiration in 2nd intercostal space mid-clavicular line of affected side is called for – *do not wait for CXR* – should be an immediate hiss and escape of air. Give 100% O_2. Insert chest drain.
Pleural effusion	Breathless and stony dullness could be fluid. Get CXR. Usually significant size if symptomatic. Controlled drainage of effusion 1–2 L at a time. Risk of pulmonary oedema. Determine cause.
Pulmonary embolism	Very common in hospital. Breathless, hypotensive, and increased RR. Raised JVP, RV heave, loud P2, signs of DVT, CXR often normal. Elevated dimers and risk factors. Anticoagulate and give IV fluids; thrombolysis in selected severe cases. Vigorous CPR may help. See *Section 12.8.*
Exacerbation of COPD	Pre-existing COPD. Smoking history. Type 2 RF on ABG. Wheezy. Sputum. Consider NIV or if progressively acidotic then discuss ITU admission with intensivists.
Acute LVF	Acute dyspnoea, bibasal crackles, triple rhythm (S3/S4), worse lying flat. CXR diagnostic. ECG to look for STEMI needing PPCI. Echocardiogram when possible.
Pneumonia	**Community acquired pneumonia**: breathless, sputum, fever, dullness, reduced air entry, pleurisy, fever, raised WCC/CRP. Consolidation on CXR may not be seen acutely. **Aspiration pneumonia:** usually those with poor airways protection, stroke and coma and bulbar paralysis. ***Pneumocystis jiroveci* pneumonia**: seen with AIDS and immunocompromised patient causes a more generalized alveolar shadowing?

Differential	Information and notes
Hypoventilating	COPD, obesity, sedation, CO_2 narcosis, respiratory muscle weakness. May not be breathless. ABG show a Type 2 RF.
Respiratory muscle weakness	High cervical cord lesion, Guillain–Barré syndrome, myopathy, motor neuron disease (MND), muscular dystrophies. Monitor FVC as well as ABG. Weakness of muscles to shrug shoulders is a sign. An FVC <1.5 L is worrying. Monitor closely. Consider ventilation.
Metabolic acidosis	Kussmaul's breathing seen with DKA, salicylate overdose, etc. Check ABG.
Hyperventilation syndrome / panic attack	Setting of stress or anxiety. Examination normal, respiratory alkalosis on ABG. Breathe from bag. Sedation.
Fat embolism	Recent fracture, coma, sickle cell, agitated, skin rash. Hypoxia.
ARDS	Non-cardiogenic pulmonary oedema. Sepsis, malignancy, lung injury, trauma, obstetric emergency. CXR changes in clinical context. Echo shows normal cardiac function.
Aspiration pneumonia / pneumonitis	Suspect if NG tube may be misplaced and feed going into bronchus. Recent stroke or neurological disease (MND) or coma. Failure to protect airway due to sedation, alcohol, drugs, anaesthesia. CXR may show usually right middle or lower lobe changes. Mixed bacterial and chemical reaction produces a pneumonitis.
Pulmonary haemorrhage	Bleeding within the alveoli and bronchioles. Goodpasture's syndrome, Wegener's granulomatosis, CXR shows alveolar shadowing, renal failure.
Cheyne-Stokes breathing	Usually a sign of significant brain damage and brainstem compression. Alternating cycles of slow and then fast respirations in a profoundly comatose patient.

Investigations

- **Bloods:** FBC, U&E, glucose, CRP. **ABG:** look for hypoxia +/– hypercarbia.
- **Cardiac troponin**: ACS, myocarditis, myocardial injury.
- **D-dimer**: elevated with DVT/PE and other causes (sensitive but non-specific).
- **ECG:** AF, STEMI, NSTEMI, tachyarrhythmias, S1Q3T3.
- **CXR:** pulmonary oedema, PTX, consolidation, pleural effusion.
- **Echocardiogram:** MI and poor LV, valve disease, tamponade.
- **CT pulmonary angiogram:** PE, unexpected other pathology.
- **Pulmonary functions tests** – obstruction/restrictive.
- **BNP** >400 pg/ml for decompensated heart failure. BNP <100 pg/ml, heart failure unlikely.

De novo in-hospital acute breathlessness or circulatory collapse without an obvious alternative explanation is usually a pulmonary embolism until proven otherwise.

Management

- **ABC and give O_2** as per BTS guidelines and reassess after ABG. If *in extremis*, cyanosed or severely hypoxic (SaO_2 <80%) then call cardiac arrest team.

- Airway obstructed and compromised – allergic laryngeal oedema with stridor – give steroids +/– IM adrenaline and consider urgent cricothyrotomy (fast bleep anaesthetics and ENT).
- Common causes, e.g. COPD, LVF, acute PE, asthma, chest infection. Any signs of DVT? Look at hospital notes. Useful signs: raised JVP (CCF, PE, tamponade), loud systolic murmur, fast AF. New drugs or blood transfusion might suggest anaphylaxis and need for nebulizers, adrenaline and steroids.
- Look for fever: raised CRP, crackles on auscultation suggesting infection. If diagnosis still unclear or needs confirmation then CXR is useful, but may take some time to arrive and get information.
- **Treat as for cause found**: it can be useful to hedge bet and treat several causes at once whilst awaiting confirmatory tests or senior advice, e.g. IV antibiotic, **FUROSEMIDE 50 mg IV** if pulmonary oedema suspected and **SALBUTAMOL 2.5 mg nebulizer**. Look for new MI or valve disease.
- If PE suspected then follow PE diagnostic pathway (see *Section12.8*). If *in extremis* consider thrombolysis.
- If new LBBB or ST elevation then give GTN/diamorphine and take cardiological advice on urgent primary PCI.
- If worsening hypoxia and acidosis may require NIPPV or intubation and ventilation. Get help early if deteriorating. Consider a chest drain for PTX or massive pleural effusion.

5.2 Respiratory failure

Acute respiratory failure

Definition: respiratory failure is a respiratory problem of inadequate arterial oxygenation such that PaO_2 <8 kPa (60 mmHg).

Pulse oximetry warning: the pulse oximeter has become intrinsic to monitoring oxygenation. However, it does not detect raised CO_2 or hypoxia due to carbon monoxide because oximetry does not distinguish between normal oxygen sats in the haemoglobin and the carboxyhaemoglobin saturation of haemoglobin.

Type 1 respiratory failure	Type 2 respiratory failure
Physiology of type 1: PaO_2 <8 kPa (60 mmHg) and normal or low CO_2. • **Ventilation/perfusion** (V/Q) mismatch: increased A–a gradient, e.g. pneumonia. • **Impaired diffusion:** increased A–a gradient, e.g. lung fibrosis/interstitial disease. • **Anatomical right–left AV shunt:** increased A–a gradient, e.g. pulmonary AV malformation. • **Hypoventilation:** normal A–a gradient, e.g. obesity, sedation, neuromuscular weakness. • **Breathing low pressure/FiO_2:** normal A–a gradient, e.g. climbing Everest, in aircraft.	Physiology of type 2: PaO_2 <8 kPa (60 mmHg) and PCO_2 >6 kPa (45 mmHg). (*Remember that pulse oximetry will not detect rising CO_2.*) • **Alveolar hypoventilation:** neuromuscular weakness, sedation. • **Lung disease:** emphysema/COPD due to V/Q mismatch. Increased dead space ventilation. • **Increased CO_2 production:** malignant hyperthermia, severe thyrotoxicosis, fever, sepsis, shivering, overfeeding from parenteral nutrition, bicarbonate administration, CO_2 insufflation (laparoscopy).

Type 1 respiratory failure	Type 2 respiratory failure
Causes: pneumonia, cardiogenic oedema, ARDS, pulmonary haemorrhage, acute severe asthma, pulmonary fibrosis, cyanotic congenital lung disease, fat embolism, high altitude.	**Causes:** COPD, central hypoventilation, obesity-related hypoventilation, progressive coma, sedation, Guillain–Barré syndrome, myasthenia, poliomyelitis, muscular dystrophies, chest wall disorders, and all of the causes of type 1 when tired/hypoventilating/V/Q mismatch.

Details

- Respiratory failure (ARF): PaO_2 <8 kPa (60 mmHg) +/– PCO_2 >6 kPa (45 mmHg).
- Hypoxia soon leads to death. ARF usually comes on over hours. It may be on the background of normal respiratory function or chronic RF. Determine pre-exacerbation respiratory and functional status.
- Patients can move between types of RF. A hypoxic patient with pneumonia, heart failure or even severe asthma can tire and hypoventilate and retain carbon dioxide moving from type 1 to type 2.
- **Pathophysiology**: respiration driven by pontine and medullary centres. Raised CO_2 is a stronger stimulus to ventilation than low PO_2. Response to raised CO_2 reduced by chronic hypercapnia and sedation.
- **Pulse oximetry**: uses light to determine the ratio of oxygenated Hb (940 nm) and deoxygenated Hb (660 nm). Measures only the pulsatile flow and subtracts background readings.
- **Capnography**: reflects alveolar and therefore arterial partial pressures of CO_2 which reflects respiration and circulation. Can help detect tube displacement. During resuscitation, recovery is evident by an abrupt increase in the CO_2 reading.
- **Clinical effects of hypercarbia**: increasing confusion, asterixis, peripheral vasodilation, anxiety, obtunded, raised ICP, coma, hypoventilation. Compensatory raised HCO_3 and raised K.

Clinical

- Typically breathless but not always, especially with hypoventilating type 2 RF.
- Cyanosis (increased deoxygenated Hb), reduced cognition, altered behaviour.
- Comatose and decreased respiratory effort. History – cough, acute onset, smoker.
- Increased effort using accessory muscles, intercostal recession, and tachycardia.
- Tachypnoea. Signs of PTX, consolidation, pulmonary oedema, fibrosis, wheeze.

Investigations

- **FBC:** polycythaemia suggests chronic hypoxia/smoking. Look for anaemia.
- **U&E:** raised urea/creatinine, AKI or pulmonary–renal syndrome.
- **CXR:** vital to show signs of pulmonary oedema (cardiogenic or non-cardiogenic), consolidation, alveolar haemorrhage, PTX, pleural effusion, collapse, tumour, bullae, fibrosis, emphysematous change.
- **ABG:** arterial hypoxia is seen. If elevated PCO_2 then type 2. With acute RF HCO_3 is normal, but with chronic hypercapnic RF with renal compensation the HCO_3 may become elevated. The pH will usually be acidotic. The exception would be early type 1 failure with hyperventilation.
- **ECG** may suggest a cardiac cause. Look for tachycardia, AF. Ischaemia. RVH.
- **Echocardiography** rarely useful in pure type 1/2 RF except perhaps to help exclude PE. May suggest pulmonary hypertension.
- **Pulmonary functions tests (PFTs):** if possible can be helpful, e.g. FVC helps determine respiratory muscle strength. Reduced FEV/FVC in obstructive lung disease.

Respiratory failure is rare in COPD when FEV_1 >1 L and in restrictive diseases when FVC >1 L.

Management

- **ABC:** airways assessment is the first step in all management of respiratory compromise, followed by breathing and circulation. Look for cause based on clinical assessment, past history, CXR and ECG findings and arterial blood gases.
- **Controlled oxygen therapy:** the ward/ITU staff should give the lowest level of oxygen (flow, mask) to hit the prescribed oxygen saturation of 94–98% or 88–92%. Allow the staff to either increase or reduce the FiO_2 to attain this. An increased O_2 demand to hit the target SaO_2 needs to be escalated and patient reassessed as can signify a deteriorating patient.

Oxygen delivery to achieve 94–98% saturation

Step	Using a Venturi mask	Using nasal specs
1	24% (2–4 L/min)	1 L/min
2	28% (4–6 L/min)	2 L/min
3	35% (8–10 L/min)	4 L/min
4	40% (10–12 L/min)	Simple face mask 5–6 L/min
5	60% (12–14 L/min)	Simple face mask 7–10 L/min
6	Reservoir mask at 15 L/min O_2	

Give 100% O_2 – cardiac/respiratory arrest or periarrest, shock, patient *in extremis*, severe type 1 RF, carbon monoxide poisoning, pneumothorax (speeds resolution), and/or prior to attempting intubation.

- **Treat causes:** reverse or stop sedation, diuresis and nitrates for cardiogenic pulmonary oedema, bronchodilation (antibiotics, steroids, controlled O_2 for COPD), and anticoagulation for acute PE, chest drain for PTX and so on. NIV in COPD with acidosis.
- **NIPPV:** see discussion below. Consider where there is COPD with progressive CO_2 retention and worsening acidosis (pH <7.25). If it fails to oxygenate then mechanical ventilation should be considered and support sought from ITU/HDU.
- **Simple actions:** simple interventions – sitting patients up or out of bed can improve lung ventilation by aiding expectoration of secretions. Chest physiotherapy. Encourage coughing. Basal atelectasis and mucus plugs can all exacerbate ventilation. Occasionally bronchoscopy to remove mucus plugs and other material.
- **Antibiotics:** tailor to the likely pathogen. Is it viral, bacterial, fungal? Is it an exacerbation of COPD or community acquired pneumonia? Is the patient immunocompromised? Could this be PCP pneumonia with undiagnosed HIV/AIDS?
- **Respiratory stimulants: DOXAPRAM** can be used to stimulate and increase breathing rate/depth and can sometimes be tried as an alternative to NIV.
- **Extracorporeal membrane oxygenation** (ECMO) used for potentially reversible RF. It can be lifesaving and considered in patients with persisting RF despite maximal therapy due to a potentially reversible pathology. Talk to local ECMO centre.
- **Hypercapnia is rarely the result of O_2 therapy.** Usually due to hypoventilation. True hypoxic drivers usually have severe COPD, polycythaemia / cor pulmonale, FEV_1 <1 L, home O_2, nebulisers, raised HCO_3, normal respiratory rate. Management is to assess for NIV or invasive ventilation.

06 Coma

Always consider hypoglycaemia and opiate excess if coma is otherwise inexplicable. Have a very low threshold for IV glucose or IV naloxone if unsure.

Answering bleep

- What is the GCS? Why are they in hospital? Are they diabetic on hypoglycaemic agents?
- What is the temperature, pulse, BP, O_2 sats, respiratory rate?
- If reduced GCS, place patient in the recovery position. Get anaesthetic review.
- Assess ABC, give oxygen and monitor sats.
- If unresponsive and with difficulty breathing then call arrest team.
- Severe difficulty breathing or severe hypoxia or cyanosed then alert arrest team.
- Look for and treat any hypoglycaemia – if comatose IV dextrose or IM glucagon.

On arrival to a comatose patient

- **ABC: high flow O_2.** Examine if breathing. If not then institute BLS/ALS. If GCS <9 place patient in recovery position. If airway unsafe, breathing difficult then place in recovery position and oro/nasopharyngeal airway. Get ITU review. Suction secretions. If there is poor respiratory effort then bag–mask ventilation manually whilst preparing for intubation. Check core temperature.
- **Perform top to toe assessment** if new patient to look for any signs of trauma or any other signs, e.g. petechiae from meningococcaemia. If any concerns of spinal injury then immobilise.
- **Check observations**: temp/HR/BP/O_2 sats, RR and ensure not hypothermic (exposure, hypothyroid) and if so treat. Quickly check bedside capillary blood glucose. If any doubts treat for hypoglycaemia (20–50 ml of 50% dextrose into large vein and flush). If alcoholism or any suggestion of dietary issues give **Thiamine IV** or as part of **Pabrinex ampoules IV**.
- **Opiate toxicity**: if any suggestion of opiate use then consider **NALOXONE IV bolus**. Beware opiate patches: search for and remove any opiate/fentanyl patches. Repeat GCS and get notes and determine potential causes. Is patient waking up or stable or worsening. Take senior advice.
- **CT head** will quickly exclude structural problem: SAH, subdural, extradural, intracerebral or cerebellar bleed, tumour, oedema, herniation syndromes, hydrocephalus and make it a medical coma rather than surgical.
- **Recent travel in malarial area**. Send films. Look for haemolysis. Recent flu-like illness before deterioration. Investigate and treat quickly if falciparum malaria considered.
- **Encephalitis/meningitis**: if CT shows no surgical cause then needs LP with opening CSF pressures to be performed – check no coagulopathy first.
- **Post-seizure or non-convulsive status:** consider IV phenytoin if ongoing/repeated seizure activity.
- **Stroke:** usually obvious on scan, e.g. large bleed with coning or malignant MCA. Bilateral thalamic and top of the basilar artery infarcts can give coma disproportionate to CT findings.
- **Toxicology screen**: thick/thin films, ketones, ABG, blood cultures.
- **IV drugs to consider** in a comatose patient – naloxone, glucose, thiamine, aciclovir, ceftriaxone, IV quinine, lorazepam/phenytoin (fitting), mannitol (raised ICP), insulin if DKA.

Clinical assessment

- **Signs of trauma and injury**: Battle's sign, panda eyes, skull lacerations or haematomas. If so consider immobilising the spine and excluding spinal injury.
- Bitten (usually the side) tongue may suggest seizure and post ictal drowsiness.

- **Eyes**: dilated pupil (cocaine, IIIrd nerve) and may suggest coning if single and fixed; constricted pupil (opiates, some brainstem strokes, Horner's syndrome). Bilateral fixed dilated is usually brainstem death but exclude hypothermia and drug toxicity. Dysconjugate gaze suggests brainstem pathology. If the head can be safely turned (no spinal injury) then usually the eye moves relative to the orbit fixated at same position. If the eyes are static within the orbit this is abnormal loss of 'Doll's eye movement'.
- **Jaundiced**: hepatic encephalopathy, falciparum malaria, and malignancy.
- Pyrexia, cold sores: HSV encephalitis.
- Check drug chart for sedatives and skin for opiate patches.
- Check skin for petechiae: ?meningococcal meningitis. DIC.
- Look for fentanyl/opiate patches. Signs of opiate addiction.
- Turn patient and check back including along spinal cord and orifices.
- Abdominal, chest and cardiac exam are needed.

Investigations

- **FBC, U&E CRP:** WCC, glucose, TSH/T4 (myxoedema coma), infection.
- **ABG**: hypoxia, hypercarbia, acidosis. For metabolic acidosis calculate anion gap.
- **Urine:** blood, protein, WCC, toxicology if overdose suspected (check blood paracetamol/salicylates).
- **CT head:** often the most discriminating test in unexplained coma.
- **Lumbar puncture:** if no SOL and raised ICP on CT and suspected meningitis or encephalitis. Consider treating for meningitis + encephalitis if any doubts and IV naloxone if opiate usage or small pupils.
- **MRI scan and EEG:** done later. Difficult to monitor sick restless patient in MRI scanner. Treat for seizures acutely if suspected.
- **IV anticonvulsant:** (consider IV phenytoin) if persisting seizures (always consider non-convulsive status).
- **Neurosurgical consult** if abnormal head CT and surgically amenable finding.

Differentials for coma

Suspected cause	Findings and causes
Obvious or occult head injury	Was there head trauma which has been missed by ED. Look for injury. Blood in ear canal. Trauma review should highlight issues. Get CT head. Look for haemorrhage, oedema. Exclude cervical spine injury? Do not accept trauma patients with 'medical' problems medically unless a full trauma survey has been done. CT may look normal if there is diffuse neuronal injury with perhaps signs of cerebral oedema.
Subarachnoid haemorrhage	Thunderclap headache, persisting headache, nausea and/or vomiting, low GCS. May be localising signs. Blood in subarachnoid space on CT and aneurysm/ AVM may be seen. Site of blood helps locate aneurysmal site. Unilateral dilated pupil (IIIrd nerve) due to raised ICP or post communicating/superior cerebellar aneurysm. Urgent neurosurgical consult. CT-negative needs LP at the earliest 12 h post event. Look for hydrocephalus.
Haemorrhagic stroke	Large haemorrhage with raised ICP (cerebellar bleeds and possibly supratentorial superficial cortical bleeds benefit from surgery). Look for and manage secondary hydrocephalus with external ventricular drainage.
Subdural haematoma	May be astonishingly little to find even with marked changes if gradual onset; even a minor TIA episode. Stop anticoagulants. CT is diagnostic. Neurosurgical referral.

Suspected cause	Findings and causes
Ischaemic stroke	Large infarct with oedema (consider hemicraniectomy). Assess for thrombolysis. Strokes generally do not cause coma unless raised ICP and pressure on brainstem, e.g. malignant MCA syndrome or large cerebral/subthalamic/cerebellar haemorrhage. The very rare exception is unilateral or bilateral thalamic strokes or top of the basilar artery stroke (if suspected get MRI) and extensive brainstem strokes.
Non-convulsive status epilepticus	May be few or no outward sign of on-going seizures except perhaps eye flickering. Needs EEG. Treat with anticonvulsants, e.g. IV phenytoin.
Post cardiac arrest	Often undergo urgent PCI and consider therapeutic hypothermia (cooled to 32–34°C for 12–24 h if rhythm was VF). Supportive management after PCI.
Severe renal failure	Uraemia can reduce GCS. Can reduce clearance of opiates. Bloods show AKI.
Drug overdose	Alcohol, ethylene glycol (specific antidote), benzodiazepines (flumazenil in selected cases), tricyclic antidepressants. This list is not comprehensive.
Opiates	Causes miosis, respiratory depression. Opiate medications, transdermal patches **NALOXONE IV stat** and repeated as half-life short if required.
CNS infections	**Meningitis:** purpura, fever, neck stiffness. Meningism. CT/LP. Give **CEFTRIAXONE IV. Encephalitis**: seizure, focal CNS signs, fever, neck stiffness, delirium. Assume HSV and give **ACICLOVIR IV**. Needs CT/LP. **Cerebral malaria**: travel in endemic area <6 months. Get blood films. **QUININE IV.**
Post ictal	Supportive ABCs if fitting has stopped. May need anticonvulsant if status epilepticus. Should gradually awaken within 2 h – if not then start to look for causes.
Raised ICP	Space occupying lesion, e.g. abscess, tumour, haematoma will be seen on CT.
Cerebral oedema	Post-hypoxic brain damage or proximal MCA stroke, tumour, vasogenic oedema, diabetic ketoacidosis, high altitude, Reye's syndrome, hypoxic injury, carbon monoxide, SIADH.
Liver failure	Jaundice, abnormal LFTs, signs of liver failure; recent paracetamol overdose – *N*-acetyl cysteine.
Encephalopathy	Drug-induced, metabolic, liver failure. One to look out for is **Sodium Valproate** which can cause profound coma and associated with raised blood ammonia.
Endocrine	**Hypothyroid**: hypothyroid appearance, thyroidectomy scar, bradycardia, Give thyroxine +/− steroids. **Hypoglycaemia**: check blood glucose, give IV dextrose or IM glucagon. Look for cause. **Hyperglycaemia**: DKA/HHS with dehydration, smell of ketones, hypernatraemia, cerebral oedema. **Addisonian crisis**: hypotension, pigmentation, hyponatraemia. **Pituitary apoplexy**: CT shows bleeding, visual loss, see *Section 13.9*.

Management

Acutely with a normal CT and no other cause consider ABC + IV Aciclovir, IV Ceftriaxone, IV Pabrinex and IV naloxone and IV glucose if opiate toxicity or hypoglycaemia not excluded.

- **Supportive:** ABC, oxygen, physiological monitoring. Ideally HDU or ITU bed. Correct positioning, skin care, recovery position. May need intubation and ventilation if airway and breathing unsafe or GCS <9. Discuss with ITU and critical care outreach team. Escalate for consultant to consultant referral if appropriate on a case-by-case basis.
- **Initial:** all patients need rapid blood glucose determination and 50 ml of **50% DEXTROSE IV** where indicated. **PABRINEX IV** (THIAMINE) if deficiency suspected. **NALOXONE IV** if opiate use suspected.
- **Differential is wide**: if unclear despite history and examination and initial bloods then a **CT brain** will help to separate potential surgical/physical causes from medical causes. A normal CT brain has its own diagnostic differential.

Causes of coma with a normal (initial) CT head

- Head injury, hypoglycaemia, sepsis
- Hyponatraemia, myxoedema
- Post-cardiac arrest, hypoxic brain damage
- Opiates/codeine/sedation
- Post seizure, non-convulsive status (EEG)
- Top of the basilar artery occlusion (dot sign only)
- Haemorrhagic/ischaemic stroke
- Encephalopathy, encephalitis
- Meningoencephalitis, cerebral malaria
- Hypoactive delirium, malingering/ psychiatric

- **Urinary catheters**: only if essential. Patients can be padded and simple suprapubic pressure can result in reflex bladder emptying. Only if retention or close does output need monitoring.
- **Seizures**: if continuing then IV Phenytoin/Fosphenytoin (see *Section 19.4*).
- **Hydration:** can be difficult to assess. Fluid replacement IV NS 2–3 L per day in all comatose patients, initially to match normal losses. If coma persists then manage feeding and nutritional issues.
- **Medications**: these will often be stopped. If they are vital then try other routes, e.g. PR for aspirin. An NG tube can be placed for vital medications. Some important medications to continue – steroids (may need to be increased) or immunosuppression, anti-Parkinsonian medications, anti-anginals, antibiotic prophylaxis, warfarin or other anticoagulants where appropriate, rate-controlling medications, e.g. digoxin (give IV or NG) or beta-blockers, HAART therapies, anticonvulsants.
- **Exposure:** avoid possible hypothermia with blankets or 'space blankets' and warmers as needed.
- **Stress ulcers:** stress ulceration – consider PPI/H2 blocker in selected patients.
- **Resuscitation status:** determine ceiling of care, particularly in patients with poor prognosis.
- Management of raised ICP: see below

6.1 Raised intracranial pressure

The brain and CSF and blood are all contained within a rigid bony box. ICP will increase linearly with added volume with some compensation until a point where ICP rises become exponential.

About

- Rising ICP can lead to coning and death. Needs rapid diagnosis and treatment.

Aetiology

- **Excess soft tissue**: benign/malignant/primary/metastatic tumour, cerebral oedema (vasogenic/cytotoxic), brain (DKA, the non-ketotic hyperosmolar state, and hyponatraemia), abscess.
- **Excess CSF:** hydrocephalus (obstructive or communicating), e.g. idiopathic intracranial hypertension, cerebral venous thrombosis, SAH with impaired ventricular drainage.
- **Excess blood**: haematoma (ICH/SDH/EDH/SAH), vasodilation (raised PCO_2).

Clinical

- **Classical triad**: headache, papilloedema and vomiting often after waking is considered indicative of raised ICP. The headache is worse with coughing, sneezing, recumbency or exertion.
- **Papilloedema**: usually indicates raised pressure. However, raised ICP may fail to cause papilloedema if the subarachnoid sleeve around the optic nerve does not communicate with the subarachnoid space.
- **Progressive coma**: fall in GCS, pupillary dilation, Cheyne–Stokes respiration, bradycardia, hypertension and additional signs with herniation syndromes.

If you see a space occupying lesion don't stop there because metastases can be multiple so look at all the slices pre- and post-contrast, always look for an SDH, subarachnoid blood and check no early signs of hydrocephalus.

Investigations

- **FBC, U&E**: may show anaemia and suggest pathology.
- **CXR**: may show a lung tumour or sarcoidosis or TB.
- **CT brain +/– contrast**: IV contrast is usually given (ensure IV access) if radiology identify a space occupying lesion during initial CT. CT may show haemorrhage or tumour and vasogenic or cytotoxic oedema. May be signs of herniation. Cerebral oedema alone may be due to DKA, traumatic injury, Reye's syndrome, hyponatraemia, fulminant hepatic encephalopathy, and other toxic and metabolic insults. CT may show obstructive hydrocephalus with enlarged temporal horns and trans-ependymal oedema (high T2 signal) or low density change on CT around the margins of the ventricles which can resemble small vessel disease. If 3rd ventricle dilated there will be outward bowing of the lateral walls. Measurement of ICP can be by direct invasive measures in a neurological ICU by inserting a probe into ventricles.

Emergency management of raised ICP

- **Decide whether treatment is appropriate:** with a massive cerebral injury (infarct or haemorrhage or tumour) and clear evidence of raised ICP then outcome is likely to be poor and palliation may be more appropriate. Take expert advice.

Ensure oxygenation, treat fever, manage BP and elevate the head of the bed. Hypothermia is sometimes used. Monitor blood sugar and attempt glucose control between 4 and 8 mmol/L but with close monitoring and avoidance of hypoglycaemia.

- **Look for definitive plans**: external ventricular drainage for hydrocephalus, burr holes or craniectomy for large SDH/EDH, hemicraniectomy for malignant MCA, and sub-occipital craniectomy for cerebellar bleed, tumour debulking by surgery or radiotherapy. Use medical measures to buy time to allow transfer to a neurosurgical centre.
- **Ensure SaO_2 94–98%:** intubation and hyperventilation to lower $PaCO_2$ <4.0 kPa reduces ICP. Typical agents include Propofol, Midazolam and Morphine.
- **MANNITOL IV** infusion should be given over 20–30 min and can be repeated.
- **DEXAMETHASONE 10 mg stat and 4 mg 4–6 hourly PO/IV** if there is a tumour with vasogenic oedema. Steroids should be avoided with ischaemic or haemorrhagic stroke or head trauma.
- **Avoid hypotension**: if SBP <100 mmHg consider inotropes/vasopressors to raise MAP to maintain cerebral perfusion pressure. Cerebral autoregulation is impaired and dependent on MAP which needs to be supported.
- **Infections**: treat any underlying cause, e.g. meningitis, encephalitis.
- In some causes of raised ICP a lumbar puncture and removal of CSF is both diagnostic and therapeutic (e.g. idiopathic intracranial hypertension) but this must only be done with expert neurological and neurosurgical advice, because if done in the wrong scenario it can precipitate a herniation syndrome.

07 Chest pain

The immediate killers are myocardial infarction, aortic dissection and pulmonary embolism. Acute diagnosis and management of these must be your first concern.

Answering bleep

- What are the patient's observations? If inpatient, why in hospital? Check if breathless, hypotensive, tachycardic, hypoxic as all need instant attention. Give O_2 as per BTS guidelines.
- If IHD then give GTN spray or equivalent unless hypotensive. Request ECG to be done immediately and attend. If peri-arrest then consider arrest team.
- On arrival think life threatening causes – quick examination. Ensure defibrillator is to hand in case of VF. Ensure IV access, bloods and consider CXR. See individual topics for more help

Differential for chest pain

Suspected cause	Findings and causes
Acute coronary syndrome	Central heavy chest pain with radiation into arms/jaw. Risk factors – smoker, HTN, lipids, diabetes. Sweating, distressed, pale. Immediate ECG is diagnostic. ECG shows STEMI then primary PCI or thrombolysis if primary PCI not possible. See *Section 11.2*.
Aortic dissection	History of HTN. Widened mediastinum on CXR. Hypertensive but appears 'shocked'. BP different in arms. Inferior MI on ECG if right coronary artery obstructed at ostia (left coronary obstruction usually fatal). Get urgent CT aortogram or TOE. BP lowering. Proximal lesion move now to cardiothoracic centre for surgery. Avoid ACS management.
Pulmonary embolism	Sudden pain plus breathlessness. Sometimes with syncope and dyspnoea. Collapse in toilet. Obvious increased RR. Hypoxic ABG. Fall in saturations. Look for risk factors. Look for DVT. Anticoagulate, consider thrombolysis with RV dysfunction or circulatory collapse. IV fluids support RV dysfunction. Needs CTPA/VQ scan.
Pneumothorax	Sudden breathlessness and chest pain may be seen. Clicking sound heard on auscultation, hyper-resonant, CXR diagnostic but can be subtle. See *Section 12.4*.
Pneumonia	Unwell, toxic, feverish with pyrexia, pleuritic pain, raised WCC, CXR changes.
Oesophageal spasm	Central chest pain lasting a few minutes. Can be very intense. Related to eating/drinking. Benign.
Oesophageal perforation	Following oesophageal instrumentation or forceful vomiting. Toxic sick patient. Avoid passing NG tubes or oesophageal instrumentation.
Costochondritis (Tietze's syndrome)	Tenderness over costochondral joints, classically the second costochondral joint. Note that chest wall tenderness can be unreliable and seen with ACS pain too. Treat with NSAID and determine if there is a physical cause.

Suspected cause	Findings and causes
Chest wall pain	Look for localised defined tenderness. X-ray for fractures of ribs and sternum. May be trauma related. Also consider bone metastases. Check ALP/X-ray.
Takotsubo cardiomyopathy	Usually indistinguishable from that of ACS. Chest pain and dyspnoea, palpitations, nausea, vomiting, syncope, and, rarely, cardiogenic shock have been reported. Stress/emotional trigger.
Acute sickling crisis	Known sickle cell disease. May be hypoxic with pleuritic type pain. See *Section 16.3.*
Pericarditis	Younger patient. Possibly viral or recent MI and Dressler's syndrome. Eased by sitting forwards, audible rub, saddle shaped ST elevation. See *Section 11.11.*
Oesophagitis	Food related, reflux symptoms, eased by antacids.
Shingles	May be unilateral dermatomal distribution chest wall pain before the distinctive band of vesicles. Immunocompromised.
Idiopathic	Despite investigations the cause may be unknown. Main need is to exclude sinister causes. Manage residual pain with analgesia.
Pleurisy	Can be secondary to infection – viral or bacterial and underlying lung consolidation or possible connective tissue disease, neoplastic or idiopathic. Always consider if the history matches a possible PE and pulmonary infarction. Listen for a pleural rub. Check FBC, ESR, CXR. Consider autoantibodies if suggestion of RA or SLE. Non sinister causes are managed conservatively with NSAID analgesia.

Caution because palpable chest wall tenderness is reported in cases of ACS.

Immediate assessment

- **Cardiac:** ACS pain is central and heavy radiating to arms or jaw, but may be atypical in elderly and diabetics. Patient may be pale, sweaty and terrified looking with a large STEMI.
- **Aorta:** could this be an aortic dissection? History of HTN, tearing pain into back. BP disparity in arms. Unfolded aorta on CXR, aortic regurgitation. If so, need urgent CT aorta and avoid any anticoagulants.
- **Lungs:** pain more likely to be pleuritic. Significant risk factors for PE + hypoxia or signs of DVT. See *Section 12.8*. Signs of chest infection, pain pleuritic? See *Sections 12.5* and *12.6*. Get a CXR to exclude PTX and consolidation or rib fracture.
- **Oesophagus:** has patient had an oesophageal stricture dilated or any procedure. Oesophageal perforation. GORD symptoms, oesophagitis.
- **Chest wall**: sternal fracture, rib fractures, Bornholm's disease.

Elderly and diabetics with MI may have minimal chest pain or just acute confusion, agitation or 'off legs'. Always look at ECG and check troponin if suspicious.

Management

- Give O_2 if needed as per BTS guidelines. Get IV access. Bed rest and telemetry. Ensure access to defibrillation. Consider likely causes and exclude ACS.

- Check ECG: ST elevation and STEMI or new LBBB: cardiology consult for primary PCI/thrombolysis. Non-specific ST/T changes suggest NSTEMI. Saddle-shaped ST elevation throughout all leads except aVr, suggests pericarditis. In PE, tachycardia and S1Q3T3 may be seen but often non-specific.
- Check FBC, U&E, troponin and dimer (if indicated). Dimer not needed if high probability of PE. Doing dimers without any PE risk assessment is not recommended.
- Check ABG if breathless or low saturations. Arrange CXR and look for oedema, mediastinal widening, consolidation, PTX, fibrosis, or apical shadowing or mass.
- If pain considered cardiac give sublingual GTN **300 mcg (1–2 spray)** if SBP >110 mmHg and reassess. If pain is severe then give **DIAMORPHINE 2.5–5 mg IV** or **MORPHINE 5–10 mg IV** with an antiemetic, usually **METOCLOPRAMIDE 10 mg slow IV**.
- If ACS possible, then consider **ASPIRIN 300 mg PO** and follow local guidance which should be for PPCI if there is a STEMI; for further management see *Section 11.2*. If aortic dissection then avoid anticoagulation and arrange CT chest (see *Section 11.9*). If PE considered and no contraindication then anticoagulate; see *Section 12.8*.

08 Syncope

The important potentially fatal causes not to miss are malignant tachy/bradyarrhythmias, aortic stenosis/HCM and a small PE that may be a precursor to something bigger. Always consider driving and give advice.

About

- Patients who present with an episode(s) of collapse with spontaneous return of consciousness. The diagnostic list includes the causes of transient hypotension as well as neurological diagnoses.
- Transient syncope suggests a global central nervous system issue such as an episode of cerebral hypoperfusion, a generalised seizure, acute hydrocephalus and others.
- In some the cause remains unknown and is labelled as a 'funny turn'. This label helps avoid premature diagnostic labelling for the sake of it, which might stop a clinician making the correct diagnosis later.

Normal physiology of standing

- Standing requires prompt physiological adaptation to gravity. There is an instantaneous descent of about 500 ml of blood from the thorax to the lower abdomen, buttocks, and legs.
- There can be up to a 25% shift of plasma volume out of the vasculature and into the interstitial tissue, which reduces venous return to the heart. The result is a transient decline in both arterial pressure and cardiac filling. This has the effect of reducing the pressure on the baroreceptors, triggering a compensatory sympathetic mediated increase in heart rate and systemic vasoconstriction.
- The assumption of upright posture results in a 10–20 beat per minute increase in heart rate, a negligible change in systolic blood pressure, and approximately 5 mmHg increase in diastolic blood pressure.
- With age, diuretics, vasodilators, dehydration and any transient obstructive element there is much more likelihood of a simple transient failure of cerebral perfusion pressure. Following gravity to the floor quickly restores cerebral perfusion.

General

- Feeling as if about to faint or buzzing ears or vision constricting, suggests a hypotensive cause with reduced cerebral flow. Bruising to the face usually suggests severe and sudden loss of consciousness. Try to get the history from a witness of the episode. This can be invaluable.
- Was there chest pain, headache (SAH) or breathlessness before? What position – standing, sitting, lying? Doing what – coughing, micturition, and exertion? What was head position – looking up? Patient getting out of a hot bath or standing up in church. Did patient use GTN? Grey colour suggests faint and hypotension. Vasovagal usually recover quickly.
- What was BP/pulse in ambulance notes? Vasovagal syncope common and often exacerbated by antihypertensives/antianginals. How long until regain of consciousness – before or after ambulance? Is patient pregnant – a very common cause of fainting.

Reduced consciousness episode

- Jerking. Not all that jerks is a potential seizure. Momentary cerebral hypoperfusion in vasovagal syncope can cause jerks lasting 5–10 s. Urinary incontinence also seen with vasovagal syncope.
- Determine real level of consciousness – ask witness if patient was 'like a dead person' and one often finds that an 'unconscious' patient was not so and was even communicating to the witness throughout.
- Truly syncopal patients will usually go to ground unless held up or supported in some way. Sitting is an active process and patients will fall out of a chair or slump on a sofa.
- Give driving advice. In the UK it is the doctor's responsibility to advise a patient with a potentially recurring cause of syncope not to drive and document it. Take senior advice where unsure. It is the responsibility of the patient who wishes to drive to inform the DVLA.
- **Secondary trauma**: exclude intracerebral haemorrhage, subdural and ruptured spleens and fractures. Non-displaced hip fracture may be missed and so not all will have classical leg shortening and external rotation. Repeated examination may be needed. Pain may not be noted until attempts to mobilise. Initial trauma surveys can miss things so have a low threshold to repeat examination and imaging if there is evidence or suspicion of possible problems. Do not get distracted by the secondary trauma and forget about the primary cause of syncope.

Post-syncope clues

- Headache, drowsiness, rapid recovery over minutes (vasovagal), gradual recovery over several hours (seizure), breathless (PE), weakness (stroke/seizure), abdominal pain (leaking AAA), sore tongue (seizure – bites side of tongue).

The difficulty is often separating causes of reduced cerebral perfusion and seizure. Potentially malignant causes of reduced cerebral perfusion are rare but need urgent specialist assessment.

Differential and initial management of syncope / presyncope

Suspected cause	Findings and causes
Acute coronary syndrome	A potential cause of syncope (elderly and diabetics may not have chest pain). ECG will show ST/T wave changes, ST elevation, CHB, other forms of heart block, LBBB, RBBB, hemiblocks, VT, etc. Paramedics may capture a non-sustained VT, or heart block, or ischaemic changes, or the cause was 'pump failure' and poor LV or even RV. Beware the rush to diagnosing ACS and starting anti-thrombotics in simple collapses unless there is chest pain and ACS-type ECG changes, or a definite ischaemic arrhythmia. Without these most do not have ACS but may have had head trauma/SAH or hip trauma on falling and they will bleed and develop ICH/SDH, etc. If unclear wait for early troponin. See *Section 11.2*.

Suspected cause	Findings and causes
Cardiac – electrical	Brady- and tachyarrhythmias can cause syncope/presyncope and falls. Ensure ECG checked and any ambulance recordings reviewed. Particularly interested in sinus pauses >3 s, CHB and VT, non-sustained VT, and ECG evidence of conduction tissue disease. Rarely, but importantly, ECG changes of Brugada syndrome or HCM or RV dysplasia, long QT syndromes precipitating VT, WPW syndrome with short PR and delta wave and SVT or AF, ACS, hyper/hypokalaemia. A 12-lead ECG is mandatory. Most malignant arrhythmias are due to IHD/cardiomyopathy and associated with poor LV function. If you suspect an arrhythmia then keep for at least 24–48 h of telemetry, Echo and OP 7 day tape and cardiology consult. If there are sufficient concerns (family history of sudden death, poor LV function, Brugada syndrome or cardiac arrest) then patient stays until decision made, e.g. some may need ICD insertion. May need 7 day tape or reveal device. If there is conduction disease or bradycardia look to see if it is drug-induced (e.g. beta blockers, verapamil) and discuss if sufficient evidence for pacemaker with cardiologist. No driving until resolved and DVLA referral. See *Section 11.1* for more information.
Cardiac – structural	Always look for murmurs of obstructive lesions: aortic stenosis, HCM, mitral stenosis or atrial myxoma. Get an Echo and ECG, telemetry and cardiology consult.
Pregnancy	A cause of hypotension and predisposition to fainting. Always consider in fertile female. Rarely ectopic pregnancy can present with collapse and abdominal pain and shock.
Vasovagal syncope	Very common. Vasodepressor (BP falls), cardio-inhibitory (HR falls). Get ECG, consider OP tilt table if repeated episodes despite simple measures and cause not apparant. Lying/sitting and standing BP. Review medications – GTN spray? Are they hypovolemic from diuretics? Consider cough syncope, micturition syncope, syncope during/after large meal +/– alcohol. Fasting, fear, heat. Note twitching and jerks and urinary incontinence may be seen and can be misdiagnosed as epilepsy. For a reliable diagnosis look for the 3 'P's – Provocation (pain, fright, etc.), Prodromal (dimmed vision and hearing for a few seconds) and Posture (when standing/sitting). If diagnosis is quite clear then driving is allowed otherwise DVLA referral.
Postural hypotension	Precipitated by dehydration, hypovolaemia, pigmented (consider Addison's disease), autonomic dysfunction (e.g. diabetes, multiple systems atrophy, amyloid), Parkinson's disease. Check medications for antihypertensives, nitrates, GTN spray, calcium antagonists, levodopa, tricyclic antidepressants, phenothiazine. Telemetry, ECG, look for and stop unneeded drugs.
Postural tachycardia syndrome	Orthostatic tachycardia in the absence of orthostatic hypotension. Complain of symptoms of tachycardia, exercise intolerance, presyncope, extreme fatigue, headache and mental clouding. Have a heart rate increase of ≥30 bpm with prolonged standing (5–30 min), often have high levels of upright plasma noradrenaline (reflecting sympathetic nervous system activation), and many patients have a low blood volume. Ensure good hydration. Water intake ++. Increase sodium intake – NaCl tablets 1 g/tablet TID with meals. Exercise.

Suspected cause	Findings and causes
Carotid sinus hypersensitivity	Pressure on neck causes syncope. Tight collars. Consider CSM whilst monitored. Looking for symptomatic pauses >3 s. May need pacemaker. It may be wise to get a Doppler before CSM as bilateral internal carotid stenosis can cause syncope and mimic hypersensitivity.
Hypoglycaemia	A diabetic on insulin or oral hypoglycaemic agents or Addison's disease or insulinoma. Recovered with glucose.
Subarachnoid haemorrhage	Can present with thunderclap headache and collapse and recovery. Needs CT +/– LP.
Pulmonary embolism	Breathlessness and collapse, tachycardia, hypoxia. Elevated dimer. DVT. Risk factors. Consider treatment dose LMWH prior to CT–PA/VQ scan. Mechanism may be a saddle embolus which disintegrates quickly.
Complex seizure	Loss of consciousness, tongue biting, slow to wake up, known epilepsy, incontinent, headache after. Get a CT head acutely. No driving and DVLA referral. Seizure advice. Referral to first fit clinic.
Aortic dissection	Tearing interscapular / chest pain plus syncope. Consider diagnosis. CXR, CT chest. Raised dimers.
Occult haemorrhage	Gastrointestinal where melena delayed, leaking AAA but pain usually. Hidden bleeding, e.g. retroperitoneal, psoas muscle particularly in those on warfarin. Coagulopathy. PV bleed in pregnancy. Patient hypotensive and syncopal.
Autonomic dysfunction	Autonomic dysfunction seen with Guillain–Barré syndrome, acute porphyria or transverse myelitis, amyloid and diabetes and rarer causes. Lose ability to sweat, and suffer bowel and bladder dysfunctions. Bloating, nausea, vomiting, and abdominal pain and impotence. Constipation will alternate with diarrhoea. HR will be at a fixed rate of 40–50 bpm with inappropriate response. Pupils dilated and poorly reactive to light.
Addisonian crisis	Occasional subtle presentation with syncopal episodes. Systemic hypotensive, pigmentation, hyponatraemia, autoimmune disease. Some may have had recent abrupt cessation of steroids. Check U&E. Short synACTHen. Give IV HYDROCORTISONE.
Colloid cyst IIIrd ventricle	CT scan is generally diagnostic and syncope is due to abrupt rises in ICP.

Answering referral

- How is the patient now? BP, HR, pulse, glucose. Unresponsive, no breaths – call arrest team. Are they protecting airway especially if GCS <9. Any injury sustained?
- Describe the events of syncope – hypotension, chest pain, breathlessness, confusion (see above).

On arrival and thoughts

- The history and witness report are key. Anything sounding like a seizure or cardiac syncope, must advise no driving until full assessment and later discussion. Look for any sign of structural cardiac disease.
- Run through typical causes. General and cardiovascular and neurological exam. Main worry is malignant arrhythmias and alarm bells should ring if ECG

abnormal, history of ACS or poor LV function or long QT syndrome, family history or Brugada. If concerned admit under cardiology and place on CCU for telemetry.

- Arrange CT head if any concerns of acute seizure, SAH, colloid cyst or any other cause of syncope. Assess any obvious secondary injury. Has there been a hip or other fracture. Is there head or scalp injury. Is intracerebral haemorrhage the cause of the syncope or the result of it? Refer accordingly.
- Always give driving advice to drivers post-syncope. If unsure acutely of cause and happy to discharge for expectant management then reasonable to advise not to drive until all results back and then you can make an assessment or suggest referral to DVLA. Very definite vasovagal syncope which does not occur whilst driving does not usually curtail driving. Eliminate any precipitant.
- If there is a convincing vasovagal syncope story with precipitant and rapid recovery, limit any causes or precipitants and consider discharge.

09 Weakness

About

- Weakness can originate anywhere from the Betz cells of the primary motor cortex to the neuromuscular junction and the muscles being assessed. Weakness can at times be functional, but this is a diagnosis of last resort made by experts.
- Weakness in the acute setting is important because early diagnosis and intervention can shorten duration and prevent long term disability – stroke, cord compression, Guillain–Barré syndrome.
- Weakness affecting respiratory muscles potentially leading to respiratory failure is an emergency and close monitoring (usually FEV) is needed with ready access to intubation and ventilation.

Assessment clues

- What is the GCS and observations? How is the patient – well or unwell?
- Where is the weakness – face, arm, and legs, which side? Unilateral weakness strongly suggests intracranial pathology. If symmetrical, e.g. both legs, this suggests a cauda equina or spinal cord lesion, or bilateral brainstem/cortical/ subcortical lesions, which are uncommon.
- Arms are supplied by C5–T1 so weak legs alone are a lesion below T1. Look for a sensory level.
- Is sensation affected (none with MND)? Asymmetrical suggests intracranial lesion or a cord or root lesion. Symmetrical distal sensory loss is either a cord/cauda equina or symmetrical peripheral neuropathy.
- What is respiratory rate, O_2 sats and BP/HR? FVC guides respiratory muscle strength.
- Are the pupils affected? Not affected with Guillain–Barré syndrome, MG, or MND, but seen with strokes, brainstem lesions, intracranial tumours and space occupying lesions, drugs.
- Is there double vision or ophthalmoplegia? Not seen with MND, but seen with stroke, MS, MG, space occupying lesions, Miller–Fisher syndrome, botulism.
- Any persisting sphincter weakness suggests suspected cord or cauda equina pathology.
- Stroke is seen in all ages but prevalence increased with age.

Weakness	
UMN	Increased tone (spasticity), hyperreflexia, clonus, upgoing plantar, upper limb extensors and abductors and lower limb flexors, no wasting other than disuse.
LMN	Reduced tone, absent/reduced reflexes, muscle wasting, absent plantar response.
Muscle end plate	Fatigability, no wasting, reflexes normal or reduced, plantar normal or reduced.
Myopathy	Proximal weakness, reduced tone and reflexes and plantar response mild wasting.

Patterns of weakness

UMN: weakness, increased tone, reflexes, extensor plantars. **LMN**: weakness, reduced tone, reflexes, absent or downgoing plantar. Acute neurological lesions may all appear LMN initially.

Anatomical level	Findings and causes
Cortical weakness (frontal lobe precentral gyrus)	C/L weakness in face/arm/leg or adjacent subset. Increased tone ('clasp knife'), extensor plantar, upper limb flexors stronger than extensors. Lower limb extensors stronger than flexors. Clues may be C/L visual and cortical function loss, e.g. right arm and dysphasia. C/L hemisensory loss too. Look for cortical stroke, trauma, tumour, abscess, and demyelination. Get CT/MRI.
Subcortical weakness	C/L weakness in face/arm/leg or subset. Increased tone, extensor plantar. No visual (usually unless affecting optic radiations) or higher cortical function loss (dysphasia/neglect/apraxia). Lacunar strokes, demyelination, tumour, PML. Get CT/MRI.
Brainstem weakness	C/L weakness in arm/leg or subset with ipsilateral cranial nerve/face weakness and cerebellar signs. Increased tone, extensor plantar. Diplopia and vertigo possible if brainstem affected. Horner's syndrome, internuclear ophthalmoplegia. Ipsilateral cerebellar signs. CT to exclude bleed/tumour/hydrocephalus acutely, but MRI best to confirm diagnosis – stroke, demyelination, tumour.
Cerebellum	Ipsilateral ataxia, no weakness, nystagmus, past pointing, dysarthria and cranial nerve lesion. CT acutely to exclude cerebellar stroke, but MRI best if available. A cerebellar haematoma should be discussed with neurosurgeons for evacuation. Causes: stroke, tumour, alcohol (usually diffuse), neurodegeneration.
Cervical spine	UMN quadriparesis. Arms innervated by C5–T1. Extensor plantars. Spastic weakness. Sensory loss below level. Horner's syndrome. Reflexes lost at compression level. High lesions cause diaphragmatic paralysis and respiratory failure. T1 supplies muscles of hand. Lesions below T1 spares upper limbs. Sensory ataxia.
Thoracic spine	UMN weakness in both legs. Extensor plantars. Sensory loss below level. Reflex lost at compression level. Sensory ataxia.
Lumbar spine	Spinal cord ends L1. Below this any destructive compressive lesion damages the roots of cauda equina. This causes LMN weakness in the legs, saddle anaesthesia (can't feel seat or bottom or touch around the anus – the lowest roots provide sensation peri-anally) and sphincter loss. Areflexia in legs.
Radiculopathy	Nerves that leave cord. Bilaterally. Carrying motor out and sensory in. Unilateral dermatomal and myotomal LMN motor weakness and sensory loss or pain and reflex lost at compression level and wasting. Usually a prolapsed disc. MRI at suspected level.
Hemisection of cord	Spastic (UMN) weakness and increased reflexes on same side, dorsal column loss, ipsilateral and pain/temp other side. MRI of cord at suspected level.

Anatomical level	Findings and causes
Symmetrical ascending polyneuropathy	Progressive distal to proximal weakness. Sensory loss. Lost ankle jerks, areflexia. Wasting if chronic. Guillain–Barré syndrome or chronic inflammatory demyelinating polyneuropathy. Weakness + ophthalmoplegia = Miller–Fisher syndrome. Needs LP and nerve conduction studies.
Muscle end plate	Fatigability, no wasting, reflexes normal or reduced, plantar normal or reduced. Tensilon test or ice cube test. Cranial motor nerves involved and skeletal.
Myopathy	Proximal weakness, reduced tone and reflexes and plantar response mild wasting. Needs EMG, CK, muscle biopsy.

Speed of onset of neurology	Findings and causes
Sudden and immediate	Dramatic. Usually vascular or electrical. Vascular (embolic stroke is sudden, thrombotic stroke tends to stutter in onset, haemorrhage can be sudden but usually slow and progressive), seizure, SAH, functional, migraine (usually over minutes).
Minutes to hours	Migrainous aura, seizure, thrombotic stroke, subdural haematoma, extradural haemorrhage.
Hours to days	Demyelination, inflammation, infections, e.g. viral encephalitis, meningitis.
Months	Creutzfeldt–Jakob disease, aggressive tumours, e.g. glioblastomas or metastases.
Years	Low grade gliomas, progressive stroke disease, neurodegenerative diseases, e.g. Parkinson's, Alzheimer's, Huntington's. Primary progressive MS, secondary progressive MS.
Recurrent	Migraine, epilepsy, demyelination, stroke, relapsing–remitting MS.

Neurological phenomena	Associated with	Cause
Positive	Tingling, flashing lights, allodynia, jerks and movements.	Migrainous aura spreads over minutes (cortical spreading depression) or a focal seizure spreads over seconds usually due to an irritative focus.
Negative	Weakness, hemianopia, loss of sensation, incoordination, deafness.	Suggests destructive pathology – inflammatory, vascular, demyelination, tumour, etc.

Differentials

Causes	Notes
Acute stroke	Comes on over seconds. Usually a unilateral deficit involving a (UMN) hemiparesis, hemisensory loss and hemianopia. Higher cortical features, e.g. dysphasia, apraxia. In ischaemia the signs match a particular vascular territory. In haemorrhage less so. Brainstem may have cranial nerve signs and ipsilateral weakness. Cerebellar will have ipsilateral cerebellar signs. See *Section 19.8*. Needs urgent CT brain if candidate for thrombolysis.

Causes	Notes
Seizure	Post-seizure Todd's paralysis. The history of a seizure-like episode is vital or a history of previous similar episodes.
Functional	Diagnosis of exclusion – can mimic any neurological disorder or none. Absence of hard signs helps and normal tests. Expert review needed. Can occur and resolve quickly or slowly. Pattern of weakness/sensory loss can mimic true pathology. Paraplegia, stroke-like, seizure-like. Give-way weakness. Lots of effort. Uneconomic gaits and postures. Contrast between exam findings and therapy findings. Positive Hoover's sign. Normal imaging. Give lots of positive support: 'You have a block'.
Ascending polyneuropathy	*Ascending inflammatory demyelinating polyneuropathy*: ascending usually symmetrical weakness of both legs over days with areflexia; can also cause weakness in arms and face and respiratory muscles. Motor, sensory and autonomic symptoms. Areflexia is a useful sign. May follow gastroenteritis or viral illness. LP shows raised protein. See *Section 19.14*. *Chronic inflammatory demyelinating polyneuropathy*: similar but slower in onset and is steroid responsive.
Space occupying lesion	Cortical lesion will cause progressive weakness, seizures similar to stroke but slowly progressive. Focal signs may be present, e.g. hemianopia, hemiparesis, cognitive and other changes. Morning headache may be present. Causes can be tumour, abscess, demyelinating plaque, haematoma, subdural haematoma.
Tick paralysis	Seen in Australia and North America. Weakness 2–5 days after tick exposure. Female tick releases a neurotoxin in saliva. Might find large engorged tick on skin (often scalp); when tick removed symptoms improve and resolve – grasp the tick as close to the skin as possible and pull in a firm steady manner ensuring all parts removed. Progressive ascending weakness like GBS.
Subdural haematoma	Contralateral weakness and signs. Always consider in anticoagulated or elderly patient post fall and get urgent CT.
Acute myelopathy or cauda equina lesion	Sudden or subacute onset of quadriplegia or paraplegia and loss of sphincter control and sensory level. Need to identify if this is a compressive lesion or medical cause, e.g. spinal stroke or transverse myelitis. Urgent MRI indicated and if non-compression then LP for CSF. Cord lesions often cause initial flaccid weakness but becomes hypertonic within 24–48 h. Pain may help identify level and suggests a more surgical compressive cause.
Myasthenia gravis	Progressive fatigable weakness: proximal limbs, face (bilateral ptosis) and diplopia and difficulty swallowing. Consider myasthenia. Check antibodies against acetylcholine receptors. Ice cube/tensilon test. Lambert–Eaton syndrome weakness gets stronger with repeated use.
Motor neuron disease	Aged 40+ (sometimes younger). Progressive weakness over weeks or longer. Mixed UMN/LMN in arms and legs, generalised hyperreflexia, **no diplopia or sensory loss or sphincter involvement**. Bulbar palsy. Sphincters preserved. Wasting fasciculation especially in hands, legs and tongue. The diagnosis may be in the mouth! Exaggerated jaw jerk. Exclude MND. Test EMG.

Causes	Notes
Multiple sclerosis	Adult. Might be remitting relapsing or progressive forms. Mixed UMN signs, cord signs, dysarthria, diplopia, painful monocular visual loss (optic neuritis), internuclear ophthalmoplegia, cerebellar signs. **No LMN signs**. Ataxia, scissors gait if spastic diplegia. Ask about previous events.
Neuromyelitis optica	Transverse myelitis with paraparesis or quadriparesis, sensory level and bladder and bowel dysfunction + optic neuritis (progressive blindness) and presence of Ab against Aquaporin4.
Paraneoplastic disorder	If the patient has disseminated malignant disease then a useful assumption is to assume any neurology is directly due to primary spread or metastases or possibly paraneoplastic until excluded.
Botulism	Progressive flaccid paralysis and weakness involving skeletal muscles and cranial nerves (diplopia, dysphagia, bulbar weakness, dry mouth) within hours after ingestion of toxin. May be associated gastroenteritis, hypotension, constipation.
Myopathy	Proximal weakness – raising hands above head or standing.
Electrolytes	Low potassium, calcium, magnesium can all cause generalised fatigue and weakness.
Periodic paralysis	Low and high potassium levels, associated with thyroid disease. Seen more in Asia. Provoked by fasting or high carbohydrate meals or exercise. Measure electrolytes.
Sleep paralysis	Transient inability to move or speak on waking. Linked to narcolepsy. May have daytime sleepiness, cataplexy, hypnagogic hallucinations, sleep paralysis.
Poliomyelitis	Causes an acute flaccid paralysis. Usually seen in non-vaccinated from endemic areas.
Peripheral neuropathy	Can be motor, e.g. Charcot–Marie–Tooth and related conditions.

10 Acute severe headache

On referral

- If thunderclap at onset then SAH is the immediate concern.
- What is the GCS and observations? How is the patient? Symptoms/signs other than headache?
- Has there been a head injury? New drugs (nitrates, dipyridamole)?
- Any meningism, fever, rash or malaise? Consider meningitis/encephalitis.

Note

- Most will be benign (even thunderclap) but all need to be taken seriously.
- The human and medicolegal cost of missing SAH is high. Keep a low threshold.
- Note red flag signs and symptoms below of serious pathology.
- Response to triptans can be seen with serious pathology and is not a useful sign.

Differential for acute severe headache

Suspected cause	Findings and causes
Subarachnoid haemorrhage	Rupture of a berry aneurysm or AVM is usually catastrophic and presents with thunderclap headache and often collapse and coma. Rapidity of onset is very useful but patients do not always give a clear history. Patients are obtunded, distressed and usually have headache and neck stiffness. There is blood on CT in 95% of those with SAH within the first 12 h. The remainder need an LP at 12 h post-headache for diagnosis. LP can be useful up to 2 weeks, looking for xanthochromia if CT negative. For SAH the main concern is a lethal or disabling rebleed or delayed ischaemia or vasospasm, and so early diagnosis and prevention is key. Refer immediately to neurosurgery once diagnosis made.
Acute stroke	Both ischaemic and acute haemorrhagic stroke can cause sudden headache but more common with haemorrhage. CT scan will be diagnostic. Particularly worrying is patient on anticoagulation or with any focal neurology. Needs urgent CT head.
Cerebral venous thrombosis	Consider this 2nd after SAH in the differential of thunderclap presentation. CT head may be normal, show clot or venous infarction with haemorrhage. Diagnose with CTV or MRV. Suspect if LP done for ?SAH shows high red cells, high opening pressure and increased lymphocytes. Diagnosis formally made by CTV or MRV (magnetic resonance venography), whichever available. Anticoagulate.
Migraine	Recurrent episodic headache with systemic symptoms. Comes on gradually, and there may be preceding aura such as tingling, weakness, and altered speech, word finding difficulties, flashing lights, scotomas or fortification spectra. Positive family history. Headache then comes on and lasts 4–72 h. Patients feel awful; usual response for severe attacks is to want to lie down and sleep. Try **IBUPROFEN 600 mg PO** if not vomiting or else **IM DICLOFENAC + METOCLOPRAMIDE**. Triptans, e.g. **SUMATRIPTAN 6 mg SC**, can also be used (C/I with IHD). If severe vomiting consider IV normal saline.

Suspected cause	Findings and causes
Space occupying lesion	Gradually increasing size or oedema or bleed into a focal lesion, e.g. tumour or abscess.
Cluster headaches; trigeminal autonomic cephalgias	Occur in repeated attacks. Severe. Restless patient pacing floor. Give 100% O_2 and **SUMATRIPTAN 6 mg SC** is recommended as the first choice treatment for the relief of acute attacks of cluster headache. Can be so severe that people commit suicide. Eye tearing. Commoner in men.
Acute infection	**Bacterial meningitis:** look for petechiae if meningococcaemia, neck stiffness, Kernig's sign, meningism. Acute delirium in elderly, pyrexia. Treat empirically if any suspicion. **Viral meningitis**: similar presentation to bacterial meningitis so investigate and treat as for bacterial meningitis until diagnosis excluded. **Encephalitis**: fever, obtunded, seizures, focal neurology, cold sores. Needs LP and antivirals: IV acyclovir if diagnosis considered.
Pituitary apoplexy	Severe headache and IIIrd nerve palsy and visual loss as severe pressure around optic nerve from haematoma. CT/MRI will show bleeding. May have known pituitary tumour. Needs neurosurgical decompression. Needs IV hydrocortisone because acute hypopituitarism is possible.
Cervical arterial dissection	Neck, retro-orbital pain or occipital pain. Associated focal neurological signs. Horner's syndrome with ipsilateral carotid dissection. Brainstem signs with vertebral dissection and may also have a Horner's from PICA thrombosis and lateral medullary syndrome.
Third ventricular colloid cysts	Headache, syncope. CT evidence. May see acute hydrocephalus.
Reversible cerebral vasoconstriction syndrome (RCVS)	Underdiagnosed syndrome with severe, often bilateral, and even daily headaches, often thunderclap and possibly seizures and focal neurological deficits. The headache, which is the dominant feature, may wane after 1–3 h leaving behind a 'background' headache. The headaches can persist almost daily for several weeks.
Temporal arteritis	Subacute headache in older patient. Check ESR or CRP. Temporal artery tenderness or polymyalgia symptoms or transient or persistent visual loss. Needs TAB.
Coital/post-coital headache	Diagnosis once SAH excluded. May be experienced with orgasm. There is a real possibility that this could be SAH but it would be less likely if it has occurred several times before without incident. In future take NSAIDs prior to sex. Exclude SAH in all cases with LP/CT. Benign form is orgasmic cephalgia once SAH safely excluded.
Exploding head syndrome	Auditory hallucination that occurs whilst falling asleep – like a gun going off in one's head. May be unable to speak or move. Benign condition – avoid extensive investigation or treatment.
Tension headache	Usually a chronic band-like headache but many variants. Rarely truly thunderclap. Often long history of similar episodes. No associated symptoms or signs beyond headache.

Suspected cause	Findings and causes
Medication overuse headache	Must be excluded in all patients with chronic daily headache (headache more than 15 d/m for more than 3 m) and those using opioid-containing medications or overusing triptans are at most risk.
Acute angle closure glaucoma	Consider in a patient with headache associated with a red eye, halos or unilateral visual symptoms. Urgent ophthalmology referral.
Carbon monoxide poisoning	CO produced when gas, oil, coal or wood do not burn fully. Cold weather. More than one person affected in shared accommodation. Check COHb levels.
Spontaneous intracranial hypotension	Marked headache on standing. Can come on suddenly. Relieved by remaining supine. Post LP or spontaneous leak. Give fluids and simple caffeinated drinks. May need blood patches (usually done by anaesthetist). Typical meningeal enhancement on MRI and cerebellar tonsilar descent. CSF opening pressure <10 cmH_2O.

Immediate assessment

- ABC, assess GCS and look for focal neurology. A fall in GCS warrants urgent CT (and LP). CT brain if thunderclap or possible head injury or on anticoagulants; neurosurgical referral if positive.
- Thunderclap encompasses headaches which proceed from nil to maximal within 4–5 min and not just those that feel like hit round the head with baseball bat.
- Cluster headache seen more often in middle aged males – responds to high flow oxygen. Ask about recent LP or epidural with low-pressure headache.
- Horner's syndrome (small pupil, partial ptosis are the main signs) – think carotid dissection or lateral medullary stroke, or lung tumour and cerebral metastases.
- Eye symptoms – for red eye with injected conjunctiva consider acute angle closure glaucoma especially in an older patient.

Investigations

- **ESR / CRP**: if temporal arteritis considered (age >50 y).
- **CT head**: will exclude bleeding and tumour (needs CT + contrast) and other causes. May be negative and if thunderclap onset needs an LP.
- **LP** if concerns of meningitis or encephalitis and no contraindications.
- **CT angiogram or MR angiogram**: if carotid/vertebral dissection or RCVS suspected.

Headache – red flags of sinister pathology

- Sudden onset severe (maximal <4 min): exclude SAH. Needs CT/LP.
- Headache with cough or bending: MRI for posterior fossa lesion.
- Persistent morning headache and nausea (exclude space occupying lesion).
- Steadily worsening severity: consider SOL.
- Postural: worse on standing: low ICP, CSF leak, colloid cyst of IIIrd ventricle.
- Headache + neurological symptoms/signs needs investigation.
- New or change in headache/visual loss with age >50 y: check ESR – ?GCA.
- Headache and immunosuppressed, e.g. steroids, HIV, ?TB, meningitis, lymphoma.
- Headache and cancer: exclude metastatic lesion.

Cardiological emergencies

11.1 Sudden cardiac death

About

Most are arrhythmogenic and unless there is early access to defibrillation (internal or otherwise) survival is poor. Manage as per resuscitation guidelines (see *Chapter 1*). Some, do survive and need ongoing management. Divide into those with a normal heart on imaging and those without.

Structurally normal heart	
Brugada syndrome	Idiopathic VF – 20% of sudden death in structurally normal hearts, sudden unexpected nocturnal death (SUND) in South-east Asian men, ST elevation in the right precordial chest leads V1–V3. ECG changes may be dynamic and concealed which can make diagnosis more difficult. Placing V1 and V2 in the 2nd rather than 4th space can help detect changes. Minority have sodium channel defect. Only ICD has been proven to help. May have self-terminating VT/VF, waking up at night after agonal respiration. Drugs used to unmask disease include Amjaline, Flecainide.
Long QT syndrome	Congenital and acquired long QT syndrome. Check family history Ca^{2+}, Mg^{2+}, drugs and other causes.
Pre-excitation syndrome	WPW with AF and an irregular fast ventricular rate over accessory pathway. ECG may show short PR interval and delta wave of pre-excitation unless the pathway is concealed.
Commotio cordis	Young adults with low-impact precordial trauma with a projectile object such as a baseball, hockey puck, fist, rubber bullet, or even a rugby ball. Early CPR and defibrillation.
Structurally abnormal heart	
Arrhythmogenic right ventricular cardiomyopathy/ dysplasia	Inherited cardiomyopathy, predisposing patients to ventricular arrhythmias (monomorphic VT/VF) and sudden cardiac death. It is characterised by structural and functional abnormalities of the right ventricular myocardium, such as fibro fatty myocardium replacement, microaneurysms or focal atrophy. ECG: T wave inversion in right precordial leads.
Ischaemic heart disease	Acute MI setting. May be arrhythmic or asystolic or LV wall rupture and tamponade.
Cardiomyopathy	Associated with poor LV, RV dysplasia. Hypertrophic cardiomyopathy.
Aortic stenosis	Critical gradient – heart failure, chest pain, syncope.
Myocarditis	Ventricular arrhythmias.

Management

- Risk assessment. Echocardiogram. Genetic studies in some. Electrophysiological studies.
- Selected groups require consideration for an ICD.

- Higher risk: poor LV <35%, cardiac arrest (VF/VT) post-MI especially post acute phase, family history of sudden cardiac death, inducible VT at EPS, dilated cardiomyopathy.

11.2 Acute coronary syndrome

Term	Pathology	Clinical
STEMI	Plaque rupture/occlusive thrombus: needs 'culprit' vessel opening (PCI/thrombolysis) + anti-thrombotics.	Chest pain or equivalent + ST elevation/new LBBB + raised troponin.
NSTEMI	Sub-occlusive flow lesion and thrombus: needs antithrombotics and antianginals to maintain patency. Some myocardial damage.	Chest pain or equivalent + ECG changes + raised troponin.
Unstable angina	Sub-occlusive flow lesion and thrombus: needs antithrombotics and antianginals to maintain patency without myocardial damage.	Chest pain/equivalent + ECG changes + normal troponin.

About

- NSTEMI patients are older, with more comorbidities and a poorer prognosis long term.

Aetiology

- Atherosclerosis – unstable plaque ruptures releasing thrombogenic material.
- Causes *in situ* thrombosis +/– vessel occlusion.
- Type A aortic dissection occluding coronary ostia.
- Severe aortic stenosis, rare causes – embolism into coronary artery – endocarditis.
- Arteritis, antiphospholipid syndrome. Vasospasm, abnormal coronary arteries.

Exacerbating factors

- Reduced coronary flow due to huge wall pressures, e.g. aortic stenosis, HCM.
- Tachycardia, e.g. AF, VT with shortened diastole will reduce coronary blood flow.
- Increased myocardial work will increase O_2 demand and ischaemia.
- Anaemia: ideal Hb is 9–10 g/dL in IHD. Treat severe hypertension.
- Increased systemic O_2 demands – sepsis, PE, hypotension, shock.

Clinical

- Chest pain, SOB, sweating, nausea, vomiting, LVF, arrhythmias.
- Take careful history of onset of symptoms and relation to exertion.
- **Rest pain** is ominous and important. Assess for HTN, pulmonary oedema.
- New mitral regurgitation, valvular heart disease (aortic stenosis), hypertrophic cardiomyopathy.
- Heart failure and pulmonary disease.
- Breathlessness without pain, delirium and confusion in the elderly.
- Falls, delirium and syncope also in elderly.
- Epigastric symptoms (inferior MI).
- Silent MI: elderly and diabetics. ECG is paramount.

Signs

- Pale, terrified and cold peripherally, pulmonary oedema and cardiogenic shock.
- An S_3, PSM of mitral regurgitation, raised JVP and some basal inspiratory crackles.
- Pulmonary oedema is a poor prognostic sign. Ventricular arrhythmias acutely.

Differentials

- Pulmonary embolism, aortic dissection, pericarditis, oesophageal spasm/reflux/ rupture, biliary tract disease, peptic ulcer disease, pancreatitis.
- Chest wall pain, pleurisy/pneumonia, sickling crisis, herpes zoster, Bornholm disease.

Poor prognosis

- On-going and recurrent ischaemia, widespread ECG changes, raised CK/ troponins, low BP.
- Mitral regurgitation with ischaemia, pulmonary oedema, cardiogenic shock.

Investigations

- **Bloods**: **FBC**: low Hb exacerbates ACS. **U&E:** renal function. **Glucose**: diabetes.
- **Electrocardiogram:** always repeat with new symptoms. Comparison with previous ECGs is valuable. ECG splits patients with a suspicion of ACS in two categories requiring different therapeutic approaches: ST-segment elevation signifies complete occlusion of a major coronary artery and immediate reperfusion therapy is usually indicated. ST elevation due to STEMI is associated with ST depression in opposing leads as well as T wave changes.

ECG in ST elevation MI

- ECG ST elevation >2 mm in V1–V6 or >1 mm in any other 2 contiguous limb leads. New LBBB now only felt to suggest STEMI in a minority of patients. Take advice.
- Consider other causes of ST elevation which bear consideration.
  (1) High take off where ST looks elevated in V2, V3. No reciprocal changes elsewhere.
  (2) Myopericarditis saddle-shaped ST elevation all except cavity leads (aVr).
  (3) Coronary spasm – Prinzmetal's angina settles with antianginals.
  (4) LV aneurysm – history of previous anterior MI. Diagnose on echo.
  (5) Brugada syndrome – rare and not really associated with ACS. ST-segment changes but without persistent ST-segment elevation or a normal ECG. Will need estimation of biochemical markers. In a small number there are undetermined ECG changes such as BBB or pacemaker rhythm.

ECG in NSTEMI

- Symmetrical T wave inversion (in leads V1–V4 can suggest LAD stenosis).
- Transient ST elevation +/– but usually dynamic ST depression.

Cardiac biomarkers

- Troponin T/I (Trop T >0.1 ng/ml or Trop I >1 ng/ml at 12 h or before suggests MI rather than ischaemia/unstable angina). CKMB/AST/LDH are historical biomarkers superseded by troponin. CKMB may be useful where suspected false positive troponin occurs.
- False positives: tachyarrhythmias, myocarditis, coronary artery spasm from cocaine, severe cardiac failure, cardiac trauma from surgery or road traffic incident, pulmonary embolus, renal failure, acute exacerbation of LVF.

Echocardiogram

- Can show wall movement abnormalities suggesting ischaemia/infarction.
- Can be useful if ECG ambiguous. Assess LV function and regional wall abnormalities.

Cardiac stress tests

- If pain settles and ECG changes equivocal and troponin negative then consider controlled different ways to cause transient measurable myocardial ischaemia. Objective evidence of ischaemia may be displayed on ECG, echo or by scintigraphy.
- Tests to assess hibernating myocardium whose viability will improve with revascularisation by PCI or CABG. Cardiac MRI or PET scan. DOBUTAMINE stress echo, thallium. Most give a sensitivity of over 90% except stress echo (70%).

Angiography in STEMI / high risk NSTEMI

- This is the definitive test and shows any occluded or stenosed vessels and can assess cardiac function. If done early it allows opening of culprit vessel and opportunity for angioplasty and stenting or thrombus aspiration. It can help select those for CABG.

Cardiac troponin (*Circulation* 2011;124: 2350, but use local assay guidance)

Cardiac troponin T at 12 h µg/L	• <0.01 µg/L unstable angina • >0.01 µg/L and <1 µg/L: unstable angina or myocyte necrosis. Some guidelines define this as MI and others unstable angina • >1 µg/L: MI
Cardiac troponin I	• <0.06 ng/ml: normal; 0.07–0.49 ng/ml: indeterminate • >0.50 ng/ml: consistent with myocardial necrosis

Note about LBBB and acute MI and Sgarbossa and Wellen syndrome criteria

Despite traditional teaching there is increasing recognition that LBBB and chest pain are associated with acute MI due to occlusive thrombotic disease in a minority. To help support the diagnosis and avoid inappropriate thrombolysis or PCI, various characteristics can help.

The three ECG criteria in order of diagnostic power for acute MI in chest pain patients with LBBB or ventricular paced rhythm (VPR) were:

(1) ST segment elevation of >1 mm that was concordant in leads with a positive QRS complex (+5)
(2) ST segment depression of >1 mm in lead V1–V3 (+3), and
(3) ST segment elevation of >5 mm that was discordant with the QRS complex (+2) (in the usual opposite direction from the QRS but of heightened amplitude; less specific than 1 & 2 but more useful in VPR)

A total score of ≥3 has a specificity of 90% and sensitivity of 36% for diagnosing MI.

Acute management of all ACS patients

Acute management for <u>all</u> ACS patients

- **OXYGEN:** as per BTS guidance. Admit to CCU. Telemetry. Treat chest pain and/or pulmonary oedema.
- **NITRATES:** if chest pain or LVF give GTN sublingual 0.3–1 mg (1–2 sprays) or buccal nitrate 2–5 mg 8 hourly unless hypotensive. Watch BP. Ongoing pain or pulmonary oedema consider IV GTN infusion. Make up GTN 50 mg in 50 ml NS and run at 2–10 ml/h through syringe driver. Titrate to pain, breathlessness and BP.
- **OPIATES:** on-going pain or pulmonary oedema give either: DIAMORPHINE 2.5–5 mg IV with anti-emetic, e.g. METOCLOPRAMIDE 10 mg IV or MORPHINE 5–10 mg IV with anti-emetic, e.g. METOCLOPRAMIDE 10 mg IV.

- **ANTIPLATELETS:** give both ASPIRIN 300 mg PO stat chew/dispersible within 12 h (25% mortality reduction) and CLOPIDOGREL 300 mg PO stat and then 150 mg for 1 week and 75 mg OD after (see below) unless CABG planned. Seek senior advice. Other alternatives to CLOPIDOGREL include prasugrel or ticagrelor based on local guidance. See below.
- **BETA-BLOCKERS:** usually given IV in STEMI and as oral drugs in unstable angina/NSTEMI. Give either STEMI: METOPROLOL 1–5 mg IV (up to 15 mg given) stop if SBP <100 mmHg or HR <60 bpm. NSTEMI: METOPROLOL 25–50 mg PO tds or oral ATENOLOL 50–100 mg OD. Avoid if asthmatic, hypotensive, LVF, HR <60, 2nd or 3rd degree heart block. Unable to take beta blockers try DILTIAZEM 60–90 mg (up to 120 mg BD) BD PO.
- **ANTICOAGULANTS:** consider one of these: ENOXAPARIN 1 mg/kg SC BD (LMWH) for 2–8 days or until revascularisation or discharge. FONDAPARINUX 2.5 mg SC OD for 2–8 days or until revascularisation or discharge. BIVALIRUDIN 0.75 mg/kg instead of heparin, plus a GPI if the patient is not on fondaparinux or a GPI and angiography is scheduled within 24 h of admission. Unfractionated HEPARIN IV bolus up to 4000 U and then 1000 U/h to give APTT 1.5–2 × control.

OTHERS

- **If diabetes or blood sugar** >11.0 mmol/L then a variable rate IV insulin infusion should be used to aim for good glycaemic control (6–10 mmol/L). Avoid hypoglycaemia.
- **High dose statin** ATORVASTATIN 40–80 mg PO ON.
- **Pulmonary oedema**: Furosemide 50–100 mg IV.
- **ACE inhibitor RAMIPRIL 1.25 mg OD** if signs of heart failure or reduced LV function.
- **IV fluids**: should be considered unless pulmonary oedema. Can help with RV failure due to inferior MI with hypotension and raised JVP.
- **Treat as STEMI** if ST elevation >2 mm in V1–V6 or >1 mm in any other two contiguous limb leads or new LBBB for urgent revascularisation.
- **GP IIb/IIIa inhibitors if patient is for PCI:** these include ABCIXIMAB, EPTIFIBATIDE, TIROFIBAN depending on local policy. These can be considered with aspirin and clopidogrel when undergoing PCI.

CLOPIDOGREL and alternatives

- **CLOPIDOGREL 300–600 mg PO stat followed by 150 mg OD for a week and then 75 mg OD for 12 months.** A higher clopidogrel loading dose (600 mg) should be considered if patients undergoing PCI within 24 h of admission.
- **TICAGRELOR 180 mg** followed by **Ticagrelor 90 mg BD** for up to 12 months may be used instead of clopidogrel in NSTEMI or unstable angina with ST/T changes and age >60 y, previous MI or CABG, CAD with stenosis >50% in at least two vessels; previous ischaemic stroke/TIA, carotid stenosis of at least 50%, or cerebral revascularisation; diabetes mellitus; peripheral arterial disease; or CKD with creatinine clearance of less than 60 ml/min/1.73 m^2 of body surface area.
- **PRASUGREL 60 mg stat followed by 10 mg OD for up to 15 months** may be used instead of clopidogrel if the patient with ACS (NSTEMI) is considered for PCI and stent thrombosis has occurred during clopidogrel treatment or the patient has diabetes mellitus.

STEMI management to urgently open the 'culprit' vessel

- **STEMI diagnosis**: chest pain + ST elevation >2 mm in two or more contiguous chest leads V1–V6, or ST elevation >1 mm in two or more contiguous limb leads, or new LBBB. If there are signs of posterior MI (tall R wave V1 and reciprocal ST changes) take immediate senior advice.
- **Primary percutaneous coronary intervention (PPCI):** PPCI within 90 min of patient arrival at hospital is preferred as superior to fibrinolysis in reducing death, stroke, and re-infarction where a skilled interventional cardiologist and catheterisation laboratory with surgical backup are available. Perform within 12 h of symptom onset. Allows angioplasty and stenting of culprit

lesion with reperfusion and salvage of viable myocardium. **PPCI** also preferred if contraindication to fibrinolytic therapy, e.g. bleeding risk or older patients (>75y; increased risk of ICH with fibrinolysis) or those with cardiovascular compromise (LVF/shock) suggesting a high risk of an infarct-related complicated medical course or death. Patients usually receive a combination of antiplatelet and anticoagulants prior to and during PCI as detailed above. GPIIb/IIIa inhibitors (GPIs) should also be considered.

- **Stenting culprit vessels – bare metal stents** (BMS) routinely used and need a minimum 3 months clopidogrel as well as aspirin. Preferred in those who cannot tolerate long-term dual antiplatelet therapy. **Drug-eluting stents** (DES) are bare metal stents coated with a drug, usually an immune suppressant to reduce inflammation or an antimitotic agent to reduce cell proliferation, and need 12 months clopidogrel and aspirin. There is a risk of stent thrombosis associated with the use of both DES and BMS, but seemingly more so with DES. **Drug eluting stents** have a small reduction in target vessel revascularisation (TVR) rates so only used in higher risk patients (diabetes/high risk lesions) and where the target artery to be treated has less than a 3 mm calibre, or the lesion is longer than 15 mm. *DES and BMS show no difference in mortality or MI rates or stent thrombosis. Avoid DES if raised bleed risk with prolonged dual antiplatelet therapy for 12 months.* (NICE 2003, TA71: Ischaemic heart disease – coronary artery stents.)

Cardiac thrombolysis (reduces hospital mortality by 25–50%)

- Those patients not suitable for PCI (or PCI not available), those who seek medical attention less than 1 h after the onset of symptoms (in whom the therapy may abort the infarction), and those with a history of anaphylaxis due to radiographic contrast material. Door to needle time should be less than 30 min.
- Offer thrombolysis to those with acute STEMI presenting within 12 h of onset of symptoms if PPCI cannot be delivered within 120 min of the time when fibrinolysis could have been given.
- If ST elevation persists for 60–90 min post fibrinolysis then reconsider PCI. Further administration of fibrinolytic is not recommended.
- **Contraindications to cardiac thrombolysis:** bleeding (gynaecological, internal, gastrointestinal, urological), acute pancreatitis, severe liver disease, oesophageal varices, recent trauma/surgery within 2 weeks, BP >200/120 mmHg, suspected aortic dissection, allergic to thrombolytic agents, brain tumour, haemorrhagic stroke at any time, ischaemic stroke within 3 months.

Thrombolytic agents

- **STREPTOKINASE**: 1.5 MU in 100 ml NS over 1 h. S/E hypotension, slowing down and give fluid challenge but no need to stop. Other agents preferred for anterior infarction. Streptokinase tends not to be reused because antibodies are formed which reduce efficacy. Anaphylaxis – hydrocortisone and chlorphenamine.
- **TENECTEPLASE** 30–50 mg IV push in 10 s.
- **ALTEPLASE** 15 mg IV push, 50 mg over 30 min and then 35 mg over 60 min.
- **RETEPLASE**: 2 × 10 unit boluses given 30 min apart.
- **ALTEPLASE, RETEPLASE and TENECTEPLASE** need IV heparin for 24–48 h and then LMWH for 4–8 days. IV heparin is not needed following STREPTOKINASE.
- **Bleeding after thrombolysis:** if bleeding is serious or life threatening give **Tranexamic acid 1 g IV over 15 min** whilst awaiting coagulation indices. If thrombin time and INR are prolonged but fibrinogen >1 g/L give 2–4 U of FFP. If thrombin time is prolonged and fibrinogen is low (<1 g/L), give 10 U cryoprecipitate.
- **Advice on agents:** alteplase/reteplase preferred over STREPTOKINASE in anterior MI or new LBBB and those who have previously had STREPTOKINASE where PPCI is not possible. Cerebral haemorrhage risk additional 4 per 1000 patients treated. Bleed risks are 0.5–1.0%.

NSTEMI risk assessment

Risk assessing the more severe NSTEMI cases for angiogram +/– PCI

TIMI risk score for NSTEMI

- Age >65 y +1; >3 risk factors for CAD +1; known CAD (stenosis >50%) +1
- ASPIRIN use in past 7 day +1; severe angina (> 2 episodes/24 h) +1
- ST changes > 0.5 mm +1; cardiac marker +1.

Use the TIMI score to risk stratify NSTEMI patients for an early angiography strategy**:** TIMI >4 is high risk with 20% risk at 14 days of all-cause mortality, new or recurrent MI, or severe recurrent ischaemia requiring angiography and urgent revascularisation.

Markers of high risk NSTEMI

- Persistent / recurrent angina, ST depression >2 mm, deep negative T waves.
- Signs of heart failure or hypotension EF <0.4, sustained VT, positive stress test.
- Diabetes mellitus, renal impairment, reduced LV function, previous CABG or recent PCI <6/12.

Diabetic patients

- Are likely to have multivessel disease and have a worse prognosis.
- They should undergo inpatient angiography if possible.

Exercise stress testing is used to risk-stratify patients except in those with severe aortic stenosis, LBBB, on-going typical chest pain, haemodynamic instability, dynamic ST changes, severe LV outflow obstruction and hypertrophic cardiomyopathy, poor mobility.
Risks of coronary angiography: death 1 in 1000 (0.1%), MI 1 in 1000 (0.1%), stroke 1 in 1000 (0.1%), significant arterial complications 1 in 500 (0.2%).
Risk of PCI (angioplasty and stenting): death 0.7%, MI (usually minor) <1%, stroke <1%, emergency CABG 1 in 200 (0.5%), significant arterial complications 1 in 200 (0.5%).

Complications	Notes
Tachyarrhythmias	AF, sinus tachycardia, ventricular ectopics, idioventricular rhythm (do not treat if not compromised), VT, VF (particularly VF/VT amendable to early defibrillation, which is key).
Bradyarrhythmias	Sinus bradycardia, heart block; may need pacing if haemodynamically compromised and both bundle branches taken out.
On-going chest pain	Escalate to look for treatable ischaemia or PCI/thrombolysis if re-infarction or failed reperfusion.
LV dysfunction	Heart failure, cardiogenic shock; poor prognosis. Needs echocardiogram. Survival LV function.
Venous thromboembolism	DVT, PE.
Myocardial rupture	VSD seen in 3% of MIs, usually in first week and seen more in elderly. Sudden loud PSM with hypotension/CCF but more right-sided failure than seen with acute myocardial rupture. Needs urgent echocardiogram and surgical assessment for repair.

Complications	Notes
Acute mitral regurgitation	Due to papillary muscle dysfunction. Day 2–7 post MI. Partial rupture – loud PSM, S3 and hypotension and CCF. Complete rupture of papillary muscle can cause rapid death, usually in first week. Surgery is associated with high risk. Echocardiogram to confirm. Rupture of free wall – usually causes cardiac tamponade and sudden cardiac death. Discuss with tertiary cardiology centre.
Ventricular septal rupture	Seen with Q wave MI affecting septum. Hypotension and PSM at the left sternal edge, but less breathless than acute myocardial rupture. Pulmonary plethora rather than oedema on CXR. Urgent referral is required, and IABP as a bridge to surgical closure. Discuss with tertiary centre.
LV aneurysm	After 2–3 months presenting with dyspnoea, hypotension and a dyskinetic parasternal pulsation and ST elevation. Take advice. Echocardiography. Some may need surgery. Rupture is main concern as well as thromboembolism and arrhythmias.
Intracardiac thrombus and cardioembolism	From akinetic cardiac apex, left atrial or LV aneurysm. Causes stroke, ischaemic limb, mesenteric ischaemia. Tends to be acute and needs anticoagulation. Warfarin should be continued for 3 months, unless AF or considered high risk when it may be continued.
Psychosocial	Depression, sexual impotence, employment issues.
Pericarditis	Early, late (Dressler's syndrome), widespread saddle-shaped ST elevation.

Post ACS management (NEJM, 2007; 356:47)

- **ANTIPLATELET:** aspirin 75 mg OD long term. CLOPIDOGREL 75 mg OD PO 1 month minimum and additional as per diagnosis and stenting, continue for 1 y after NSTEMI.
- **ACE inhibition**: ramipril 1.25–5 mg PO 12 hourly or enalapril 10 mg PO 12 hourly for all non-hypotensive patients can help reduce ventricular remodelling in the first 4–6 weeks. Continue long term for those with impaired LV function.
- **Statin:** atorvastatin commencing at 80 mg at night for at least 3 months, then the choice of statin to be selected by the GP on their review. Reduces cholesterol and mortality. Aim to get total cholesterol <4 mmol/L and LDL-C <2 mmol/L.
- **Nitrates:** for on-going chest pain or pulmonary oedema. IV nitrate or buccal nitrate 2–5 mg 8 hourly.
- **Beta-blocker:** long term, e.g. Metoprolol or Bisoprolol 2.5–10 mg PO OD especially with impaired LV function.
- **Eplerenone** (aldosterone antagonist): used for heart failure. Start Eplerenone 25 mg OD after the initiation of the ACE within the first 3–14 days post MI if there is poor LV function.
- **Warfarin/NOAC** for AF, Warfarin for LV thrombus, PE, DVT.
- **ICD:** if VT/VF >48 h after the initial MI or cardiac arrest and poor LV.
- **Antihypertensive:** aim for BP <140/90 mmHg.
- **Other:** smoking cessation; cardiac rehabilitation; diabetic control: HbA1c <7%; annual influenza vaccination.

11.3 Arrhythmias

ECG interpretation of arrhythmias

- Heart rate = 300/R to R interval squares. ECG is a graph:
  - X axis (horizontal) is time at 25 mm/s; each small square is 40 ms.
  - Y axis (vertical) is millivolts at 1 mV = 1 cm; each small square is 0.1 mV.
- Normal PR interval is 120–200 ms (3–5 small squares); normal QRS is <120 ms (3 small squares).
- QT (measured from the start of the QRS to the end of the T wave); correct for rate (QTc) to 60 beats/min using the equation: QTc = (QT)/(square root of RR,) where RR is the RR interval in seconds.
- Normal between 0.35 and 0.43 s (9–11 small squares).
- Irregular: measure RR interval and it changes beat to beat. Broad complex QRS >3 small squares.

ECG	Diagnosis	Management
Slow ventricular rate	CHB	If rate has caused the associated hypotension and circulatory collapse consider repeated atropine 0.5 mg IV and Isoprenaline. IV Glucagon if on beta-blockers. External pacing as a bridge to transvenous pacing. See *Chapter 1*.
Irregular broad complex	Fast AF	Treat as fast AF. Consider IV Amiodarone. However, if there are delta waves or WPW suspected **avoid IV Digoxin or Verapamil**. If unwell consider low voltage DC cardioversion.
Regular broad complex	VT or aberrantly conducted SVT	Treat with IV Amiodarone 150–300 mg IV over 20–60 min. Consider carotid massage if safe (aged <50 and no suggestion of TIA/Stroke/Bruit) and/or adenosine if you think it's aberrantly conducted SVT. DC cardiovert if falling BP. **Do not give IV Verapamil**.
Narrow complex regular	AVRT or AVNRT or atrial flutter 2:1, 3:1 or 4:1 block	Can settle spontaneously. Usually benign unless in context of other cardiac disease. Consider CSM. IV adenosine is very useful. IV beta blockade. If very unwell consider low voltage DC cardioversion. **If AVRT and WPW avoid Digoxin or Verapamil.**
Narrow complex irregular	Fast AF	Consider IV amiodarone or IV beta-blocker or IV Digoxin. If very unwell consider low voltage DC cardioversion if anticoagulated or very recent onset (<24–48 h).

Differential of a narrow complex tachycardia

Regular	Irregular
Sinus tachycardia	Atrial fibrillation
Paroxysmal SVT	Atrial flutter with variable block
Atrial flutter with 2:1, 3:1 or 4:1 block	Atrial tachycardia with variable block
Atrial tachycardia with consistent conduction	Multifocal atrial tachycardia
AV reciprocating (orthodromic) tachycardia (WPW)	

11.4 Ventricular tachycardia

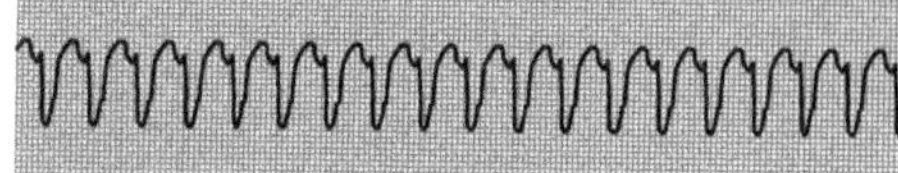

About

- All fast unstable rhythms should be considered for urgent DC cardioversion. Most broad complex regular tachycardias are VT especially if there is evidence of IHD. But some are simply SVT with a BBB.
- VT can be well tolerated and then decompensate depending on LV function, rate and ischaemia. Ensure immediate access to defibrillation.

Aetiology

- Increased automaticity, circus entry pathways, channelopathies.
- Broad complex and regular >3 small squares or 120 ms QRS complexes.

Note

- VT can degenerate quickly into pulseless VT or VF. Patients must be monitored constantly to enable rapid access to defibrillation. Broad complex regular (QRS >120 ms (3 small squares)) HR >120/min.
- Differentiate from an SVT with aberrant conduction. Prognosis very much related to LV function.

Differential of a regular broad complex tachycardia

- (Accelerated) idioventricular rhythm (HR 100–120/min) seen post MI.
- Monomorphic ventricular tachycardia: regular wide complex.
- Polymorphic VT (Torsades de pointes) seen with long QT.
- SVT / atrial flutter or atrial tachycardia with aberrant conduction.
- WPW syndrome with retrograde conduction of an AVNRT / atrial flutter.
- Motion artefact, pacemaker syndromes (consider turning off pacemaker with a magnet).

Findings suggestive of VT (must treat as VT if unsure)

- Fusion beats, capture (narrow) beats.
- Ischaemic heart disease or known structural heart disease.
- Absence of RS wave in V1–V6.
- Presence of AV dissociation (Cannon 'a' waves).
- RBBB pattern >140 ms; LBBB pattern >160 ms.
- Extreme LAD, extreme R to R regularity.

Causes of VT

- **Cardiac disease**: IHD especially with LV dysfunction, cardiomyopathy (hypertrophic cardiomyopathy, dilated, restrictive), arrhythmogenic RV dysplasia, myocarditis, sarcoidosis, haemochromatosis.
- **Drug induced,** e.g. TCA overdose, digoxin, antiarrhythmics, hypo- or hyperkalaemia, hypomagnesaemia, hypocalcaemia, cocaine, phaeochromocytoma.
- **Channelopathies:** Brugada syndrome, long QT syndromes, drugs causing long QT.
- **Others**: chest trauma, idiopathic, structural congenital disorders.

Clinical

- Some tolerate VT very well, others develop angina, pulmonary oedema, cardiac arrest. Depends on LV function, rate and coronary perfusion.
- Palpitations, breathlessness, pulmonary oedema.
- Hypotension, chest pain, Cannon 'a' wave in JVP (AV dissociation).
- Status depends on ventricular rate and underlying LV function.

Investigations

- **Bloods**: check FBC, U&E, cardiac troponin, Mg, Ca.
- **Serial ECGs**: ensure capture 12-lead of the arrhythmia if possible.
- **Echocardiogram**: for LV systolic and diastolic function and structural disease.
- **Coronary angiogram**: to look for treatable coronary artery disease.
- **Electrophysiology studies**: provoke arrhythmias, mapping.

Management

- If pulseless then ALS algorithm. Otherwise IV access and O_2 as per BTS guidelines.
- **IV DIAMORPHINE OR MORPHINE** for chest pain if present.
- **Revascularisation** (PCI / thrombolysis) if STEMI or severe ischaemic basis suspected.
- **Correct electrolytes**. Keep K^+ >4 mmol/L.
- Consider **IV MAGNESIUM** especially if low (alcoholics/diuretics).
- **AMIODARONE** IV or **LIDOCAINE** IV may be considered (see *Chapter 30*). If not responding to drugs or hypotension or persisting, then consider **synchronised DC cardioversion** (see *Chapter 1*).

Prevention

- Follow up with a cardiologist specialising in arrhythmias. Needs echocardiogram, angiography and electrophysiological studies and Holter monitoring and cardiac MRI.
- Treatment of underlying cause, e.g. treat IHD – drugs, PCI, CABG.
- Antiarrhythmics: **SOTALOL** usually when LV function is good, **AMIODARONE** when LV function is impaired. ICD implantation + SOTALOL/AMIODARONE.

11.5 Torsades de pointes (polymorphic VT)

About

- Torsades de pointes (TdP) is a polymorphic VT where the axis constantly changes.
- Associated with acquired and congenital long QT syndromes.

Aetiology

- Prolonged ventricular repolarisation (QT duration).
- Precipitated by antiarrhythmic drugs that cause a long QT interval.
- Note usually when QTc >500 ms. It does not correlate with risk.

Drug causes of long QT – check all drugs taken in *BNF*

- Amiodarone, erythromycin, terfenadine, TCA, quinidine.
- Methadone, class I and III antiarrhythmics, lithium, phenothiazine.
- Hypokalaemia, hypomagnesaemia, hypocalcaemia, congenital syndromes.

Congenital long QT syndromes

- Genetically driven. Long QT due to various channelopathies.
- Beta blockade advocated for congenital long QT syndromes.
- Some may require ICD.

Investigations

- **Bloods**: check FBC, U&E, troponin, Mg, Ca.
- **Serial ECGs** and ensure capture 12-lead of the arrhythmia if possible.
- **Echocardiogram** for LV and valves or structural disease.
- Electrophysiology studies may be useful.

Management

- **Exclude drug cause**: avoid amiodarone or other antiarrhythmics because they can lengthen QT. Stop any drugs which may be to blame (check *BNF*).
- Check and correct electrolytes and K/Ca/Mg. Give **IV Magnesium 8 mmol over 15 min then 72 mmol over 24 h**.
- **Pacing**: temporary atrial or ventricular pacing increases ventricular rate which can terminate and reduce the episodes of TdP until the QT normalises.
- **Isoprenaline** can also be used to increase rate but *not in those with congenital long QT syndromes*.
- **ICD for high risk patients,** i.e. QT >500 ms and high risk genotypes with congenital long QT syndromes
- If unstable then give Magnesium and consider **synchronised DC cardioversion** (see *Chapter 1*).

11.6 Supraventricular tachycardia

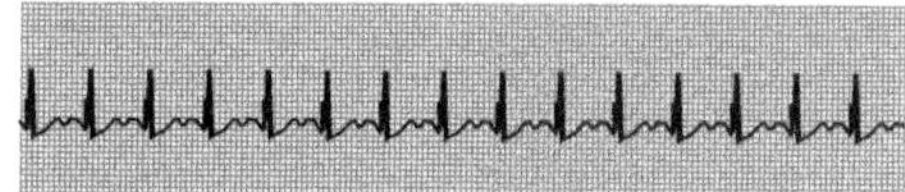

About

- SVT (excludes AF and flutter). Usually AVNRT or AVRT.
- A benign but troublesome arrhythmia not typically associated with cardiac death.
- Hospital admission if there is structural heart disease or severe symptoms.
- Seen in 3 in 1000 often young females but can occur at any age.
- The heart is usually structurally normal. The cure is ablation.

ECG

- QRS complex width <120 ms (assuming no IV conduction defect).
- QRS complexes are regular, HR >100 bpm, AVRT or AVNRT are 150–200/min. P wave buried in QRS.

Differential of fast regular narrow tachycardia

- Sinus tachycardia, atrial tachycardia.
- Atrial flutter 2:1 or 3:1 block (vagal stimulation will show flutter waves).

AVNRT

- Circus re-entry pathways around the AV node. Two pathways: one fast conduction but a long refractory period and one slow conduction and shorter refractory period.
- Usually anterograde (A to V) conduction is through the slow side and retrograde through the fast, then it is a slow–fast AVNRT, and vice versa. Often induced by an ectopic atrial beat when the fast side is still refractory. Captures the slow path and conducts back along the fast pathway.

- Retrograde activated P waves seen in the QRS. Retrograde ventricular conduction is fast with slow–fast and so this is a short RP form as the atria is stimulated very quickly. Fast–slow are long RP forms. The rarest form is slow–slow.

AVRT

- Accessory pathway joins atria and ventricles electrically.
- Seen with WPW syndrome or Lown–Ganong–Levine.
- Accessory pathways can conduct anterogradely or retrogradely.
- They are not always evident on the resting ECG and may be 'concealed'.
- Dangerous when patient develops AF and has an accessory pathway that allows rapid anterograde conduction. See also *Section 11.8*.

Clinical

- Palpitations, dizziness, light headed even syncope, mild hypotension but not cardiac arrest unless coexisting cardiac disease. Post palpitation polyuria due to release of ANP.
- AVNRT may cause heart failure if poor LV or other structural heart disease, e.g. mitral stenosis.

Electrocardiogram

- Narrow complex QRS rates of 150–250 bpm and a regular rhythm.
- AVNRT + aberrancy with a wide complex tachycardia. P waves are not seen hidden within the QRS complex. Onset with an atrial premature complex, which conducts with a prolonged PR interval.
- Fast–slow has a P wave before the QRS complex.
- Slow–slow AVNRT can occur with a P wave mid-diastole.
- Abrupt termination occurs retrograde P wave +/– brief asystole or bradycardia.

Investigations

- **Bloods:** FBC, U&E, TFT, CXR, CRP.
- **Echocardiogram**: exclude structural disease and show LV function.
- **Troponin** only if IHD suspected, e.g. chest pain and ECG changes.
- **Electrophysiology** studies as precursor to ablation and other therapies.

Management

- **ABC**: rarely indicated. If the patient is stable then simply trying some vagal manoeuvres or adenosine is usually successful.
- **Vagal manoeuvres**, e.g. valsalva, cold water on the face – diving reflex, carotid sinus massage. In a younger person this is fairly safe. In an older person aged >50 or with a history of TIA or a bruit then best avoided because it may cause TIA/stroke.
- **ADENOSINE IV** is excellent at terminating re-entrant tachycardias, e.g. AVRT and AVNRT, or slowing atrial flutter. **ATENOLOL IV** or other beta-blocker is very reasonable if not asthmatic. If asthmatic then **VERAPAMIL** slow IV is useful if there is no concern about poor LV function and the rhythm is definitely narrow complex.
- **AMIODARONE IV** over 20–60 min is another possibility.
- **Synchronised DC cardioversion** is the management for any tachycardia if hypotensive or unwell (see *Chapter 1*).
- Most patients can go home following resumption of sinus rhythm for outpatient cardiology referral to discuss ablation therapy to prevent further arrhythmias. Exclude thyrotoxicosis.

11.7 Symptomatic bradycardia

About

- BP is more important than HR – determine quickly if patient is compromised.
- A young and fit athlete may have a resting HR of 40 bpm.
- Second-degree heart block can suggest impending CHB/asystole.

Sinus bradycardia

- Normal P wave and QRS complex at rate <60 bpm. Intrinsic rate is 100/min. Vagal tone can slow the heart to 70/min or <50/min when sleeping.
- High vagal tone, e.g. post vasovagal syncope 'faint', cholestatic jaundice.
- Excess beta blockade, conduction tissue disease, hypothyroidism. Raised intracranial pressure.

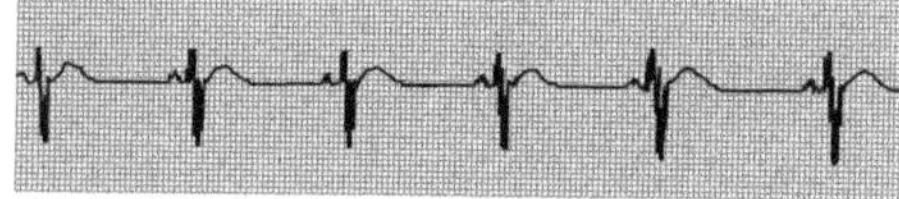

Sinus pauses/arrest

- Normal P QRS T wave then no P wave for 3 s or longer.
- Stop any exacerbating drugs. May need to be paced if symptomatic.

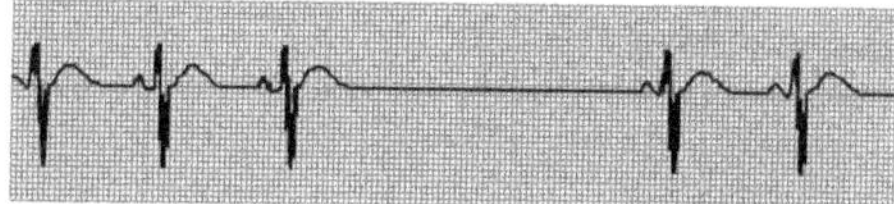

Slow atrial fibrillation

- Irregular QRS complex, absent P wave. Natural rate 90–100 bpm.
- May suggest excess digoxin/beta blockers or AV nodal disease.

Tachy–brady syndrome

- The bradycardia side can be sinus pauses, sinus bradycardia.

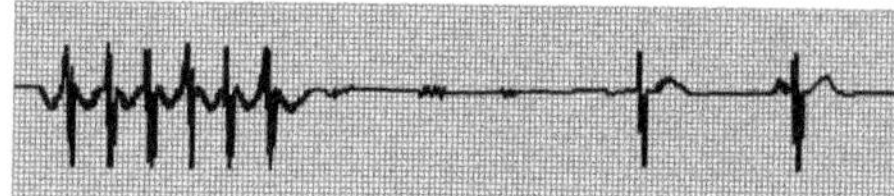

1st degree heart block

- Long PR >200–220 ms; each P wave followed by a delayed QRS complex.
- Overall ventricular HR unaffected unless other disease. Rarely needs intervention.

2nd degree heart block – Mobitz Type I

- P wave and lengthening PR until a P wave fails to be followed by a QRS complex.
- Wenckebach phenomenon is due to a block at AV nodal level.
- May be physiological or seen at rest or sleeping or in athletes.
- Pacing rarely needed except if symptomatic bradycardia.

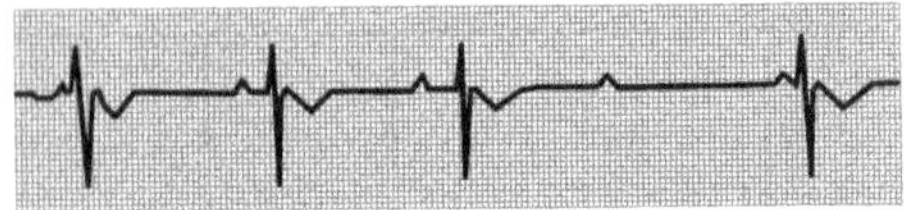

2nd Degree heart block – Mobitz Type II

- QRS is intermittently dropped but not preceded by a progressively lengthening PR interval. Damage is infranodal and is a more significant arrhythmia with lower threshold to pace than Mobitz I.
- Pace if permanent or intermittent, regardless of the type or the site of the block, with symptomatic bradycardia. Consider pacing in setting of acute MI. Risk of asystole.

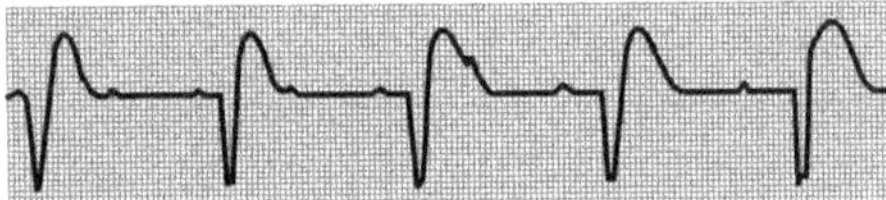

2nd degree with 2:1 or 3:1 block

- Every 2nd or 3rd beat is blocked and does not conduct to ventricles.
- Disease may be at AV node or below. Pace if symptomatic or acute MI.

3rd degree complete heart block

- Complete failure of communication between atria and ventricles. Ventricles beat at intrinsic rate which may be 30-40 bpm. Cannon 'a' waves are seen with complete heart block
- Nearly always requires pacing. Risk of asystole.

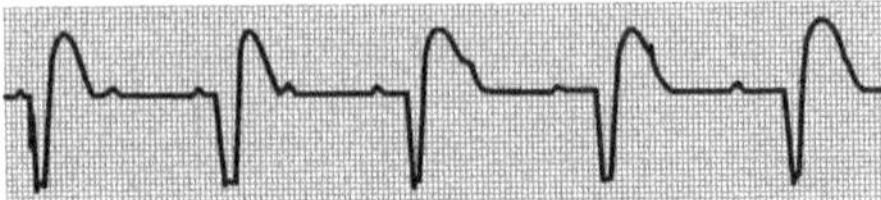

Clinical

- May be pale, shocked, low BP, HR <60 bpm. Obtunded.
- Some patients, e.g. bed-bound elderly, can tolerate CHB quite well.
- **Stokes–Adams attacks** are due to short periods of asystole or very slow CHB.

Investigations

- U&E, FBC, cardiac troponin if ACS suspected.
- ECG, echocardiogram to assess LV.

Management

- ABC O_2, IV fluids, IV access, ECG monitor.
- If BP <90/60 mmHg and HR <60 bpm consider **ATROPINE 0.5–1 mg IV** to a maximum dose of 3 mg.
- Persisting hypotensive bradycardia try **ISOPRENALINE infusion or ADRENALINE or DOPAMINE infusion. GLUCAGON infusion** has classically been recommended for beta-blocker induced bradycardia.
- **Transvenous cardiac pacing** if hypotensive due to bradycardia.

- **AV block and acute MI:** a branch of the RCA supplies AV node. May cause transient AV block with an escape rhythm and if patient well no treatment needed. May improve with reperfusion. Can give atropine. If worsens then temporary pacing. AV block tends to resolve in approximately 1 week. AV block in anterior MI suggests significant damage to bundle branches, and 2nd or 3rd degree AV block carries risk of asystole and should be paced.

Indications for a permanent pacemaker

Absolute

- Sick sinus syndrome, symptomatic sinus bradycardia, tachycardia-bradycardia syndrome.
- AF with sinus node dysfunction, complete AV block (third-degree block).
- Chronotropic incompetence (inability to increase the heart rate to match a level of exercise).
- Prolonged QT syndrome, cardiac resynchronization therapy with biventricular pacing.

Relative

- Cardiomyopathy (hypertrophic or dilated).
- Severe refractory neurocardiogenic syncope.

Complications of pacing: pneumothorax, pericarditis, infection, skin erosion, haematoma, lead dislodgment, venous thrombosis.

11.8 Fast atrial fibrillation

Most morbidity in AF is caused by stroke which embolises from clot in the LA appendage. Assess stroke risk from CHA_2DS_2VaSc or similar scoring system and consider anticoagulation.

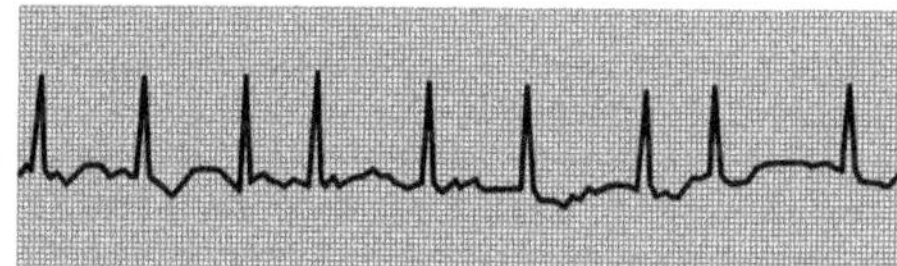

About

- AF due to uncoordinated atrial activation with atrial mechanical dysfunction.
- It is a major risk factor for ischaemic stroke. Assess with risk score.

Aetiology

- Atrial fibrosis and loss of atrial muscle mass.
- Increased automaticity or multiple re-entrant wavelets.
- Atrial 'rate' of AF is 400–600/min but the ventricular response that matters.
- Ventricular rate held in check by AV node at <200/min.
- An accessory bundle (WPW) can allow faster rates to conduct AV causing VF.

Haemodynamics

- Increased HR shortens diastole and limits LV filling and coronary perfusion.
- LV filling already compromised by loss of atrial systole.
- Rate control with drugs, treat failure and DC shock if needed.
- Impaired LV function or mitral stenosis makes things much worse.

Clinical

- Often asymptomatic, palpitations, chest pain as can provoke ischaemia.
- Cardioembolic stroke, mesenteric emboli, limb emboli, dyspnoea.
- Fatigue and worsening heart failure, syncope, presyncope.
- Hypotension with fast/slow AF, irregularly irregular pulse. Pulse deficit.
- Murmurs suggesting valve disease, signs of thyroid disease, hypertension.

Causes of atrial fibrillation

- Ischaemic heart disease; valvular/rheumatic heart disease
- Hypertensive heart disease; cardiomyopathy; post cardiac surgery
- Thyrotoxicosis; alcohol – acute binge or chronic; sick sinus syndrome
- Congenital heart disease; pulmonary embolism; pneumonia
- Sarcoidosis; amyloidosis; haemochromatosis
- Lone AF (idiopathic); pericarditis; myocarditis

Classification of atrial fibrillation

- Persistent: lasts >7 days
- Paroxysmal: more than 2 episodes self-terminating lasting <7 days
- Permanent: lasts >1 year and fails to cardiovert
- Lone AF: aged <60 y, no hypertension, normal echo, no risk factors

Investigations

- **Bloods:** FBC anaemia, raised WCC with sepsis, U&E, Mg, Ca, K, TFT thyrotoxicosis, LFTs, alcohol, haemochromatosis.
- **CXR:** cardiomegaly, pulmonary oedema, infection, post cardiac surgery effusion.
- **Troponin:** raised with ACS or myocarditis and minor rise with DC shock.
- **ECG:** absent 'P' waves – no organised atrial activity, fibrillatory waves that vary in amplitude, shape, and timing, QRS complexes which are irregularly irregular. **Aberrantly conducted AF** – wide complex and fast but irregular. **Pre-excited AF:** QRS 160–300/min and slurred up or down stroke of delta waves seen giving wide complex appearance but very irregular; the irregularity means that it is not VT.
- **Transthoracic echocardiogram:** assess LV function, valve disease, LA size.
- **Transoesophageal echocardiogram**: closer inspection of valves, mitral disease, ASD, endocarditis, LA thrombus may be seen and can help assess risk of thromboembolism.
- **Coronary angiography**: if IHD suspected.

Management: compromised = hypotensive, pulmonary oedema, chest pain.

- **ABC + give O_2** as per BTS guidelines and reassess after ABG.
- IV fluids cautiously if at all in LVF or fluid overloaded.
- **Treat any cause**: chest infection, thyrotoxicosis, ACS, PE, infection, etc.
- **Treat any pulmonary oedema – FUROSEMIDE 50–100 mg IV stat** +/– Diamorphine.
- **Newly diagnosed AF and well:** rate 60–120 and haemodynamically well. Determine and manage cause.
- **Fast AF and compromised:** needs O_2, IV access and **AMIODARONE 150–300 mg IV** over 10–20 min through a large bore cannula or preferably a central line. If this is not working quickly then perform emergency DC cardioversion. Further amiodarone infusions require a central line. Give LMW heparin.
- **Fast AF and not compromised (fast AF >110/min):** consider **IV/PO DIGOXIN 500 mcg** infusion or orally and then **DIGOXIN 250–500 mcg orally** 6 h later, and then **125 mcg**

once daily. Reduce dose with renal failure. Many would suggest beta-blocker first line, e.g. Bisoprolol, Atenolol or Metoprolol are reasonable, especially if angina or hypertension. Consider anticoagulation as above.

- **Fast AF and not compromised and known onset <2 days:** consider chemical cardioversion, e.g. **Flecainide** when there is no evidence of structural heart disease or IHD, but usually requires an echo. If any doubt then some might give oral loading of **AMIODARONE.** Anticoagulate.
- **Pre-excited AF and WPW syndrome:** the treatment of choice is **IV PROCAINAMIDE** but if not available then Sotalol or Flecainide or Amiodarone and if this is unsuccessful then immediate DC cardioversion should be considered. **DO NOT GIVE DIGOXIN TO AF IN WPW.**
- Urgent synchronised DC cardioversion if persisting or unstable: (*see Chapter 1*).
- **Anticoagulation:** consider in all whose AF lasts more than 24/48 h or PAF. Determine CHA_2DS_2VaSc score and HAS-BLED score and assess risk/benefits of anticoagulation. If non-valvular AF (those with severe MS or AS or with a metal valve must have warfarin) then consider Warfarin or one of the novel oral anticoagulants. In those who cannot take warfarin, e.g. allergy or pregnant then LMWH should be considered. High CHA_2DS_2VaSc score needs either LMWH or a new oral anticoagulant rather than to wait for an outpatient warfarin clinic during which they have a stroke.

11.9 Aortic dissection

> If suspected then arrange urgent CT aorta and if Type A dissection found you must reduce the BP whilst getting the patient to a cardiothoracic centre immediately.

About

- Aorta consists of the layers intima, media and adventitia. Dissection involves separation of the media and intima often with intramural bleeding with haematoma which can dissect distally or sometimes proximally (into pericardium) powered by the pulsatile force of the aortic flow.

Aetiology

- Blood can track under the intima and into the media. There can be bleeding from vasa vasorum causing intramural thrombus. The intima can tear distally and lead to a double lumen. On CT or other imaging there can be a 'true lumen' and 'false lumen'
- There may be a connective tissue problem such as cystic medial degeneration, Marfan's and Ehlers–Danlos syndrome. May also be seen with blunt thoracic trauma causing a tear in the arterial wall.
- Intima tears within a few centimetres of the aortic valve, usually on the right lateral wall of the aortic arch where shear stresses are high. Distal dissections occur beyond left subclavian artery. Obstruction of RCA more common. Occlusion of LCA usually instantly fatal. Dissection can therefore be accompanied by MI.

Causes

- HTN, aortic atherosclerosis, cystic medial degeneration.
- Marfan's syndrome, cystic medical degeneration, Ehlers–Danlos syndrome.
- Loeys–Dietz aneurysm syndrome, Turner syndrome.

- Trauma – sudden deceleration, cocaine, phaeochromocytoma, heavy weightlifting.
- Pregnancy, coarctation of the aorta, bicuspid aortic valves, aortitis – Takayasu's arteritis.
- Syphilis, aortic valve replacement, familial – autosomal dominant.
- Iatrogenic aortic manipulation (including angiography and stenting).

Stanford classification

- **Stanford Type A** [PROXIMAL] (60%) – any involvement of ascending aorta. Mortality 80% in first 48 h and related to time to surgery. High risk rupture, tamponade, acute MI, stroke, acute AR and cardiogenic shock, innominate compromised (60–70%): involves proximal aorta and arch usually requires urgent surgery. Most tears are seen in upper right lateral wall of the ascending aorta.
- **Stanford Type B** [DISTAL] (30–40%): not involving ascending aorta, usually distal to left subclavian artery and may extend down as far as the iliac vessels and have better outcome; management is medical.

Clinical

- Sudden anterior (root and ascending aorta) or interscapular (descending aorta) chest wall pain or even abdominal pain. Some pain may radiate into the back. Syncopal or presyncopal episode with tearing/stabbing/sharp interscapular pain.
- **Aortic regurgitation**: dissection can shear the aortic valve. Look for new early diastolic murmur suggesting AR of proximal disease and may be associated with acute LVF. Look for a Marfanoid appearance. History of bicuspid valve or hypertension. May be shocked if there is blood loss or tamponade.
- **Aortic arch**: dissection may shear off vessels in the proximal aorta (right brachiocephalic gives off right subclavian and carotid, left common carotid and left subclavian). Causes stroke. Reduced pulsation or reduced BP because the arm supplied by the subclavian/brachiocephalic artery is obstructed.
- **Coronary artery obstruction**: left main stem = death because of massive LV infarction; right coronary artery: inferior MI with additional chest pain.
- **Right brachiocephalic**: obstruction will cause reduced flow to right subclavian, right common carotid and right vertebral and is usually devastating if complete with a right TACI with right hemiparesis and potential posterior circulation signs and right arm ischaemia.
- **Left subclavian:** ataxia (vertebral) and arm ischaemia and low BP left arm and posterior circulation symptoms and signs.
- **Left common carotid**: most striking will be a left TACI stroke with right hemiparesis.
- **Anterior spinal artery:** paraplegia affecting legs with preserved dorsal columns.
- **Coeliac axis:** ischaemic bowel. **Renal artery:** anuria, haematuria and AKI.

Differential

- See *Chapter 7* but consider ACS and PE and oesophageal causes.

Investigations

- **Bloods:** U&E, FBC, LFTs, troponin, group and cross-match.
- **D-dimer**: raised dimer (can lead to misdiagnosis as PE hopefully with dissection diagnosed on CTPA).
- **CXR:** unfolded aorta, widening of mediastinum (>6 cm), left pleural effusion may be exudate from an inflamed aorta. Widening mediastinum 80% of acute dissection.
- **ECG:** arrhythmias. Inferior MI if RCA involved. Longstanding LVH. Can be normal.

- **CT AORTOGRAM:** the diagnostic test. Shows false lumen and true lumen of dissection. Defines the operative anatomy and involvement of branch vessels. False lumen can have a greater cross-sectional area. False lumen beaks are often filled with low attenuation thrombus. Outer wall calcification is present in true lumen. It is important to determine the luminal origins of branch vessels before surgery. The beak sign is the cross-sectional imaging manifestation of the wedge of haematoma that cleaves a space for the propagating false lumen and that is present microscopically in all dissections. May be picked up incidentally on CTPA.
- **Transthoracic echo**: suprasternal views may be useful.
- **Transoesophageal echo**: gives detailed views of aorta and valve. Main advantage is anatomical AND a functional assessment of aortic valve. Where available it is used instead of CT in high-risk patients.

Complications

- Aortic rupture, ischaemic stroke – TACI-like presentation if brachiocephalic occluded.
- Subclavian obstruction may cause a possible posterior circulation event but collateral opposite vertebral.
- Cardiac tamponade (blood) – drainage can precipitate more bleeding and death.
- Acute aortic regurgitation and LVF, spinal cord infarction. Mesenteric/renal ischaemia.
- Left pleural haemothorax – ominous sign on CXR, sudden death, distal limb ischaemia.

The mortality of untreated type A dissections is approximately 1% per hour in the first 24 hours, peaking with an overall in-hospital mortality of 58% and 26% for those who undergo surgery.

Acute management

- **ABC resuscitation:** O_2 as per BTS. Good IV access × 2. If haemorrhage or tamponade death is usually imminent. Group and cross-match according to local policy because if cardiothoracic centre is in another hospital they may not accept blood cross-matched elsewhere. Cross-match will be for perioperative blood loss. Acute dissection of the ascending aorta is highly lethal with a cumulative mortality rate of 1–2% per hour early after the onset of symptoms so rapid stabilisation and transfer is needed.
- **Get ECG and CXR to exclude differentials** for acute chest pain. Avoid anticoagulation/antithrombotic if dissection considered. Thrombolysis will delay any urgent surgery and may provoke fatal bleeding. If suspicious for dissection then discuss now with radiology for CT aortogram.
- **Pain relief: DIAMORPHINE 2.5–5.0 mg IV** or **MORPHINE 5–10 mg IV** for chest pain may help reduce preload and pulmonary oedema.
- **Blood (pulse) pressure**: reduce driving pressure of dp/dt BP and pulse pressure with **LABETALOL IV and/or IV NITROPRUSSIDE** in Type A. In those with Type B dissection these agents can be used acutely and then patient managed onto oral medication. Consider aiming for SBP <110 mmHg.
- **Cardiac tamponade**: emergency pericardiocentesis of an acute Type A aortic dissection complicated by cardiac tamponade can result in sudden deterioration and should be avoided if possible; every effort should be made to proceed as urgently as possible to the operating room for direct surgical repair of the aorta with intra-operative drainage of the haemopericardium.

- **Cardiothoracic surgery for Type A** involves replacement of proximal aorta by a tube graft – may require resection and replacement of the aortic valve and sewing in of coronary vessels and repair of the coronary sinus. Surgery is done using cardiopulmonary bypass and the patient cooled to 22°C. Endovascular treatment involving the insertion of stents is still a research area but is used in some centres. Mortality rate with surgery for Type A dissection is 26% and for those treated medically is 58%. Patients need to move immediately to a cardiothoracic centre. Contact and discuss urgent transfer. Delay increases mortality.
- **Long-term management:** both Type A and B require long term BP control. Beta-blocker-based therapy is the foundation of long-term medical management. ACE inhibitors may be beneficial. Lifelong imaging of the entire aorta at regular intervals for further problems by either CT or MRI is advocated. Uncomplicated Type B dissection has an in-hospital mortality rate of 10%.

Reference: Braverman (2010) Acute aortic dissection: clinician update. *Circulation*, 122:184.

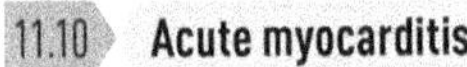

11.10 Acute myocarditis

About

- Acute myocarditis and preserved LV ejection fraction have a good prognosis with a high rate of spontaneous improvement without sequelae.

Aetiology

- Inflammation of the myocardium. Can present with arrhythmias and acute heart failure.
- Can result in end-stage cardiac failure, thromboembolism and arrhythmias.
- Regarded as a precursor of dilated cardiomyopathy (DCM).

Causes

- **Idiopathic:** all investigations negative; 50% presumably viral but unproven.
- **Viral infection**: parvovirus B19 (PVB19) and human herpesvirus 6. Coxsackie A (mild), Coxsackie B (severe) and influenza; echovirus; adenovirus; HIV; CMV.
- **Non-viral infection:** Chagas disease (*Trypanosoma cruzi*), toxoplasmosis. Rickettsial: Scrub typhus, Rocky Mountain spotted fever, Q fever, Lyme disease causes temporary conduction block. Bacterial: leptospirosis, diphtheria, TB, brucella.
- **Drugs and toxins**: doxorubicin, herceptin, cyclophosphamide, penicillin, phenytoin, methyldopa, cocaine abuse. Heavy metals: arsenic, cobalt, mercury exposure.
- **Miscellaneous:** radiation, peripartum cardiomyopathy, post cardiac transplant rejection.
- **Inflammatory:** sarcoidosis, Kawasaki disease, SLE, Wegener's granulomatosis, thyrotoxicosis, rheumatoid arthritis, rheumatic fever.

Clinical

- Occasionally presents with acute LVF and VT.
- Ask about recent viral illness and drug usage.
- Chest pain, coexisting pericarditis, malaise, dyspnoea, heart failure.
- Murmurs of MR, S4, etc., arrhythmias, e.g. AF, VT, pericardial effusion, tamponade.

Investigation

- **FBC:** raised WCC, raised CRP, and raised ESR.
- **Others:** check ANA, dsDNA, ASO titres, TFTs. HIV test.

- **ECG**: AF, ST/T wave changes even mimicking STEMI/NSTEMI; those with Q waves or LBBB are a poor prognostic group; ectopics, VT, VF, heart block.
- **CXR**: cardiomegaly, pulmonary oedema.
- **Cardiac biomarkers**: raised CK and CKMB, raised troponin in proportion to damage.
- **Echocardiogram**: no specific features. May see LV and RV dysfunction, enlarged chambers, thrombus, pericardial effusion, and valve regurgitation. Useful to exclude other causes, e.g. HCM.
- **Cardiac MR**: non-invasive and valuable clinical tool for the diagnosis of myocarditis. Initial changes in myocardial tissue can be seen on T2-weighted oedema imaging.
- **Myocardial biopsy:** rarely done but is the gold standard for diagnosis. It may show lymphocytic infiltration and myocyte necrosis.
- **Serology and PCR**: influenza or Coxsackie serology and Parvovirus.
- **Coronary angiography**: if CAD suspected.

Complications

- Some develop a dilated cardiomyopathy and end-stage heart failure.
- VT / VF. Heart block needing pacing. Sudden cardiac death, thromboembolism.

Management

- **Supportive:** bed-rest, treat heart failure and arrhythmias as usual. Usually in CCU with telemetry depending on presentation and presence of heart failure and arrhythmias. Ensure access to early defibrillation.
  Balloon pumping for heart failure not responding to usual medications. Standard heart failure regime including beta-blockers, diuretics, ACE inhibitors or angiotensin-II receptor blockers (ARBs) should be initiated.
- **VTE prophylaxis** and full anticoagulation, especially if AF or LA / LV thrombus.
- **Steroids** have been used with mixed results. No trials showing a benefit from immunosuppression.
- **Avoid exercise** during acute period and convalescence.
- **Heart transplant** in those with dilated CMP and end-stage cardiac failure.

Reference: Kinderman *et al.* (2012) Update on myocarditis. *J Am Coll Cardiol*, 59:779.

11.11 Acute pericarditis

Saddle-shaped ST elevation in all 12 leads other than aVr is likely to be pericarditis and not ACS. Avoid ACS anticoagulants as risk of haemopericardium.

About

- Seen in 5% of CCU chest pain admissions. Usually benign – exclude dissection, ACS, PE.
- Often found in association with acute myocarditis and both have similar aetiologies.

Aetiology

- **Idiopathic** is commonest (presumably viral).
- **Infectious**: bacterial: TB, *Coxiella burnettii*, pneumococcus, meningococcal. Viral: increasing role for parvovirus B19, echovirus, coxsackie, influenza, CMV, EBV, adenovirus, HBV, HCV, etc. HIV: often causes effusion. Fungal: histoplasmosis. Pyogenic post-op pericarditis or post pneumonia.
- **Inflammatory**: post myocardial injury (Dressler's syndrome), autoimmune disorder (SLE/RA/Behcet's), drug-induced lupus (hydralazine, procainamide), familial

Mediterranean fever, rheumatic fever (with associated pancarditis and murmurs, rash, joint aches).

- **Malignancy:** lymphoma, lung or breast cancer, melanoma, leukaemia.
- **Miscellaneous**: metabolic (uraemia – end-stage kidney disease), hypothyroid/ myxoedema (large chronic effusion but rarely compromising).

Clinical

- Fever, malaise, myalgia, post-viral syndrome, myocarditis symptoms (see *Section 11.10*).
- Pleuritic type chest pain eased by sitting forwards, worse lying flat and on inspiration. Pain referred to shoulder or scapula.
- Auscultation friction rub (very useful sign worth looking for) with a systolic (ventricular filling) and atrial systolic component.

Diagnostic criteria: presence of all 4 makes diagnosis probable:

(1) typical chest pain associated with pericarditis
(2) pericardial friction rub on auscultation
(3) gradual changes in the ECG such as diffuse ST elevation
(4) new or increased pericardial effusion.

Differential

- Acute coronary syndrome, aortic dissection, pulmonary embolism, oesophageal disease.

Investigation

- **FBC**: raised WCC, raised ESR and raised CRP may be seen with infective and inflammatory causes.
- **U&E**: AKI or chronic kidney disease with uraemic pericarditis.
- **TFT**: raised TSH diagnoses hypothyroidism.
- **Tuberculin testing and CXR**: for TB if suspected.
- **HIV test:** where suspected. Other viral studies where indicated.
- **ECG**: shows **saddle-shaped ST elevation** in all leads **except aVr and V1** which look into the cavity of the heart where there is therefore an inverted lead, showing ST depression. Eventually ST and PR normalise and there is T wave inversion, which then normalises. May be AF or other atrial arrhythmias. ECG may be low voltage if effusion.
- **CXR**: usually normal but any cardiac enlargement or globular heart is suggestive.
- **Echocardiogram**: to look for pericardial fluid, LV function (as ever very important), tamponade. Pericardial effusion may be classified into 3 groups according to diastolic distance between the pericardium and the ventricle: (1) <10 mm, (2) moderate 10–20 mm, (3) severe >20 mm. The incidence of cardiac tamponade secondary to severe pericardial effusion is about 3%. Right ventricular dysfunction seems to be the greatest predictor of mortality and cardiac transplantation.
- **CK and troponin**: usually negative except where there is an associated myopericarditis.
- **Diagnostic pericardiocentesis**: exclude TB and diagnose malignancy where appropriate.

Management

- **Acute treatment**: aspirin or NSAIDs are given. If unwell with perhaps associated myocarditis or significant effusion, or arrhythmias, then hospitalise, but other cases can be managed with ambulatory care and repeat echo where needed. Reassurance is sufficient in most cases especially if troponin negative. Therapeutic pericardiocentesis if evidence of tamponade.

- **Risk assessment**: those in a higher risk group needing admission for initial expert evaluation would be those with fever above 38°C, subacute onset, immunosuppression, anticoagulation treatment, caused by trauma, myopericarditis, severe pericardial effusion, cardiac tamponade, or no anti-inflammatory response after 1 week. Again manage with high dose aspirin/ NSAID + PPI. Colchicine has been used for recurrent events. Avoid exercise, bed to chair existence whilst symptomatic. Weigh up risks of low dose VTE and haemorrhage into pericardium. In severe cases steroids, e.g. prednisolone 40 mg OD for 2 weeks may be used.
- In those with pericarditis post acute MI then cautions with NSAID or steroids. They could impair ventricular remodelling. NSAID can worsen renal and platelet function. Ibuprofen is probably the safest choice +/– PPI.
- Pericarditis may be seen post pneumonia and may require IV antibiotics depending on the likely organism. Any suggestion of a purulent effusion will need urgent consideration for drainage.
- Any concerns about effusion settled with echocardiogram. Where diagnosis is unclear and pain continues and risk of IHD high then angiography may be required to exclude ACS.
- Patients should be given clear advice on readmission if there are new or on-going symptoms. The main worry is fluid collection and tamponade.

Reference: Freixa (2010) Evaluation, management, and treatment of acute pericarditis and myocarditis in the emergency department. *Emergencias*, 22:301.

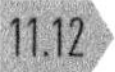

11.12 Pericardial effusion / tamponade

Cardiac tamponade is uncommon even when the effusion is large. Caution with drainage if proximal aortic dissection as can cause haemodynamic collapse.

About

- Note: consider bleeding into pericardial space if on anticoagulants or trauma or cardiac intervention or cardiac rupture post STEMI or dissection.
- Tamponade is uncommon even with large pericardial effusions. It causes obstructive shock. Small effusions are often found at routine echocardiogram.

Aetiology

- Fluid/blood collects in pericardial space. Volume of fluid present usually less than 50 ml. Parietal pericardium inelastic and pericardial space normally holds 20–50 ml of fluid. Chronic accumulation of fluid over months can produce up to 500–1000 ml without significant compromise as pericardial sac stretches.
- In cardiac tamponade, the pericardial pressure may reach 15–20 mmHg, leading to an equalisation of pressures into the cardiac chambers and to a huge decrease in the systemic venous return.
- Acute accumulations of even 100 ml may be enough to cause haemodynamic collapse as increased volume and pressure leads the right atrium and then the right ventricle to collapse in diastole.

- **Beck's triad** can be detected with low BP, reduced heart sounds and raised JVP with prominent *x* descent and absent *y* descent. Slow collections tolerated well. If diastolic cardiac filling compromised then tamponade.

Causes of effusion more likely to cause tamponade

- Neoplastic disease, idiopathic pericarditis, renal disease, tuberculosis.
- Haemopericardium – warfarin, NOAC, heparin, DIC, trauma, uraemia.
- Post MI and ventricular rupture, Type A aortic dissection proximally.
- Post procedure – cardiac catheterisation or pacemaker insertion, transeptal catheter.

Clinical (signs of effusion and likely causes)

- Asymptomatic if small, pericarditis-type symptoms (see *Section 11.11*).
- Cough, fever, malaise and systemic symptoms. Muffled heart sounds.
- Right heart failure with peripheral oedema and hepatomegaly.
- Cachexia and weight loss may suggest malignancy, TB or HIV.
- **Acute tamponade**: can cause bradycardia due to pericardial stretch followed by hypotension and marked fall in pulse pressure such that radial pulse becomes impalpable. Marked fall in BP of over 10 mmHg with inspiration.
- **Pulsus paradoxus** or the radial pulse may become impalpable on inspiration.
- Jugular venous pressure: markedly raised JVP (RA pressure raised) which rises with inspiration. **Kussmaul's sign** and **loss of *y* descent**.
- Heart sounds are quiet and area of cardiac dullness increases.

Differential

- Acute coronary syndrome, aortic dissection, pulmonary embolism, oesophageal disease.

Investigation

- **FBC:** raised WCC, ESR and raised CRP may be seen.
- **APTT/PT:** coagulation screen if on anticoagulants
- **ECG**: low voltage QRS complexes, AF, evidence of pericarditis or recent MI. Electrical alternans.
- **CXR:** shows cardiac enlargement (cardiomegaly or effusion needs echo to differentiate) or may show underlying neighbouring malignancy. Large effusions present as globular cardiomegaly with sharp margins. If the effusion develops during catheterisation, it may also be identified by the development of lucent lines in the cardiopericardial silhouette or so called epicardial halo sign or fat pad sign. Straightening and immobility of the left heart border. CXR may show TB or lung malignancy.
- **Echocardiogram**: look for pericardial fluid and assess cardiac function. Pericardial effusion may be classified into 3 groups according to diastolic distance between the pericardium and the ventricle: (1) <10 mm, (2) moderate 10–20 mm, (3) severe >20 mm. The incidence of cardiac tamponade secondary to severe pericardial effusion is about 3%. **Tamponade:** diastolic collapse of RA and free wall of RV are serious signs of incipient circulatory compromise. RV collapse is the most specific echo finding. Also look for fall in mitral inflow velocity or aortic velocity by 25% with inspiration. Invasive monitoring would show a fall in aortic pressure and rise in RA pressure. Echo can be used to guide pericardiocentesis.
- **Cardiac MRI** is useful for detecting pericardial effusion and loculated pericardial effusion and thickening.
- **Cardiac troponin I/T**: usually negative except where there is an associated myopericarditis or ACS.

- **Check clotting:** if coagulopathy or warfarin and haemopericardium suspected.
- **Diagnostic pericardiocentesis** if TB or malignancy. Exudate suggests an infective/ inflammatory or malignant process. Assess protein, **LDH, Hb, WCC, viral, bacterial, TB cultures.**

Management

- **If acutely compromised then ABCs**. Resuscitation, O_2. Good IV access. Give IV fluids **0.5–1.0 L NS** to ensure filling pressures. Volume resuscitation and catecholamines are temporary but the only remaining effective treatment in tamponade is urgent **needle pericardiocentesis**, except where a Type A proximal aortic dissection is suspected which can cause circulatory collapse – needs cardiothoracic advice. If anticoagulated suspect bleeding into pericardial space – stop and reverse any anticoagulation / coagulopathy.
- **Volume loading:** may be beneficial and repeated trials of 250–500 ml of NS should be assessed for improvement of haemodynamics. **Catecholamines** and **IV NITROPRUSSIDE** to reduce afterload and/or **IV DOBUTAMINE** may also be of benefit in some patients.
- **Therapeutic pericardiocentesis**: consider transfer to tertiary centre with access to expert cardiological and cardiothoracic surgical expertise.

References:

Bodson *et al.* (2011) Cardiac tamponade. *Curr Opin Crit Care*, 17:416.

Maisch *et al.* (2004) Guidelines on the diagnosis and management of pericardial diseases: executive summary. *Eur Heart J*, 25:587.

11.13 Severe (malignant) hypertension

About

- Less common now as screening and treatment so much better.
- BP causes end organ damage over years.
- Acute rises should be gradually reduced in most circumstances.
- Evidence base for acute hypertensive emergency management is lacking.
- Malignant hypertension by definition requires fundoscopy to see Grade 3/4 retinal changes.

Aetiology

- Untreated/undiagnosed essential hypertension; failure to take medication.
- Phaeochromocytoma or other secondary cause.
- Acute cocaine, severe anxiety, pain, acute urinary retention, preeclampsia.

Clinical

- Asymptomatic to mild malaise, mild headache, anxiety, distress.
- Breathless with pulmonary oedema, microangiopathic haemolytic anaemia.
- Renal failure, stroke (ischaemic or haemorrhagic).
- Fundoscopy – retinal haemorrhages and papilloedema, confusion.
- Delirium – encephalopathy, look for clues in history and examine.
- Phaeochromocytoma, renal bruits, radiofemoral delay.
- Renal masses, examine drug chart – NSAID, ciclosporin.

Malignant hypertension

- High BP + retinal haemorrhages + papilloedema + nephropathy or chest pain.
- Beware watershed cerebral infarction with rapid lowering.

Secondary causes of hypertension

- Conn's syndrome, Cushing's syndrome, steroids, oral contraceptive pill.
- Aortic coarctation 0.25%, renal artery stenosis 0.5%.
- Polycystic kidney disease, preeclampsia, CKD.
- Cocaine usage, alcohol, amphetamines, ciclosporin, NSAIDs.

Investigations

- **FBC, U&E** (CKD, hypokalaemia with Conn's syndrome).
- **ECG:** AF, LVH, LAD, LBBB, ST/T wave changes. R plus S greater than 35 mm.
- **CXR**: cardiomegaly, rib notching with coarctation of the aorta.
- **Echocardiogram:** LVH, diastolic dysfunction, assess LV (exclude coarctation).
- **Renal USS**: small kidneys with CKD, polycystic kidneys, difference in size with RAS. Adrenal mass.
- **Urine** for proteinuria, cocaine, amphetamines.
- **Others:** urinary catecholamines, dexamethasone suppression, renin/aldosterone levels.
- **CT/MRI head**: if new neurology, e.g. haemorrhage or infarct, tumour or posterior reversible encephalopathy syndrome.

Indications for emergency BP reduction: Acute BP lowering is not risk-free and risks vs. benefits need to be evaluated. Rapid precipitous drops must be avoided as they can lead to myocardial and cerebral hypoperfusion.

- **Acute pulmonary oedema**: lower to level that helps resolves oedema. Preference for starting ACEi, IV furosemide + IV nitrates.
- **Acute MI**: (raised BP increases myocardial work and ischaemia) preference for IV nitrates + start small dose ACE inhibitor.
- **Acute aortic dissection**: BP target will be 120/80 mmHg or lower if tolerated especially for proximal dissection. Use IV labetalol.
- **Eclampsia** (seizures, pregnancy): use hydralazine, labetalol, and nifedipine and IV magnesium.
- **Acute intracerebral haemorrhage:** very gradually (over 12–24 h) lower to approximately 185/110 mmHg. If safe consider lowering further – depends on baselines, size of bleed. Consult.
- **Hypertensive encephalopathy**: (headache, confusion, seizures, symptoms + papilloedema) use IV labetalol though no real preference.
- **Stroke thrombolysis**: lower BP to <185/110 mmHg **if safe to do so within the thrombolysis time frame**. A rapid drop in BP and cerebral blood flow might cause watershed infarcts and do more harm than thrombolysis benefits. Likely to be more at risk if significant cerebral atherosclerosis.
- **Cocaine induced HTN:** use IV nitrates, calcium antagonists and diazepam. Avoid beta blockers.
- **Phaeochromocytoma-induced hypertension**: there is elevated urine catecholamines and metanephrines and plasma catecholamines. Tumour usually seen on CT abdomen though 10% are extra-adrenal (in sympathetic chain from neck to bladder) and 10% malignant and bilateral. **Ensure alpha blockade before beta blockers added for BP control**. If acute need to treat then Phentolamine 2–5 mg IV bolus. If stable then Phenoxybenzamine 20–80 mg daily initially in divided doses followed by Propranolol (120–240 mg daily). Alternatively start Doxazosin 2–4 mg daily in divided doses. Also consider IV nitrates, calcium antagonists and diazepam. If perioperative management there can be a huge fall in circulating

catecholamines once the tumour is removed and sudden fall in SVR needing rapid volume replacement.

Management

- **General measures:** a quiet room, good nursing care and a good bedside manner can often help reduce BP, especially when patients get onto a quiet ward rather than the busy ED. No smoking, no coffee. In an asymptomatic patient with BP >220/120 mmHg then rest, relief of pain, agitation and simple observation and commencing one or more oral agents for a few hours may suffice, and follow up within days may be reasonable. A higher BP may warrant admission for on-going assessment, especially with evidence of end-organ damage or any symptoms, but ambulatory care should be sufficient. In the admitted or in an inpatient look for and treat any agitation, pain or acute urinary retention. In those without urgent need to reduce BP then lower BP in a slow controlled manner over hours and days to acceptable levels (e.g. to <180/110 mmHg) using slow onset oral agents. Sharp drops in BP may be harmful. Hypertensive damage is caused much more by chronic long-term hypertensive changes than acute rises in BP. Most of these patients have simply had undiagnosed untreated hypertension for years. Target a gradual reduction to a normal BP over days rather than minutes or hours unless complicated.
- **Urgent reduction**: general measures + oral drugs – lower BP over hours unless urgent indications (see above). No evidence base for which drugs to use. Suggest oral nifedipine TABLETS (**NB: not capsules or sublingual preparation**) 10–20 mg or ATENOLOL 25 mg, or other beta blocker can be used if phaeochromocytoma very unlikely (no history of sweating ++, palpitations, headache). Set a target BP with an escalation policy because it means that BP is better controlled and hopefully neither over- nor undertreated – the nursing and medical staff will then have a value to aim for. Set a target that is perhaps 10–20% lower than the current BP, e.g. 180/110 mmHg. But immediate aim is not to achieve a BP of 120/80 mmHg. If precipitated by stopping usual BP meds and no adverse effects with these then consider reintroduction slowly perhaps one by one until controlled.
- **Emergency BP reduction:** severe cases as described above or, if BP sustained at >220/120 mmHg despite other measures, then consider (if no history of bronchospasm/asthma) **LABETALOL IV 20 mg over 1 min** which is easy to simply draw up and give initially as a bolus or infusion. An alternative, especially if angina or pulmonary oedema, is **IV GLYCERYL TRINITRATE**. The nitric oxide donor **IV NITROPRUSSIDE** can also be considered. No need to treat BP in ischaemic stroke unless sustained BP >220/120 mmHg, or patient is for thrombolysis. Reduce BP slowly. With haemorrhagic stroke aim for cautious slow controlled reduction to just below 185/110 mmHg, but useful evidence is lacking. Again very gradually.
- **Additional steps:** if agitation or delirium or aggression is a driver to the BP consider **DIAZEPAM 2–5 mg PO/IV** or **HALOPERIDOL 1–2 mg PO/IV** which can be given orally or IM/IV. Beta blockers avoided if phaeochromocytoma suspected.
- Give **FUROSEMIDE IV or GTN** for pulmonary oedema.
- Manage AKI and exclude renal causes – check urine for blood and protein and nephritis and renal parenchymal causes (see *Section 18.3*). Consider a urinary catheter if you really need to assess urine output or exclude obstruction. Always double check (especially in older confused patient) that you haven't missed urinary retention or untreated pain with its usual pressor response. Patients can be significantly volume depleted and may need volume expansion once BP is controlled with IV NS.

11.14 Infective endocarditis

About

- Infection of cardiac valves/endocardium. Underlying structural cardiac defects.
- Rheumatic heart disease less common so now seen in older patients and those with prosthetic valves. Mortality 15–20%.

Pathology

- Infective vegetations form on heart valves containing fibrin, platelets, and microorganisms.
- High pressure jet of blood on endocardium or valve. Vegetations can embolise.
- Rheumatic heart disease, congenital heart disease or other lesions.
- Seen with mitral valve prolapse, aortic sclerosis, and bicuspid aortic valves.

Organisms

- **Pacemaker endocarditis:** early cases caused by *Staph. aureus* and late cases by *Staph. epidermidis.*
- **Native valve endocarditis:** *Strep. viridans* 40%, *Staph. aureus* 20%, *Enterococcus* spp. 10%, others are streptococci, coagulase-negative staphylococci, Gram-negative bacilli, fungi.
- **Early onset prosthetic valve endocarditis (<60 days post-op):** *Staph. epidermidis* 40%, *Staph. aureus* 9%, *Enterococci* 6%, Gram-negative bacilli 4%, fungi 11%, others.
- **IV drug users:** tricuspid valve endocarditis with *Staph. aureus/epidermidis.*
- **Bicuspid aortic valve** – aortic valve endocarditis.

Microbiology

- ***Staph. aureus:*** most common pathogen and causes a more aggressive acute endocarditis type disease of normal valves or may be post-operative. Affects those with IV lines and central lines and IV drug users. Causes early and late prosthetic valve endocarditis and pacemaker endocarditis.
- ***Strep. viridans*:** a low virulence organism seen where there is a history of rheumatic fever. An oral commensal. Causes a subacute clinical picture.
- **Coagulase-negative staphylococcus:** usually causes early PVE. Occasionally pacemaker endocarditis. They may produce a biofilm on prosthetic surfaces, which also promotes adherence.
- **Fungal endocarditis:** prolonged antibiotics or parenteral nutrition. Often immunocompromised. Usually *Candida albicans* or *C. parapsilosis.*
- **HACEK group:** Gram-negative bacteria. Fastidious. *Haemophilus, Actinobacillus, Cardiobacterium, Eikenella,* and *Kingella* species. May be ill for months. Painful embolic lesion to an extremity.
- **Q fever endocarditis:** *Coxiella burnettii* is an example. May be no fever. Valvular heart disease and on immunosuppressive therapy. Vegetations rare on echo. Organism isolated from buffy coat cultures. Serological studies are reasonably specific.

Cardiac disease and risk of endocarditis

- **High risk:** previous endocarditis, aortic valve disease, rheumatic heart disease, prosthetic valves, mitral regurgitation or AR, VSD, ductus arteriosus, aortic coarctation, acyanotic congenital heart disease.
- **Medium risk:** aortic stenosis, HCM, mitral valve prolapse (MVP) with MR, isolated mitral stenosis, tricuspid disease, pulmonary stenosis.
- **Low risk:** secundum ASD, IHD, previous CABG, MVP without MR.

Clinical

- Fever, malaise, joint pains, stroke/TIA-like episodes if emboli.
- Peripheral emboli – gangrene/ischaemic bowel, finger clubbing is rare.
- Osler's nodes – painful, tender nodules on the pulps of fingers.
- Janeway lesions – small (<5 mm) flat painless red spots seen on palms and soles.
- Roth's spots – retinal haemorrhage and micro-infarction.
- New or changing murmurs. Splenomegaly.
- Splinter haemorrhages – also seen in manual workers, labourers.

Investigations

- **FBC:** anaemia, raised WCC, **ESR and CRP**. U&E. Urinalysis – microscopic haematuria.
- **ECG**: new AV block, increased PR interval suggests aortic valve involvement.
- **CXR:** evidence of cardiomegaly, mitral stenosis.
- **Echo (transthoracic) findings**: mobile intracardiac mass (vegetation), root or valve abscess, partial dehiscence of prosthetic valve, new valve regurgitation.
- **Transoesophageal echo**: TOE indicated if transthoracic echo negative and suspicion or with prosthetic valve. A normal echo does not exclude the diagnosis.
- **Blood cultures**: at least 6 from multiple sites spaced in time before antibiotics started. Use fastidious care to avoid contaminants. Do not start antibiotics until multiple cultures from multiple sites have been taken over 12–24 h period unless the organism is known and the infection is proven and severe.

Complications

- Valve failure with heart failure (and cardiogenic shock).
- Septic emboli, e.g. stroke (avoid anticoagulation).
- Glomerulonephritis, aortic root abscess, valvular abscess.
- Pericarditis, death, conduction defects.

Modified Duke criteria for diagnosis: 2 M or 1 M + 2 m or 5 m minor criteria

MAJOR CRITERIA (M criteria)

- Supportive lab evidence: typical microorganism from two separate blood cultures, e.g. *Strep. viridans* and the HACEK group OR persistent bacteraemia from 2 blood cultures taken >12 h apart or 3 or more positive blood cultures where the pathogen is less specific, e.g. *Staph. aureus* and *Staph. epidermidis* OR positive serology for *Coxiella burnettii*, *Bartonella* species, or *Chlamydia psittaci*, OR positive molecular assays for specific gene targets.
- Evidence of endocardial involvement – echo supportive of infective endocarditis showing oscillating structures, abscess formation, new valvular regurgitation or dehiscence of prosthetic valves.

MINOR CRITERIA (m criteria)

(1) **Risk:** predisposing heart condition or intravenous drug use.
(2) **Fever:** >38.0°C.
(3) **Vascular phenomena**: major arterial emboli, septic pulmonary infarcts, mycotic aneurysm, intracranial haemorrhage, conjunctival haemorrhages, Janeway lesions.
(4) **Immunological phenomena**: glomerulonephritis, Osler's nodes, Roth spots, +ve rheumatoid factor.
(5) **Positive blood culture** not meeting major criterion as noted previously (excluding single positive cultures for coagulase-negative staphylococci and organisms that do not cause endocarditis) or serologic evidence of active infection with organism consistent with infective endocarditis.
(6) **Raised** inflammatory markers: CRP >100 mg/L, raised ESR.

Management

- **Involve cardiology and microbiology** for advice on clinical assessment, diagnosis and management. Those with haemodynamic compromise should be referred to local cardiothoracic centre cardiologists.
- **Starting antibiotics**: if patient stable and endocarditis uncomplicated can wait 1–2 days to get multiple cultures before starting antibiotics. Complicated endocarditis should receive empirical antibiotic as soon as 3–6 sets of blood cultures taken. Review antibiotics as soon as aetiological agent is identified. Duration of therapy depends on the organism, microbiology advice and whether native or prosthetic valve.
- **Empirical antibiotic therapy**:
  - **indolent presentation**: BENZYLPENICILLIN IV for 4 weeks + GENTAMICIN IV for 2 weeks (modified according to renal function – see *Chapter 29*).
  - **acute presentation**: FLUCLOXACILLIN IV for 4 weeks + GENTAMICIN for 3–5 days.
  - **prosthetic heart valve, MRSA carrier or penicillin allergy**: IV vancomycin (modified according to renal function for 6 weeks, see *BNF* Appendix 3) + RIFAMPICIN + IV GENTAMICIN for 2–6 weeks (modified according to renal function, see *BNF* Appendix 4).
- **Valve surgery**: if heart failure due to valve destruction, large vegetations on left side with embolic concerns, abscess formation, failing antibiotic therapy.

12 Respiratory emergencies

12.1 Adult respiratory distress syndrome

About

- Acute lung injury (ALI) and ARDS are seen acutely.
- A complication of trauma, sepsis, tissue damage and other severe illnesses.

Aetiology

- Type 1 respiratory failure without evidence of significant cardiac dysfunction.
- Pulmonary oedema due to increased permeability of the alveolar capillary membrane with resulting stiff boggy poorly compliant lungs.

Clinical

- Breathlessness, cyanosis, basal inspiratory crackles.
- Tachycardia, severe hypoxia in the context of critical illness.

Causes of ARDS/ALI

- **Primary**: burns and smoke inhalation, pneumonia, pneumonitis from aspiration, high altitude, fat or air embolism, near drowning, oxygen toxicity.
- **Systemic**: sepsis, trauma, eclampsia, acute pancreatitis, heroin, barbiturates, transfusion-associated lung injury, malignancies, cardiopulmonary bypass.

American–European Consensus Conference: definition for ARDS and ALI

- Acute onset of respiratory symptoms within 72 h of hypoxaemia and bilateral opacities on chest imaging not explained by other pulmonary pathology.
- Pulmonary artery wedge pressure (PAWP) <18 mmHg (no left heart failure).
- ALI: PaO_2/FiO_2 ratio <300 mmHg (40 kPa).
- ARDS: PaO_2/FiO_2 ratio <200 mmHg (26 kPa). Severe ARDS: ≤100 mmHg (≤13.3 kPa).

Investigations

- **Arterial blood gases**: PO_2 < 8 kPa despite high FiO_2.
- **FBC**: anaemia, raised neutrophils.
- **U&E / LFT lactate**: AKI may be seen, raised lactate, deranged LFTs.
- **CXR:** pulmonary oedema. **Chest CT**: ground glass appearance.
- **Echocardiogram**: normal LV function typically.
- **Right heart catheterisation**: normal pulmonary capillary wedge pressure.
- **Blood cultures**: sepsis.
- **Coagulopathy:** e.g. DIC may develop with raised APTT, PT and low platelets.

Management

- **Determine and manage the cause.** Admit to care of intensivists in a HDU/ITU setting. **Cautious fluid management** and use of diuretics to minimise pulmonary oedema without impairing LV filling. Generate a negative fluid balance. Haemofiltration may be used.
- **Supportive care**: including enteral nutrition. Treat any obvious cause and manage other organ failure. Steroids have no evidence base.
- **Intubation and ventilation** (PEEP – positive end-expiratory pressure): required when hypoxaemia despite high FiO_2 and/or worsening radiological changes. Lung protective ventilation strategies that limit tidal volumes, plateau pressures,

or both have been developed. The goal of ventilating a patient with ARDS is to maintain adequate gas exchange while minimising ventilator-induced lung injury. Mechanical ventilation and prone positioning may be advocated. Neuromuscular blockade for 48 h may help.

- **ITU care**: inhaled nitric oxide is often tried as well as aerosolised surfactant and prostacyclin.
- Death is primarily due to multi-organ dysfunction.

References:

de Haro *et al.* (2013) ARDS: prevention and early recognition. *Annals Int Care*, 3:11.

Ferguson *et al.* (2005) Development of a clinical definition for ARDS using the Delphi technique. *J Crit Care*, 20:147.

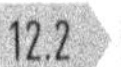

12.2 Acute exacerbation of COPD

About

- COPD is a chronic illness punctuated with acute exacerbations, some infective.
- Community teams can help reduce hospital admissions.

Cause of worsening

- **Irritants**, e.g. cigarette smoke, noxious particles and SO_2, NO_2, ozone.
- **Viral:** 50% rhinoviruses, coronaviruses, influenza, parainfluenza, adenovirus, RSV.
- **Bacterial:** *Haemophilus influenza, Strep. pneumonia, Moraxella catarrhalis, Pseudomonas aeruginosa, Chlamydia pneumonia.*

Clinical

- Increased breathlessness, expiratory wheezes and cough which may be productive. Malaise, cachexia. Pursed lips breathing, barrel-chested, use of accessory muscles – tripod position.
- New onset cyanosis, peripheral oedema, nicotine staining and signs of smoking.
- Bounding pulse, drowsy, tremor and headache can suggest CO_2 retention.
- Determine best baseline exercise function – useful guide of overall function and goals. Ask about pets and allergies, occupation, asbestos. Home oxygen.

MRC dyspnoea scale	
Grade 0	No breathlessness except with strenuous exercise
Grade 1	Breathlessness hurrying on level or walking up a slight hill
Grade 2	Has to walk slower than contemporaries on level ground due to breathlessness or stop for breath
Grade 3	Stops for breath after 100 yards or few minutes on level ground
Grade 4	Too breathless to leave house. Breathless with dressing/undressing

Oxygen management in COPD: in severe COPD start with a 28% Venturi mask at 4 L/min in prehospital care or a 24% Venturi mask at 2–4 L/min in hospital settings. Target saturation of 88–92% pending urgent blood gas results. Until ABG results are known the oxygen dose should be reduced if the saturation exceeds 92%.

Investigations

- **FBC:** raised WCC and raised CRP suggest infection. Steroids increase WCC.
- **U&E:** may be dehydrated with raised urea/creatinine. Hyponatraemia.
- **CXR:** hyper-expanded dark lungs typical of emphysema and may be patchy shadowing. Look for PTX which may be difficult to differentiate from bullae (if unsure CT may be useful). There may be pneumonic changes or possible lung malignancy. Suspect a lung malignancy in all smokers.
- **ECG:** sinus tachycardia, AF, P pulmonale, RVH, ST/T wave changes.
- **ABG**: low PO_2 <8 kPa and raised PCO_2 >6 kPa, pH <7.25. A raised HCO_3 suggests a more chronic COPD respiratory acidosis. Try to find out from past admissions and A&E notes what worst and best ABG was as a guide.
- **Pulmonary function tests**: try to determine FEV / FVC when possible.
- **Consider troponin and risk assess if PE considered for dimer**: if suspicion this is ACS / PE. Exacerbations of COPD can be LVF or PE and these diagnoses should be sensibly considered.

Management

- **General:** diagnostic care because patients with COPD also have PEs, heart failure and pneumothoracies. Getting patient sitting up supported and so not having to use energy on posture and to allow use of accessory muscles is useful and can raise the O_2 saturation a few points. Chest physiotherapy to aid expectoration and IV fluids can be useful for those too tired to drink.
- **Controlled O_2 as per BTS guidance** is given, usually 24–28% initially to achieve O_2 saturation of 88–92% and PO_2 >8 kPa with <1.5 kPa rise in PCO_2. Venturi mask initially 28% at 4 L/min O_2 preferred because this allows accurate amounts of O_2 to be given. Repeat ABG 30 min after altering FiO_2. If the PCO_2 is normal then increase target O_2 saturation to 94–98% and repeat ABG after 30 min. Rising PCO_2 and acidosis suggests respiratory support initially NIV.
- **Bronchodilator therapy**: nebulised SALBUTAMOL 2.5–5 mg 4–6 times per day. Nebulised IPRATROPIUM BROMIDE 500 mcg qds (Atrovent). Nebulisers should be driven by air and not oxygen.
- **Steroids**: **HYDROCORTISONE 100–200 mg IV** initially then **PREDNISOLONE 30–40 mg OD**. Steroids continued for 7–14 days and then stopped.
- **IV AMINOPHYLLINE**: loading dose if not on theophyllines or else maintenance dose as per formulary.
- **Antibiotics: IV / PO Augmentin** or other antibiotics if infection suspected, e.g. fever, sputum, raised WCC or CRP. CXR changes suggesting infection.

Non-invasive ventilation

- **NIV is recommended** in an acute exacerbation of COPD if respiratory acidosis **pH <7.35 and PCO_2 >6 kPa** despite treatment with controlled oxygen: nebulised bronchodilators, oral/parenteral steroids and antibiotics.
- **NIV should be considered in all such patients within 1 h of admission.** It reduces the need for intubation and ITU admissions, improves blood gases and reduces the work of breathing and also reduces infective complications and hospital stay. Avoid in drowsy uncooperative patients, severe acidosis, unstable haemodynamics.
- Patients should be conscious and cooperative and able to protect their airway. A full-face mask should be used initially. Start with low pressures to allow patient to get used to the feeling but then escalate to therapeutic pressures.

- NIV is discussed in more detail in *Section 5.2*. Start with IPAP of 10 cmH_2O and EPAP of 5 cmH_2O. Increase IPAP by 5 cmH_2O every 5–10 min to a target of 20 cmH_2O (max 25).
- Ensure ABG checked 1 h after all changes in settings and this can be reduced once stable to 4 hourly or less if improving. Watch respiratory rate and heart rate.
- Give nebulisers as needed. NIV can be gradually weaned down to 16 h on day 2 and 12 h on day 3 with 6–8 h overnight adjusted to the patient's condition. Discontinue day 4 as appropriate.
- A tiring worsening hypoxic hypercarbic acidotic patient may benefit from ITU admission and full intubation and ventilation. Senior medical staff should discuss with ITU and family and patient if possible. There may be an advance directive. In some cases NIV will be the ceiling of respiratory support.

Respiratory stimulants

- **IV Doxapram** should be considered and is a respiratory stimulant in the tiring patient. May aid expectoration. May be considered in those in whom NIV is not tolerated or possible (see *Section 3.3* for NIV).

Other considerations

- **VTE prophylaxis**: standard LMWH and early mobilisation.
- **Chest physiotherapy:** can be useful to aid expectoration and respiratory effort and to help with posture and maximise position of comfort to aid respiratory effort.

Prevention

- Involvement of the respiratory team can allow the patient to be visited at home and look at preventative strategies. Providing patient with steroids and antibiotics for acute exacerbations with purulent sputum. Inhaled steroids and long-acting bronchodilator therapy and Tiotropium.
- Encouraging smoking cessation and pulmonary rehabilitation (exercise, smoking and nutritional advice).
- Assessment for long term O_2 therapy which can prevent pulmonary hypertension. Requires 15+ hours per day. Long term O_2 therapy: aim to keep SaO_2 >90 % and PaO_2 >8 kPa. These patients become accustomed to worsening disease and hospital admissions.
- **Palliation and setting ceilings of care**: it is becoming more common to ask patients with end-stage disease to discuss end of life plans with regard to interventions such as ventilation prior to this in the non-acute phase. Patient expectations need to be carefully balanced with the potential futility of some treatments.

References:

Soo Hoo (2012) Noninvasive ventilation. *MedScape*, 1–20 (http://emedicine.medscape.com/article/304235-overview [accessed 12 Feb 2014]).

Royal College of Physicians (2008) NIV in COPD: management of acute type 2 respiratory failure. *National Guideline* Number 11.

12.3 Acute severe asthma (status asthmaticus)

No asthmatic patient who gets to hospital breathing should die. If hypoxic give high FiO_2 (over 60%), steroids and nebulisers. Ensure accompanied at all times, e.g. in X-ray dept. Crash team if they are deteriorating. Senior medical and anaesthetic input early.

About

- Immediately assess severity, ensure appropriate treatment and rapid escalation.
- Close observation and early senior input and liaison with ITU are key.

Aetiology

- In some there is a potentially lethal mixture of tiredness and bronchoconstriction.
- Exacerbated by mucus plugging and V/Q mismatches.
- In fatal asthma, extensive mucus plugging of the airways is found at autopsy.

Assessing asthma severity

Acute severe asthma ⟶	Life threatening asthma ⟶	Near fatal asthma
• Unable to complete sentence in one breath, respiratory rate >25/min • HR >110 bpm • PEFR 33–50% best/predicted	• Silent chest, confusion, tiring, comatose, hypotension • Poor respiratory effort, unable to blow a PEFR (PEFR <33% expected/usual, or at all) • HR >120 bpm or <60 bpm • SaO_2 <92% or PaO_2 <8 kPa, pH <7.35 or elevated $PaCO_2$ >4.6 kPa • Pulsus paradoxus is an unreliable sign and the other signs suffice in determining severity	• $PaCO_2$ >6 kPa • Needing ventilation

Investigations

- **ABG**: hypoxia +/− hypercarbia. **FBC**: raised WCC, CRP suggests infection.
- **Eosinophilia:** consider aspergillus, parasites, drugs, Churg–Strauss syndrome.
- **U&E**: ensure normal and check CRP. **ECG:** sinus tachycardia.
- **CXR:** is indicated in all but the mildest cases to exclude pneumonia or pneumothorax.
- **PEFR**: difficult in acute severe asthma. Compare with baseline.
- **Pulmonary function tests**: can be done later if diagnosis unclear.
- **Echo/BNP/D-dimer**, etc. if diagnostic uncertainty, e.g. PE.

Management (liaise closely with ITU)

- **General:** most need only oxygen, steroids, nebulised salbutamol and Atrovent, support and time. It's the steroids that matter most. Reassurance, hydration, encourage slower and deeper respirations – a positive confident competent attitude from staff can help greatly because patient is working hard and *in extremis* and is often terrified. Ask anaesthetists to review EARLY any patient not rapidly improving. Antibiotics only if clear evidence of infection.
- **Direct observation:** patient must be accompanied and monitored at all times as rapid deterioration is possible, e.g. in X-ray department.
- **Oxygen**: ABC high FiO_2 initially then adjusted to deliver sats of 94–98% or 88–92% if severe COPD and reassess after ABG. If sats <85% then high flow 10–15 L/min with non-rebreather mask and get urgent anaesthetic help (patient is in peri-arrest).
- **IV fluids** to avoid dehydration as patient too breathless to drink. Ensure patient sitting up and as comfortable as possible.
- **Bronchodilator**: nebulised SALBUTAMOL 2.5–5 mg repeated every 15–20 min initially and then 2 hourly + IPRATROPIUM BROMIDE (Atrovent) 0.5 mg 4 hourly.

- **PREDNISOLONE 40–60 mg stat** PO and/or **IV HYDROCORTISONE 100–200 mg IV stat.** Once you get to this point take stock. Are things improving?
- **IV MAGNESIUM SULPHATE** which may help to improve FEV_1 if unresponsive to other treatments. Small improvements.
- **IV loading dose AMINOPHYLLINE**. Omit loading dose if on AMINOPHYLLINE already. Maintenance dose thereafter. Ensure ECG monitoring if patient not already on theophylline. The therapeutic window is narrow and macrolides and ciprofloxacin can cause toxicity. Watch serum levels.
- **IV SALBUTAMOL** with ECG monitoring if unresponsive to other treatments. However, has been associated with Type B lactic acidosis and severe agitation and tachycardia. Use with caution.
- **Intubation and ventilation:** 1–3% require intubation. Bag valve–mask ventilation is very difficult due to severe airway obstruction. Rapid sequence induction is used.
- **IM ADRENALINE** may be used *in extremis* as per anaphylaxis. IV adrenaline is generally avoided because of lethal arrhythmias and even ST changes.
- **Pregnancy:** treat as in non-pregnant. Asthma can seriously complicate pregnancy. Real risk is undertreatment. In 33% asthma improves, in 33% asthma worsens and in 33% there is no change; those with more severe asthma worsen. Ensure patients know to continue medications to ensure good asthma control. Uncontrolled asthma is associated with many maternal and fetal complications, including hyperemesis, hypertension, pre-eclampsia, vaginal haemorrhage, complicated labour, fetal growth restriction, preterm birth, increased perinatal mortality, and neonatal hypoxia. Advise women who smoke to stop smoking. Anti-asthma drugs are safe to use in pregnancy and during breastfeeding. Give O_2 / salbutamol IV or oral steroids / oral or IV theophyllines / IV magnesium as needed. However, IV adrenaline (epinephrine) should be avoided in the pregnant patient. Leukotriene antagonists may be continued in women who have demonstrated significant improvement in asthma control with these agents prior to pregnancy, not achievable with other medications. In labour – if anaesthesia is required, regional blockade is preferable to general anaesthesia. Prostaglandin E_2 may safely be used for labour inductions. However, use prostaglandin $F_2\alpha$ with extreme caution in women with asthma because of the risk of inducing bronchoconstriction. Women receiving steroid tablets at a dose exceeding prednisolone 7.5 mg per day for more than 2 weeks prior to delivery should receive parenteral hydrocortisone 100 mg 6–8 hourly during labour.

Post recovery

- **Discharge:** those with a PEFR <50% should be admitted. Consider discharge if PEFR >75% of baseline. Mild cases which are responsive can go home after a few hours observation with a short course of oral steroids. Very mild cases go on inhaled steroids and salbutamol. On discharge give a peak flow meter with instructions and show how to use it.
- **Advice:** always advise the patient and family to return if deterioration by calling 999. Be aware that those who do badly tend to come from more difficult social environments and it may be wise to hold on to them longer; send home those who are sensible and who have someone to assist them if there are any problems. Flare-ups can be unpredictable and it is important to give clear instructions on what to do if they occur. Patients are often experienced in self-management and should be involved in their discharge timing decision.

References: Guide (2008) British Guideline on the Management of Asthma. *Thorax*, 63(Suppl 4):1.

12.4 Pneumothorax and tension pneumothorax

All patients with underlying lung disease and PTX should be admitted for inpatient observation

About

- Air within the pleural space.
  Primary pneumothorax (PTX) occurs in those with normal lungs.
- Secondary PTX occurs in those with underlying lung disease and all with PTX need to be admitted as they are higher risk.
- Severe symptoms and haemodynamic collapse suggests tension PTX.

Primary PTX

- Tall thin males aged 20–40 with no known lung disease. Increased risk and commoner on right side. Commoner in smokers who possibly have subclinical lung disease. Increased stresses on the lung apices in tall people cause a predisposition to subpleural bleb formation, which can later cause a PTX.
- Most often recur within 1st year especially in those who are tall and continue to smoke (40% in 2 years).

Secondary PTX (spontaneous / traumatic / iatrogenic / chronic lung disease)

- **Trauma:** especially penetrating chest trauma, iatrogenic trauma – pleural biopsy. Lung biopsy, central line insertion, high PEEP ventilation.
- **Infection:** lung abscess, PCP pneumonia (AIDS), cystic fibrosis.
- **Others:** asthma, emphysema, idiopathic pulmonary fibrosis, sarcoidosis. Endometriosis / catamenial PTX – occurs within 72 h of menses. Oesophageal rupture. Lymphangioleiomyomatosis, lung carcinoma, histiocytosis X, eosinophilic granuloma, Marfan's syndrome, and homocystinuria.

Size

- **Small PTX** rim <2 cm. **Large PTX** rim >2 cm (suggests >50% lung volume loss).
- Measure gap between lung margin and the chest wall (at the level of the hilum).

Tension PTX

- Ventilated patients on ICU, trauma patients, resuscitation patients (CPR).
- Lung disease – acute presentations of asthma and COPD; blocked, clamped or displaced chest drains; patients receiving NIV or hyperbaric O_2 treatment.

Clinical

- Small PTX: may be asymptomatic or mild dyspnoea.
- Larger PTX: causes mild to severe dyspnoea. Depends on size and lung function. Cyanosis when a large PTX. Localised chest pain and even a click or added sounds.
- Affected side hyper-resonant with reduced breath sounds.
- Tension PTX: trachea pushed away, *in extremis*, tachycardia and hypotension. Suspect in ventilated patient who suddenly deteriorates.

Investigations

- **FBC, U&E, CRP:** raised WCC, infection, anaemia, inflammatory/infectious.
- **ABG**: if breathless and suspicion of RF. CXR: a standard departmental PA chest.
- **CXR (PA +/– lateral):** is the standard and shows an absence of lung markings between the ribs and a line demarcating the edge of the lung. New imaging systems may make it more difficult to see a lung edge than the old X-ray film so

care must be taken. Expiratory films no longer advocated. Lateral CXR or even CT may help if PTX suspected and PA chest not definitive. **CXR (PA)**: measure and use distance b at level of hilum (see *figure*).

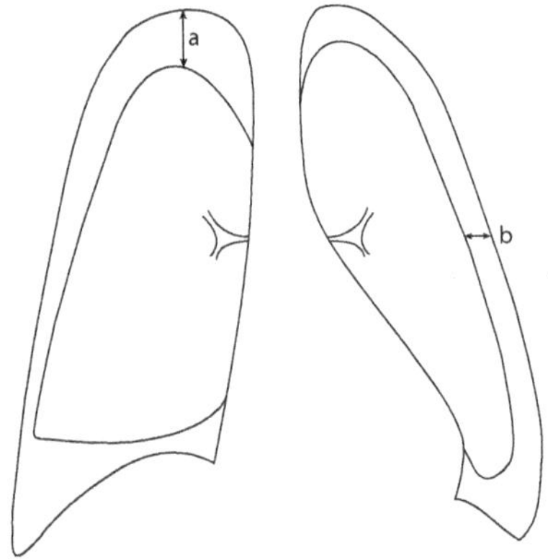

a = apex to cupola distance – American Guidelines
b = interpleural distance at level of the hilum – British Guidelines

- **Chest CT:** can be useful especially to differentiate bullae from PTX and to determine any underlying parenchymal pathology. Can also aid decisions on best place to position drain in complex cases and in detecting small pneumothoracies.
- **Other:** in selected cases HIV test in at-risk groups, ACE and calcium for sarcoidosis, bronchoscopy and lung biopsy, etc.

Smoking cessation reduces recurrence rate and is an important part of PTX management and prevention.

Management

- **General points:** O_2 as per BTS guidance; however, there is an argument to giving higher O_2 because it helps resorb the pleural cavity air and this should be assessed on a case by case basis. PA CXR film should be taken in the department if at all possible. Much better quality than on the ward with a portable machine.
- **Tension PTX:** give high flow O_2. Usually too ill to wait for CXR so proceed on clinical findings. Patient critical then **immediate needle decompression in the 2nd intercostal space in mid-clavicular line on the affected side**. Identify space and mark it. Prepare the area as best one can. If time allows, wash hands, put on sterile gloves, clean area, strict asepsis if possible but need to be quick. Get venflon and insert in marked space. There should be a 'hiss' as it decompresses and BP should rise. Remove the inner metal needle and leave it to decompress. Then insert chest drain.
- **Determine if primary or secondary:** if age >50 and significant smoking history or evidence of underlying chronic lung disease in history, examination or on CXR, then treat as secondary PTX. Symptoms often more pronounced in secondary. Mortality is higher. Patients with pre-existing lung disease tolerate a PTX less well.
- **Primary PTX management:** if CXR shows >2 cm rim of PTX **and/or** patient is breathless, then aspirate with 16–18G cannula up to 2.5 L and repeat CXR. If success (<2 cm and less breathless) then observe for 4–6 h and consider discharge and review in respiratory clinic in 4–6 weeks or sooner. If, however,

after aspiration PTX is not <2 cm and breathlessness not improved then chest drain with size 8–14Fr and admit. Discharged patients should return by calling 999 if new SOB.

- **Secondary PTX management**: if CXR show >2 cm rim of PTX **and/or** patient is breathless then chest drain with size 8–14Fr and admit. If CXR shows 1–2 cm rim of PTX **and** patient is not breathless then aspirate with 16–18G cannula up to 2.5 L and repeat CXR. If size now <1 cm then admit and high flow O_2 (unless O_2 sensitive) and observe for 24 h. If after aspirating PTX is still >1 cm then chest drain with size 8–14Fr and admit. Those on positive pressure ventilation require chest drain insertion as positive pressure maintains the air leak. All are admitted.
- **Flying and diving post PTX**: patients should be cautioned against flying until CXR shows complete resolution and most airlines suggest flying acceptable after 6 weeks of full resolution or a definitive surgical procedure. Risk is significant for a year and some may prefer to wait. Suggest expert individual advice. Never allow to scuba dive unless bilateral pleurectomies and specialist approval.
- **PTX and pregnancy**: PTX recurrence is more common in pregnancy and poses risks to the mother and fetus. Requires close cooperation between chest physicians, obstetricians and thoracic surgeons. PTX that occurs during pregnancy can be managed by simple observation if the mother is not dyspnoeic, there is no fetal distress and the PTX is small (<2 cm). Otherwise aspiration can be performed, chest drain insertion being reserved for those with a persistent air leak. Because of the risk of recurrence in subsequent pregnancies, a minimally invasive *video-assisted thoracoscopic surgery (VATS)* should be considered after convalescence.
- **PTX and AIDS/HIV infection:** the combination of PTX and HIV infection requires early intercostal tube drainage and surgical referral, in addition to appropriate treatment for HIV and *Pneumocystis jiroveci* infection. *Pneumocystis jiroveci* pneumonia (previously *Pneumocystis carinii* pneumonia) causes a severe form of necrotising alveolitis in which the subpleural pulmonary parenchyma is replaced by necrotic thin-walled cysts and pneumatoceles. They have more prolonged air leaks, treatment failure, recurrence and higher hospital mortality. More aggressive intervention indicated.
- **PTX and cystic fibrosis:** this requires early and aggressive treatment with early surgical referral. Pleural procedures, including pleurodesis, do not have a significant adverse effect on the outcome of subsequent lung transplantation.
- **Pleural aspiration for PTX:** infiltrate local anaesthetic down to the pleura, in the 2nd ICS in the mid-clavicular line (the axillary approach is an alternative). Using a cannula (French gauge 14–16), enter the pleural cavity and withdraw the needle. Connect both the cannula and a 50 ml syringe (Luer lock) to a three-way tap, so that aspirated air can be voided. Aspiration should be discontinued if resistance is felt or the patient coughs excessively, or more than 2.5 L (that is, 50 ml removed 50 times) is aspirated. Repeat CXR in inspiration (an expiration film is unnecessary) in the X-ray department. If PTX is now only small, or resolved, the procedure has been successful. Note that failure to aspirate further may be due to the cannula being inadvertently withdrawn from the pleural cavity, or becoming kinked. If this is suspected, another attempt at aspiration should be considered; aspiration should not be repeated unless there were technical difficulties. If this fails then a small-bore (<14Fr) chest drain insertion is recommended (see *Section 27.3*).

Reference: Macduff *et al.* (2010) Management of spontaneous pneumothorax: British Thoracic Society pleural disease guideline. *Thorax*, 65(Suppl II):18.

12.5 Pneumonia

About

- Infection and inflammation of the air spaces and substance of the lung, which are normally sterile.
- Lobar – restricted to the whole of one lobe, exclude a bronchostenotic lesion.
- Bronchopneumonia affects lobules and bronchi. CURB-65 scoring for community-acquired pneumonias.

Aetiology: different locations and different organisms: bacterial, viral or fungal

- **Community-acquired (CAP)**: symptoms + signs of consolidation. Often healthy, young patients.
- **Hospital (HAP) or institutional**: acquired – onset >48 h after admission. These patients have significant co-morbidities. Difficulty swallowing. Poor nutrition. More likely to have aerobic Gram-negative infections, e.g. *Pseudomonas, E. coli,* anaerobes and *Staph. aureus.*
- **Ventilator-acquired pneumonia**: same organisms as HAP.
- **Aspiration pneumonia**: gastric acid into lungs + foodstuff. Goes to right mid zone or apex of right lower lobe. Co-Amoxiclav is suitable.

Risks

- Young and elderly. Co-morbidities – renal disease, HIV, diabetes, heart disease.
- Lung disease: COPD, cystic fibrosis, bronchiectasis, old TB, bronchostenotic lesion.
- Others: smoker, alcohol excess, IV drugs, steroids.

Causative organisms: vary by study, age, location, co-morbidities, exposure

- *Strep. pneumoniae* 39%, *Haemophilus influenzae* 5.2%, *Chlamydophila pneumonia* 15%. Influenza virus A/B 10%, *Mycoplasma pneumonia* 10%, *Moraxella catarrhalis* (COPD) 2%. *Chlamydophila psittaci* (avian) 2.6 %, *Coxiella burnettii* 1.2%.
- *Legionella* virus like illness. Low sodium and WCC. Confusion. Diarrhoea.
- *Staph. aureus* 1.9% (post influenza), *Pneumocystis jiroveci* pneumonia (HIV).
- Tuberculosis not usually included as a cause of community-acquired pneumonia but is a cause of pulmonary infection.

Types

- **Community-acquired pneumonia** – at-risk groups: aspiration (stroke/motor neuron disease), alcohol, diabetes, steroids and immunosuppression. Smokers. COPD. Nursing home residents.
- **Hospital-acquired** – same as community-acquired. Elderly, immunosuppressed, respiratory disease, post-operative, ITU. Usually Gram-negative enterobacteria – pseudomonas. *Klebsiella* and anaerobes.
- **Atypical pneumonias** have unusual presentations, e.g. with headache and a viral meningitis picture; diarrhoea, vomiting, abdominal pain, myalgia and the chest symptoms may take time to appear clinically and radiologically.

Pathology stages

(1) Congestion and vascular engorgement and alveolar bacteria.
(2) Red hepatisation – alveolar spaces full of polymorphs and fibrin and red cells.
(3) Grey hepatisation – RBC breakdown, fibrin and suppurative inflammation.
(4) Resolution – exudate removed by macrophages.

Clinical

- Fever, sweats, rigors, dry cough initially, malaise, delirium (elderly and *Legionella*).

- Breathlessness, cyanosis, tachycardia, hypotension, pleuritic-type chest pain.
- Cough, rusty sputum (*Pneumococcus*) yellow/green sputum, haemoptysis.
- Flare up of herpes simplex (*Pneumococcus*), atypical diarrhoea.
- Myalgia, headache, reduced air entry and expansion and dullness to percussion.
- Increased vocal resonance, stony dull if effusion/empyema.

Complications

- Lung abscess, exudative pleural effusion, parapneumonic effusion.
- Empyema, bacteraemia, sepsis, cerebral abscess, meningitis.
- ARDS, respiratory failure, cardiac failure, multi-organ failure, death.

Investigations

- **Sputum/blood cultures:** Gram stain and culture and sensitivity.
- **FBC: raised** WCC. Low WCC with *Legionella*.
- **U&E:** AKI. Low Na with *Legionella*.
- **Blood film**: red cell agglutination suggests cold agglutinins and *Mycoplasma*.
- **ESR/CRP elevated** with pneumonia and empyema.
- **LFT:** raised with *Legionella*, blood cultures and sensitivities.
- **CXR**: patchy consolidation with bronchopneumonia. More defined consolidation with lobar pneumonia. Cavitation may be seen. Parapneumonic effusion. Changes often lag behind clinical changes.
- **ABG:** Type 1 and possible Type 2 respiratory failure with V/Q mismatch.
- **Serology**: *Mycoplasma*, *Chlamydophila*, *Coxiella*, influenza, adenoviral, RSV, *Legionella*, urinary pneumococcal antigen and *Legionella* antigen test.
- **Bronchoscopy** in some cases to look for any bronchostenotic lesions or remove foreign bodies or mucus plugging.
- **CT chest**: to look for and exclude other related pathology.
- **Others**: always consider HIV test and ask about risk factors.

Differentials of pneumonia

- PE, pulmonary oedema, ARDS, pulmonary haemorrhage.
- Cryptogenic organising pneumonia, lung cancer, acute extrinsic allergic alveolitis.

CURB scoring is used to define severity and advise clinical management

If age >65 score +1 point for each feature present:

- confusion: MTS <8 or new disorientation in person, place or time +1 point
- urea >7 mmol/L +1 point
- respiratory rate >30/min +1 point
- blood pressure (SBP <90 mmHg or DBP <60 mmHg) +1 point

CURB score:

- 0/1: probably suitable for home treatment
- 2: admit – options may include short inpatient stay or hospital-supervised outpatient
- 3/4+: manage in hospital as severe pneumonia. Consider ICU admission if CURB-65 score = 4+.

Additional evidence of severity

- **WCC** >20 or <4. **CXR**: multilobe involvement. **Albumin** <35 g/L.
- **Microbiology**: positive blood culture.
- **Others**: stroke, COPD, cardiac disease, diabetes.

Clues to causative agents

- ***Strep. pneumoniae***: cold sore, rusty sputum, consolidation/cavities (serotype 3).
- ***Chlamydophila pneumoniae***: epidemics, raised AST.

- **Viral pneumonia**: influenza A and B, parainfluenza, measles, RSV in infants. Varicella can cause severe pneumonia with miliary nodular shadows, which may calcify.
- ***Mycoplasma pneumoniae***: younger patients, autumnal, erythema nodosum and multiforme, myocarditis, pericarditis, meningoencephalitis, Guillain–Barré syndrome, haemolytic anaemia, bullous myringitis, cold agglutinins in 50%, headache, otalgia, transverse myelitis, pancreatitis, lymphadenopathy, splenomegaly.
- ***Legionella pneumoniae***: older patients. From showerheads and air conditioning. Headache, malaise, myalgia, high fever, dry cough, nausea, vomiting, diarrhoea, confusion, hepatitis, low sodium, low albumin, abnormal LFTs, high CK.
- ***Haemophilus influenzae***: 3% bronchopneumonia.
- ***Staph. aureus***: winter. Post-influenza/viral pneumonia. CXR cavitation and abscess.
- ***Chlamydophila psittaci***: sick bird. Malaise, low-grade fever, hepatosplenomegaly.
- ***Coxiella burnettii***: animal contact. Chronic influenzal illness with dry cough, conjunctivitis, hepatosplenomegaly, endocarditis. CXR: multiple segmental shadows.
- ***Klebsiella pneumonia***: widespread consolidation (upper lobes). High mortality.

Slow resolution – consider empyema, underlying neoplasm or antibiotic resistance or is it the wrong diagnosis.

Management

- **ABC and FiO_2** to deliver sats of 94–98% or 88–92% if severe COPD. Check ABG.
- **IV fluids**: hydration important. May need CPAP, BIPAP or ITU if worsening respiratory failure. Aspirate pleural effusions. Chest drain for empyema. Chest physiotherapy. VTE prophylaxis. Nutrition.
- **Consider ITU admission** if pH <7.26 or PO_2 <8 kPa or rising PCO_2 or breathless and tiring patient.
- **Prevention**: influenza and pneumococcal vaccination should be considered.

Antimicrobial management

- **Community treated non-severe pneumonia** (CURB-65 score = 0): treat for 5–7 days with AMOXICILLIN IV/PO. Penicillin allergic: CLARITHROMYCIN PO/IV.
- **Community-acquired non-severe pneumonia** (CURB-65 score = 1–2): treat for 5–7 days with AMOXICILLIN IV/PO plus CLARITHROMYCIN PO/IV.
- **Community-acquired severe pneumonia** (CURB-65 score = 3–5): treat for 7–10 days or 7–14 days for *Mycoplasma*, *Legionella* and *Chlamydophila* or severe disease. Contact microbiology if no improvement in 24 h. Discuss duration with microbiology in case of Legionnaires disease. BENZYLPENICILLIN IV plus CLARITHROMYCIN PO/IV. Switch to oral AMOXICILLIN and CLARITHROMYCIN PO/IV when clinically appropriate. Penicillin allergic (severe): TEICOPLANIN plus CLARITHROMYCIN PO/IV.
- **Hospital-acquired pneumonia**: defined as infection occurring after ventilation or >3 days of hospital stay. TAZOCIN IV tds. If penicillin allergic (severe/anaphylaxis): TEICOPLANIN plus GENTAMICIN IV (see *Chapter 29*). If evidence of aspiration add METRONIDAZOLE. Contact microbiology if MRSA-positive or if no improvement in 24 h.
- **Acute bronchitis/acute exacerbations of COPD**: AMOXICILLIN or DOXYCYCLINE PO. Treat for 5–7 days. If severe, or if resistant bacteria isolated, discuss with Consultant Microbiologist. Suspect *Staph. aureus*: IV FLUCLOXACILLIN +/– SODIUM FUSIDATE. Anaerobes – consider adding IV metronidazole. Aspiration

pneumonia (mainly chemical but may be super-infection). Hospital-acquired – add IV metronidazole if aspiration and ensure cover for Gram negatives. Observe local antibiotic policies. Avoid causing *Clostridium difficile* associated colitis.

12.6 Pneumocystis pneumonia

Patients desaturate on exercise which can be a useful sign. Seen in immunosuppressed, e.g. HIV with CD4 <200/mm^3, post-transplantation, methotrexate, long term steroids.

About

- Infection by *P. jiroveci* (formerly *P. carinii*). Seen in immunocompromised.
- Seen in untreated HIV infection or in those on immunosuppression.

Aetiology

- Infection damages alveolar epithelium, impedes gas exchange and leads to Type 1 respiratory failure.

Clinical

- Breathless, PTX, fever, dry cough, fine crackles. Check O_2 sats on mild exertion.
- Signs of AIDS, e.g. oral candida, Kaposi's sarcoma, hairy leukoplakia, herpes zoster, etc.

Investigations

- **FBC and U&E**: low WCC.
- **ABG**: PaO_2 <8 kPa on air defined as severe PCP. Desaturation with exercise is a useful clue.
- **HIV test**: CD4 cell counts (usually <200/mm^3) and HIV viral load measurements.
- **CXR:** normal or bilateral infiltrates, cavitation, cysts, TB in AIDs, nodules or PTX.
- **HRCT:** characteristic ground-glass appearance, cysts, nodules, PTX.

Management

- **ABC** + O_2 adjusted to deliver sats of 94–98% or 88–92% if severe COPD.
- **ITU:** CPAP or intubation and ventilation if persisting refractory RF. Watch out for PTX which is seen with pneumocystis pneumonia.
- **High dose CO-TRIMOXAZOLE** (trimethoprim + sulphamethoxazole) 120 mg/kg/day (of the TMP component) IV or PO daily in three or four divided doses for 14–21 days. Alternatives to co-trimoxazole include **IV PENTAMIDINE** (4 mg/kg per day) **and Dapsone and Clindamycin.** Take expert help.
- **Steroids:** give steroids if severe (PaO_2 <9.3 kPa on air). **PREDNISOLONE** 80 mg/day for at least the first 5 days, tapering off over the next 2–3 weeks. In severe disease, **IV HYDROCORTISONE** should initially be used.
- **AIDS:** will need specialist review for commencement of highly active antiretroviral therapy (HAART) if confirmed AIDS. Check CD4 count. Not usually started acutely. Take expert advice.
- Smoking cessation is advocated.
- **PCP prevention**: CO-TRIMOXAZOLE 960 mg PO daily.

12.7 Lung abscess

About

- Formation of an infected pus-filled cavity within lung parenchyma.

Aetiology

- Post pneumonia usually *Staph. aureus*, *Klebsiella*, Gram negatives, anaerobes.
- Infected cavity, TB, aspiration pneumonia, bronchiectasis.
- Trans-diaphragmatic spreads from amoebic abscess.
- Distal to endobronchial obstruction, e.g. inhaled foreign body or tumour.

Clinical

- Fever, malaise, weight loss, breathlessness, pain, foul breath.
- Clubbing may be seen with chronic untreated suppurative disease.

Investigation

- FBC: raised WCC, ESR, CRP. Sputum/blood cultures.
- CXR and HRCT: demonstrates any infected cavity or tumour, and lymph nodes and lung parenchyma.

Management

- Prolonged IV antibiotics and surgical or percutaneous drainage.
- Bronchoscopy to remove any foreign body or biopsy endobronchial lesion.

12.8 Pulmonary embolism and DVT

About

- Deep vein thrombosis (DVT) and pulmonary embolism (PE) are all part of same disease. Clots arise in the deep veins of the legs and thigh and pelvis and pass to the lungs and occasionally to the left atrium and systemic circulation if septal defects.
- Reduce by early mobilisation and low dose LMWH or equivalent in those at increased risk. Untreated mortality is 30% (not all PEs are the same), which falls to 3–8% with treatment. However, data come from a time when only larger PEs were detectable.
- Can expect 500 per DGH per year. 65–90% emboli from legs. Rivaroxaban is now licenced to treat DVT/PE and other new oral anticoagulants (NOACs) will come on line soon.
- Many small DVTs and even PEs are potentially benign. Anticoagulation has risks and these need to be balanced. Need better algorithms to select those in whom risk of VTE exceeds that of anticoagulation.

Aetiology

- Most thrombi originate in the proximal veins of the lower leg and pelvis. Consider a thrombophilia disorder in those under 45 without a clear precipitant.
- DVT can embolise across a right/left shunt (e.g. PFO/ASD) and cause an embolic stroke. Most emboli are multiple to lower lobes and 10% cause infarction.
- Autopsies show high incidence of undiagnosed VTE as a cause of death.

Clinical (a useful way to think of PE)

- **Deep vein thrombosis**: pain, redness, swelling, increased circumference, can extend to the calf or the whole leg swollen in large proximal thrombosis.
- **Small emboli/small vessel occluded**: initially asymptomatic but over time multiple recurrent thromboembolism leads to progressive breathlessness and ultimately cor pulmonale and pulmonary hypertension. Single small emboli may be subtle and non-specific, e.g. causing confusion especially in elderly.

- **Medium sized or moderate vessel or vessels occluded**: dyspnoea, tachypnoea, haemoptysis, pleuritic chest pain, pleural rub, transient collapse, syncope or presyncope.
- **Large vessel or multiple vessels occluded**: there is acute right heart failure with marked dyspnoea, tachypnoea, presyncope or syncope. Urge to defecate (often collapse in toilet), chest pain, tachycardia, raised JVP and loud P2 on auscultation, hypotension.
- **Massive PE/saddle embolism:** embolism obstructing one or both pulmonary arteries – sudden cardiac death, obstructive shock.

Risks

- Previous DVT/PE, malignancy, immobility, obesity, perioperative event, stroke, severe illness, spinal injury, Guillain–Barré syndrome, trauma, HHS, localised trauma.
- Phlebitis, post-MI, pregnancy and postpartum, pelvic tumour, polycythaemia, sickle cell disease, hyperviscosity, protein C and S deficiencies, smoking, combined OCP, HRT, and recent long haul travel.

Wells clinical model for predicting pre-test probability of DVT

- Active cancer (treatment within last six months or palliative): +1 point
- Calf swelling >3 cm compared to asymptomatic calf (measured 10 cm below tibial tuberosity): +1 point
- Collateral superficial veins (non-varicose): +1 point
- Pitting oedema (confined to symptomatic leg): +1 point
- Swelling of entire leg: +1 point
- Localised tenderness along distribution of deep venous system: +1 point
- Paralysis, paresis, or recent cast immobilisation of lower extremities: +1 point
- Recently bedridden >3 days, or major surgery requiring regional or general anaesthetic in the previous 12 weeks: +1 point
- Previously documented DVT: +1 point
- Alternative diagnosis at least as likely as DVT: –2 points

Clinical probability of DVT: score of 2 or higher – DVT is 'likely'; score of less than 2 – DVT is 'unlikely'

Wells clinical model for predicting pre-test probability of PE

- Previous PE/DVT: + 1.5 points
- Heart rate >100 bpm: +1.5 points
- Recent surgery/immobilization (<30 days): +1.5 points
- Clinical signs of DVT: +3 points
- Alternative diagnosis less likely than PE: +3 points
- Haemoptysis: +1 point
- Cancer treated <6 month ago: +1 point

Clinical probability of PE

Score: low 0–1; intermediate 2–6; high ≥6. Others interpret as score >4 suggests PE likely and a score ≤4 PE less likely. Check D-dimer.

Revised Geneva scoring system for PE

- Age >65: +1 point
- Previous DVT/PE: +3 points
- Recent fracture/surgery <1 month: +2 points
- Active malignancy: +2 points
- HR >75–94 bpm: +3 points; >94 bpm: +5 points
- Pain on leg deep vein palpation or unilateral oedema: +4 points

Clinical probability of PE

Score: low 0–3; intermediate 4–10; high >10

Differential diagnosis for DVT

- Leg trauma +/− haematoma, internal derangement of the knee.
- Muscle tear and damage, ruptured Baker's cyst, cellulitis, obstructive lymphadenopathy.
- Lymphoedema, drug-induced oedema (amlodipine, etc.).

Investigations

- **Bloods:** FBC, U&E, LFTs, CRP, ESR typically normal unless reflecting underlying cause, e.g. malignancy.
- **ABG:** medium to large PE can cause a reduced PO_2 and reduced/normal PCO_2 (Type 1 RF). *In extremis* may be acidotic.
- **D-dimer:** >500 ng/ml in nearly all patients with DVT/PE, and false positives in others. Only those patients classified as low or intermediate risk of PE should undergo quantitative D-dimer testing. If the D-dimer level is below your local lab cut-off level and the patient is classified as low probability then the diagnosis of PE can be excluded. D-dimer test is sensitive but not specific for PE. D-dimer unhelpful in pregnancy, infections, sepsis, anticoagulated, post-op. It is a degradation product of cross-linked fibrin. Don't bother if high probability.
- **Compression ultrasonography (Doppler) of lower limb veins:** is the preferred diagnostic test. It is non-invasive, relatively inexpensive and readily available. It has replaced contrast venography as the modality of choice. It is particularly useful for pelvic and iliofemoral clots.

The superficial femoral vein is a deep vein and thrombosis requires treatment. To avoid confusion it has been renamed the distal femoral vein.

- **ECG findings:** tachycardia, new AF. Others include S1Q3T3 pattern. Right ventricular strain. New incomplete RBBB. Alternatively, the ECG may be normal.
- **CXR:** a normal CXR is entirely compatible with a large PE. Segmental wedge collapse, pleural effusion, area of lung infarction, raised hemidiaphragm, prominent pulmonary artery and a localised absence of vascular markings.
- **Cardiac troponin and BNP levels** elevated in large PEs and are associated with a worse outcome.
- **Echocardiogram:** right atria and right ventricle dilated, tricuspid regurgitation, right heart strain, pulmonary hypertension. Diagnostic in massive PE but less helpful in sub-massive PE. RV hypokinesis has been shown to be associated with double the 30-day mortality.
- **Ventilation–perfusion (V/Q) scanning** is used in many centres as the preferred initial imaging, especially in pregnancy or the young with a normal CXR or renal failure or allergy to IV contrast. Ventilation scan by inhaling radioactive xenon gas. Perfusion using radiolabelled albumin macro-aggregates. Then look for areas of ventilation but low perfusion. Lots of unsatisfactory low or intermediate probability results which will require CTPA or Doppler of legs to properly risk assess.
- **CT pulmonary angiography (CTPA):** multislice helical CTPA is perhaps the commonest test these days and involves giving IV contrast. It is useful for identifying pulmonary emboli and other lung pathology. It is quick and can be done out of hours. Current fear of overdiagnosis.
- **Pulmonary angiography** is the gold standard but rarely done nowadays. When CTPA or V/Q scan not desired, e.g. pregnant or not possible, then the finding of thrombus on USS legs may be used as a surrogate marker for PE, when there is

DVT and appropriate chest symptoms and a decision to anticoagulate is straightforward.

- **General comments**: CTPA is sensitive and easy to obtain, but for clinically stable patients alternative tests reduce exposure radiation, cost less, and are less likely to lead to overdiagnosis. V/Q scans may be preferable in younger patients (less radiation), patients with normal lungs (a definitive result is more likely), and patients with renal dysfunction (no nephrotoxic contrast). Detection of DVT by ultrasonography of the legs when PE is suspected makes subsequent lung imaging unnecessary because patients need anticoagulation anyway. There is no single pathway. Depends on access to tests, availability of ambulatory testing and this is a complex and difficult area. Take advice.
- **Thrombophilia testing:** consider testing for antiphospholipid antibodies in patients who have had an unprovoked DVT/PE or if it is planned to stop anticoagulation treatment. Consider testing for hereditary thrombophilia in patients who have had unprovoked DVT or PE and who have a first-degree relative who has had DVT or PE if it is planned to stop anticoagulation treatment. **Do not** offer thrombophilia testing to patients who have had a provoked DVT or PE. **Do** offer thrombophilia testing to first-degree relatives of people with a history of DVT or PE and thrombophilia.
- **Cancer screening**: for unprovoked DVT/PE in those who are not already known to have cancer, the following investigations for cancer are suggested: should have a full history and appropriate physical examination, CXR, FBC, U&E, Ca, LFTs and urinalysis.

Diagnostic algorithm

- **DVT**: if predictive scoring (see above) says DVT likely then patient should have a proximal vein USS and LMWH if this is not carried out within 4 h. If the scan is positive then continue/start treatment. If scan negative then do not treat. If two level Wells score suggests DVT unlikely then check D-dimer. In negative non-treated patients seek help and follow up if any further symptoms.
- **PE**: if predictive score suggests PE likely then CTPA or V/Q scan and treat if positive. If Wells score suggests PE unlikely then check D-dimer. If D-dimer positive then CTPA and V/Q scan; if scan negative then no treatment but seek help and follow up if any further symptoms. Give interim anticoagulation until all results known.

Management

- **ABC high FiO_2** initially then adjusted to deliver sats of 94–98% or 88–92% if severe COPD and reassess after ABG. Cardiac monitoring of BP, HR, O_2 saturation. Commence **1 L IV crystalloid** to ensure adequate right-sided filling, especially if hypotensive.
- **Cardiac arrest then CPR:** give up to 30 min CPR +/− thrombolysis in event of cardiac arrest with suspected PE.
- **Thrombolysis for PE:** should be considered in a patient with a large compromising PE where there is hypotension/signs of severe RV dysfunction. See *Chapter 29*.
- **Thrombolysis for DVT:** discuss with vascular team. **Catheter-directed thrombolytic therapy** for patients with symptomatic iliofemoral DVT who have symptoms <2 weeks and good functional status and a life expectancy of 1 year or more and a low risk of bleeding. There is risk of limb ischaemia and postphlebitic syndrome.

- **Pulmonary embolectomy:** may be available in some centres and there is no clear guidance on patient selection, though those who are moribund may be the most suitable. Discuss with surgeons according to local pathways. Some research has been done on extending use to those with anatomically extensive PE and concomitant moderate to severe right ventricular dysfunction despite preserved systemic arterial pressure; requires cardiac bypass and heparinisation (Circulation, 2002;105:1416.)
- **LMWH or Fondaparinux:** all patients should receive (normal renal function) on the basis of clinical suspicion and this should be stopped if subsequent tests are negative. If a PE is identified then **ENOXAPARIN** is continued indefinitely or if warfarinised until INR >2.0 for at least 5 days.
    - **DVT and PE: ENOXAPARIN** 1.5 mg/kg SC OD is recommended by the *BNF*. American College of Chest Physicians (*Chest*. 2012;142:1074) recommends 1.5 mg/kg SC OD or 1 mg/kg SC bd. Treat as soon as there is high clinical suspicion and stop when PE has been disproved. Take advice.
    - Fondaparinux 5 mg (body weight <50 kg), 7.5 mg (50–100 kg), or 10 mg (>100 kg) SC OD.
    - **Tinzaparin:** DVT or PE: 175 U/kg daily.
- **Management of below knee DVT:** consider repeating USS after 5 days to see if there is extension above the knee of any clot if the diagnosis is unclear. The management of isolated calf vein thrombosis is controversial. Those undergoing orthopaedic procedures, those with malignancy, and those that were immobile had a higher risk of propagation. Risk of PE and other complications seems very low as over 90% of PEs arise from above the knee thrombus. Mortality rate of proximal DVT is greater than distal DVT. There is no consensus on whether to treat, observe or not treat. Full dose anticoagulation is not without risk. Follow local expert guidance.
- **Warfarin** for 3–6 months for a first idiopathic PE/DVT is routine. A 12 week course where there is an identifiable temporary precipitant. There should be an overlap of Warfarin and heparin for 5 days because a transient pro-coagulant condition can exist. Advice is to offer treatment for confirmed unprovoked proximal DVT or PE within 24 h of diagnosis and continue for 3 months. At 3 months, assess the risks and benefits of continuing Warfarin treatment. May continue treatment for a full 6 months in total. At this stage do thrombophilia testing in the young or those with a family history.
- **Rivaroxaban** is now recommended (NICE, 2013, TA287) as an option for the acute treatment of PE and preventing recurrent DVT and PE in adults. Dosage of **Rivaroxaban is 15 mg BD for the first 21 days followed by Rivaroxaban 20 mg OD** for continued treatment and prevention of recurrent venous thromboembolism. Other NOACs are undergoing evaluation.
- **IVC filters** may be used where there is a high risk of VTE and anticoagulation is not possible in the short term or when PEs still recur despite anticoagulation. IVC filters are effective for 12 days. There is no difference in mortality and recurrence may be higher in the filter groups. Patients should eventually be started on Warfarin. Newer retrievable filter devices can be removed after 6 weeks. The filters tend to clot off and can cause leg oedema.
- **PE and known cancer**: standard practice is to offer LMWH to patients with active cancer and confirmed proximal DVT or PE, and to continue the LMWH for 6 months. At 6 months, assess the risks and benefits of continuing anticoagulation.
- **Warfarin is not harmless**: CTPA can detect isolated small subsegmental pulmonary emboli which are not clinically important and so where the real risks of

anticoagulation may outweigh benefits – take expert advice. Interestingly, the higher resolution of CTPA versus V/Q scan diagnosis increases the number of PEs diagnosed, but detecting small PEs does not alter overall outcome.

- **Other tests:** a new PE without obvious precipitant may be a sign of an occult malignancy and a full history and examination and targeted investigations should be considered. Some would consider focused clinical examination, CT chest, abdomen pelvis, basic bloods and tumour markers.
- **Ambulatory care of suspected PE**: exclusion criteria as follows: studies have shown that for selected low risk patients with acute symptomatic PE outpatient treatment with LMWH is not inferior to inpatient treatment in terms of effectiveness and safety. Those who are sent home must be a very well, stable, independent group who can readily seek help.

Ambulatory care management of PE – those not suitable include

- Breathless at rest, O_2 sats <97%, PO_2 <10 kPa on air.
- HR >100 bpm or SBP <100 mmHg, CKD necessitating IV heparin therapy.
- Other illnesses requiring admission, difficult social circumstances.
- Thrombocytopenia precluding heparin therapy (platelet count <70 × 10^9/L).
- Active bleeding or high bleeding risk, acute anaemia.
- History of heparin-induced thrombocytopenia, suspected PE on anticoagulation.
- Current alcohol/illicit drug abuse, psychosis, dementia, or homelessness.
- Pregnancy, ECG RV strain, pain requiring IV opiates.

PE and pregnancy

- PE is a leading cause of pregnancy-related mortality. Clinical diagnosis is difficult as signs and symptoms resemble physiological changes of pregnancy. The tests are imperfect and must be gauged with clinical findings. **D-dimer** is often mildly elevated and so a raised value must be corroborated with other investigations. Involve senior obstetricians, radiologists and respiratory team urgently if patient compromised or peri-arrest. If clinically likely **treat as such with LMWH or IV heparin** whilst tests awaited.
- **You should do a CXR.** It is appropriate and may identify and rule out other pathology (?PTX, effusion, consolidation, pneumonia) and involves a tiny radiation dose and the fetus can be shielded. Useful evidence from **USS Doppler of leg veins for a DVT** (ask radiologist to screen from calf veins to inferior vena caval bifurcation as there are often large pelvic thrombi) will indicate a need for anticoagulation without radiation. **Echocardiogram** may show right heart changes. The **perfusion (Q) only part of V/Q scanning** may be used. **CTPA may be considered,** especially where there has been preceding lung disease. The theoretical concern is CTPA irradiating pregnant breast tissue with long-term breast cancer risks, but misdiagnosis kills mother and fetus and the radiation risk is tiny compared with the risk of misdiagnosis and not treating. If there is diagnostic suspicion and Q scan and echo/doppler equivocal/unhelpful then CTPA.
- Standard treatment is LMWH. Warfarin is contraindicated. **IV heparin preferred if imminent delivery being contemplated and should be stopped 4–6 h before.** In extreme situations thrombolysis, and catheter and surgical embolectomy have been performed. Take local expert advice because protocols vary. Manage with obstetric input at all stages. After delivery warfarin can be started and is safe in breastfeeding. Continue anticoagulation at least 6–12 weeks post-delivery.

References and further reading:

NICE (2012) Venous thromboembolic diseases, CG144.

Task Force for the Diagnosis and Management of Acute Pulmonary Embolism of the European Society of Cardiology (2008) Guidelines on the diagnosis and management of acute pulmonary embolism. *Eur Heart J*, 29:2276.

Wiener *et al*. (2013) When a test is too good: how CT pulmonary angiograms find pulmonary emboli that do not need to be found. *BMJ*, 347:f3368.

12.9 Massive haemoptysis

About

- Haemoptysis is reasonably common but massive life threatening haemoptysis is rare. Death is from hypoxia rather than exsanguination, so keep the non-bleeding lung uppermost to protect airway.
- Sedation and palliation may be more appropriate with advanced lung cancer.

Aetiology

- The lungs are supplied by the bronchial arteries under systemic pressure, e.g. 120 mmHg. The pulmonary arteries are under much lower pulmonary artery pressure, e.g. 25 mmHg. Severe bleeding is more likely from the bronchial arterial vessels. Bronchial vessels can be embolised in severe haemorrhage.

Causes

- Primary lung cancer or pulmonary metastases (smoker, weight loss, clubbing).
- Pneumonia or bronchiectasis (cough + purulent sputum).
- Chronic bronchitis (chronic cough), lung abscess (with pus).
- Pulmonary tuberculosis (weight loss, calcification and consolidation and lymphadenopathy).
- Pulmonary oedema (bat wing alveolar oedema, Kerley B lines, cardiomegaly).
- Alveolar haemorrhage (WG/Goodpasture's alveolar shadowing and cavitation).
- Hereditary haemorrhagic telangiectasia, pulmonary AV fistula, pulmonary artery aneurysms.

Clinical

- Distressed, breathless, cyanosed, clubbing and weight loss if underlying tumour.
- Expectorating bright red frothy blood, hypoxic, hypotensive.
- Listening over chest may hear gurgling from affected side.
- Upper zone blood may gravitate to lower lobes depending on position.
- Consider metastases, e.g. renal, testicular, gastrointestinal.
- Overseas/HIV makes TB more likely.

Investigations

- **FBC**: raised WCC, ESR, CRP infective, inflammatory or malignancy.
- **U&E**: AKI with Wegener's granulomatosis or Goodpasture's syndrome.
- **Blood cross match**: if anaemic or bleeding is significant.
- **Coagulation screen**: APTT, prothrombin time (PT), INR, platelets, fibrinogen.
- **ECG**: non-specific unless cardiac disease or acute PE.
- **Sputum for culture**, AFB and cytology.
- **CXR:** is valuable because it lateralises the cause and helps diagnose the lesion causing the bleeding.
- **CT chest:** may provide more information if possible.
- **CTPA and/or V/Q:** if PE considered.

- **Antibodies to C-ANCA (proteinase 3)** for Wegener's granulomatosis and **anti-GBM** (anti-glomerular basement antibody) for Goodpasture's syndrome if indicated. Check urine for blood and protein.
- **Echocardiogram** if cardiac disease or PE suspected. **Cardiac troponin** if cardiac disease suspected.

Management: (death is from hypoxia rather than exsanguination)

- **ABC FiO_2** as per BTS guidelines. Sedation may be useful in a distressed patient.
- Start IV fluids and group and cross match and transfuse blood as needed. Treat any coagulopathy.
- **Positioning**: protect the good lung – keep the patient lying on side with bleeding side down and unaffected side uppermost.
- **Nebulised adrenaline**: can be used (5–10 ml of 1 in 10 000 adrenaline).
- **Intubation:** consider intubation if tiring or there is on-going bleeding and risk of asphyxiation, falling SaO_2. Use large bore tube which may be single or double lumen.
- **Bronchoscopy** has long been considered by chest clinicians to be the primary method for diagnosis and localisation of haemoptysis, but can be difficult with acute bleeding in visualising the bleeding source. Case by case assessment.
- **Bronchial artery angiography and embolisation** is indicated from interventional radiology (side-effects include cord ischaemia/infarction if anterior spinal artery compromised).
- **Tamponade:** where the bronchial balloon of a double lumen tube, or a 4 French 100 cm Fogarty embolectomy catheter, or Arndt endobronchial blocker, inserted via a single lumen tube, can be used for tamponade and left inflated for 24 h before deflation and observation. There is a theoretical risk of mucosal ischaemia with this approach.
- **Lavage:** use of saline cooled in ice in 50 ml aliquots down the bronchoscope with volumes up to 1 L is well described, and can arrest bleeding.
- **Topical coagulants:** thrombin and fibrinogen concentrates have been topically instilled, with anecdotal success. Laser, diathermy, or cryocautery. These are possible through a rigid bronchoscope and can be applied to, for example, a bleeding endobronchial tumour.
- **Surgical management:** may be applicable in some cases where a more conservative approach is not sufficient. In some cases emergency pulmonary resection provides an effective treatment with acceptable morbidity and mortality in patients with massive haemoptysis.
- **Palliation** where the patient has a known terminal lung malignancy and bleeding cannot be stopped is appropriate. Consider morphine and palliative care team.

12.10 Pleural effusion

About

- Pleural effusions may be signs of local or systemic pathology.
- When very large they can impair respiratory function.
- May become infected and if so need to be drained. Check a drug history.

Aetiology

- Collection of fluid within the pleural space can restrict lung function.

Clinical

- Signs of RA, SLE, heart failure, clubbing, malignancy. Assess symptoms.

- Depends on size, rate of accumulation and underlying cardiorespiratory function.
- Increased SOB, pleuritic chest pain, reduced wall movement, vocal resonance, and breath sounds.
- Stony dull to percussion, deviation of the trachea/mediastinum away if large.

Investigations

- **FBC**: anaemia, raised WCC infective or inflammatory, malignant cause.
- **U&E CRP**: raised AKI, raised **LFTs:** albumin, raised CRP/ESR, raised ALP, ALT (metastases) PT.
- **Chest imaging: PA CXR:** useful to show size. The meniscus is an optical illusion due to curvature of chest wall. Hilar enlargement, cardiomegaly, pulmonary oedema, malignancy, TB, breast shadowing.
- **Echocardiogram or BNP**: poor LV function.
- Adenosine deaminase (ADA) to rule out TB.
- **High resolution CT** with contrast: identify local causes and lung parenchyma.
- **USS**: can identify good aspiration site. Helpful if fluid loculated.
- **Pleural aspirate, protein, glucose, LDH, culture:** see fluid on CXR and diagnostic aspiration. Needs >300 ml to be clinically detectable. This can be done with a fine bore (21 G) needle and a 50 ml syringe. Inspect appearance and send aspirate for cytology: protein, lactate, glucose, LDH. A low glucose (<3.3 mmol/L) suggests infection, tumour, RA, mesothelioma. Aspiration should be avoided for bilateral effusions in a clinical setting strongly suggestive of a transudate and CCF, unless there are atypical features or they fail to respond to therapy.
- **Pleural fluid inspection:** bloody fluid can be confirmed by measuring haematocrit. Milky fluid suggests a chylothorax which may be due to damage to the thoracic duct. In this situation measure pleural fluid triglyceride and cholesterol levels.
- **Aspirate cytology:** malignant effusions show pleural fluid cytology in about 60% of cases.
- **Aspirate amylase**: if oesophageal rupture or pancreatic disease suspected.
- **Aspirate pH useful** where infection suspected; a pH <7.2 with a suspected parapneumonic effusion indicates the need for tube drainage.
- **Aspirate glucose**: <1.6 mmol/L in RA.
- **Percutaneous pleural biopsy** under image guidance for pleural thickening on CT.
- **Thoracoscopy**: considered for an exudative pleural effusion where a diagnostic pleural aspiration is inconclusive and malignancy is suspected.

Causes of pleural effusion by Light's criteria

Transudate	Exudate
Those not fulfilling Light's criteria for exudate	Pleural protein >50% of serum protein, pleural LDH >60% serum LDH, pleural LDH >66% upper limit of normal for serum
Failures: cardiac failure, nephrotic syndrome, liver failure **Miscellaneous**: myxoedema, hypo-albuminaemia Meigs's syndrome with ovarian tumour and right pleural effusion	**Infection**: pneumonia; tuberculosis; empyema **Cancer:** (blood stained) bronchogenic, mesothelioma, lung metastases, ovarian tumours **Cardiac/vascular**: pulmonary infarct (bloody), post-MI; constrictive pericarditis **Gastro**: pancreatitis, oesophageal rupture (both raised amylase)

Transudate	Exudate
	Connective tissue disease: SLE, RA, FMF **Drugs:** methysergide, nitrofurantoin **Miscellaneous:** radiotherapy; trauma; post-cardiac surgery; asbestosis (blood stained); yellow nail syndrome

Management

- **ABC high O_2** adjusted to deliver sats of 94–98% or 88–92% if severe COPD. Depends on determining the likely cause and managing that through simple investigations. If the effusion is causing compromise then drainage required. Otherwise a diagnostic tap can be performed as suggested above. Drainage requires 1–2 L to be taken off.
- **Diagnostic aspiration** is useful. Light's criteria should be used to help diagnosis. Infections and empyema and haemothorax and malignancy all have their particular specialist management.
- Outpatients: if stable, not breathless on minimal exertion or at rest, and mobile, consider referral of selected patients to a **pleural effusion clinic**. Advise to return if worse. Some can have on-going investigations, e.g. CT chest and investigation for secondary causes as an outpatient.

Reference: British Thoracic Society Pleural Disease Guideline Group (2010) BTS Pleural Disease Guideline.

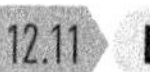

12.11 Empyema

About

- Pus in the pleural space usually post-bacterial pneumonia.
- It requires effective drainage and systemic antibiotics.

Aetiology

- Parapneumonic effusion after bacterial pneumonia becomes infected.
- Associated with diabetes, alcohol abuse, IV drug use, GORD.
- Post trauma or a complicated lung abscess or thoracic surgery or infected draining catheter.

Clinical

- Purulent cough, pyrexia, dyspnoea after recent pneumonia.
- Weight loss, pleurisy and fever, night sweats, clubbing.

Investigations

- **FBC**: raised WCC and CRP. **U&E**: AKI. **CXR:** pleural effusion.
- **If suspected then pleural aspiration:** shows a purulent or turbid/cloudy pleural fluid exudate which may be neutrophil-rich and viscous with raised protein and white cells. Empyema – glucose <2.2 mmol/L, pH <7.2 OR pH >7.8 suggests *Proteus*. Ensure all pleural fluid analysed in blood gas machine has been heparinised. **LDH**: >1000 IU/L.
- **Blood cultures** for aerobic and anaerobic bacteria performed.
- **Chest CT/USS:** to help locate drain optimally because the cavities may become loculated. CT is ideal to define the anatomy. Gas may strongly suggest an empyema.

Management

- **ABC O_2** as per BTS guidelines. Ensure adequate nutrition in patients with pleural infection. Abstain from alcohol/smoking. Identify any immunocompromise.
- **Ensure VTE prophylaxis** as high risk and give LMWH.
- **Chest drain**: if diagnosis confirmed by aspiration then insert a drain large enough to drain the fluid. A small bore catheter 10–14 Fr will be adequate for most cases of pleural infection. Occasionally viscid and difficult to drain but in many cases a small tube inserted by Seldinger method is adequate. The small catheters can be placed using either ultrasound or CT scans. Previously streptokinase to cause localised fibrinolysis has been used but less so now as data have not been positive. If parapneumonic effusion not confirmed by aspirate then do not drain but continue antibiotics and watch CRP and reassess and take advice. *Pleural procedures should not take place out of hours except in an emergency.*
- **IV antibiotics**: take microbiology advice – usually same antibiotics as pneumonia. Aminoglycosides are inactivated by low pH. May need to cover anaerobes and pseudomonas. Get results of culture and adjust accordingly.
- **Involve chest team** and they may need to involve thoracic surgery (thoracotomy and decortication) in difficult cases. Decortication involves the removal of all fibrous tissue from the visceral pleura and parietal pleura, and the evacuation of all pus and debris from the pleural space.

Reference: British Thoracic Society Pleural Disease Guideline Group (2010) BTS Pleural Disease Guideline.

13 Endocrinology and diabetes emergencies

13.1 Primary hypoadrenalism (Addisonian crisis)

About

- Acutely reduced adrenocortical function (glucocorticoids, mineralocorticoids).
- Insidious and subtle or acute and life threatening, provoked by illness, e.g. infection. Some are due to cessation of medically prescribed steroids.

Aetiology

- Adrenally produced cortisol and mineralocorticoids needed for life.
- Increased demand during stresses (infection, trauma, illness).
- Cortisol released in response to pituitary ACTH (adrenocorticotrophic hormone).
- Aldosterone released in response to angiotensin II.
- Loss of the adrenal medulla has no known clinical sequelae.

Types

- Primary due to adrenal disease, with glucorticorticoid/mineralocorticoid loss.
- Needs 90% adrenal destruction before detectable.
- Secondary disease with pituitary disease and ACTH insufficiency.
- Tertiary due to removal of exogenous/endogenous steroid excess.

Causes

- Abrupt cessation of medically prescribed steroids +/– physiological stress (sepsis or surgery).
- **Autoimmune adrenalitis**: 70% (lymphocytic infiltration) often with autoimmune disease (Grave's disease, Hashimoto's thyroiditis, pernicious anaemia, hypoparathyroidism or Type I diabetes or vitiligo).
- **Infections**: TB both adrenals (may calcify on AXR), HIV, CMV adrenalitis. Progressive disseminated histoplasmosis. Waterhouse–Friederichsen syndrome (adrenal haemorrhage) associated with meningococcaemia.
- **Malignancy**: breast and lung and melanoma and lymphoma.
- **Genetic**: adrenoleukodystrophy – inborn error of fatty acid metabolism.
- **Miscellaneous**: amyloidosis, post-bilateral adrenalectomy, polyglandular autoimmune syndromes.
- **Secondary adrenocortical insufficiency**: pituitary haemorrhage, Sheehan's syndrome.

Pathophysiology

- Adrenal failure causes low glucocorticoids and mineralocorticoids and aldosterone.
- Failure to retain salt and water causes hypotension.
- Pituitary releases increased ACTH/MSH with pigmentation.

Clinical

- Subacute with fatigue, anorexia, weight loss, tiredness, diarrhoea, vomiting.
- Abdominal pain, generalised weakness, precipitated by sepsis, surgery.
- Postural hypotension, tachycardia, shocked, confusion, hypoglycaemia.
- In secondary disease (pituitary) mineralocorticoid function is unimpaired.
- Loss of axillary and pubic body hair in females (loss of adrenal androgens).
- Pigmentation in gums, buccal mucosa, skin, pressure points, skin creases, scars.
- Hypoglycaemia is more common in secondary adrenal insufficiency.

Investigations

- **FBC:** raised neutrophils, **U&E** Low Na^+, high K^+, low HCO_3, low Cl^-, low glucose, low urea, high Ca^{2+}
- **ABG or venous gas**: low HCO_3 mild metabolic acidosis.
- **ACTH** >80 ng/L at 0900 with a low/low–normal cortisol confirms diagnosis.
- **Short synACTHen test** shows low rise in 30 min cortisol to ACTH.
- **Aldosterone**: low and renin is high.
- **Adrenal antibodies:** seen in autoimmune disease.
- **CXR/AXR:** to look for active TB disease and classically small heart. Calcification.
- **CT abdomen**: may show enlarged necrotic glands with calcification.
- **Adrenal biopsy** in selected cases.

Short synACTHen test

- Baseline cortisol. Give synthetic ACTH (synacthen) 250 mcg IV (1 vial) and check 30 min cortisol. Adrenal insufficiency excluded by additional rise in cortisol of >200 nmol/L and a 30 min value >600 nmol/L. Treat on clinical evidence because result may take 2–3 days to come back. This can always be done later if not done acutely. Initially one should at least send a baseline cortisol.
- Some patients may have relative adrenal insufficiency, which only becomes apparent with stress-haemorrhage, infection, and surgery/trauma. A short synACTHen may show a muted response. Have a low threshold to treating possible adrenal insufficiency in critical care.
- Steroid equivalence roughly is Hydrocortisone 100 mg = Methylprednisolone 125 mg = Dexamethasone 4–5 mg = Prednisolone 40–50 mg.

Management

- **ABC and O_2** as per BTS guidelines. 1 L NS IV over 30–60 minutes + 50 ml 50% dextrose if hypoglycaemic. Send random cortisol 10 ml in a heparinised tube.
- **Steroids:** hydrocortisone 100 mg IV initially then IM every 6 hours. If able to take oral then start hydrocortisone 20 mg TDS and gradually wean down to 30 mg per day in divided doses usually with a larger morning dose. Fludrocortisone not needed acutely as the raised hydrocortisone dose has sufficient mineralocorticoid activity.
- **Inotropes:** dopamine may be considered in severe cases to support the circulation.
- **Determine cause**: treat for TB or HIV.
- **Long term steroids**: once stabilised can reduce and give oral steroids such as **HYDROCORTISONE 10 mg am and 5 mg at midday and 5 mg at 6pm** as well as **FLUDROCORTISONE 0.1 mg/day** if adrenal disease with postural hypotension.
- **Sick day rules**: double steroid dose if unwell. Family should be aware. Patients should carry a steroid card to alert staff. Recommended to have an ampoule of hydrocortisone for IM administration in the event of being unable to take oral.
- **Prior to operative procedures** patients should be given hydrocortisone 100 mg IM before and a further 50–100 mg IM 6 hourly until back on oral therapy.

13.2 Hypoglycaemia

Starvation in those not on insulin or oral hypoglycaemics or with acute alcohol rarely, if ever, causes significant hypoglycaemia. Be sceptical about diagnosing light-headedness and funny spells as hypoglycaemia unless there is clear evidence, e.g. a laboratory glucose reading.

About

- Prolonged hypoglycaemia causes brain injury and death.
- Check capillary blood glucose and send lab sample in any confused or comatose patient.
- Treat any symptomatic blood glucose <4.0 mmol/L.

Aetiology

- Causes neuroglycopaenia and neuronal dysfunction and increased sympathetic drive.
- Neurons do not need insulin to allow glucose to enter cells.
- High metabolising brain is dependent on a steady supply of glucose/ketones. Any shortfall in supply quickly leads to neuronal dysfunction.

Clinical

- Sweating, trembling, palpitations, anxiety, blurred vision, hunger, headache.
- Lack of coordination, ataxia, stroke mimic – hemiparesis, confusion, aggression.
- Loss of inhibitions, convulsions, coma, brain damage, death, violence, agitation.
- Morning headache, night sweats, vivid dreams suggest nocturnal hypoglycaemia or nocturnal seizures.

Causes

- Drugs: Insulin, Sulphonylurea, Meglitinides (not metformin), Pentamidine, Quinine, Salicylates, acute alcohol, Propranolol.
- Endocrine: Addison's disease, growth hormone (GH) deficiency, hypopituitarism.
- Liver failure, insulinoma, chronic pancreatitis with a loss of glucagon activity.
- Worsening renal function increases insulin sensitivity.

NOT USUALLY CAUSED BY

- Metformin, Glitazones, Thiazolidinediones, DPP-4 inhibitors, GLP-1 analogues.
- Starvation: those in fasts or famines or hunger-strikes do not usually succumb to acute hypoglycaemia.

Impaired awareness of hypoglycaemia (IAH)

- Acquired syndrome with insulin treatment. Diminished warning symptoms of hypoglycaemia. Increases vulnerability to severe hypoglycaemia.
- Prevalence increases with duration of diabetes and seen T1DM > T2DM.

Investigations

- High morning glucose may suggest overnight hypoglycaemia with stress response. Measure overnight 16 hour fast levels of glucose and insulin to look for low glucose and high insulin suggestive of insulinoma.
- U&E, LFTs, cortisol, C-peptide which mirrors endogenous insulin production.
- Test if overnight blood glucose <4 mmol/L. Urine sulphonylurea screen in rare unexplained cases.

Management

> Be careful: there may be a marked disparity between arterial and venous blood glucose which can lead to misdiagnosis of hypoglycaemia based on symptoms and misleadingly low venous levels when arterial levels are actually normal.

- **Hypoglycaemia symptoms:** blood glucose >4 mmol/L treat with a sugary soft drink or sugary tea or juice (not diet drink) or small carbohydrate snack only. Adults who are conscious but uncooperative but can swallow can give a small snack or 1.5–2 tubes Glucogel/Dextrogel squeezed into the mouth. **If ineffective or oral intake unsafe** or impossible then consider **GLUCAGON 1 mg IM** which may be less effective in patients prescribed sulphonylurea therapy.

- **Adults who are unconscious or fitting** then check ABC + O_2 and give **20–50 ml IV 50% dextrose** through a large vein and place in recovery position and manage as for status epilepticus (see *Section 19.4*). If no venous access or no IV dextrose then **GLUCAGON 1 mg IM**. Glucagon may take up to 15 min to take effect because it mobilises glycogen from the liver and so it will be less effective in those who are chronically malnourished (e.g. alcoholics) or in patients who have had a prolonged period of starvation and have depleted liver glycogen stores, or in those with severe liver disease. In this situation, or if prolonged treatment is required, IV dextrose is better. Once normoglycaemic, assess cause and make changes to diabetic regimen if needed.
- If there is any suspicion of adrenocortical insufficiency then **HYDROCORTISONE 50–100 mg IV tds** should be given after a cortisol level has been quickly sent. An insulin and C-peptide assay can be done where hypoglycaemia is unexplained and deliberate or accidental misuse of insulin suspected. Exogenous insulin causes a rise in insulin but not C-peptide. Endogenous insulin release is accompanied by C-peptide release. If hypoglycaemia confirmed with no obvious cause, then one should consider admission for further tests, e.g. a prolonged fast and other assessments of endocrine function.

13.3 Hyperkalaemia

Medical emergency if K^+ >6.5 mmol/L or ECG changes then give 10 ml of 10% calcium gluconate or chloride slow IV.

Clinical

- Asymptomatic, arrhythmias, muscle weakness, cramps, paraesthesia.
- Hypotension, bradycardia, cardiac arrest.

Severity

- **Mild** (K^+ 5.5–6.0 mmol/L) or **moderate** (K^+ 6.1–6.5 mmol/L).
- **Severe** (K^+ >6.5 mmol/L) or if **ECG changes** or symptoms.

Investigations

- **U&E**: repeat sample in case it is false, especially if ECG normal and hyperkalaemia inexplicable. AKI.
- **FBC/LDH:** haemolysis. **CK:** rhabdomyolysis.
- **Venous/arterial blood gases**: metabolic acidosis.
- **ECG signs:** peaked 'tented' T waves, widened QRS, sine waves, agonal rhythm and VT/VF.

Causes (most commonly drugs – check drug chart)

- False result: haemolysed sample, laboratory or sampling error.
- Acute kidney injury, CKD, digoxin poisoning (poor prognostic sign).
- Rhabdomyolysis, vigorous exercise, haemolysis, blood transfusion.
- Drugs: ACE inhibitor, angiotensin II blockers, Spironolactone, Eplerenone, Amiloride, NSAIDs, Ciclosporin, depolarising muscle relaxants.
- Acidosis, Addison's disease, Type 4 renal tubular acidosis (diabetes), hyperkalemic periodic paralysis.

Further management

- **ABC. Assess ECG changes.** Stop all potentially offending drugs or infusions immediately. This is easily overlooked. Ensure IV access, repeat any sample if surprise result. Start IV fluids. Potassium >6.0 mmol/L and ECG changes needs telemetry and defibrillator available.
- Severe (K^+ >6.5 mmol/L or ECG changes) then cardioprotect with 10 ml 10% CALCIUM GLUCONATE/CHLORIDE and 50 ml of 50% dextrose with 10 units of SOLUBLE INSULIN (moves K^+ into cells) and SALBUTAMOL repeated 5 mg nebulised. Furosemide initially 10–20 mg IV may be considered if not dehydrated. U&E needs to be repeated every 2 h and capillary blood glucose for 6–12 h. The remainder need ECG and underlying cause to be found and close monitoring.
- **CALCIUM RESONIUM 30 g initially and then 15 g QDS.** PR route is possibly more effective than PO. When given rectally the calcium resonium must be retained for 9 h followed by irrigation to remove resin from the colon to prevent faecal impaction. Bowel perforation can be a rare complication.
- **Consider IV $NaHCO_3$ 1.26%** if pH < 6.9. No evidence that it works as a potassium-lowering agent in this context. Can cause sodium overload.
- **AKI assess and manage cause**: renal referral needed. If AKI/CKD and refractory/severe hyperkalaemia despite treatment then discuss suitability for haemodialysis/haemoperfusion.
- Adopt a 'low potassium diet', e.g. avoid chocolate, fruit juices. Ensure that any AMILORIDE, SPIRONOLACTONE, ACE inhibitor, ARB or similar has been stopped.

Reference: Clinical Resource Efficiency Support Team (2005) Guidelines for the treatment of hyperkalaemia in adults.

13.4 Hypokalaemia

About

- Major intracellular cation. In cardiac patients aim for a K^+ of 4.0–5.0 mmol/L.
- Beware – rapid administration of IV potassium can cause lethal arrhythmias.
- The IV rate of KCl administration should not exceed 20 mmol/h.

Aetiology

- The daily intake of potassium in the western diet is between 80 and 120 mmol.
- Low K^+ reduces muscle and nerve excitability and enhances digoxin toxicity.

Causes

- Thiazides and loop diuretics, Conn syndrome, Cushing syndrome.
- Severe diarrhoea (potassium-rich mucus from colonic adenoma, fistulas, laxatives or a VIPoma can cause hypokalaemia with metabolic acidosis). Alcohol abuse and magnesium depletion.
- Renal tubular acidosis 1 and 2, nephrotoxic drugs, severe vomiting with metabolic alkalosis.
- Insulin therapy in setting of DKA, IV/nebulised salbutamol.
- Familial (hypokalaemia) periodic paralysis, amphotericin B, gentamicin, levodopa.
- Congenital adrenogenital syndromes, Liddle syndrome.
- Bartter syndrome (alkalosis, hypocalciuria) and Gitelman syndromes.

Clinical

- Mild: lethargy, weakness, paralysis, diarrhoea (as a cause).
- Muscle pains, rhabdomyolysis, paralytic ileus, palpitations (ectopics).

- Hypertension (Conn syndrome, Cushing syndrome).
- Check drugs: loop diuretics, thiazides.

Investigations

- **U&E:** K^+ <3.5 mmol/L (severe K^+ <2.5 mmol/L) with normal K^+ 3.5–5.0 mmol/L.
- **ECG**: atrial/ventricular ectopics, arrhythmias, ST changes, U wave, T wave flattening.
- **TFT**: raised T_4 and low TSH if hyperthyroid. **HCO_3** is low in RTA
- **Endocrine testing** for Cushing syndrome, Conn syndrome.
- **Blood gases** may show a metabolic alkalosis

Management

- **Mild (3.0–3.4 mmol/L):** give 50–100 mmol over 24 h. Oral/NG replacement Sando-K 2 tablets (i.e. 24 mmol KCl) tds or Kay-Cee-L 25 ml tds (75 mmol/day) for 24–48 h and then recheck level.
- **Moderate (2.5–2.9 mmol/L):** give 100 mmol over 24 h. Consider oral/NG Sando-K 2 tablets (i.e. 24 mmol KCl) qds or Kay-Cee-L 25 ml qds for 24–48 h and then recheck level.
- **Severe (<2.5 mmol/L)**: replace IV with IV plus oral. Replace in total 100–200 mmol over 24 h. Give 20–40 mmol of potassium in 1 L and infuse over 4 h. Suggested rate is 10 mmol/h. Maximal rate is 20 mmol/h. This can be repeated 2–3 times per day with at least monitoring twice daily.
- **Replacement:** One Sando-K tablet = 12 mmol KCl, 25 ml Kay-Cee-L = 25 mmol KCl. **Avoid solutions more concentrated than 40 mmol in 1 L** as they can cause phlebitis and pain. Use the largest peripheral vein available. Give by central line with close monitoring. Potassium-containing solutions should be given by infusion pump to avoid accidental high flow rates. Treat any magnesium deficiency.
- **NPSA recommends:** a second practitioner should always check for correct product, dosage dilution, mixing and KCl concentrate and other strong potassium solutions.

References:

Rastergar & Soleimani (2001) Hypokalaemia and hyperkalaemia. *Postgrad Med J*, 77:759.

National Patient Safety Agency (2002) Potassium chloride concentrate solution. *Patient Safety Alert*.

13.5 Hypercalcaemia

90% of hypercalcaemia is due to primary hyperparathyroidism or malignancy.

About

- Normal Ca^{2+} 2.15–2.50 mmol/L. Corrected calcium <2.50 mmol/L.
- Total calcium (bound and free) is measured typically.
- Severe hypercalcaemia is a corrected calcium of >3.5 mmol/L or severe symptoms.

Severity of corrected calcium

- <3.0 mmol/L: often asymptomatic and does not usually require urgent correction.
- 3.0–3.5 mmol/L: can be well tolerated. If symptomatic then prompt treatment is usually indicated.
- >3.5 mmol/L: requires urgent correction due to risk of dysrhythmia and coma.

Aetiology

- Free ionised Ca^{2+} is biologically active but difficult to measure. Total calcium is measured routinely. Unionised calcium is carried bound to albumin, citrate and phosphate.
- Low albumin gives a falsely low calcium and vice versa and correction is needed. The amount of free calcium also depends on acid/base balance.
- Acidosis reduces protein binding sites and increases the amount of ionised Ca^{2+}. Alkalosis increases protein binding sites and ionised Ca^{2+} is lower, so that signs of hypocalcaemia may develop with, for example, a respiratory alkalosis and a normal measured total calcium.
- Body contains 1–2 kg calcium, almost all of which is in bone. This store increases blood levels of calcium where there is any hypocalcaemia via action of PTH (parathyroid hormone).

Causes

- **Primary and tertiary hyperparathyroidism**: raised PTH and calcium often in an otherwise well patient. Symptoms may be minimal and patients otherwise appear well.
- **Malignancy (low PTH):** if undiagnosed often unwell with weight loss and other malignancy symptoms. Due to bone metastases (lung, breast, renal, thyroid and myeloma) or PTH-related peptide (squamous cell lung). Needs CXR. Symptoms usually marked. Myeloma screen.
- **Sarcoidosis:** raised ectopic $1{,}25(OH)_2D_3$ seen with many granulomatous diseases, TB, Lymphoma.
- **Drugs:** thiazides, calcium, vitamin D, lithium.
- **Endocrine:** Addison's disease, hyperthyroid, phaeochromocytoma, acromegaly, MEN I / II
- **Familial hypercalcaemic hypocalciuria:** autosomal dominant with increased PTH – it is important to identify patients with familial hypocalciuric hypercalcaemia to prevent a wrong diagnosis of primary hyperparathyroidism.
- **Milk-alkali syndrome:** was seen with milk + excess antacids.
- **Paget's disease:** with immobilisation. Usually calcium normal in Paget's disease.
- **Tertiary hyperparathyroidism:** secondary hyperparathyroidism which has become autonomous. Usually seen in those with CKD.

Clinical

- Constipation, nausea and vomiting, confusion, depression, delirium even psychosis and coma. Polyuria and/or polydipsia, hypotonia, hyporeflexia, weakness +/– hyperreflexia and tongue fasciculation.
- Long-standing hypercalcaemia may cause band keratopathy. Peptic ulcer disease.
- Renal stones, pancreatitis. Can cause seizures and arrhythmias.
- Look for malignancy: weight loss, neck, respiratory, abdomen, breasts, lymph nodes, finger clubbing, chest signs.

Investigations

- **FBC** and **U&E**: raised urea, ESR (myeloma/malignancy). **TFT**: ?hyperthyroid.
- **Corrected calcium**: measured serum calcium + (40 – serum albumin) × 0.02.
- **Phosphate:** raised in tertiary hyperparathyroidism.
- **ECG**: a short QT interval and risk of dysrhythmias.
- **CXR:** squamous cell carcinoma, sarcoidosis, TB.
- **PTH level**: a normal or high PTH in the setting of a raised calcium is suggestive of primary hyperparathyroidism. A low PTH suggests malignancy or sarcoid or other cause. Measure **PTH reactive protein** in malignancy.

Management

- **IMMEDIATE**: if corrected calcium level >3.2 mmol/L and symptoms should get **IV rehydration** with at least 3–6 L NS per day. NS titrated to degree of fluid depletion (HR/BP). It may require HDU admission and central line insertion to avoid fluid overload and the risks of oedema in the elderly. In some patients with mild to moderate hypercalcaemia (corrected calcium <3.5 mmol/L) then admission may not be needed and if no heart or renal issues advise the person, provided there are no contraindications, to maintain good hydration by drinking 3–4 L of fluid per day. Encourage mobilisation and return if symptoms worsen. Monitor closely.
- **DRUGS**: stop any calcium/vitamin D medication (this is often forgotten).
- **Bisphosphonates IV**: *after rehydration* if the corrected calcium is >3.0 mmol/L and renal function is normal (rehydrate first for 12 h and repeat calcium) then **IV PAMIDRONATE 60–90 mg given in 500 ml NS over 90 min**. Lower dose in renal failure and GFR <20 ml/min. Alternatives include **IV ZOLEDRONIC ACID 4 mg over 15 min.**
- **FUROSEMIDE IV**: will clear calcium. Should not be used until the patient is fully volume replaced.
- **CALCITONIN**: 200 units every 6–12 h until calcium falls. Rarely used.
- **PREDNISOLONE** may be required to treat hypercalcaemia related to lymphoma, myeloma and sarcoidosis. Steroids inhibit 1,25(OH)D_3 production. Start at prednisolone 40 mg daily.
- **Parathyroidectomy**: for primary and tertiary hyperparathyroidism. Indications in primary disease is for those with stones, renal impairment, bone disease, Ca >3.0 mmol/L and in younger patients. Monitoring maybe appropriate for older patients with Ca 2.65–3.00 mmol/L.

References:

NICE (2010) Hypercalcaemia, CKS.

Society for Endocrinology (2013) Acute hypercalcaemia. www.endocrinology.org/policy.

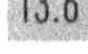

13.6 Hypocalcaemia

About

- Normal Ca 2.15–2.50 mmol/L. Total (bound and free) Ca^{2+} <2.05 mmol/L.

Aetiology

- For calcium homeostasis, see *Section 13.5*.

Causes	Notes
Hypoalbuminaemia	Low albumin which normally binds calcium and so gives a low total calcium but ionised should be normal; CKD 5 usually (failure of renal hydroxylation of vitamin D).
Parathyroid loss	Surgery/neck irradiation, Di George syndrome (hypoparathyroid with thymic aplasia).
PTH resistance	Pseudohypoparathyroidism.
Hyperphosphataemia	Phosphate binds calcium.
Vitamin D deficiency or resistance	Coeliac disease, Crohn's disease, short bowel syndrome, CF or chronic pancreatic insufficiency.

Causes	Notes
Miscellaneous	Acute pancreatitis, hypomagnesaemia (diuretics, alcohol abuse), cinacalcet, tumour lysis syndrome, multiple blood transfusions, rhabdomyolysis, sepsis/toxic shock syndrome, hungry bone syndrome post correction of primary hypoparathyroidism; bisphosphonates, foscarnet.

Clinical

- **Mild:** asymptomatic, unless **chronic:** cataracts, basal ganglia calcification, dry skin, pruritus.
- **Moderate:** numbness, paraesthesia, mild muscle weakness, wheezing. Positive Chvostek sign – tapping over facial nerve causes facial muscles to contract. Positive Trousseau sign – inflate BP cuff to 20 mmHg above SBP for 3–5 min – causes muscle spasm, and flexion of the wrist and metacarpal phalangeal joints can be observed with extension of the interphalangeal joints and adduction of the thumb (carpal spasm). More specific but less sensitive than the Chvostek sign.
- **Severe:** delirium, seizures, papilloedema, movement disorders, tetany, refractory hypotension, or arrhythmias (needs IV calcium + magnesium).

Investigations

- **FBC, U&E**: AKI, CKD. Determine estimated glomerular filtration rate (GFR).
- **Corrected calcium:** measured serum calcium + (40 – serum albumin) × 0.02. The finding of a serum calcium level lower than 2.05 mmol/L. Magnesium, hypocalcaemia and elevated phosphate suggests hypoparathyroidism or pseudohypoparathyroidism. In critically ill patients or those with acid–base disorders and suspected hypocalcaemia, measure ionised calcium on a blood sample obtained without a tourniquet.
- **Vitamin D level:** low 25(OH)D <50 nmol/L with vitamin D deficiency.
- **PTH:** low in hypoparathyroidism, elevated in all other causes.
- **Phosphate:** high with hypoparathyroidism and CKD.
- **Magnesium:** Mg <0.5 mmol/L typically results in symptomatic hypocalcaemia.
- **Alkaline phosphatase, PSA. PTH** level will be high unless hypoparathyroidism.
- **X-ray** for Looser zone and osteomalacia. Short 4th metacarpals in pseudohypoparathyroidism.
- **ECG**: a long QT interval. **Amylase** if pancreatitis considered.

Management

- **Severe hypocalcaemia**: give 20 ml of calcium gluconate 10% IV over 15 min. Calcium gluconate is preferred over calcium chloride because it causes less tissue necrosis if extravasated. Calcium for infusion diluted in saline or dextrose solution. The infusion should not contain bicarbonate or phosphate because this can form an insoluble calcium salt. If indicated a separate IV line should be used.
- **Treat any coexisting hypomagnesaemia**: acutely give with IV magnesium 2 g (8 mmol magnesium sulphate in 100 ml) given over 20 min until the patient's symptoms have cleared. Magnesium avoided in CKD. Should be given into a large vein; take care in patients with renal insufficiency because they cannot excrete excess magnesium.
- **Commence oral calcium and vitamin D replacement** (at 750–1000 mg per day). Monitor calcium levels. Replacement 750–1000 mg per day.
- Referral to endocrinology for complex patients e.g. PTH resistance should be managed by specialists.

Reference: Hannan & Thakker (2013) Investigating hypocalcaemia. *BMJ* 346:f2213.

13.7 Myxoedema coma

Consider hypothyroidism in every older patient with hyponatraemia, hypothermia, bradycardia and delirium. Mortality can exceed 20% even with optimal treatment.

About

- May complicate long-standing often undiagnosed/untreated hypothyroidism.
- May be precipitated by an acute physiological stress event.

Risk factors

- Mostly older females (mean age = 75) usually during winter.
- Usually long-standing primary thyroid failure but rarely pituitary failure.
- Previous thyroidectomy.

Causes

- Hashimoto's disease, post-thyroidectomy, radioactive iodine or antithyroid drugs.
- Drugs – lithium, amiodarone, iodine deficiency.

Precipitants

- Look for infection/sepsis (chest/urine/encephalitis), GI bleed. Drugs – alcohol, sedatives, tranquilisers, narcotics (drug metabolism is slowed so toxicity ensues), amiodarone, lithium, beta-blockers. Lung disease, stroke, CCF, ACS, upper GI bleed, acute trauma/surgery/burns.
- Hypothermia, hypoglycaemia, noncompliance with thyroid replacement.

Clinical

- Fatigue, increased weight, constipation and cold intolerance.
- Psychosis with delusions and hallucinations ('myxoedema madness').
- Hypothermia, generalised oedema, cool dry rough skin, sparse hair, macroglossia.
- Seizures, coma, bradycardia, hypotension, hypoventilation.
- Abdominal distension/pain. Paralytic ileus, megacolon, old thyroidectomy scar. Goitre with Hashimoto's disease.

Investigations

- **FBC U&E**: macrocytic anaemia, leukopenia, hyponatraemia, decreased GFR.
- **Glucose**: may be low, elevated **CK/LDH**, hyperlipidaemia.
- **TFT**: raised TSH >10 μU/ml (low if pituitary disease), low T_4 and T_3.
- **Thyroid autoantibodies** (thyroid peroxidase antibody) in Hashimoto's disease.
- **ABG**: Type 2 respiratory failure may be seen.
- **CSF:** pressure is low (some say high) and elevated protein content.
- **Abdominal X-ray:** ileus and distended bowel and faeces.
- **ECG**: bradycardia, flattened T-waves, low QRS. Torsades de pointes.
- **CXR**: cardiomegaly, pericardial and pleural effusion.

Management

- **Supportive:** look for precipitant. Admit to ITU to manage haemodynamic and any hypoventilatory status. Treat hypoxia and hypotension with O_2 and fluids/inotropes. Gradually rewarm if hypothermic but generally avoid active warming as may vasodilate and drop the BP. Watch for arrhythmias and monitor electrolytes and ABG. Interpretation impaired if hypothermic.
- **SEPSIS**: have a low threshold for IV antibiotics as signs of sepsis may be concealed by hypothyroidism, e.g. fever and tachycardia.

- **LEVOTHYROXINE** (T_4) 100–500 mcg IV once followed by 50–100 mcg OD IV until tolerating PO or via NG tube. T_4 (a prodrug converted to T_3) may provide a smoother and more gradual though slower onset of action than T_3. Lower doses of T_4, e.g. 25–50 mcg OD, may be advocated in elderly or those with cardiac disease.
- **Parenteral T_3** is available and may be the choice of some. Recommended doses range from 2.5 to 20 mcg 8 hourly. Give **T_3 10 mcg bolus IV** and then **10 mcg 8–12 hourly for 24–48 h** and then start oral T_4. Lower doses may be advocated in elderly or those with cardiac disease.
- **HYDROCORTISONE 100 mg IV and then IM 8 hourly** given for first few days and the tapered off. The rationale being possible hypopituitarism and adrenal insufficiency.
- **Hypoglycaemia:** glycogen is often depleted so hypoglycaemia may be seen and so glucose should be monitored. A glucose infusion should be considered.
- **Poor prognosis associated with** hypothermia, advanced age, bradycardia, hypotension, MI/CCF. No indication for prescribing T_4 or any preparation containing thyroid hormones to patients with thyroid blood tests within the reference ranges.

Reference: Wall (2000) Myxoedema coma: diagnosis and treatment. *Am Fam Physician*, 62:2485.

13.8 Thyroid storm / thyrotoxic crisis

About

- Rare and life threatening condition due to excess T_3/T_4.
- 2% of those with hyperthyroidism. Mortality is quoted as 10–20%.

Aetiology

- Grave's disease by the far the commonest pathology.
- Toxic adenoma or multinodular goitre, thyroiditis, post-partum thyroiditis.
- Excessive T_4 ingestion – deliberate or accidental.
- Recent amiodarone or intravenous iodinated contrast.
- Chronic tachycardia causes a cardiomyopathy.

Precipitant

- Recent minor/major illness or post radioactive iodine treatment.
- Post thyroid surgery or stopping treatment, e.g. carbimazole or propylthiouracil.

Clinical

- Tachycardia, palpitations, AF, heart failure, weight loss, tremor, lethargic.
- Sweating and agitation, fever, hypo- or hyperactive delirium.
- Apathetic (more like hypothyroidism) in elderly, abdominal pain.
- Grave's eye disease: proptosis, lid lag, chemosis, acropachy.
- Pretibial myxoedema, tender gland suggests thyroiditis.

Differential

- Hyperactive or any form of delirium, septic shock, anticholinergic toxicity.
- Delirium tremens, acute pulmonary oedema, apathetic cases can be subtle.

Investigations

- **Bloods**: FBC, U&E, ESR/CRP: raised Ca^{2+}.
- **ECG**: SR, sinus tachycardia, AF, ST/T wave changes, especially if IHD.

- **TFT**: raised T_3 and T_4 and TSH <0.05 mU/L. Thyroid peroxidase, thyroglobulin antibodies and TSH receptor antibodies in Grave's disease.
- **CXR** if infection suspected. **Blood cultures** and **CSF** if obtunded.
- **ECHO:** may show a transient rate-induced cardiomyopathy and reduced LV function.

Management

- **Manage ABCs** and give O_2 as per BTS. Consider ITU/HDU.
- **IV fluids** as per clinical status (500 ml NS over 2–4 h to start) and correct electrolytes.
- Avoid **aspirin** as it can displace Thyroxine from its protein binding and may increase its biological effects.
- **Exclude sepsis:** blood/urine/CSF (if indicated) and manage pyrexia with **paracetamol.**
- **Sedation** with HALOPERIDOL or LORAZEPAM or DIAZEPAM as needed.
- **Beta-blocker:** blockers IV or orally **PROPRANOLOL** to rate control tachycardia/AF.
- **Antithyroid:** therapy can be started – **CARBIMAZOLE** or **PROPYLTHIOURACIL (PTU)**. PTU is frequently initiated at a dose of 100–200 mg tds, depending on the severity of the illness and is preferred in pregnancy. Pregnant women suffering from thyrotoxicosis should be managed with obstetric consultation, also give PTU and then after 1 h give **IODIDE**. PTU may be preferred because it reduces T_4 to T_3 conversion.
- **POTASSIUM IODIDE:** blocks organification of iodine and reduces peripheral T_4 to T_3 conversion and is given once antithyroid drugs have been given. This is the Wolff–Chaikoff effect.
- **HYDROCORTISONE 100 mg 8 hourly** IV and then IM prevents T_4 to T_3 and suppresses the autoimmune process.
- **Plasmapheresis** has been used to treat thyroid storm in adults.
- **Thyroid eye disease** in 10–25%. More commonly in smokers – must stop. Can occur after treatment with radioactive iodine. Proptosis, swelling and oedema. Monitor visual acuity and specialist ophthalmology referral. Tape eyes closed overnight, artificial tears for gritty eyes. May require high dose steroids and even decompression surgery if sight is at risk. Ophthalmic emergency.

13.9 Pituitary apoplexy

Needs urgent neurosurgical referral to preserve vision and steroids for any secondary adrenal insufficiency.

About

- Pituitary macroadenoma (>1 cm) undergoes haemorrhagic infarction.
- Seen in 1% of pituitary tumours. Blood seen on CT.

Clinical

- Consider especially when pre-existing adenoma and severe headache +/– eye signs, coma. Hypotensive shocked with secondary hypoadrenalism.
- Ophthalmoplegia, bitemporal hemianopia and loss of vision or varying visual symptoms.
- Subarachnoid haemorrhage. Misdiagnosis reported as stroke, SAH, syncope, sepsis. May be precipitated by anticoagulants or surgery.

Aetiology

- Rapidly growing tumour outgrows blood supply or compresses its own blood supply. Expanding mass arising from the sella turcica can compress optic nerve and chiasma.
- Compresses nerves II, III, IV and VI and ophthalmic branch V_1 which lie laterally in the cavernous sinuses.
- Pituitary vascular supply from the inferior hypophyseal branch of the internal carotid artery.
- Result is hypopituitarism and hypoadrenalism.

Investigations

- **FBC, U&E**: anaemia.
- **Hormones:** cortisol, prolactin, FT_4, TSH, GH, LH, FSH and testosterone in men, oestradiol in women. Commonest tumours secrete prolactin or growth hormone.
- **CT head:** within first 24 h acutely will show a hyperdense lesion consistent with blood in an existing pituitary tumour, local haemorrhage or subarachnoid bleed and haemorrhage within the tumour.
- **MRI pituitary**: more sensitive after 24 h showing blood, tumour and necrosis. Hypopituitarism.
- **Preoperative CT** is preferable to show bony anatomy.
- **MRA / CTA pituitary**: shows pituitary and vascular structures better.

Management

- **HYDROCORTISONE 200 mg IV bolus** and then 100 mg IM qds to manage acute period.
- **IV fluid replacement.** Look out for cranial diabetes insipidus (polyuria).
- **Urgent MRI (or CT if MRI not possible) and referral to local neurosurgical/endocrine team** for rapid and effective transphenoidal surgical decompression to preserve vision and reduce pressure on local structures. Complications include damage to local structures, especially the carotid arteries laterally.
- **Formal visual fields assessment** (liaise with ophthalmology) must be undertaken when the patient is clinically stable, preferably within 24 h of suspected diagnosis.
- **Medical management** *may be sufficient* in non-visually impaired prolactinomas where a trial of dopamine agonists may be considered. This will be decided by a neurosurgeon with endocrinologist. Acutely also stop and reverse any coincidental anticoagulation. Long-term pituitary hormone replacement.

Reference: Rajasekaran *et al.* (2011) UK guidelines for the management of pituitary apoplexy. *Clinical Endocrinology*, 74:9.

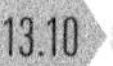

13.10 Hyponatraemia

Low serum Na reduces osmolality, causes cellular swelling and cerebral oedema.

About

- A low serum Na with low serum osmolality causes cerebral oedema, progressive coma and seizures.
- Rapid uncontrolled normalisation can lead to spastic paraparesis.

Pathophysiology

- Normal plasma osmolality is 275–295 mOsm/kg.
- Any rise in osmolality leads to ADH release and free water retention.
- ADH raises urine osmolality. ADH acts on renal V2 receptors.

Different scenarios

- **Salt level fixed and water excess:** syndrome of inappropriate release of ADH (SIADH) with excessive water resorption, excess 5% dextrose infusions, drinking excess water, water from prostate irrigation, ADH released due to pain, opiates, surgery.
- **Salt loss and water loss**: diuretics, tubular disorders, surgical drains.
- Hyponatraemia leads to movement of water into cells and cerebral oedema.
- Natural compensation: brain physiologically compensates but this takes time.

Clinical

- **Mild**: 125–130 mmol/L: symptoms of lethargy.
- **Moderate:** 115–125 mmol/L: headache, nausea, cramps, confusion.
- **Severe:** <115 mmol/L: confusion, seizure, delirium, coma, cerebral oedema and brain herniation.
- Assess if patient is hypervolaemic, euvolaemic or hypovolaemic/dehydrated:
  - **Dehydrated**: oliguria, low lying/standing BP, heart rate, thirst, poor skin turgor, weight.
  - **Fluid overloaded**: peripheral and/or pulmonary oedema, basal crepitations S3, raised JVP.
- **Other clues**: fluid balance shows excessive IV 5% dextrose. Surgical drains and NG tube shows excessive losses associated with hypovolaemia. Euvolaemic and meningitis, brain injury or small cell lung tumour or pneumonia suggests SIADH.

Assessment of hyponatraemia		**Management**
Hypovolaemic (reduced ECF) Low BP, dehydrated Renal or GI losses or Overdiuresis	**Renal losses** (urine Na >20 mmol/L): diuretics (renal salt loss + ADH stimulation and free water retention), salt-losing nephropathy, RTA, cerebral salt wasting (SAH), Addison's disease. **Non-renal losses** (urine Na <10 mmol/L: gastrointestinal losses, burns, pancreatitis, 3rd space losses. Avoid Na retention and so urine Na <10 mmol/L, and the urine may be low volume and hyperosmolar.	**Need fluid and Na replacement** if normal renal function then salt retention will be possible so correction should be simpler. Manage underlying cause of losses. Well patient: increase salt intake with slow sodium 80 mmol/day. If vomiting then simply match losses with IV NS and 5% dextrose with 20 mmol KCl per litre. If slow to respond or encephalopathic then consider 500 ml of 3% over 6–12 hours depending on urgency and response to replacement. Test and treat for any concerns of adrenal insufficiency. Try to limit improvements to less than 10 mmol/day.
Euvolaemic (increased ICF and ECF no oedema)	Thiazide diuretics, SIADH, hypothyroidism, acute porphyria, adrenal insufficiency, Guillain–Barré syndrome.	Dilutional hyponatraemia. Avoid excessive hyponatraemic water intake (runners, ecstasy users, potomania). Correct cause. Increase salt intake with slow sodium 80 mmol/day Consider IV NS. Give 3% NS if urgent correction needed but bring levels up slowly. IV hydrocortisone if hypoadrenalism. Stop thiazides. Try to limit improvements to less than 10 mmol/day.

Assessment of hyponatraemia		Management
Hypervolaemic (increased ICF and ECF, oedema) Ascites, raised JVP	CCF, cirrhosis, nephrotic syndrome, renal disease: hyperaldosteronism, diuretic induced renal salt loss.	Dilutional hyponatraemia so the key is fluid restriction to 500–1000 ml per day and diuresis of free water by inducing diabetes insipidus or blocking ADH. In exceptions 3% NS 500 ml over 6–12 h may be given. Saline may be given with furosemide 40 mg to aid water loss. Democlocycline 300 mg BD or Tolvaptan 15 mg OD may be used to get rid of free water by inducing a nephrogenic diabetes insipidus.
Spurious (normal osmolality)	High triglyceride, protein or glucose.	
(adapted from *Postgrad Med J* 2007;83:373)		

- **Diagnosis criteria of SIADH**: hyponatraemia with low serum osmolarity (<270 mOsm/L) and an inappropriately high urine osmolarity of >100 mOsm/kg in a euvolaemic patient in whom hypopituitarism, hypoadrenalism, hypothyroidism, renal insufficiency and diuretic use have been excluded.
- **Central pontine demyelination now called osmotic demyelination syndrome**: manifests after 2–3 days as brainstem symptoms of dysarthria, dysphagia, seizures, coma, quadriparesis and can be seen on MRI. Classically seen in malnourished alcoholic with rapid correction. Exact treatment regimens are difficult because multiple factors are involved, but an effort to increase serum osmolality with either NS, or hypertonic saline if volume must be restricted, must be done carefully and cautiously with regular checking of status and bloods; if seizures and coma then more urgency may be applied. Comatose or fitting hyponatraemic patients are best managed in an HDU/ITU setting. It is certainly a time to enlist expert experienced help.

Investigations

- **FBC, U&E, urine Na** excretion, glucose, urine and plasma osmolality. In acute correction the U&E should be checked every 2–4 h.
- **TFT:** check TSH and **cortisol levels. CXR:** infection/tumour.
- **Short synACTHen** if adrenal failure considered (low BP, hypotensive, pigmentation).
- **SIADH:** urine inappropriately concentrated and often >100 mOsm/L with hyponatraemic plasma osmolarity. **Osmolality** = 2 Na + glucose + urea (all in mmol/L).

Rises in Na should be limited to 10–12 mmol/24 h or 18 mmol/48 h. Acute hyponatraemia can usually be corrected more quickly and more safely than chronic hyponatraemia.

Management

- **Supportive**: if fitting or comatose then should be on an ITU with full support. Manage seizures as per status epilepticus. CT scan if any concern as to cause of coma. General principles depend on likely cause and volume status as per the table above.

- **Principles of management:** what is the volume status? Has the low Na^+ been present for more than 48 h, i.e. chronic rather than acute? Are there signs of cerebral oedema that necessitate treatment with hypertonic saline? Assess fluid balance, osmolality and urinary osmolality, volume and salt loss. Try to break it down into hypo/eu/hypervolaemia, though some have multiple pathologies. Those with chronic hyponatraemia should have the sodium corrected much more slowly. A target of 120 mmol/L should resolve acute symptoms.
- **SIADH**: there is excessive free water retention. Low serum osmolality and urine osmolality inappropriately concentrated (>100 mOsm/kg) and urine Na >30 mmol/L. Check and stop any causative drugs and look for other causes (malignancy, Ecstasy (MDMA is often combined with excess water intake), CNS disorders, drugs, lung disease, nausea, postoperative pain, HIV, infections, Guillain–Barré syndrome, acute porphyria). Fluid restriction to 800 ml/day is needed. See above for managing severe hyponatraemia. **Demeclocycline** if euvolaemic: Demeclocycline 150–300 mg qds can be given to induce a nephrogenic diabetes insipidus and lose free water. **Conivaptan** or **Tolvaptan may also be used.** They are vasopressin V2-receptor antagonists; there are arguments for giving an ADH receptor antagonist although experience is limited in those with SIADH and some with hypervolaemic/euvolaemic hyponatraemia, e.g. Tolvaptan 15 mg (up to 60 mg/day) administered once daily. Need to watch for rapid rises in Na which can result in neurological sequelae. Uses should be for specialists only. Fluid status should be monitored frequently and the patient should be encouraged to drink freely.
- **Adrenal insufficiency** should be treated as per Addisonian crisis with IV NS and steroids. See *Section 13.1* for more information.

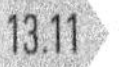

13.11 Hypernatraemia

Most often due to an impaired access to water or loss of free water greater than can be replaced by drinking or other routes.

About

- Most often free water loss or no access to water. Occasionally excessive salt.
- Mild hypernatraemia Na >145 mmol/L; severe hypernatraemia >160 mmol/L.
- Mortality can be up to 50% in elderly patients. Correct slowly at <12 mmol/day.

Aetiology

- Raised serum osmolality causes water to leave cells and cells shrink.
- A small rise in osmolality detected by osmoreceptors causes desire to drink.
- Hypernatraemia occurs where there is limited access to water, e.g. desert or stuck in a side room and too confused or comatose to drink, or water not to hand.

Causes

- Water/hypotonic fluid loss or impaired water intake.
- Polyuria with excess free water loss unmatched by water intake: hypercalcaemia, hypokalaemia, cranial and nephrogenic diabetes insipidus, diabetic ketoacidosis, HONK.
- Simple dehydration + fever especially older people + impaired access to water.
- Water losses due to burns, sweat, vomiting, severe diarrhoea.
- Renal fluid losses: nephropathy, myeloma, obstructive uropathy, adult polycystic kidney disease.

Excessive sodium intake

- Mild hypernatraemia with Conn syndrome/Cushing syndrome.
- Salt poisoning, ingestion of seawater, salt tablets, IV $NaHCO_3$, hypertonic saline.

Clinical

- Dehydration, thirsty, agitation, ataxia, progressively obtunded and comatose.
- Hypotension, thready pulse, sunken eyes, low BP, coma and seizures.

Investigations

- **FBC, U&E, Ca, K, glucose:** exclude AKI, high glucose, high Ca, hypokalaemia.
- **Raised** serum and urine osmolality (>600 mOsmol/kg) unless renal concentrating issue or diabetes insipidus.
- **CT/MRI head** if suspect cranial diabetes insipidus.

Management

- **Determine cause:** this is fundamental and key. Investigate for free water loss. Assess renal concentrating function and serum and urine osmolality and look for high glucose and calcium or hypokalaemia which can cause polyuria. May just be failure to match normal losses as listed above in *Causes*.
- **Fluid replacement**: no definite treatment plan. Cautious rehydration if cardiac disease or elderly. Treat and look for a cause if not obvious. Consider 0.18 saline (with 4% glucose) or dextrose 5% IV slowly with administration guided by plasma Na and urine output. This can be alternated with NS, to avoid too rapid a fall in plasma osmolality which can cause cerebral oedema. Can use a mixture of both. Volume replacement may be up to 4 L/day. Titrate to clinical response. Do not change [Na] by more than 12 mmol/day. Oral fluids may be given as long as losses are replaced and fluid balance maintained.
- **Risk of VTE:** administer VTE prophylaxis with clexane or equivalent.
- **Diabetes insipidus** (urine has low osmolality)**:** nephrogenic diabetes insipidus: fluid replacement, look for cause, e.g. lithium, correct electrolytes and paradoxically may need to give thiazide diuretics. Cranial diabetes insipidus: look for cause, replace losses. Consider Desmopressin given as nasal spray or tablets.

13.12 Disorders of magnesium and phosphate

Magnesium (normal 0.75–1.0 mmol/L)	
Low magnesium	Malnourished patients or (loop) diuretics, alcoholism, diarrhoea, laxative abuse, pancreatitis Gitelman's syndrome, DKA. **Clinical:** irritability, tremor, carpopedal spasm, ataxia, increased reflexes, adrenal insufficiency, confusion, fits, Torsade de pointes. Daily intake is 15 mmol. **Investigations:** U&E: low Mg, ECG: 1st degree heart block, T wave flattened, widened QRS, ventricular arrhythmias, TdP. [1g $MgSO_4$ = 4 mmol $MgSO_4$.] **Management: severe symptomatic give 2 g (8 mmol) IV $MgSO_4$ over 15–30 min.** Replace with IV Mg 50 mmol (12 g) in 1 L of NS or 5% dextrose in the first 24 h. This can be repeated until levels in normal range. Oral Mg often not adequate. Treat any cause.

High magnesium	Seen where there is impaired renal excretion or excessive infusion. There are reduced reflexes, weakness, even cardiac arrest in severe cases. **Investigations:** U&E: AKI/CKD, symptomatic Mg >2 mmol/L. **Management:** give 10 ml of 10% calcium gluconate. Haemodialysis for renal failure. Dextrose and insulin can also be given (same as for hyperkalaemia).
Phosphate (normal 0.8–1.4 mmol/L)	
Low phosphate	Common in the critically ill, treatment for DKA, refeeding syndrome, malabsorption, vomiting or renal loss, respiratory and muscle weakness, ileus, cardiac failure. For mild loss replace orally with Phosphate-Sandoz tablets up to 6 tablets per day. More severe deficiency then replace with IV phosphate (9 mmol given over 12 h). Watch serum calcium. Treat any vitamin D deficiency. May precipitate hypocalcaemia.
High phosphate	Due to renal failure, hypoparathyroidism, tumour lysis syndrome, rhabdomyolysis. Usually causes calcium deposition. Treat with gut phosphate binders such as calcium carbonate.

13.13 Lactic acidosis

About

- Acidosis due to increased lactic acid caused by tissue hypoperfusion.

Aetiology

- Impaired glycolytic metabolism increases lactate and reduces pH.
- L-lactate is endogenous; D-lactate from gut bacteria.

Types

- **Type A lactic acidosis** (tissue hypoxia): severe sepsis, diabetes, pancreatitis, malignancy, shock, LVF, renal and liver failure, respiratory failure, carbon monoxide, severe anaemia, local hypoperfusion, e.g. limb ischaemia or bowel ischaemia.
- **Type B lactic acidosis** (no tissue hypoxia): alcohol, iron, salicylates, isoniazid, metformin, Zidovudine. Inborn errors of metabolism, thiamine deficiency, pyruvate dehydrogenase dysfunction, cyanide, exercise, seizures.

Clinical

- Kussmaul's breathing, hypotension, signs of sepsis, shock, hypoxia.
- Do they have AIDS and on HAART. Check drugs.

Investigations

- **FBC, U&E:** anaemia, AKI, **lactate** >4 mmol/L with sepsis/metabolic acidosis.
- **ABG**: hypoxia, hypercarbia may be seen.
- **Metabolic acidosis:** low HCO_3 may not be seen even with a modest rise in lactate.
- **Anion gap:** is increased [Na+K] – [Cl+HCO_3] >12 mmol/L.

Management

- Determine and treat cause. Stop causative drugs. Lactate in many conditions is a useful marker of poor prognosis requiring expert and rapid intervention.
- Manage as per shock guidance or sepsis guidance. Dialysis can be considered in severe cases. Get expert help before considering an infusion of 500 ml isotonic 1.26% bicarbonate.

13.14 Acute porphyria

About

- Deficiency of an enzyme in the heme biosynthesis pathway with overproduction of porphyrin precursors. Heme made from succinyl-coA + glycine by 8 enzymic steps in cytoplasm and mitochondria.
- Drugs can induce some of the initial steps in the pathway precipitating acute attacks. Acute attacks may occur with: acute intermittent porphyria, variegate porphyria, hereditary coproporphyria.

Clinical

- Diagnosis often known. Often a family history is available.
- Episodes of neuropathic abdominal pain, back pain, constipation.
- Tachycardia, hypertension. Women > men aged 20–40.

Precipitants

- Fasting, infection, surgery, drugs: Sulfonamides, Rifampicin, OCP, anaesthetic agents, Barbiturates, Alcohol, some ACE inhibitors, Carbamazepine, Dapsone, Furosemide, Methyldopa, Theophylline, some NSAIDs. Check any new drug in *BNF*.

Investigations

- **FBC, U&E:** urea raised **LFTs:** bloods as indicated with signs.
- **Increased PBG and ALA:** urine darkens to port wine on standing and goes pink with Ehrlich's reagent, which remains despite chloroform. Referral to specialist for individual enzyme assays and further tests. *Urine porphobilinogen (PBG) analysis* to confirm an acute attack of porphyria or for monitoring known patients can be carried out at UK Porphyria centres. Collect a random 10 ml urine sample in a plain tube, check the tube is labelled with patient details, and protect from light by wrapping in foil or a brown envelope. Sample request card should state 'urine for porphobilinogen quantitation' for a patient with known porphyria, or 'urine for porphobilinogen screening test' for a patient without a previous diagnosis of porphyria. Refrigerate the sample prior to analysis. Send by first class post to local National Acute Porphyria Service laboratory.

Management

- **Supportive:** hydration, pain relief, rest, increased carbohydrate intake.
- **Acute attacks**: **IV haem arginate infusion**, a blood product. Shortens duration of attacks with less risk of complications. National Acute Porphyria Service (NAPS) can help obtain haem arginate.
- **Prevention**: avoid precipitating drugs and alcohol, stopping smoking.

Reference: National Acute Porphyria Service (NAPS) section for Medical Professionals

13.15 Diabetes emergencies and care

Increasing numbers of diabetic patients. Increased risks with critical illness and surgery. These risks are heightened if patient has had diabetes for an extended period of time, there is poor control or brittle (have difficulty controlling glucose level) diabetes. Diabetic patients often have co-morbidities.

Introduction

- Best management policy for diabetic emergencies is prevention.

- Many are due to issues with less than satisfactory self or medical care.
- Need to know and understand management of hypoglycaemia, DKA and HHS.

Diagnosis of diabetes

Diagnosis	Fasting sugar	GTT (75 g in 2 h)
Normal	<6.1 mmol/L	<7.8 mmol/L
Impaired fasting glucose	5.6–6.9 mmol/L	
Impaired glucose tolerance		7.8–11 mmol/L
Diabetes	>7.0 mmol/L	Random or 2 h post GTT >11.1 mmol/L

General principles of acute diabetic glycaemic control

- Insulin (from endogenous pancreatic B cells or exogenous IV/SC/IM) allows glucose to enter cells for ATP generation and lowers blood glucose. Excess insulin or sulphonylurea or Meglitinides can cause hypoglycaemia which, if prolonged or severe, can cause brain injury and death.
- Absence of insulin, e.g. Type 1 diabetes, leads to hyperglycaemia. Cells starved of glucose which leads them to burn fats causing acidosis and ketonaemia/ketonuria which can be measured. Those with Type 2 diabetes have some but not enough insulin to manage their blood glucose. DKA does not occur, but hyperglycaemia and severe fluid loss can, which can cause HONK.
- Physiological stress, e.g. illness, surgery, physical trauma or even pregnancy can cause a state of hyperglycaemia which causes polyuria, dehydration and volume loss. This is controlled by insulin release normally, but the diabetic patient needs to have their insulin dose increased. If there is an absence of insulin + stress then the result will be a rapid development of DKA. DKA kills, mainly through circulatory collapse and cerebral oedema.
- In diabetic patients you must supply the correct amount of insulin to match the physiological needs, ideally maintaining blood glucose, but this can be difficult as physiological demands vary as well as calorific intake and other factors. The primary aim is to avoid severe hypoglycaemia and severe hyperglycaemia (>20 mmol/L). **If the blood glucose is high you must give more insulin. If low you give less.** Insulins come in various formats to change the half-life, but the active molecule is the same. The formulation just alters the half-life so that it can be short acting or long acting. Hospital is the safest place to adjust insulin if monitoring is frequent and hyperglycaemia and hypoglycaemia can be quickly detected and treated. Hypoglycaemia can develop silently in comatose or obtunded patients, e.g. stroke, and so monitoring must be frequent if patients are on insulin or oral hypoglycaemic drugs.

Types of commercial insulin

- **Fast acting short half-life**: *Actrapid* or *Humulin S* (soluble/short). These act within a half hour and peak at 2–4 h. Their duration is short at about 6 h in total. They are used to make up sliding scales.
- **Intermediate acting**: *Humulin I* or *Insulatard*, which are normally given in BD doses pre-breakfast and pre-evening meal.
- **Long acting**: *Glargine* or *Detemir*. These have a much longer period of activity and can be given either once or twice daily. They can mimic the basal level of insulin.
- **Combined insulins**: fast and intermediate acting insulins can be combined and so can mimic the basal level and there is a short acting insulin which can deal

with mealtime hyperglycaemia. Twice daily and three times daily insulins are prescribed, usually before meals.
- In most cases the potential problems can be discussed and control improved preoperatively and discussed at the preoperative assessment. There is no such opportunity to optimise diabetic control prior to emergency surgery. Before, during and post-op the aim is to keep the blood glucose level within the range 6–10 mmol/L at all times.

13.16 Diabetic ketoacidosis

Patient education is key. Patients need strict advice to never stop their insulin even if ill. If unable to eat/drink then they must come to hospital immediately for IV hydration and insulin. A failure to take insulin + acute illness + nil by mouth will rapidly result in life threatening DKA.

About
- Manage with a defined well-documented and communicated plan.
- 10% of DKA is with new diabetes, 15% from known diabetes, often provoked.
- Seen in Type 1 diabetics with intercurrent illness who reduce/stop insulin.
- Severe deficit of water, insulin and potassium.

Note of caution
- DKA is most commonly seen with Type 1 DM but can be seen with 'ketosis-prone Type 2 DM' especially in the non-white population. Treat them as DKA but ketosis-prone Type 2 DM may not need insulin long term,
- Treat all with insulin initially and arrange expert outpatient follow up and measurement of C-peptide which is preserved with Type 2 DM.

Definition
- Ketonaemia ≥3 mmol/L or significant ketonuria (>2+ on standard urine sticks).
- Hyperglycaemia: blood glucose >11 mmol/L, or known DM.
- Metabolic acidosis: bicarbonate <15 mmol/L and/or venous pH <7.3.
- Diabetic pregnant patients can develop DKA with normal blood sugars.

Aetiology
- Glucose (and K^+) enters cells by the actions of insulin on the insulin receptor. Insulin deficit leads to cell starvation despite being surrounded by a sea of excess glucose. Switch to burning fatty acids and beta-oxidation of fats creates acidic products which lower the pH. Ketone bodies include acetone, 3-beta-hydroxybutyrate (main one) and acetoacetate.
- Dehydration due to profound osmotic diuresis as a result of severe hyperglycaemia. Increased cortisol, adrenaline, glucagon, and growth hormone cause hepatic gluconeogenesis and glycogenolysis. Vomiting can compound the fluid losses. All adds to a perfect storm leading to spiralling metabolic derangement.
- Rhinocerebral mucormycosis due to increased iron availability as a result of a change in tissue pH.

Recent key recommendations
- Crystalloid: 0.9% NS is the recommended fluid of choice. Cautious replacement in young adults with concerns over cerebral oedema. Measure venous HCO_3 and pH, use blood ketone meters for near patient testing.

- If already on long-acting analogue insulin this should be continued, e.g. Levemir or Lantus. In DKA insulin is given at a fixed rate IV infusion calculated on body weight. Avoid priming dose (bolus) of insulin. HCO_3 or phosphate administration is not recommended routinely.

Clinical

- Progressive polyuria, polydipsia, tachypnoea, Kussmaul's respiration to blow off CO_2, acetone 'nail varnish' smell on the breath (not all of us can smell it), dehydration, hypotension.
- Cold peripheries, delayed capillary return, sunken eyes, hypotensive, vomiting, tachycardia, oliguria.
- Look for sepsis, chest and urine or and other acute illness, e.g. ACS, meningitis, acute abdomen.

Investigations

- **FBC, U&E**: elevated WCC, CRP may suggest infection, AKI U&E: may show mild uraemia and hypernatraemia. Initially raised K^+ due to acidosis but potassium levels fall with insulin administration.
- **Glucose**: usually >20 mmol/L at presentation.
- **Ketonuria** 3+ and glycosuria and high glucose. Treatment depends upon the suppression of ketonaemia. Measurement of blood ketones now represents best practice in monitoring the response to treatment.
- **Acidosis**: venous blood gas is now preferred over arterial for testing. A low HCO_3 (<15 mmol/L) indicates metabolic acidosis. Low pH is less than 7.30 as can be <7.10 in severe cases. Increased anion gap.
- **Cardiac troponin** if suspected ACS. **CXR** if chest disease, e.g. breathless, fever, cough.
- **CT head** scan if comatose to exclude other diagnoses.

Severity

- **Mild**: blood pH 7.25–7.30, HCO_3 15–18 mmol/L; the patient is alert.
- **Moderate**: pH 7.00–7.25, HCO_3 10–15, mild drowsiness may be present.
- **Severe:** pH below 7.00. HCO_3 <10; stupor or coma may occur.

Treatment goals (see table below)

- The key aims are restoration of circulatory volume, clearance of ketones and correction of electrolyte imbalance, particularly potassium, and insulin replacement. Set clear goals and expectations of therapy. Ensure treatment plans are well documented. Ensure good handover between doctors on shifts.

Immediate assessment

- Check ABC, get good IV access and start IV NS. Assess basic RR, heart rate, BP, O_2 sats aim for 94–98%, and temperature and GCS. Examine for infection – urine, chest, CNS, skin and soft tissue. Monitor oximetry. Establish if pregnant.
- Send: blood ketones, capillary blood glucose, venous plasma glucose, U&E, VBG, FBC, blood cultures (not done via venflon because of high rate of false positives), ECG, CXR, urinalysis and culture.
- Insulin causes a marked drop in K^+ which must be managed. Clinical and biochemical review.

Markers of severe DKA: (needs HDU level 2 bed and CVP/intra-arterial line)

- Blood ketones >6 mmol/L.
- HCO_3 <5 mmol/L, venous/arterial pH <7.0.
- K^+ on admission <3.5 mmol/L.
- GCS <12 or abnormal AVPU score.
- O_2 sats on air <92%, SBP <90 mmHg.
- HR <60 bpm, HR >100 bpm.
- Anion gap: [Na+K] – [Cl+HCO_3] >16.

Treatment goals (CBG = capillary blood glucose)

- Reduce venous blood ketones by 0.5 mmol/L/h.
- Increase the venous HCO_3 by 3 mmol/L/h.
- Reduce CBG by 3 mmol/L/h.
- Maintain K^+ between 4.0 and 5.0 mmol/L.
- Lower glucose cautiously to avoid hypoglycaemia.
- Start 10% glucose if CBG <14 mmol/L.

The first hour (NS = 0.9% normal saline)

- Commence NS solution (use large bore cannula) via infusion pump.
- Commence a fixed rate IV insulin infusion (IVII) (0.1 unit/kg/h based on estimate of weight).
- Infusion: 50 units soluble insulin (Actrapid or Humulin S) in 50 ml NS.
- If patient normally takes long acting insulin analogue (Lantus or Levemir) continue at usual dose and time.

Assess patient

- Resp rate; temp, BP, pulse; O_2 sats, GCS, full clinical examination, CBG and laboratory glucose, venous BG, U&E, FBC, blood cultures, ECG, CXR, MSU.
- Establish monitoring regimen. Check hourly CBG, capillary ketone measurement if available, venous HCO_3 and K at 60 min, 2 h and 2-hourly thereafter, 4-hourly plasma electrolytes.
- Continuous cardiac monitoring if required.
- Continuous pulse oximetry if required.
- Find and treat any precipitating causes.

Fluids

- Systolic BP (SBP) below 90 mmHg. Likely to be due to low circulating volume, but consider other causes such as heart failure, sepsis, etc. Give 500 ml of NS over 10–15 min. If SBP remains below 90 mmHg repeat whilst requesting senior input. Most patients require between 500 and 1000 ml given rapidly. Consider involving the ITU/critical care team. Once SBP above 90 mmHg give 1000 ml NS over next 60 min. Addition of potassium likely to be required in this second litre of fluid.

1–6 hours (see treatment goals above)

Re-assess patient, monitor vital signs

- Hourly blood glucose (lab blood glucose if meter reading 'HI'), hourly blood ketones if meter available.
- VBG for pH, bicarbonate and potassium at 60 min, 2 h and 2-hourly thereafter.

Potassium

- Insulin will shift K^+ into the intracellular space causing hypokalaemia. Add 20 mmol K^+ per litre from the 2nd bag.
- Check U&E regularly; hourly initially then every 2–4 h when stabilised or more if needed.
- K^+ >5.5 mmol/L: add none; K^+ 3.5–5.5 mmol/L: give 40 mmol/L; K^+ <3.5 mmol/L: senior review as increased K^+ needed.

Fluid replacement

- 1 L NS + KCl over next 2 h.
- 1 L NS + KCl over next 2 h.
- 1 L NS + KCl over next 4 h.
- Add 10% glucose 125 ml/h if blood glucose falls below 14 mmol/L.

More cautious fluid replacement in young people aged 18–25 years, elderly, pregnant, heart or renal failure (consider HDU and/or central line).

Insulin infusion rate may need review if:

- ketones not falling by at least 0.5 mmol/L/h.
- venous HCO_3 not rising by at least 3 mmol/L/h.
- plasma glucose not falling by at least 3 mmol/L/h.

Continue fixed rate IVII until ketones less than 0.3 mmol/L, venous pH over 7.3 and/or venous bicarbonate over 18 mmol/L.

If ketones/glucose not falling as expected always check the insulin infusion pump is working and connected and that the correct insulin residual volume is present (to check for pump malfunction).

The first hour (NS = 0.9% normal saline)

- SBP on admission >90 mmHg give 1000 ml NS over first 60 min.

Potassium level (mmol/L)

Potassium replacement mmol/L of infusion solution

>5.5: nil

3.5–5.5: 40 mmol/L

<3.5 senior review – additional K^+ required

1–6 hours (see treatment goals above)

If equipment working but response to treatment inadequate, increase insulin infusion rate by 1 unit/h increments hourly until targets achieved.

Additional measures

- Regular obs and Early Warning Score (EWS).
- Accurate fluid balance chart.
- Target minimum urine output 0.5 ml/kg/h.
- Consider urinary catheterisation if incontinent or anuric (not passed urine by 60 min).
- Nasogastric tube with airway protection if patient obtunded or persistent.

Other considerations

- **Acidosis**: adequate fluid and insulin therapy will resolve the acidosis in DKA and the use of HCO_3 is not indicated, though some consider treatment with a pH <7.0 and give 500 ml of sodium bicarbonate 1.26% plus 10 mmol KCl – take local expert advice if considered.
- **Urinary catheter**: if anuric or oliguric and concerns about renal function or fluid balance. Oxygen as per BTS guidance. **Consider NG tube** if vomiting. Give **VTE prophylaxis** usually LMWH as high risk.
- **Exclude sepsis**: CXR and urinalysis, soft tissue (look for boils, abscesses), consider meningitis. Always ask why DKA occurred in this patient.
- An acute abdomen or even meningitis could also present as DKA. DKA can present with abdominal pain. Surgical consult if you suspect acute abdomen. Amylase can also go up × 4 in DKA.

At 6–12 h: at 6 hours check venous pH, HCO_3, K, capillary ketones and glucose

- Ensure clinical and biochemical parameters improving. Continue IV fluid replacement. Avoid low glucose and start 10% glucose if BG <14 mmol/L.
- Continue IV fluid via infusion pump at reduced rate of 1 L NS + KCl over 4 h and then 1 L NS + KCl over 6 h.
- See advice above to watch for fall in GCS that could suggest cerebral oedema. Review all bloods at 6 h. Resolution is suggested by pH >7.3 or ketones <0.3 mmol/L.
- If not improving (see treatment goals above) then repeat review. Check insulin infusion is working and line is not blocked and that it contains insulin and no errors with making it up.

12–24 h: check venous pH, HCO_3, K, capillary ketones and glucose

- Resolution is defined as ketones <0.3 mmol/L, venous pH >7.3. Ensure targets are hit and progressive improvement. Ketonaemia and acidosis should have resolved.
- Request senior review if not improving. Continue IV fluid replacement if not eating and drinking. If ketonaemia cleared but not eating and drinking move to a variable rate IVII as per local guidelines.
- Look for complications of treatment, e.g. fluid overload, cerebral oedema and continue to treat precipitating factors. Transfer to subcutaneous insulin if patient is eating and drinking normally.

After 24 h and discharge planning and follow up

- If DKA not resolved determine why. It suggests possible failure to get enough insulin or fluids. Are the IV lines working? Does the insulin infusion contain insulin? Get expert review.
- Transfer to subcutaneous insulin when biochemical resolution (capillary ketones <0.3 mmol/L, pH >7.3) and the patient is ready and able to eat. Give subcutaneous insulin and then after 30 min stop IV insulin as there should be some overlap.
- Conversion to subcutaneous insulin should be managed by the Specialist Diabetes Team. If the team is not available use local guidelines.
- If the patient is newly diagnosed it is essential they are seen by a member of the specialist team prior to discharge. Arrange follow up with specialist team.

Complications

- Cerebral oedema (suspect if fall in GCS – more common in young).
- Arrhythmias (potassium), circulatory collapse/shock, acute kidney injury.
- Hypoglycaemia with over-treatment, aspiration pneumonia.
- Acute respiratory distress syndrome, myocardial infarction.
- Rhinocerebral mucormycosis – destructive lesions affecting face and nose.

Prevention: ensure patient educated about 'sick day rules': patients need strict advice to never stop their insulin even if ill. If unable to eat/drink then they must come to hospital immediately. Diabetic team should reinforce this message.

Pregnancy: an inherently ketosis-prone state and is a high-risk time for DKA in women with T1DM.

Reference: Joint British Diabetes Societies Inpatient Care Group (2013) *The Management of Diabetic Ketoacidosis in Adults*, 2nd edition.

13.17 Hyperosmolar hyperglycaemic state (HHS)

About

- Previously called hyperglycaemic hyperosmolar nonketotic coma (HONK).
- Mortality 10–20% compared with 3–10% for DKA. Seen in the elderly.
- Minimal ketosis or acidosis. Increased risk of VTE so give LMWH.

Precipitated by

- *De novo* presentation of Type 2 DM or Type 2 DM + stress, steroids, surgery, thiazides, infection.

Clinical

- Thirst, polydipsia, polyuria and mental clouding and delirium and coma.
- Usually known Type 2 diabetic. Exacerbated by high sugar drinks or water restriction.

Investigations

- **FBC, U&E**: raised WCC, hypernatraemia often >150 mmol/L, AKI.
- **Serum glucose:** >30 mmol/L without significant ketonaemia/acidosis.
- **Serum osmolarity:** (normal 285–300 mOsm/kg) high (>320 mmol/L), 2 × [Na+K] + urea + glucose.
- **Ketones:** usually <3 mmol/L. **Lactate** may be elevated.
- **ABG/VBG:** pH >7.3 and HCO_3 >15 mmol unless lactic acidosis.

Management

- **ABC**, O_2 as per BTS guidance. Get good venous access × 2. May need ITU/HDU if in coma/moribund and airway protection needed.
- **Urgent rehydration** as significant fluid losses with osmotic diuresis due to glycosuria; may use NS. With significant hypernatraemia 0.45% saline may be needed to prevent Na overload. Aim for net output of 3–6 L by 12 h.
- **Commence an insulin infusion** as with DKA and adjust dose. Patients need lower doses of insulin than DKA and may be sensitive to large doses. Safer to use a smaller dose, e.g. 2–4 units/h (0.05 units/kg/h). Long-term insulin usually not needed but review diabetes management.
- **VTE:** give at least prophylactic dose of LMWH as high risk of VTE. Consider looking for and treat cause, e.g. sepsis, MI, pneumonia. Observe for cerebral oedema/central pontine myelinolysis.

13.18 Diabetic foot infections

About

- Neurovascular compromise can lead to significant soft tissue damage.
- Beware as infection in the feet of diabetic patients can extend through to bone.
- Beware because pain perception, and so local protective reflexes, impaired.

Clinical

- May be painless, ulceration, necrosis, loss of pulses, claudication.
- Inspect foot, toes and sole of feet, peripheral neuropathy, Charcot's joint.
- Neuropathy: painless, high arch, clawed toes, warm good pulses, painless plantar ulcers.
- Vascular: cold feet, poor pulses, rest pain, hair loss over shin, ulcerated heels and toes.

Investigations

- **Bloods**: FBC, U&E, glucose, CRP. Swabs as available. HbA1c, albumin.
- **Plain X-ray**: may show bony involvement.
- **MRI scan**: can show bone involvement.
- **Vascular studies**: ankle brachial pressures may be required.
- **Femoral angiography:** if considered for vascular surgery.

Management

- **Team approach**: multidisciplinary care involving specialist podiatrist, diabetic team, vascular surgery. Debridement and removal of dead tissue and appropriate dressings and good glycaemic control. Ulceration but no infection: uninfected/colonisation: no antibiotics needed. Monitor and dress. Smoking cessation.
- **Mild:** check previous MRSA status, if negative use Co-Amoxiclav 625 mg tds PO. In penicillin-allergic Clindamycin 300 mg qds PO. Duration: 7–10 days.
- **Moderate**: check previous MRSA status, if negative use Co-Amoxiclav 1.2 g IV tds. For penicillin allergy, contact consultant microbiologist.
- **Severe:** blood cultures, swabs from wound. Check previous MRSA status.
- **Antibiotics:** MRSA negative **TAZOCIN IV** + **GENTAMICIN** IV stat (if hypotensive). If MRSA positive, add **TEICOPLANIN** × 3 doses and then OD (adjust dose to renal function). For penicillin allergy (severe/anaphylaxis), **TEICOPLANIN** × 3 doses and then OD + **GENTAMICIN IV** + **METRONIDAZOLE IV** tds. See *Chapter 29* for dosing and monitoring.

13.19 Diabetes and surgery

Non-insulin treated diabetics and minor surgery

- **Preoperatively**: random blood sugar on admission <10 mmol/L – give normal medication until day of op. However, if random glucose >10 mmol/L follow as for major surgery (see below).
- **On day of operation** omit oral hypoglycaemics. Check blood glucose: 1 h pre-op and at least once during op (hourly if op >1 h long) and post-op 2 hourly until eating. Postoperatively, restart oral hypoglycaemics with first meal.

Insulin-treated diabetics and minor surgery

- This regime only suitable for patients whose random sugar is <10 mmol/L on admission, will only miss one meal pre-op and are first on the list for very minor surgery, e.g. cystoscopy.
- Preoperatively, normal medication. **Day of operation**: no breakfast, no insulin, place first on list. Blood glucose: 1 h pre-op and at least once during op (hourly if op >1 h long) postop 2 hourly until eating then 4 hourly. Postoperatively, restart normal subcutaneous insulin regime with first meal.

Diabetes and major surgery or critical illness

- Applies to all diabetics who are poorly controlled (blood glucose >10 mmol/L) irrespective of whether on insulin or not at baseline. **Pre-op:** give normal medication until day of operation. **Day of operation**: omit oral hypoglycaemics and normal SC insulin.
- Check capillary blood glucose (and potassium) 1 h pre-op then 2 hourly from start of infusion at least once during operation (hourly if op >1 h long) at least once in recovery area, and 2 hourly postoperatively.
- One combination is 16 U of soluble insulin + 10 mmol of KCl in 500 ml of 10% glucose. Infusion rate of 100 ml/h with glucose checked every 2 h.
- Alternatively, a variable rate insulin infusion is used, especially in the emergency setting and will allow insulin to be administered IV and titrated to the capillary blood glucose (CBG).

13.20 Diabetes / blood glucose management

Variable rate intravenous insulin infusion

- The term variable rate intravenous insulin infusion (VRIII) replaces the term Sliding scale. No one size fits all VRIII; they must be tailored to a patient. Insulin response to a particular blood glucose depends on many physiological factors.
- A VRIII is an attempt to plan and direct glucose control when insulin demand is unpredictable and varying. Use only as long as is necessary.
- Convert to an insulin regimen as soon as requirements stable. Before stopping a VRIII prescribe appropriate insulin therapy. In comatose patients, e.g. stroke, very tight control will lead to hypoglycaemia and coma with few symptoms and signs and further damage may occur.

CBG – check every 1–2 h	Rate of delivery of soluble insulin at 1 unit/ml/h – use the larger dose if insulin resistance suspected (e.g. obese)
<4.0 mmol/L	0.5 or none if on long acting insulin; treat hypoglycaemia
4–6.9 mmol/L	1–2

CBG – check every 1–2 h	Rate of delivery of soluble insulin at 1 unit/ml/h – use the larger dose if insulin resistance suspected (e.g. obese)
7–9.9 mmol/L	2–4
10–14.9 mmol/L	3–6
15–19.9 mmol/L	4–8
>20 mmol/L	5–10 check line. Ensure insulin was added. Seek medical review

- **Preparation:** use an insulin syringe/pen to draw up 50 units of a short acting insulin e.g. Actrapid. Add to a 50 ml syringe containing 49.5 ml of NS giving 1 unit/ml. Always ensure lines and IV access working. Some patients need 100 units per day and others 30 units so the VRIII doses needs to reflect this. Basal insulin needed will escalate with physiological stress, surgery, sepsis and insulin resistance.
- The insulin is given alongside IV fluid, which must be administered using a **volumetric infusion pump**. This should be 0.45% saline with 5% glucose and 0.15% **or** 0.3% KCl. Omit KCl if K >4.5 mmol/L. The amount of KCl depends on the most recent U&E. For patients with renal impairment and hyperkalaemia 0.45% saline with 5% glucose **without** KCl should be used. In hyponatraemia NS may be used.
- Set the fluid replacement rate to deliver the hourly fluid requirements of the individual patient. The rate must not be altered thereafter without senior advice. Insulin must be infused at a variable rate to keep the blood glucose 6–10 mmol/L (acceptable range 4–12 mmol/L).
- Stopping the VRIII: for Type 2 DM **oral hypoglycaemics:** restart when oral intake possible at normal pre-op doses. Reduce or stop sulphonylurea if oral intake likely to be reduced. Metformin avoided if eGFR <50 ml/min. **Restarting insulin**: wait until normal oral intake possible. Restart normal dose but adjust down if oral intake reduced or increase if on-going sepsis or infection or postop stress. Aim for a level of 4–12 mmol/L. Involve diabetic specialist team for optimising control. Ensure that the VRIII/IV insulin infusion overlaps the giving of SC insulin by 30–60 min.

General rules for acute control in known diabetic

- If blood glucose >12 mmol/L then check capillary ketone levels using an appropriate bedside monitor if available. *If capillary blood ketones are greater than 3 mmol/L or urinary ketones greater than +++ then follow DKA guidelines* (see *Section 13.16*) and contact the on-call medical/diabetes specialist team for advice. For all others with known diabetes see as follows.
- **Type 1 diabetes: always need insulin**. Give SC rapid acting analogue insulin (i.e. Novorapid, Humalog) and assume that 1 unit of insulin will drop blood glucose by 3 mmol/L BUT wherever possible determine baseline needs. Recheck the blood glucose 1 h later to ensure it is falling. If control is still unsatisfactory discuss with medical/diabetic team. Consider VRIII.
- **Type 2 diabetes**: use SC rapid acting analogue insulin (i.e. Novorapid, Humalog). Assess using capillary blood glucose (CBG) measurement. Always recheck blood glucose 1 h later to ensure it is falling. If worsening or unsatisfactory then contact medical/diabetic team and consider VRIII.
- **New diabetes**: determine if Type 1 (young, thin, may be ketotic) will usually need insulin therapy and a VRIII is reasonable initially and an estimate of insulin needed can be made. Involve diabetic team. At earliest reasonable opportunity

commence insulin regimen. Older, obese diabetics will usually be Type 2 and dietary advice and oral medication can be considered.

- It is advisable to use your own hospital's protocol where available. The important level is to ensure enough insulin to render normoglycaemic without any ketones. If this is for DKA, continue insulin at all times (to switch off ketone production, and so reduce acidosis). If for other reasons (e.g. control peri-operatively) <4 mmol/L should stop insulin. Hypoglycaemia should be treated as usual.

14 Gastroenterology emergencies

14.1 Acute diarrhoea

Answering bleep/taking referral

- Is there known IBD? Is or was the patient on antibiotics?
- Is the patient pyrexial, tachycardic, unwell, dehydrated?
- How many times have bowels opened today and is it bloody?
- Use the Bristol stool chart to characterise diarrhoea (Type 6/7).
- Suspected infective causes need isolation and stool culture.
- Need to wash hands with soap and water. Alcohol hand washes are insufficient.

Causes of acute diarrhoea: stool weight >250 g/day

Causes	Findings and causes
Bacterial infective	*Salmonella* and *E. coli* usually cause a sudden onset gastroenteritis which can be bloody with a toxic patient. Usually with fever and abdominal pain. *Shigella* – bloody diarrhoea.
***Clostridium difficile* diarrhoea**	Caused by enterotoxins A and B. Associated with antibiotic usage that alters gut flora. Can lead to pseudomembranous colitis, megacolon and perforation and even death. Needs urgent metronidazole 500 mg tds PO or Vancomycin 125 mg qds and surgical consult if abdominal pain.
Viral infective	Norovirus must be isolated quickly. Sick, nausea and vomiting. Spreads quickly. Alarm bells if patient/staff in proximity complain of same.
Acute colitis	Known IBD may be on treatment. Bloody stools, fever. Needs stool chart and gastroenterology review and steroids.
Ischaemic colitis	Abdominal pain, vascular risks, AF, diarrhoea.
Amoebic	Caused primarily by the amoeba *Entamoeba histolytica*. Bloody, mucous.
Laxatives	Overuse.
Autonomic	Stasis and small bowel bacterial overgrowth.
Constipation with overflow	Rectum full of hard stools with liquid stool emerging.
Osmotic diarrhoea	In hospital commonly seen starting NG or PEG feeding regimens, can cause an osmotic diarrhoea which can be reduced by slowing feed temporarily and stopping laxatives.
Neoplastic disease	Colorectal malignancy is certainly a cause of on-going altered bowel function. However, more altered bowel habit than diarrhoea.
Carcinoid syndrome	Causes flushing, diarrhoea, wheezing. Measure urine 5-hydroxyindoleacetic acid (5-HIAA) and liver USS shows metastases. Give OCTREOTIDE.
Malabsorption	Pancreatic insufficiency, pale bulky stools or an osmotic diarrhoea with lactose intolerance.

Causes	Findings and causes
VIPoma	Severe watery diarrhoea and hypokalaemia due to vasoactive intestinal peptide.
Thyrotoxicosis	Increased frequency rather than diarrhoea.
Toxic shock syndrome	Diarrhoea, rash in patient who may have an infective source, e.g. simple skin wound or tampon.

Answering bleep

- Why are they in hospital? When did it start? Frequency? Bristol stool chart scale.
- Abdominal pain or vomiting, recent antibiotics, excessive laxatives.

On arrival

- Review notes and drug chart particularly antibiotics and laxatives and stop them if possible. Discuss with microbiology if need for antimicrobials.
- Abdominal examination including PR – may be hard stools with overflow.
- Check basic bloods if concerned about dehydration. If severe diarrhoea or poor oral intake then IV fluids.
- Caution with loperamide if any suggestion of infective cause. Hand washing. Isolate patient and send stool cultures if infected cause suspected.
- If suspected acute severe colitis (bloody diarrhoea) consider adding steroids.

Investigations

- **Bloods**: FBC, U&E, TFT, CRP.
- **Stool culture**: cysts, ova and parasites and *C. difficile* toxins A and B.
- **AXR**: features of IBD, toxic megacolon if pseudomembranous colitis.
- **Sigmoidoscopy:** rectal biopsy if diarrhoea persists.

General management

- Isolation if an infective cause suspected to prevent spread. Gown up and wear gloves which should be placed in bin in patient's room. Ensure hands washed with soap and water to remove any *C. difficile* spores.
- See individual cases above, but all patients need to maintain adequate hydration either orally or IV depending on losses. Monitor fluid balance and U&E and general observations.
- Codeine 30 mg tds or Loperamide can be useful for symptomatic reduction of diarrhoea if infective causes suspected. Use with caution, concern is that they may delay resolution. Best avoided if suspected *C. difficile* and pseudomembranous colitis. Surgical review if acute abdomen.

14.2 Constipation

Answering bleep

- Has there been dietary intake? When did bowels last open? Is patient in pain or discomfort?
- Patient taking opiates or dehydrated or bed bound or Parkinson's disease or hypothyroid?

On arrival

- Review notes, observations and drug chart. Assess patient and usual bowel frequency. Once a week may be normal for some.

- Is it physical/psychological, e.g. having to use bed pan or commode. Is patient in pain, e.g. anal fissure or haemorrhoids will make patient avoid defecation. Needs stool softeners.
- If not obstructed and mild may simply require improved hydration, high fibre diet and oral laxatives.
- If constipated (AXR may show stool ++) an enema, e.g. Microlax enema or if that does not work a Picolax (sodium picosulphate) enema, can be very effective.
- If there are signs of bowel obstruction then nil by mouth, bloods and AXR and surgical consult.

Causes

- A poor dietary intake or lack of dietary fibre, immobility or dehydration.
- **Drugs**: opiates, anticholinergic, diuretics, CCBs.
- **Electrolyte disturbances**, e.g. low K or Mg. Hypercalcaemia/hyperglycaemia and dehydration.
- Subacute obstruction – ileus, colorectal tumour, hypercalcaemia, hypothyroid.
- Acute porphyria, spinal cord disease, Hirschprung's disease.
- Parkinson's disease, depression, dementia.

Assessment

- Abdominal examination: tenderness, bowel sounds, peritonism, masses.
- PR examination: anal pain or discomfort, rectal tumour or impacted faeces.
- Spinal cord disease or multiple sclerosis usually already known.
- Hirschprung's disease usually from childhood.
- Myxoedema: look for clinical signs, raised TSH.

Management

- Hydration and high fibre diet and early mobility and provide time and access to optimal toileting conditions with as much privacy as can be provided. Make use of gastrocolic reflex – toileting patient after eating.
- On-going or new constipation for several weeks warrants consideration to exclude a colorectal malignancy. Try stool softeners (e.g. **sodium docusate 200 mg tds**), bulking agents (e.g. **Fybogel one sachet BD**), stimulants (e.g. senna 1 tab BD is useful especially if stools are large soft and bulky).
- Osmotic laxatives (e.g. lactulose 10–20 ml BD) really are to be avoided if possible, except to improve stool output with hepatic encephalopathy. Movicol (e.g. contains polyethylene glycol or codanthramer). Enemas (e.g. Glycerin suppository or Picolax enema) useful for distal stool.
- Occasionally all fails and you may be asked to perform a manual evacuation, which is digital removal of rectal faeces. Be sure to wear two pairs of gloves and have lots of pads. Constipation is common but significant complications are very rare, but include faecal impaction where the rectum fills with 'rocks' of hard stool with soft stool leaking around sides and overflow diarrhoea.
- Can even cause intestinal obstruction and perforation and megacolon leading to sigmoid volvulus. Rectal prolapse can be seen. It may provoke urinary retention and UTI.

14.3 Upper gastrointestinal bleeding

With a suspect GI bleed first make sure there are at least two good wide bore IV lines before all peripheral venous access disappears.

About

- Upper is defined as bleeding from above the ligament of Trietz. Think oesophagus, stomach and duodenum. Not all cirrhotic GI bleeding is variceal. Can be multiple simultaneous causes, e.g. varices and gastritis and a duodenal ulcer. Epistaxis and swallowed blood can mimic GI bleed.
- Get good venous access immediately and protect it. In a big bleed without venous access death will be quick. If the physicians can't stop life threatening bleeding it's a surgical problem.
- About 90% of non-variceal bleeds and 50% of variceal bleeds will stop spontaneously. Mortality for an acute upper GI bleed is around 10%, rising to 26% in patients who bleed during admission to hospital for other reasons. Use the Rockall score to assess patients.

Causes

Cause	Findings
Peptic ulcer disease	Usually lesser curve of stomach or duodenal bulb where an ulcer can erode into a large vessel. *H. pylori* +ve, NSAIDs. Multiple ulcers with Zollinger–Ellison syndrome. Needs OGD and endoscopic therapy and PPI and HP eradication. Rarely surgery.
Oesophageal ulcer/ severe oesophagitis	Pain on swallowing, dysphagia, GORD symptoms. In HIV, infections with candida, CMV, HSV. Local ulceration with bisphosphonates and NSAIDs.
Oesophageal cancer	Progressive dysphagia to solids then liquids. Weight loss, bleeding, adenocarcinoma.
Coagulopathy	Patient on warfarin or liver disease or severe thrombocytopenia with any other gastric pathology.
Oesophageal varices	Check for alcohol history and look for signs of chronic liver failure and Caput medusae. Splenomegaly suggests portal hypertension. Consider other causes of chronic liver disease that can result in cirrhosis and portal hypertension. Needs OGD + TERLIPRESSIN + endoscopic management + antibiotics, Sengstaken tube and TIPS.
Aorto-enteric fistula	Previous AAA surgery with fistula with 3rd part of duodenum causing severe GI bleeding.
Mallory–Weiss tear	History of retching and often alcohol misuse. Linear mucosal tear found near the oesophagogastric junction. Mucosal tear can be injected with ADRENALINE. If this fails haemoclips or band ligation.
Acute gastritis/erosions	NSAIDs make this more likely. Alcohol.
Gastric vascular ectasias	May be found and also seen with hereditary haemorrhagic telangiectasia, arteriovenous malformation and other vascular lesions.
Gastric malignancy	Chronic blood loss more usual.
Dieulafoy's lesion	A large calibre arteriole, which lies just below the mucosa and causes an arterial bleed through a pinpoint mucosal lesion. Most commonly on the lesser curve.

Cause	Findings
Spurious	Swallowed epistaxis blood or from nasopharynx can cause haematemesis and melena. Ask about these. Epistaxis can be severe with swallowed blood but the history should be clear if asked.
Right colonic bleed	May cause melena-type stools but this is rare.

Clinical history / risk factors

- Ask about liver disease, peptic ulcer disease, alcohol intake, aspirin usage, NSAIDs, warfarin, steroids.
- A history of bleeding problems – dental extractions, etc.

Examination

- Signs of liver disease and portal hypertension suggest varices, e.g. ascites, jaundice, gynaecomastia, Dupuytren's contracture, clubbing, spider naevi, Caput medusae, palmar erythema, etc.
- Signs of liver decompensation, e.g. jaundice, encephalopathy, asterixis. Liver flap.

Evidence for bleeding

- Upper GI bleeding manifests as either vomited bright red or altered blood 'coffee grounds' called haematemesis, or altered blood products passed PR as melena. Normal dark bile often mistaken for coffee grounds. 'Coffee grounds' and melena show bleeding that occurred minutes to hours before.
- Huge amounts of GI bleed will pass quickly and cause bright red blood passing within minutes. The GI protein load of blood and the anaemia and hypotension can cause agitation and delirium. Bleeding may, however, be occult with just progressive signs of anaemia.

Evidence of significant blood loss

- Look for postural fall in BP >20 mmHg and postural HR increase >30 bpm (lying and then sitting upright – there is no need to ask a potentially hypotensive patient to stand) before the patient is clinically shocked.
- Signs of shock and haemodynamic compromise. Thready pulse, thirst, poor skin turgor, cold nose. Increased capillary refill time. Oliguria – consider catheter if shocked and poor urinary output. Rectal examination if melena not evident.

Investigations

- **FBC:** initially often normal and misleading because haemodilution yet to take place. Check platelets.
- **U&E:** raised urea may suggest GI blood loss and protein load in gut. Target Hb 80 g/dL. Recent evidence suggests that higher Hb targets associated with increased mortality.
- **LFT and coagulation screen**: at baseline and repeat as needed. INR/prothrombin time vital.
- **Blood group and cross-match** 2–4 units depending on estimated losses.
- **Upper GI endoscopy**: usually within 24 h or sooner.

> If shocked and *in extremis* with obvious active witnessed extreme bleeding consider **universal donor O negative blood**.

Management

- **Get good IV access and protect it**: if hypotensive and raised HR or melena or witnessed haematemesis then need good venous access with **2 GREY VENFLONS IN**

EACH ANTECUBITAL FOSSA. If difficult IV access get help from registrar or anaesthetist – don't waste time if difficult. A central line is too long and fine bore for good flow and not good for giving volume quickly.

- **Give crystalloids and blood**: start 1 L NS over 20 min. O_2 as per BTS guidance. Once access gained send bloods FBC, U&E, LFT, clotting, and group and cross-match 2–4 units or more if needed. See massive transfusion protocol (*Section 4.1*).
- Start oral proton pump inhibitor (PPI), e.g. 30 mg lansoprazole, and give IV only if cannot take PO.
- If patient dying in front of you from obvious active witnessed bleeding consider **universal donor O negative blood** and send someone to fetch it.
- **Observations**: repeat frequent assessments of BP, HR and JVP and titrate volume and blood replacement with these. Take care not to volume overload the frail and elderly and those with poor cardiac function. A urinary catheter can be the poor man's central line because it can give some measure as a surrogate marker of renal and general perfusion. If you can get the patient to an HDU bed with arterial monitoring and 1:1 nursing then that is ideal for the shocked bleeder.
- **Calculate Rockall score** and discuss with gastroenterologists who may proceed urgently to upper GI endoscopy if shocked or liver disease. Gastroenterologists may suggest IV omeprazole or other PPI if endoscopic evidence of bleeding.
- **Surgical liaison:** if bleeding continues despite endoscopy then surgeons and anaesthetists will be involved, as laparotomy may be the only way to stop the bleeding. The patient becomes a surgical rather than a medical emergency.
- **ITU/HDU:** patients may be best on HDU/ITU especially if need for intubation or ventilation or inotropic support or multi-organ failure. Speak to ITU team and involve them early in a deteriorating patient.

Rockall score (*Gut*, 1999;44:331)

- **Age:** <60 (+0), 60–79 (+1), >80 (+2).
- **Shock:** HR <100 SBP >100 mmHg (+0), HR >100 SBP >100 mmHg (+1), SBP <100 mmHg (+2).
- **Co-morbidities:** none significant (+0), IHD/CCF or other major co-morbidity (+2), liver failure/ kidney failure/metastatic cancer (+3).

Post endoscopy findings

- **Endoscopic diagnosis**: Mallory–Weiss tear (+0), all other diagnosis (+1), gastrointestinal malignancy (+2).
- **Bleeding at endoscopy:** none or dark spots only (+0), blood, spurting vessel, adherent clot (+2).

Calculate total

NB: pre-endoscopy score out of 7 used to risk assess. Helps gastroenterologists to select those for urgent endoscopy. Post-endoscopy score out of 11. Those with an additional low score may not require urgent endoscopy and some may be managed as outpatient.

Score: very low risk: 1–2 can be considered for instant discharge and OP OGD and PPI and follow up. **Low risk** <3: 0% expected mortality and 5% rebleed – good prognosis; consider discharge, outpatient endoscopy on PPI. **Intermediate 3–8**: monitor as inpatient. **High risk** >8: high (41%) mortality and (42%) rebleed – consider urgent endoscopy.

Warnings

- Elderly patients decompensate early; healthy younger patients (under 50) decompensate late and quickly so take care and don't be lulled into a false sense of security.
- GI blood loss by its nature is occult initially. Assume things may be worse than you see. Be careful with those on beta-blockers where normal tachycardia response may be muted.

Diagnosis specific management

Coagulopathy

- **Warfarin induced bleed**: needs IV vitamin K 10 mg and prothrombin complex concentrates, e.g. OCTAPLEX or BERIPLEX. Target INR <1.5. REVERSE WARFARIN EVEN IN THOSE WITH METAL HEART VALVES WITH MAJOR BLEED. Thromboembolic risk from temporary reversal of anticoagulation for several days is tiny compared to risk of exsanguination in those with genuine signs of significant haemorrhage.
- **Other coagulopathy** (discuss with haematology): requires fresh frozen plasma (FFP) and cryoprecipitate. Give FFP at 15 ml/kg (each unit is about 150 ml). If the fibrinogen is <1 mg/L give cryoprecipitate (2 units) as per transfusion policy. Give platelets if $<50 \times 10^9$/L especially if also on ASPIRIN or CLOPIDOGREL or PRASUGREL or equivalent. Withhold these agents actively if active bleeding. Take senior advice. Patients with critical coronary artery disease or bare metal or drug-eluting stents should be discussed with cardiology prior to next dose. Uncontrolled bleeding and anaemia will lead to MI and worse.

Severe oesophagitis

- Oral Omeprazole 40 mg OD. Manage blood loss. Consider also **Sucralfate 1 g qds.**

Oesophageal variceal bleed

- **Active management**: 40% will not settle conservatively and need active treatment to control bleed. Admit ITU/HDU. Target Hb 80 g/L. Risk factors for bleeding include: severity of cirrhosis, raised hepatic vein pressure, variceal size, tense ascites, endoscopic appearance, e.g. haematocystic spots, diffuse erythema, bluish colour, cherry red spots, or white-nipple spots.
- **TERLIPRESSIN IV 4 hourly for 48 h** (not if IHD); mesenteric/splanchnic vasoconstrictor decreases portal venous inflow. 34% reduction in mortality for variceal bleed. Give immediately prior to endoscopy if varices likely. Alternative is **OCTREOTIDE (somatostatin analogue)** infusion for 3–5 days (can be used in those with IHD).
- **ANTIBIOTICS:** 25% reduction in mortality (Cochrane Review, 2009) and 2–3 times less likely to rebleed. **CIPROFLOXACIN PO** for 7 days or **TRIMETHOPRIM PO** for 7 days or 3rd generation cephalosporin.
- **LAXATIVES: reduce risk of encephalopathy**: 30–50 ml lactulose BD and phosphate enemas to get 2 or more bowel motions per day.
- **Oesophageal banding or sclerotherapy**: rubber band placed around varix. More successful than injection sclerotherapy.
- **Balloon tamponade:** Sengstaken tube with gastric and oesophageal balloons. Placed in intubated patient. Gastric balloon placed in stomach via mouth and filled with 200–300 ml of water as per instructions. AXR to check position. Gentle retraction pressure on balloon can stop bleeding – usually the weight of a 500 ml or 1 L bag of fluids. Oesophageal balloon rarely needs filling. Sedation, intubation and ventilation will aid airway protection and tolerance of the procedure.

- **Transjugular intrahepatic porto-systemic shunt** (TIPS): if persistent bleeding. Radiological guidance. Guide wire inserted into internal jugular to IVC to hepatic vein into liver. Stent passed over wire to create communication, allows high-pressure portal veins to shunt into systemic veins. This drops portal pressure, reducing bleeding and shunts portal venous blood bypassing liver to IVC, but can worsen encephalopathy. Local gastroenterologists will suggest when appropriate. Usually done at tertiary centre.
- **Long term:** beta-blockers for varices decrease rebleed by 40%. Re-banding for varices until obliterated. Liver transplantation.

Peptic ulcers

- **Reduce bleeding and rebleeding:** rebleeders are large ulcers over 2 cm and lesser curve gastric ulcers and posterior wall duodenal ulcers. Visible clot and visible bleeding increase bleed risk.
- **Urgent endoscopic therapy**: visible clot removed and bleeding vessel injected with adrenaline which tamponades and vasoconstricts vessels. Addition of a second endoscopic treatment following adrenaline injection (thermal coagulation or clips) improves outcome in high risk bleeding ulcers.
- **IV OMEPRAZOLE 80 mg bolus followed by infusion of 8 mg/h for 48–72 h** if there is evidence of severe bleeding. This raises gastric pH and aids clot stability and haemostasis. Continue for 3 days when rebleeding most common. Low risk patients can start oral PPI, e.g. omeprazole post-endoscopy. PPIs should be used for at least 4 weeks to heal ulcers, e.g. omeprazole 20 mg OD.
- **Angiography** combined with selective vessel embolisation or selective intra-arterial VASOPRESSIN may be used where available if bleeding persists.
- **Surgery:** when all modalities fail and bleeding persists then direct ligation of bleeding vessel needed. Uncommon event nowadays. Declining surgical experience. Liaise quickly if deteriorating.
- **HP eradication:** all should have CLO test and *H. pylori* eradication if positive. Early pre-endoscopy PPI can reduce sensitivity of *H. pylori* detection at endoscopy.

Others

- **Gastritis/duodenitis:** oral PPI therapy and *H. pylori* eradication if CLO test positive.
- **Gastric/oesophageal cancer:** treat much the same as peptic ulcer disease. Argon laser or other comparable interventions may be tried. Some may need surgery.
- **Dieulafoy's lesion:** cautery or angiographic embolisation. Surgical over-sewing if other management fails.
- **Upper GI bleeding and stent or metal valves**: risk of bleeding usually is the more pressing and anticoagulation/antiplatelets should be stopped or reversed acutely.

14.4 Lower gastrointestinal bleeding

About

- Bleeding from beyond the ligament of Treitz. May be from small bowel or colorectal.
- If source unclear do OGD. A torrential upper GI bleed can cause fresh PR bleeding.

Note

- A history of pain and weight loss in combination with bleeding suggests a colorectal cancer.

Causes

- Diverticular disease, ischaemic colitis, haemorrhoids, colorectal cancer.
- Ulcerative/Crohn's colitis, ischaemic colitis, pseudomembranous colitis.
- Angiodysplasia, colorectal polyps, Meckel's diverticulum.
- Radiation enteropathy, e.g. for gynaecological malignancies.

Clinical

- Signs of shock and volume loss/anaemia.
- A history of pain and weight loss and altered bowel habit suggests cancer.
- Check if patient on warfarin, clopidogrel, aspirin or new oral anticoagulants.
- Evidence of coagulopathy – liver failure.
- Gynaecological malignancies and bowel irradiation (radiation proctitis).
- Perform digital rectal examination and proctoscopy.

Investigation

- **FBC, U&E, coagulation** if coagulopathy suspected or warfarin.
- **Group and cross-match** 2–4 units or more as needed.
- **Colonoscopy:** usually with good bowel prep to help visibility is the investigation of choice and can visualise entire colon. Often difficult to see source when bleeding acutely.
- **OGD**: do if source unclear. A torrential upper GI bleed can cause fresh PR bleeding. May be multiple sources.
- **Sigmoidoscopy:** may be used for a distal lesion. Proctoscopy is useful to identify haemorrhoids.
- **Mesenteric angiography:** for angiodysplasia for an occult bleeding lesion. The yield is low and therefore usefulness in question.
- **Technetium-labelled red cell scan**: for occult bleeding.
- **CT and CT angiography** may localise underlying pathology.

Markers of poor prognosis

- **Age**: acute lower GI bleeding occurs most often in the elderly.
- **Acute haemodynamic disturbance**: tachycardia, hypotension, shock.
- **Gross rectal bleeding** on initial examination (× 2.3–3).
- **Co-morbidity**: 2+ conditions doubles the chance of a severe bleed.
- **Aspirin or NSAIDs**: increased risk of severe lower GI bleeding × 1.8–2.7.
- **Inpatients**: (any cause) who bleed after admission have a mortality rate of 23% compared with 3.6% in those admitted to hospital because of rectal bleeding.

Management

- **Supportive**: ABC, high flow O_2 if shocked and resuscitate with initial 1–2 L IV NS and blood. Correct any coagulopathy and transfuse and replace fluids as required. Most cases settle conservatively with supportive measures. In the acute stage, colonoscopy can be difficult if there is marked bleeding, however, colonoscopic haemostasis is an effective means of controlling haemorrhage from active diverticular bleeding or post-polypectomy bleeding, when appropriately skilled expertise is available.
- **Surgery:** massive on-going bleeding (>5 units in 24 h) requires surgical intervention. Involve surgeons early if bleeding does not settle quickly. Localised segmental intestinal resection or subtotal colectomy is recommended.
- **Catheter mesenteric angiography** and embolisation may be attempted (note that the quantity of evidence on which this practice is based is limited).

Reference: SIGN (2008) Management of acute upper and lower gastrointestinal bleeding: a national clinical guideline. SIGN Guideline 105.

14.5 Gastric outlet obstruction / pyloric stenosis

About

- Weight loss, food regurgitation.

Causes

- Pancreatic or gastric malignancy.
- Peptic ulcer disease with scarring and oedema of pylorus.
- Gastric polyps, duodenal malignancy, cholangiocarcinoma.

Clinical

- Fullness and vomiting immediately postprandial which is non-bilious.
- Weight loss, succussion splash if NBM for 2–3 h.
- Palpable abdominal mass and gastric dilation.
- Malnutrition is seen late. Aspiration pneumonia.
- Supraclavicular lymph nodes. Hepatomegaly and jaundice if liver metastases.

Investigations

- **FBC, U&E**, raised urea and creatinine, low K^+ develops later after 2–3 weeks.
- **LFT**: raised ALP or bilirubin may suggest malignancy.
- **USS abdomen**: liver metastases, obstructive jaundice.
- **Imaging:** abdominal ultrasound or CT abdomen: define any masses.
- **ABG:** hypochloraemic (eventually hypokalaemic) metabolic alkalosis.
- **Upper GI endoscopy**: may still be food residue in stomach and difficulty passing probe. A lesion may be seen and biopsies taken. A stent may be passable.

Management

- IV rehydration and fluid and electrolyte replacement and nutrition.
- Manage electrolytes and acid–base disturbances.
- Specific management depends on cause.
- Stenting may be possible depending on circumstances.
- Surgical referral in appropriate cases.

14.6 Acute severe colitis

Stool frequency of >8 or raised CRP >45 on day 3 of admission predicts an 85% likelihood of requiring a colectomy during that admission.

About

- Combined medical/surgical approach is key to best care.

Causes

- **Inflammatory bowel disease:** ulcerative colitis, Crohn's disease, **c**olitis of **u**ndetermined **t**ype and a**e**tiology (CUTE)
- **Infection,** e.g. *Shigella* and certain *E. coli* (risk of HUS). Pseudomembranous colitis (PMC): recent antibiotics. Amoebiasis. CMV colitis can mimic ulcerative colitis.
- **Others:** radiation colitis, ischaemic colitis (older, AF, vascular disease).

Clinical

- Diarrhoea, mucus, bloody often 10–20/day and urgency.
- IBD flare up can be provoked by infection, stress, NSAIDs, antibiotics.
- Crampy abdominal pain, weight loss, fevers.
- Silent rigid abdomen suggests perforation.

- Rebound suggests peritonism. Distension, vomiting suggests obstruction.
- Look for signs of sepsis an volume depletion.
- Enquire if infective source – chicken, contact with livestock, salads.

Findings suggesting IBD (most will have a known diagnosis)

- Mouth ulcers, eye disease – conjunctivitis, iritis, episcleritis.
- Erythema nodosum – painful red lesions usually over the lower legs.
- Joint pain – large joints, migratory, asymmetrical.
- Enclosing spondylitis seen with Crohn's disease, sacroilitis – low back pain.
- Pyoderma gangrenosum pustule, expands as a large ulcer with violaceous margins.

Pathology

- Ulcerative colitis: starts distally and confined to colon and rectum (proctitis). Contact bleeding.
- Crohn's disease: skip lesions, perianal involvement, colitis/proctitis, transmural inflammation.
- Pseudomembranous colitis: adherent surface membrane, *C. difficile* toxin.

Supporting evidence for severe colitis (can be used for inflammatory and infective colitis)

- Bloody stool frequency >6/day
- Fever temp >37.5°C
- HR >90 bpm
- ESR >30 mm/h
- Hb <10 g/dL
- Albumin <30 g/L

Investigations

- **FBC:** low Hb. Microcytic if Fe loss, macrocytic if B12/folate deficient.
- **CRP and ESR and low albumin**: acute phase response with any flair up.
- **U&E:** raised urea and creatinine. **pANCA** positive in ulcerative colitis.
- **LFTs:** low albumin. Raised ALP and AST with liver disease.
- **Stool culture and *C. difficile* toxin testing** if suspected.
- **Abdominal film**: look for megacolon with colonic diameter >6 cm, perforation, no faeces, mucosal oedema, mucosal islands, thumb printing. Extent of disease can be assessed with reasonable accuracy by the distal extent of faecal residue visible on a plain abdominal radiograph. Should be repeated daily whilst the patient fulfils the criteria for severe colitis and with any evidence of worsening such as an increase in pulse rate, temperature or stool frequency.
- **Small bowel imaging:** is needed with suspected Crohn's disease and abdominal symptoms.
- **Flexible sigmoidoscopy:** confirms diagnosis and shows erythematous inflamed, even haemorrhagic, mucosa and allows biopsies.
- **Colonoscopy:** can also be done to show extent of disease and to exclude malignancy in longstanding colitis. In reality it is best avoided in the acute episode. Bowel preparation is distressing and potentially dangerous since it can provoke megacolon.
- **Barium enema:** may show loss of haustral pattern and featureless colon. Avoided during acute flare-up. Biopsies – goblet cell depletion, inflammatory, mucosal ulcers, crypt abscesses.

Management of inflammatory bowel disease related colitis

- **General**: severe cases need to be admitted with daily senior review at least. AXR to exclude toxic megacolon (>6 cm), stool for culture, frequent CRP. Fluid and electrolyte (K^+) balance and stool chart is required. If dehydrated and volume depleted then ensure IV access and volume replacement and transfusion as required to match losses to maintain Hb >10 g/dL. Maintain adequate fluid balance and electrolytes. Potassium losses can be significant and need replacing at up to 60–100 mmol/day.

- **Other causes**: *Campylobacter* and other infections can mimic severe colitis. Ischaemic colitis can cause bloody diarrhoea associated with abdominal pain, usually in older patients, with AXR appearance and hypotension and AF and atherosclerosis and urgent surgical consult is needed. If *C. difficile* is suspected then avoid steroids and manage supportively with oral METRONIDAZOLE and/or Vancomycin.
- **Mild to moderate colitis:** (<4 stools/day, non-toxic, systemically well): can be treated with oral prednisolone 20 mg OD and management as an outpatient with close liaison with GI team, IBD specialist nurses, and regular review. This can be combined with a 5-ASA (aminosalicylic acid) such as ASACOL MR (MESALAZINE) 2.4 g/day in divided doses. As disease is often distal this can be combined with steroid enemas (PREDSOL 20 mg at bedtime) for 2–4 weeks. Mild and moderate cases may go home on steroids if sensible, coping and knowing to return if worsens. Direct telephone access to IBD nurse specialists.
- **Moderate colitis:** (4–6 stools per day) then PREDNISOLONE 40 mg per day and MESALAZINE or equivalent and STEROID ENEMAS. Admission initially for senior assessment especially if unwell. Oral steroid course is needed for 2–4 weeks and is titrated by the colitis team to match the response.
- **Acute severe colitic disease:** IV HYDROCORTISONE 100 mg 6-hourly × 5 days followed by oral steroids which may be given where the presentation is of suspected inflammatory bowel disease. Failure to respond, perforation or toxic megacolon all demand urgent surgical review. *Typical clinical signs of perforation may be minimal, because patients are being treated with steroids*. Response rate to IV steroids in acute severe colitis is 40%. Oral steroids, e.g. Prednisolone, can be used and continued as an outpatient.
- **Surgery**: a colorectal surgeon should be aware from admission of any patient with acute severe ulcerative colitis and should be involved in clinical decision-making. Colectomy for IBD-related acute severe colitis can be lifesaving for those who are failing to respond to acute medical therapy. Early input can help prepare the patient for possible colectomy and introduce them to a stoma therapist.
- **Steroid-sparing agents**: IV Ciclosporin and other agents have been used for severe acute disease in those who may need a colectomy.
- **Biological agents**: consider a single dose of infliximab (antibody to TNF-alpha) for those with a poor response to steroids with acute severe colitis. It has been shown to reduce need for colectomy. Risk of infection and disseminated TB. This is for specialist use only.
- **Enteral feeding**: should be continued as long as tolerated, often in conjunction with other agents including biologicals. Nutrition is fundamental to a good outcome.
- **LMWH** should be given for VTE prophylaxis because this is a prothrombotic period even with mild to moderate bloody stool but watch Hb.
- **A word of caution**: care must be taken to ensure you are treating an acute colitis flare-up rather than a Crohn's flare with infective complication before starting steroids. In ulcerative colitis it is usually evident but with Crohn's disease there may be abdominal pain, and systemic illness and complex transmural bowel-penetrating disease with localised abscess formation, and in these cases steroids

should be withheld and antibiotics, abscess drainage (surgical or USS guidance) and liquid formula diet instituted as appropriate. In most cases where colitis is the dominant feature steroids are appropriate. Crohn's' complications include stricture and abscess, fistula formation, infection. Take expert advice; these patients should ideally be under the care of a specialist from day 1.

Reference: Jakobovits & Travis (2006) Management of acute severe colitis. *Br Med Bull* 75–76:131.

14.7 Acute colonic pseudo-obstruction

About

- Appearance of obstruction usually in elderly but no obstructive lesion. Motility disorder. Also known as Ogilvie syndrome.

Complications

- Perforation (usually of caecum), peritonitis, death.
- Risks of perforation higher with caecal diameter >14 cm, delayed compression, and elderly.

Clinical

- Abdominal distension, colicky pain and vomiting, constipation.
- Measure abdominal circumference.

Causes

- Co-morbidities, e.g. CCF, sepsis, renal and respiratory failure, spinal injury.
- Drugs – TCA, codeine, electrolyte abnormalities.

Investigations

- **FBC**: anaemia, WCC. **U&E**, Ca, Mg, TFT.
- **AXR:** may show massive dilation of the lower bowel. Measure caecal diameter. Look for evidence of perforation.
- **Abdominal CT scan:** can be considered but contrast enema or colonoscopy best to exclude physical colonic obstruction.
- **Water-soluble contrast enema**: can exclude lesion and break up hard faeces.
- **Colonoscopy**: can exclude obstructive lesion and aid decompression.

Management

- **Supportive:** treat any identifiable cause and exclude a physical obstructive cause. Stop any responsible medication and seek and correct any electrolyte disturbance and ensure hydration. NBM and NG tube to allow decompression from above.
- Consider Prucolapride (used off-licence for ACPO) 1–2 mg PO OD. If no response then **Neostigmine 2 mg IV over 5 min** and watch for bradycardia. This can be repeated; take specialist advice. Treats 85–90% of cases. If any significant bradycardia give atropine 0.3–1.0 mg.
- **Earlier mobilisation** and positioning of patients – get them out of bed.
- **Nutrition:** if prolonged may need Total Parenteral Nutrition (TPN).
- Flexible sigmoidoscopy for decompression or simple insertion of a flatus tube should be considered if caecal diameter >9 cm. Consider if medical management fails; repeat as many times as needed.
- **Surgical caecostomy** if not settling conservatively.

14.8 Acute pancreatitis

About

- Significant morbidity and mortality. Usually managed by surgeons with gastroenterology.

Causes

- **Gallstones**: a gallstone in ampulla of Vater can allow bile reflux into pancreatic duct activating enzymes.
- **Alcohol:** chronic alcohol for several years or occasional binge.
- **Hypertriglyceridaemia**: look at fundi for lipaemia retinalis.
- **Hyperparathyroidism**: check Ca, pancreatic cancer, post ERCP complication.
- **Miscellaneous:** trauma, snake bite, HIV, CMV, EBV.
- **Drugs**: steroids, thiazides, azathioprine, sulphonamide.

Aetiology

- Activation of trypsin, lipase and amylase and autodigestion.
- Leads to an inflamed oedematous/haemorrhagic pancreas.
- On-going tissue damage can activate complement.
- Progressive systemic inflammatory response syndrome.

Types

- Acute/mild/oedematous pancreatitis which settles.
- Acute/severe/haemorrhagic with longer course and complications.
- Pancreatic phlegmon-inflammatory mass seen by radiology/surgery.
- Sterile pancreatic necrosis – pseudocyst with fluid in the lesser sac.
- Pancreatic abscess – contains pus and may be drained percutaneously.

Clinical

- Tachycardia, hypotension, shock from sepsis, haemorrhagic pancreatitis.
- Severe epigastric pain to back eased with sitting up and forwards.
- Peritonitis with guarding, signs of causes, e.g. gallstones, alcoholism.
- Shocked, sepsis – generalised, pneumonia, anaemia.
- Bruising in flanks – Grey–Turner's sign.
- Periumbilical bruising – Cullen's sign (haemorrhagic pancreatitis).
- Coagulopathy from DIC. Cyanosed, dyspnoea from ARDS.
- Oliguria from AKI and/or hypovolaemia.

Ranson criteria for severity and prognosis

At admission or diagnosis	First 48 hours
• Age >55 • WCC >16 000/mm^3 • Glucose >11 mmol/L • LDH >350 IU/L or AST >250 IU/L	• Hct fall >10%, Ca <2 mmol/L • PaO_2 <8 kPa • Base excess >–4 mmol/L • Urea increase >1.8 mmol/L • Fluid needs >6 L
First 48 h prognosis: 0–2 criteria <5% mortality, 3–4 criteria 20% mortality, 5–6 criteria 40% mortality, 7–8 criteria 100% mortality.	

Investigations

- **FBC**: low Hb with haem pancreatitis; raised MCV with alcohol. **U&E:** AKI, low Ca, raised triglycerides (familial hypertriglyceridaemia).

- **CRP**: >100 on day 5 high risk of complications, e.g. infection, pseudocyst, abscess formation.
- **Amylase** (× 3–5 upper limit is diagnostic) usually >1000 IU/ml (levels up to 10 000 may be seen). Mild elevations >200 IU/ml not unique to pancreatitis but may also be seen in abdominal pain due to perforation of a viscus, small bowel obstruction, leaking AAA, ectopic pregnancy. A level of >1000 is more diagnostic, *but there is not a close correlation between amylase level and clinical severity*. Very rarely a normal amylase may suggest previous pancreatic damage with little pancreatic tissue left.
- **Pancreatic lipase**: has a higher sensitivity and specificity than amylase.
- **Erect CXR/AXR**: exclude perforation, small bowel obstruction. Left pleural effusion may be seen. Look for calcification and sentinel loop. Bowel gas is seen in small bowel in centre of abdomen.
- **USS abdomen**: pancreatic mass, gallstones, pseudocyst, liver disease.
- **Arterial blood gases**: metabolic acidosis, hypoxia in severe cases. **Elevated lactate.**
- **CT/MRI abdomen**: determine degree of pancreatic necrosis, but full changes take several days, and the presence of any fluid. CT may show fat-stranding surrounding the inflamed pancreas. Fluid may be aspirated to detect infection. Necrotic pancreas is identified by failure to opacify when CT with contrast is carried out. Gas bubbles may suggest infection.
- **ERCP**: may be diagnostically important when aetiology unclear and may show a cause, e.g. ampullary tumour, stricture, gallstones, pancreas divisum and may allow sphincterotomy.

Complications

- **Pancreatic pseudocyst**: can form around the pancreatic mass and may need laparoscopic drainage.
- **Necrotising pancreatitis**: more than 50% of gland necrosed on imaging. Can lead to infection and abscess formation and needs antibiotics and occasionally surgery. Malabsorption, recurrent acute pancreatitis.
- **Systemic**: ARDS, AKI, DIC, multiorgan failure, generalised or local sepsis, secondary diabetes.

Management

- **ABC** and O_2 as per BTS guidance. Give **IV fluids,** crystalloids (NS or Hartmann's solution) and close management of fluid balance is necessary in all but the mildest cases with CVP monitoring if needed, urinary catheter and clinical assessments of hydration, oxygenation, etc. There may be significant 'third space' losses, which will need to be accounted for. ITU admission for severe cases. All patients who are vomiting require an NG tube. May be some degree of gastroparesis.
- **Analgesia for severe pain**: TRAMADOL 50–100 mg IV tds is preferred. Alternatives are MORPHINE 5–10 mg IV + CYCLIZINE 50 mg. Pethidine is avoided.
- **Variable rate insulin infusion** if hyperglycaemic or known diabetes.
- **Broad-spectrum antibiotics** given where sepsis is suspected and not routinely. Fever is usually related to the inflammatory nature of the disease. If infection considered then **TAZOCIN IV or MEROPENEM IV** if penicillin allergic.
- **Nutrition:** nasogastric/nasojejunal or oral feeding recommended once diagnosis made and no contraindications. If on-going enteral nutritional support not possible and on-going nutritional needs then consider TPN.

- **ERCP +/− sphincterotomy** should be considered, usually within 72 h where there is a cholangitis or jaundice and a common duct stone, which requires removal. A sphincterotomy may be performed and/or stone removed.
- **CT-guided aspiration** of pancreas to establish presence of infection may be considered and may help decide if surgery needed.
- **SURGERY** may be required where there is a severe necrotizing pancreatitis or if there is an abscess or pseudocyst. A pancreatic necrosectomy involves removing dead pancreatic tissue, which may be done by laparoscopy. Infection increases the indication for necrosectomy.

14.9 Acute cholecystitis

About

- Commoner in women. Gallstones are seen in 10% of the population.

Aetiology

- Lithogenic bile, raised insoluble cholesterol and insufficient bile acids.
- Obstruction of the gallbladder neck or cystic duct by a gallstone.
- Inflammation is more likely chemical rather than infective as bile is usually sterile.

Clinical

- Constant pain in epigastrium and/or RUQ and upper abdomen. Fever.
- Murphy's sign is positive – pressure on RUQ catches patient on inspiration.
- Jaundice if a stone blocks the common bile duct.
- Rigors suggest infection and cholangitis.

Investigation

- **FBC and U&E**: elevated WCC, CRP.
- **LFT**: raised bilirubin and ALP, GGT (esp. if common bile duct blocked) and mild increase in ALT and AST.
- **Abdominal USS**: enlarged hydropic gallbladder with a thickened wall in the region of maximum tenderness. Gallstones in gallbladder and/or cystic duct or common bile duct.
- **ERCP with cholangiogram** may be needed for ductal stones.

Complications

- Biliary sepsis and cholangitis, empyema (pus) of the gallbladder.
- Perforation and peritonitis.

Management

- **Supportive:** ABC and O_2 as per BTS guidelines + IV access + nil by mouth. Commence 1 L crystalloids (NS or Hartmann's) over 2–4 h and assess volume needs and replace.
- **Pain relief**: MORPHINE 5–10 mg IV + CYCLIZINE 50 mg.
- **Antibiotics**: TAZOCIN IV for 7–10 days or IV CEFUROXIME/METRONIDAZOLE.
- **Laparoscopic cholecystectomy** should be carried out urgently or within 5 days of onset of symptoms otherwise the patient is prone to further episodes.
- **Surgery,** e.g. **open cholecystectomy** is only indicated in those with at least clinical evidence of gallstones causing symptoms. 90% of gallstones are symptom-free and do not warrant any action. Once symptoms develop and they are attributable to gallstones then cholecystectomy should be considered as there is then a high chance of recurrence with risk of complications.

- **Acalculous cholecystitis** can occur with no stones seen but a typical acute cholecystitis picture. Prognosis is worse. Seen with diabetes, fasting, TPN, sepsis, trauma, burns, opiates, IHD. Treat with antibiotics and supportive management. Gangrene and perforation are more common. Urgent cholecystectomy may be indicated

14.10 Acute cholangitis

Aetiology

- Bacterial infection of the biliary tree usually due to stones or impaired drainage.

Causes

- Gallstones, strictures, Sclerosing cholangitis, chronic pancreatitis, HIV-related cholangiopathy.

Clinical

- Charcot's triad of non-colicky RUQ pain to right shoulder, jaundice and fever.
- Biliary obstruction – dark urine and pale stool.

Investigation

- **FBC and U&E**: raised WCC, bilirubin and ALP and GGT.
- **Abdominal USS**: enlarged hydropic gallbladder with a thickened wall and stones.
- **Abdominal CT:** can be useful to see obstruction and measure common bile duct. Can also exclude pancreatic carcinoma/other pathologies.
- **Magnetic resonance cholangiopancreatography (MRCP):** can visualise biliary tree anatomy and stones. Not possible if patient has pacemaker, etc.

Management

- **Supportive:** IV fluids, crystalloids and basic ABC + O_2 as per BTS guidelines.
- **Antibiotics: CEFUROXIME IV + METRONIDAZOLE IV or TAZOCIN IV.** For penicillin allergy take advice – possibilities include **MEROPENEM IV.** Treat for 7–10 days.
- **ERCP +/– sphincterotomy** can allow biliary drainage and passage of a stone +/– spontaneously or pulled out with a basket device. If there is a malignant lesion or stricture a stent can be placed.
- **Consider cholecystectomy** at 6–12 weeks for gallbladder stones and is commonly done laparoscopically nowadays.

Complications: sepsis, ARDS, multiorgan failure.

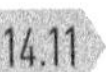

14.11 Acute abdomen

About

- Rapid onset of abdominal pain, vomiting, pyrexia and possibly hypotension.
- This is a surgical emergency potentially requiring operative management.
- Do not admit under medicine.

> Atypical presentations seen in: elderly, immunocompromised, recent high dose steroids as patients may have diminished symptoms and signs but may be gravely ill and septic.

Frequency

- Acute appendicitis 30%, acute cholecystitis 10%, small bowel obstruction 5%.
- Perforated peptic ulcer 3%, pancreatitis 3%, diverticular disease 2%.
- Urgent senior review needing resuscitation and possible surgery:

  - Severe haemorrhage (hypotension, tachycardia, anaemia appears late with ruptured AAA or ectopic pregnancy or splenic rupture).
  - Perforation or rupture of a viscus (toxic appearance, rigid abdomen, absent bowel sounds, *in extremis*, air under diaphragm), ascending cholangitis (jaundice, rigors, RUQ pain).
  - Viscus necrosis, e.g. ischaemic bowel from atherosclerosis, embolism or strangulated hernia, pancreatitis, intussusception, volvulus.

Clinical

- **Historical clues:** previous surgery – adhesions suggest causes of obstruction. Known IBD. Peptic ulcer disease and perforation: use of NSAIDs, steroids. Previous appendectomy excludes appendicitis. Warfarin – psoas/retroperitoneal haematoma. Known AAA. Immunosuppression.
- **Volume status**: look for tachycardia, low BP or low BP on sitting or standing suggests significant hypovolaemia, e.g. acute haemorrhage and blood loss (GI bleed, leaking AAA) or volume loss into obstructed bowel.
- **Abdominal pain:** examine abdomen carefully looking for area of maximum tenderness. Pain tends to come on suddenly or sub-acutely. Mechanism is either peritonitis with well-localised pain that is painful on coughing and movement and patient lies still with guarding and a rigid abdomen. Pain may also be colicky in nature and patient moves about and suggests a more obstructive luminal mechanism, e.g. intestinal obstruction. Associated nausea and vomiting.
- **Position**: sitting bending forward – chronic pancreatitis, lying still – perforation, restless – renal colic.
- **Visible peristalsis and distension**: suggests obstruction.
- **Radiation of pain:** to shoulder – diaphragmatic irritation, to the back – consider AAA or acute pancreatitis or posterior perforation. To umbilicus – acute appendicitis.
- **Guarding:** reflex contraction of abdominal muscles and discomfort on light abdominal palpation.
- **Rebound tenderness:** increase in severe pain and discomfort when the doctor abruptly stops pressing on a localized region of the abdomen or on percussion suggests peritonitis (25% don't have it).
- **Rigid abdomen:** contraction of abdominal muscles. Abdomen feels hard like a wooden board. Suggests perforation.
- **Fever: temperature** >38°C suggests infective or inflammatory process.
- **Jaundice:** common bile duct obstruction, liver failure, gallstones, haemolysis.
- **Dehydration:** peritonitis, small bowel obstruction, DKA, hypercalcaemia.
- **Ascites**: bulging flanks, abdominal distension with shifting dullness. Bowel floats and ascites gravitates to lowest point. Consider spontaneous bacterial peritonitis in liver disease.
- **Murphy's sign:** palpation over RUQ causes acute severe pain stopping inspiration. Acute cholecystitis.
- **Don't forget:** check groin and all hernial orifices as well as scrotal sac and contents.
- **Per rectum examination** – tenderness, induration, mass, frank blood.
- **Per vaginum examination** where indicated - bleeding, discharge, cervical motion tenderness, adnexal masses, and tenderness, uterine size.
- **Bowel sounds**: listen for 2 minutes to ensure absent. May be high pitched and tinkling.
- **Check hernial orifices**, e.g. strangulated femoral hernia, and the testes of men for a testicular torsion or hernia. Can identify cause of bowel obstruction.

Causes: those with potential surgical management:

- **Cholecystitis:** gallstones, RIF pain, Murphy's sign, fever, jaundice if stone in common bile duct.
- **Acute appendicitis:** pain begins periumbilical and moves to RIF as becomes more peritonitis.
- **Leaking abdominal aortic aneurysm (AAA):** midline pulsatile expansile mass, low BP, may have lost a femoral pulse.
- **Acute pancreatitis:** history of gallstones or alcohol and raised amylase.
- **Adhesions causing bowel obstruction:** previous surgery, abdominal scars and old incisional wounds.
- **Incarcerated or strangulated hernia:** bowel obstruction and tender hernial orifices.
- **Pelvic inflammatory pain:** may have similar history, vaginal discharge, history of STDs.
- **Acute diverticulitis:** left iliac fossa pain, older patient.
- **Abdominal wall haematoma**: on warfarin.
- **Gastrointestinal malignancy:** stomach, pancreas, small bowel, colonic.
- **Budd–Chiari:** prothrombotic, RIF pain, jaundice.
- **Inflammatory bowel disease:** Crohn's disease predominantly a small bowel obstruction picture. Ulcerative colitis mainly a colitis picture. Watch for toxic megacolon.
- **Testicular torsion**: testicular pain.
- **Ureteric colic/renal stones.**
- **Meckel's diverticulum:** pain in RIF. May perforate. Seen in adolescents and young adults. Can mimic appendicitis.
- **Gynaecological**: endometriosis: recurrent pain. Ectopic pregnancy: positive pregnancy test and abdominal pain. Acute salpingitis: on right can mimic appendicitis. Ovarian torsion: on right can mimic appendicitis. Mittleschmerz: ovulation mid-cycle pain. May need urgent gynaecological consult and urgent surgery.

Causes: those with non-surgical management:

- **Gastroenteritis:** vomiting and diarrhoea predominate with vague pain and tenderness; gradually settles.
- **Myocardial infarction** (diaphragmatic/inferior): ECG – ST/T changes and troponin.
- **Lower lobe pneumonia**: fever, breathless, chest signs, CXR signs may be delayed.
- **Pyelonephritis**: positive urinalysis, tender renal angle, female.
- **Addisonian crisis**: pale, pigmented creases and scars, hypotensive.
- **Diabetic ketoacidosis**: hyperglycaemic, ketotic.
- **Sickle cell crisis**: Afro-Caribbean origin, similar past history, anaemia. Hyposplenism.
- **Herpes zoster**: rash may not be seen early on – pain affecting abdominal dermatome does not cross midline.
- **Acute porphyria**: variegate and acute intermittent porphyria, hereditary coproporphyria.
- **Familial Mediterranean fever**: Turkish/Middle Eastern. Mesenteric adenitis: viral type illness – younger patients. Mimics appendicitis.
- **Tabes dorsalis**: as part of tertiary syphilis.

Pain and localisation is not an exact science and there is much variability, e.g. late pregnancy.

- **RUQ:** cholecystitis, gallbladder empyema, hepatitis, liver abscess, duodenal ulcer, pneumonia, subphrenic abscess, hepatic flexure of colon.

- **LUQ:** gastroenteritis, splenic disease (infarction/rupture), splenic flexure of colon, subphrenic abscess, perinephritis, acute pancreatitis.
- **Epigastrium:** oesophageal/gastric disease (perforation, gastric ulcer or duodenal ulcer), ruptured AAA, acute pancreatitis, myocardial infarction, PE, pancreatic cancer.
- **Right flank:** ureteric colic (loin to groin), pyelonephritis (renal angle), retrocaecal appendix, muscle strain, perinephric abscess.
- **Periumbilical:** early appendicitis, small bowel disease – obstruction and inflammatory bowel disease, gastroenteritis, pancreatitis, ruptured AAA, ischaemic bowel.
- **Left flank:** ureteric colic (loin to groin), pyelonephritis (renal angle), muscle strain, perinephric abscess.
- **RIF:** appendicitis, mesenteric lymphadenitis, perforated duodenal ulcer, caecal obstruction, Meckel's diverticulum, ectopic pregnancy, ovarian pathology, terminal ileal disease (Crohn's/*Yersinia* pseudotuberculosis) or very rarely RLQ diverticulitis, biliary colic with low lying gallbladder, acute salpingitis.
- **LIF:** sigmoidal diverticulitis, constipation, ectopic pregnancy, ovarian pathology, ischaemic colitis, rectal cancer, irritable bowel syndrome, ulcerative colitis.
- **Suprapubic:** cystitis, UTI, acute urinary retention, testicular torsion, pelvic inflammatory disease, ectopic pregnancy, uterine disease, diverticulitis.

Investigations

- **Bloods**: FBC, CRP, U&E, amylase. LFT and INR if any suggestion of liver disease or gallstones. Group and cross-match if suspected AAA, ectopic pregnancy or laparotomy or frank bleeding.
- **Erect CXR** and **erect abdominal films** can help exclude pathology. Perforation of viscus with free air visible under the diaphragm or between viscera and subcutaneous tissue on lateral decubitus. Distended small bowel proximal to small bowel obstruction with air-fluid levels. Small bowel more central. Thickened oedematous valvulae conniventes span entire wall of small bowel unlike colonic haustra. Renal stones may be seen best with AXR or IVU. Normal AXR does not exclude ileus or many other pathologies. Toxic megacolon if diameter >7 cm in midtransverse colon. Pancreatic calcification may suggest acute or chronic pancreatitis.
- **CT abdomen:** imaging important but does not substitute for good clinical assessment – appendicitis shows inflamed appendix fluid-filled with fat stranding and a hyperattenuated wall with IV contrast. Uncomplicated sigmoid diverticulitis can show fat stranding and focal thickening of the colonic wall in an area with diverticula. Abscess formation or fistulas may or may not be seen. Colonic cancers may be seen.
- **USS:** imaging of choice for cholecystitis with gallstones and thickened wall hydropic gallbladder. A stone may be seen blocking cystic duct. Sludge or stone material may be seen in the gallbladder. Gallstones may also suggest pancreatitis.
- **Urinary catheter**: urinalysis.
- **Pregnancy test** in all fertile women.

General management

- **Supportive**: ABC + give O_2 as per BTS guidance. Get good IV access and protect it. Start IV crystalloid fluids with good IV access and monitor physiology. Give 1 L Hartmann's or NS over 1–2 h as needed. Most patients are dry. **Analgesia**: IV morphine 5–10 mg + Cyclizine 50 mg.

- If tachycardic, hypotensive or bleeding then get senior help urgently.
- Fertile female consider ectopic pregnant for all acute abdominal pain and/or hypotension.
- Full monitoring BP, HR, temperature and urinary output. Catheterise.
- FBC, U&E, clotting if liver disease, amylase, group and hold/cross-match if haemorrhage or laparotomy.
- Severe haemorrhage – give O negative blood.
- Suspect sepsis then start IV antibiotics and fluid resuscitation. See *Section 4.6*.
- Maintain NBM until senior review decides otherwise.
- Normal important meds can sometimes be given with sip of water.
- Diabetic patients need to be started on a VRIII and keep CBG 4–12 mmol/L.
- AXR is helpful and depending on findings may need abdominal CT.
- Laparoscopy may reduce rate of unnecessary laparotomy and improve diagnostic accuracy.

14.12 Acute diverticulitis

About

- Diverticulae are protrusions of mucosa and submucosa through muscular wall of large bowel.

Aetiology

- Pouches of mucosa and submucosa herniate through the muscular wall of the bowel at points of weakness.
- Tends to affect sigmoid colon. Possibly high intraluminal pressures.
- There may be a local neural problem. Low fibre Western diets may play a role.

Clinical

- Diverticulae are clinically silent in 90% and very common.
- Diverticulitis can cause left-sided iliac fossa pain – classical symptom.
- Fever, nausea, vomiting, constipation or diarrhoea.
- Frank bleeding PR which can be significant.
- Fistula to bladder or vagina with subsequent UTI and foul discharge.

Investigations

- **FBC:** raised ESR, CRP and WCC. **U&E**: AKI.
- **Abdominal USS**: useful to show mucosal thickness and exclude an abscess and pericolic fluid.
- **Barium enema**: may demonstrate the presence of diverticulae.
- **Flexible sigmoidoscopy and colonoscopy** can show diverticulae but are not done acutely with risk of perforation.
- **Spiral CT of abdomen or CT colonograpy:** can show diseased sections, narrowing of lumen and thickening of bowel wall and lack of clarity of pericolic fat.

Management

- **Supportive:** ABC and O_2 as per BTS guidance. If unwell start IV fluids, e.g. 1 L NS and consider IV antibiotics if signs of infection. Associated haemorrhage usually managed conservatively. Surgical involvement especially if any signs of **bowel perforation or peritonitis. Perforation can lead to fistula formation.** Mild attacks may be managed with oral antibiotics as an outpatient.
- Laparoscopic surgery may be considered. An open Hartmann's procedure may be needed.

Complications

- Diverticulitis, pericolic abscess. Perforation and peritonitis and/or fistula formation to bladder, uterus, small intestine. Local narrowing and stricture formation and intestinal obstruction.

14.13 Re-feeding syndrome

About

- Restarting nutrition after a period of starvation.
- Need to manage low potassium, phosphate, magnesium and give thiamine.

> Re-feeding (whether it's oral, enteral or parenteral nutrition) triggers a switch from fat to carbohydrate metabolism, with consequent insulin release, and increased uptake of K, phosphate, Mg and water into cells.

Screening for those at risk – any 2 of:

(1) BMI <18.5 kg/m^2.
(2) Unintentional weight loss >10% in past 3–6 months.
(3) Little or no nutritional intake for over 5 days.
(4) History of alcohol excess or chemotherapy.

Clinical

- Wernicke's encephalopathy – encephalopathy, ataxic gait, oculomotor dysfunction, ophthalmoplegia.
- Cardiac and respiratory failure, arrhythmias, rhabdomyolysis, seizures, coma, death.

Investigations

- **FBC, U&E:** low K, Mg and phosphate. Check lactate and venous blood gases.

Management

- Prevention by monitoring phosphate and starting refeeding slowly at 25% normal requirement to minimise rise in insulin. Close involvement of dietitian. Watch K/P/Mg prior to and for the first few days of feeding. **IV fluids as required.**
- **Potassium**: K^+ 3.0–3.5 mmol/L give Sando K (12 mmol each) – 2 tds. K^+ 2.5–2.9 mmol/L IV KCl 40 mmol in 1 L NS (0.9%) or 5% dextrose over 8 h. Concentration must not exceed 40 mmol/L peripherally. Maximum infusion rate is 20 mmol/h unless via a central line with ECG monitoring.
- **Phosphate:** level 0.5–0.8 mmol/L give Phosphate Sandoz (16 mmol each) – 2 tds. Level 0.3–0.49 mmol/L give 25 mmol PO_4 Polyfusor (250 ml) over 12 h peripherally. Level <0.3 mmol/L give 50 mmol PO_4 Polyfusor (500 ml) over 24 h peripherally, measuring PO_4 at 12 h.
- **Thiamine**: 100 mg orally or crushed via feeding tube three times daily for 10 days or if enteral route not possible then IV thiamine (B1) (best given as IV Pabrinex which contains thiamine and other nutrients) before giving any carbohydrate.
- **Magnesium:** level: 0.5–0.7 mmol/L Magnaspartate – 1 sachet bd (10 mmol/sachet). Level: Mg <0.5 mmol/L give IV $MgSO_4$ 35–50 mmol in 1 L NS or 5% dextrose over 12–24 h peripherally.

15 Hepatology emergencies

15.1 Fulminant hepatic failure

About

- Severe hepatic failure in which encephalopathy develops in under 2 weeks in a patient with a previously normal liver.
- Prothrombin time is a useful marker of synthetic function.
- Most commonly due to drugs, toxins or viruses.
- In the UK commonly paracetamol overdose.
- Take an accurate drug history including over the counter and herbal remedies.

Synthetic function

- Procoagulant: fibrinogen, prothrombin, factors V, VII, IX, X and XIII.
- Anticoagulant proteins C and S. NOT gammaglobulins.
- Antithrombin, transferrin and caeruloplasmin. Albumin half life about 20 days.
- Glucose homeostasis – controlling blood sugar.

Causes	Details and notes
Infectious	**Viral hepatitis:** 40–70%: hepatitis A, hepatitis B, hepatitis B + D, hepatitis C is a very rare cause of FHF, hepatitis E viruses, CMV, EBV, VZV, yellow fever. Patients with known or suspected herpes virus or varicella zoster as the cause of ALF should be treated with acyclovir. Viral hepatitis A and B (and E) related ALF must be treated with supportive care because no virus-specific treatment has been proven effective. **Bacterial:** leptospirosis, severe bacterial infections. **Protozoal**: amoebic infection.
Paracetamol overdose (50% of cases in UK)	Within 4 h of presentation give activated charcoal just prior to starting *N*-acetyl cysteine. *N*-acetyl cysteine should be used promptly in all patients where paracetamol-induced liver injury is anticipated or there is concern of such and may be given acutely even if cause is unclear. See *Section 20.4* for paracetamol overdose protocol.
Other drugs and toxins	Halothane, isoniazid, phenytoin, sulphonamides, amiodarone, propylthiouracil, Ecstasy, herbal remedies. *Amanita phylloides* mushroom, carbon tetrachloride. Enquire about all drugs and environmental toxins including over the counter and herbal and natural remedies. Tetracycline, valproate and nucleoside reverse-transcriptase inhibitors can cause fatal liver disease.
Inherited	**Wilson's disease**: autosomal recessive. Copper studies should be performed. Serum copper and caeruloplasmin reduced or normal. Urinary copper is usually increased. Treat with Penicillamine.
Vascular	**Venous thrombosis: Budd–Chiari syndrome:** acute ascites, USS diagnostic with thrombosed hepatic vein. Consider thrombolysis and TIPS. Hepatic failure is an indication for liver transplantation, provided underlying malignancy is excluded.

Causes	Details and notes
Pregnancy	Acute fatty liver of pregnancy, HELLP syndrome with haemolysis, elevated liver enzymes and low platelet count. Expeditious delivery needed.
Reye's syndrome	Inhibition of beta-oxidation and uncoupling of oxidative phosphorylation in mitochondria. Acute encephalopathy with fatty infiltration of the liver. Precipitated by aspirin ingestion and viral infections.
Mushroom poisoning	ALF patients with known or suspected mushroom poisoning. Consider administration of **penicillin G and silymarin (III)** and should be considered for urgent orthoptic transplantation, the only lifesaving option.
Autoimmune hepatitis	Patients with ALF (usually a biopsy is done) due to autoimmune hepatitis should be treated with corticosteroids (prednisolone, 40–60 mg/day). In ALF patients with evidence of ischaemic injury, cardiovascular support is the treatment of choice.
Malignancy	Hepatoma: check USS and alpha-fetoprotein.
Miscellaneous	**Others**: idiopathic: viral, ischaemia: severe RHF, non-alcoholic steatohepatitis.

Clinical

- History of drug/toxin exposure key.
- Encephalopathy: flapping tremor, poor concentration.
- Reversal of day/night cycle, jaundice usually but not always, bleeding and coagulopathy.
- Hypoglycaemia, fetor hepaticus, look for Kayser–Fleischer rings.
- RUQ tenderness, NO splenomegaly or ascites, exception is Budd–Chiari syndrome.

Investigations

- **FBC:** raised WCC, ESR, CRP, low platelets (alcohol, HELLP). Haemolysis in Wilson's disease.
- **Prothrombin time:** increased. **Bilirubin:** elevated unconjugated.
- **LFT:** raised AST, ALT often >1000 (transaminases fall eventually).
- **U&E:** AKI with paracetamol toxicity or hepatorenal syndrome.
- **ABG**: metabolic acidosis and raised arterial lactate.
- **Viral serology**: anti-HAV IgM, HBsAg, anti-HBc IgM, anti-HEV, anti-HCV(rare cause).
- **Others**: paracetamol level, caeruloplasmin and 24-h urine copper, ammonia levels.
- **USS doppler**: liver size and pathology, and hepatic veins for Budd–Chiari syndrome.
- **Miscellaneous**: pregnancy test. ANA, anti-smooth muscle, immunoglobulin, HIV status.
- **NB:** focal neurology not typical and suggests need for CT brain.

Management

- **Stop all potentially implicated drugs.** Regard all as potentially hepatotoxic if no other evident cause.
- **Supportive: resuscitate:** ABCs and O_2 to get and maintain sats >92% and admit to an HDU/ITU environment. **Hypovolaemia:** replace with 4.5% serum albumin IV to elevate CVP to 10 cmH_2O or until clinically euvolaemic. **Hypotension:** consider inotropes to raise MAP >60 mmHg.

- **Hypoglycaemia:** treat with 50% IV dextrose and regular testing. Persisting may need 10% glucose infusion. Glucagon has limited effectiveness.
- **Low K^+, phosphate, magnesium:** replace as needed (see *Section 14.13*).
- **Hyponatraemia:** may need hypertonic 3% saline. See *Section 13.10.*
- **IV thiamine** 100 mg or a course of Pabrinex if alcoholic or malnourished. Give before any nutrition/IV glucose.
- **Cerebral oedema:** nurse at 20° head elevation. Hyperventilation. Mannitol: 20% mannitol (1 g/kg bodyweight) IV infusion over 30–60 min.
- **Stress ulcer prevention**: start IV PPI or RANITIDINE PO or IV.
- **Antibiotics:** low threshold to treat any infection. Bacterial and fungal. Impaired immunity.
- **Coagulopathy:** vitamin K 2–5 mg slow IV, 2–4 units FFP, platelets if <50 × 10^9/L and bleeding. Vitamin K replaces any deficit so any resulting coagulopathy is entirely due to reduced liver function.
- **Hepatic encephalopathy**: avoid the use of FFP unless actively bleeding. FFP renders the PTT (a vital prognostic marker) less useful; see *Section 15.8* for further management.
- **Ascites and spontaneous bacterial peritonitis**: see below for further management.
- **Acidosis**: take expert advice and consider IV $NaHCO_3$. A pH <7.3 at >24 h after paracetamol overdose is a poor prognostic indicator.
- **Consider** *N*-acetyl cysteine infusion where indicated.
- **Renal failure** may require haemofiltration or haemodialysis (see *Section 15.7*).

Criteria for considering Liver Unit admission (liaise before this)

- INR >3.0.
- Hepatic encephalopathy.
- Hypotension despite resuscitation.
- Metabolic acidosis.
- Prothrombin time (seconds) > time from overdose (hours).

Kings College criteria for liver transplant

Paracetamol-induced liver failure	Non-paracetamol-induced liver failure
• An arterial pH <7.3 at 24 h after ingestion	Prothrombin time >100 sec **or** 3 out of 5:
• A prothrombin time >100 sec	(1) drug induced
• Creatinine >300 µmol/L	(2) age <10 or >40
• Grade III or IV hepatic encephalopathy	(3) >1 week between jaundice and encephalopathy
	(4) prothrombin time >50 sec
	(5) bilirubin >300 µmol/L

15.2 Alcoholic hepatitis

About

- Acute liver dysfunction in known alcoholic. Poor prognosis.
- Discriminant function >32 implies >50% mortality at 1 month.

IV thiamine given empirically to prevent Wernicke–Korsakoff encephalopathy.

Causes

- Acute exacerbation in known alcohol abuser. Look out for spontaneous bacterial peritonitis.

Clinical

- Pyrexia, tachycardia, jaundice, encephalopathy, anorexia.
- Hepatomegaly (tender), abdominal discomfort, nausea, worsening ascites.

Aetiology

- Infiltration by polymorphonuclear leucocytes and hepatocyte necrosis in zone 3.
- Mallory bodies are found but are non-specific.

Investigations

- **FBC, U&E, LFT: raised** WCC, CRP, bilirubin, AST, ALT (limited to <500 U).
- **Abdominal USS:** hepatomegaly, coarse edge, increased echogenicity, free fluid.
- **Ascitic tap**: if spontaneous bacterial peritonitis suspected – neutrophil count >250 cells/mm^3.

Severity scorings to determine need for steroids

- **Discriminant function** (Maddrey score) = (4.6 × [prothrombin time – control PT]) + (serum bilirubin); >32 implies >50% mortality at 1 month.
- **Lille model:** (*Hepatology*, 2007;45:1348) www.lillemodel.com/score.asp.
- **Glasgow alcoholic hepatitis score:** a score >9 is associated with a poor prognosis.

Glasgow alcoholic hepatitis score

Score	1	2	3
Age	<50	>50	
WCC (× 10^9/L)	<15	>15	
Urea (nmol/L)	<5	>5	
Bilirubin (μmol/L)	<125	125–250	>250
INR	<1.5	1.5–2.0	>2.0

Poor prognosis = total score >9.

Management

- **Supportive management**. Avoiding and long-term abstinence from alcohol. Nutrition must be maintained with enteral feeding if required. Manage withdrawal, complications of portal hypertension, ascites, encephalopathy, variceal haemorrhage. Pabrinex IV × 2 + IV Vitamin K + Vitamin B PO + thiamine 200 mg PO OD. Chlordiazepoxide PO for DTs as needed.
- **Active treatment**: Maddrey Score >32 associated with a high short-term mortality is an indication to consider treatment. Choices are either **Prednisolone** 40 mg/d for 28 days or **Pentoxifylline** 400 mg tid for 28 days **which reduces** mortality in selected cases. Screen first and treat any sepsis.
- Early transplantation may be considered for patients with severe alcoholic hepatitis because it reduces mortality, though some will go back to alcohol.

Reference: European Association for the Study of the Liver (2010) EASL clinical practice guidelines on the management of ascites, spontaneous bacterial peritonitis, and hepatorenal syndrome in cirrhosis. *J Hepatol*, 533:97.

15.3 Alcoholic ketoacidosis

About

- Seen in those with severe alcoholic liver dysfunction + alcohol and/or starvation.

Causes

- Acute exacerbation in known alcohol abuser due to sepsis, starvation.
- Look out for spontaneous bacterial peritonitis.

Clinical

- Signs of advanced alcoholic liver disease, tachycardia, dehydration.
- Jaundice, alcoholic hepatitis, ascites, coagulopathy, encephalopathy.
- Anorexia, nausea, vomiting may be prominent. May follow 2–3 days after a binge.
- Ketones detectable in breath, Kussmaul's respiration.

Investigations

- **FBC, U&E, LFT**: low urea or AKI. Raised LFTs. Anaemia. Measure Mg, Ca, phosphate.
- **Glucose**: hypoglycaemia. **Urine:** ketones.
- **ABG:** raised anion gap metabolic acidosis with raised ketones (beta-hydroxybutyrate), but may be mixed picture with a combined metabolic alkalosis from vomiting.
- **Ascites:** test as may have SBP – always aspirate.

Management

- Supportive as for advanced alcoholic liver disease: IV fluids and IV dextrose and IV thiamine.
- Replace electrolytes and phosphate and magnesium as needed.

15.4 Alcohol abuse

- **About:** alcohol misuse is common. Take an alcohol history from all patients. Recommended target of 14 units/ week (females) and 21 units/ week (males). 1 unit = 8 g alcohol = small glass of wine or half pint of beer.
- **Aetiology:** alcohol is a colourless odourless liquid. Additives give the associated smell. CNS depressant and sudden withdrawal can cause hyper-excitability, delirium and seizures.
- **Screening for those at risk:** assess intake per week. What is told to the doctor is often an underestimate. Family estimate useful. Empty bottles per week. When is first drink taken – mornings, drinking all day or binging? Does person have responsibilities, e.g. to children, then it may become a social services issue of child safety and care. Is patient drink driving? What role does alcohol play in their life?

CAGE questionnaire is recommended

Alcohol problem very likely if 2 or more positive answers to the following:

- Have you felt you should CUT down on drinking?
- Have you been ANGERED by suggestions you cut down?
- Have you felt GUILTY about drinking?
- Have you used alcohol as an EYE opener in the morning?

Sudden acute alcohol withdrawal can lead to DTs 1–3 days later and is potentially lethal. Patients should be encouraged to gradually reduce their alcohol intake over time.

Clinical presentations of alcohol abuse

- **Alcoholic hepatitis**: jaundiced, toxic, unwell, elevated ALT.
- **Progressive liver failure:** jaundiced, coagulopathy, encephalopathy, ascites.
- **Delirium tremens**: agitated, fever, sweating, picking at bedclothes (now is the time to treat), hallucinations, e.g. rats, terrified – can progress to acute seizure.
- **Suicide:** often seen combined with alcohol abuse. High rate of suicide and needs psychiatric review.
- **Trauma:** involved in violent assaults, head injuries as well as road traffic accidents and simple falls.
- **Alcoholic cerebellar ataxia:** chronic cerebellar disease with ataxia.
- **Social:** spending one's life focused on obtaining and consuming alcohol leads to unemployment, divorce, homelessness, malnutrition, violence.
- **Cancer risk:** hepatoma, pancreatic cancer, various other cancers, e.g. of oesophagus.

Medical complications of alcoholism

- Head injury – falls, assaults, road traffic accidents, seizures, overdoses, suicidal attempts, self harm.
- Cerebral haemorrhage, hypothermia, meningitis and chest infections, cardiomyopathy.
- Ketoacidosis, pneumococcal infections, low potassium, magnesium and calcium.
- Renal failure, Wernicke's and Korsakov's psychosis and B1 deficiency.
- Variceal haemorrhage and liver disease, peptic ulcer disease.
- Peripheral neuropathy, cerebellar degeneration, atrial fibrillation.
- Social and family break up, poverty, violence.

15.5 Delirium tremens

About

- A cause of seizures and coma. Exclude subdural, meningitis, drugs.
- Best predictor is a past history of alcohol-related delirium tremens.

Aetiology

- Withdrawal symptoms 1–3 days after last drink. Mortality from DTs is about 15%.
- Alcohol is a central depressant. Withdrawal leads to a hyper-adrenergic state and seizures.
- Causes of death are respiratory failure, arrhythmias, and iatrogenic over-sedation.

Clinical

- Nausea, indigestion, coarse tremor and hyperactive delirium within 24 h.
- Fever, visual hallucinations and seizures occur after 24 h peaking at 50 h.
- Signs of advanced alcoholic liver disease, tachycardia, dehydration.
- Jaundice, alcoholic hepatitis, ascites, coagulopathy, encephalopathy.

Differential

- Opiate or cocaine use, hypoglycaemia, head injury (SDH/stroke/skull fracture).
- Sepsis, hepatic encephalopathy, psychotic illness.
- Encephalitis, non-convulsive status.

Investigations

- **FBC, U&E and LFT, CRP**: exclude infection and liver failure.
- **CXR**: exclude tumour, infection, TB, aspiration, perforation.

- **Sepsis screen:** chest, urine, aspirate ascites to exclude spontaneous bacterial peritonitis.
- **ECG**: exclude MI, AF. Coagulation screen if possible liver failure.
- **CT head**: if concerned about head injury or stroke or sub-dural haematoma, or some other pathology. Have a low threshold to scan if concerned.
- **LP** if suspected meningitis (pneumococcal seen in alcoholics).

Management

- **Supportive:** manage in a well-lit and friendly area, involve family or known trusted carers to reduce anxiety. Again, if significant sedation is needed and GCS and airway issues become an issue then patient is best on a HDU/ITU environment. Watch for low glucose, Mg and K and dehydration and treat accordingly.
- **Agitated confused patient**: start **a reducing dose regimen** of chlordiazepoxide or other benzodiazepine. When was last drink? Fits tend to classically occur about 48–96 h later. Titrate the dose to the level of agitation.
- **Seizure**: manage alcohol withdrawal seizures as you would status epilepticus. If patient becomes very drowsy watch GCS and ABCs and take advice on airways management if GCS <9. Have a low threshold to CT head if any concerns about other diagnosis, e.g. meningitis, haemorrhage and hepatic encephalopathy. In the case that you are unable to convince the patient to take medications then IM/IV LORAZEPAM 1–4 mg could be considered. The key is to identify and sedate patients likely to 'go off' early when they are compliant and to prevent seizures. Consider the fixed dose schedule below which should be started as soon as any hyperactive features appear or in a patient with previous DTs and now off alcohol. Watch for over-sedation. Consider HDU/ITU.
- Give **IV thiamine** or with other nutrients as Pabrinex. Risk of Wernicke–Korsakov syndrome if not treated. Or thiamine 200 mg PO OD + multivitamins one tab OD.
- **Prophylactic anticonvulsants:** no real evidence base but some may consider temporarily in high risk patients.

Fixed dose schedule: (consider higher doses in very agitated and those with high body weight; watch for over-sedation):

- Day 1–2: Chlordiazepoxide 10–30 mg 6 hourly.
- Day 3–4: Chlordiazepoxide 10 mg 8 hourly.
- Day 5–6: Chlordiazepoxide 10 mg 12 hourly and stop.

15.6 Ascites and liver disease

About

- Liver dysfunction with ascites. 15% inpatients with ascites.
- Spontaneous bacterial peritonitis (SBP) develops in 25% of patients within 1 year.

Clinical

- Symptoms and signs are frequently absent in patients with SBP.
- May be mild to severe abdominal pain, ascites and generalised tenderness and signs of liver disease.

Investigations

- **FBC, U&E, LFT:** anaemia, AKI, **raised** AST, ALT, alpha-fetoprotein.
- **Liver USS:** liver size, coarse edge, increased echogenicity, free fluid throughout abdomen.
- **Serum/ascites albumin gradient:** >11 g/L suggests aetiology is portal hypertension.

- **Aspirate of ascites**: a 10 ml aspirate should be taken on all patients with ascites to exclude SBP: **raised** WCC and CRP. Aspirate neutrophil count >250 cells/mm^3 and low pH of ascitic fluid. Gram stain and culture. Measure ascitic protein because SBP more common with ascitic albumin <15 g/L and may need antibiotic prophylaxis.

Cirrhotic patients with low ascitic fluid protein concentration (<10–15 g/L) and/or high serum bilirubin levels are at high risk of SBP so consider prophylactic antibiotics.

Management

- **Sodium restriction:** moderate restriction of salt intake to sodium of 80–120 mmol/day, which corresponds to 4.6–6.9 g of salt/day. No added salt diet with avoidance of pre-prepared meals.
- **Ascites:** dietary salt restriction to 90 mmol/day (5.2 g). Lowers diuretic requirement and increases resolution of ascites and shorter hospital stay.
- **Spironolactone**: start at 100 mg OD. There is a 3–5 day lag before natriuresis (urine Na > K) then add a loop diuretic (Furosemide 40–160 mg/d). If Na >126 mmol/L, no need for H_2O restriction and continue diuretics if renal function stable. If Na <125 mmol/L consider stopping diuretics, especially if Na <121 mmol/L if creatinine rising (>150 µmol/L), volume expansion maintaining renal function is crucial. The maximum recommended weight loss during diuretic therapy should be 0.5 kg/day in patients without oedema and 1 kg/day in patients with oedema.
- **Large volume paracentesis:** recommended with large ascites. **Give 8 g albumin** IV per litre removed. Failure to volume expand risks circulatory dysfunction + renal failure. Albumin better than artificial plasma expanders. Ascites recurs in 90% of patients if diuretics not begun and in 20% despite diuretics. Do NOT leave drain *in situ* overnight.
- **Antibiotics**: a diagnosis of SBP should initiate IV antibiotics. Consider IV augmentin, 3rd generation cephalosporins or quinolones such as ciprofloxacin. Resolution is seen in 90%. Those who survive an episode of SBP should be considered for liver transplantation.
- **Transjugular intrahepatic portosystemic shunt** (TIPS) for refractory ascites. 25% risk encephalopathy. Can cause heart failure.

References:

European Association for the Study of the Liver (2010) EASL clinical practice guidelines on the management of ascites, spontaneous bacterial peritonitis, and hepatorenal syndrome in cirrhosis. *J Hepatol*, 533:97.

Wiest *et al.* (2012) Spontaneous bacterial peritonitis: recent guidelines and beyond. *Gut*, 61:297.

15.7 Hepatorenal syndrome

About

- AKI in patient with advanced and severe liver disease – presents with oliguria.

Aetiology

- HRS represents the end-stage of a sequence of reductions in renal perfusion.
- There is severe afferent renal vasoconstriction with normal kidneys.
- Exclude prerenal hypovolaemia by a trial of volume expansion.

With hepatorenal syndrome – renal failure is usually irreversible unless liver transplantation is performed.

Causes

- 40% of patients with cirrhosis and ascites develop HRS during the natural history of their disease.
- Shock, sepsis, ATN, pre-renal disease, nephrotoxic drugs, renal obstruction or parenchymal renal disease.
- Exclude SBP complicated by AKI which may be reversible in 30% of cases.

Risk factors

- Low mean arterial blood pressure (<80 mmHg).
- Dilutional hyponatraemia.
- Urinary sodium retention (urine sodium <5 mmol/L).

Differential to exclude

- Hypovolaemia and shock, nephrotoxic drugs.
- Parenchymal renal disease (proteinuria/haematuria, abnormal renal USS).

Classification

- **Type 1**: rapid progressive renal impairment often precipitated by spontaneous bacterial peritonitis (25% of patients) characterized by diuretic-resistant ascites. Most die within 10 weeks.
- **Type 2**: moderate and stable reduction in the GFR median survival of 3–6 months.

Criteria for diagnosis of hepatorenal syndrome in cirrhosis

- Cirrhosis with ascites.
- Serum creatinine >130 μmol/L.
- Absence of shock and hypovolaemia as defined by no sustained improvement of renal function (creatinine decreasing to <130 μmol/L) following at least 2 days of diuretic withdrawal (if on diuretics), and volume expansion with albumin at 1 g/kg/day up to a maximum of 100 g/day.
- No current or recent treatment with nephrotoxic drugs.
- Absence of parenchymal renal disease as defined by proteinuria <0.5 g/day, no microhaematuria (<50 red cells/high powered field), and normal renal ultrasonography.

Clinical

- Fatigue, malaise, progressive uraemia with oliguria without significant proteinuria.
- Chronic liver disease, ascites, jaundice, encephalopathy.

Investigations

- **FBC, U&E, LFTS, PT:** creatinine >130 μmol/L.
- **Urine protein:** proteinuria <500 mg/d. **Renal USS:** normal.

Management

- Exclude other causes of AKI by volume expansion with IV albumin for at least 2 d and withdrawal of diuretics and other nephrotoxic drugs. These patients need specialist care.
- **IV TERLIPRESSIN** (IV 1–2 g qds) and human albumin solution (40 g/day) is safe and effective.
- **Low-dose dopamine** (2–5 mcg/kg/min) but no evidence base exists.
- **Liver transplantation** is usually needed in most cases of Type 1 and 2 HRS.

References:

European Association for the Study of the Liver (2010) EASL clinical practice guidelines on the management of ascites, spontaneous bacterial peritonitis, and hepatorenal syndrome in cirrhosis. *J Hepatol*, 533:97.

Ginès & Schrier (2009) Renal failure in cirrhosis. *N Engl J Med,* 361:1279.

15.8 Hepatic encephalopathy

About

- Spectrum of potentially reversible neuropsychiatric abnormalities in patients with liver dysfunction.
- Exclude unrelated neurologic and/or metabolic abnormalities.

Aetiology

- Associated with arterial NH_4 levels and other protein breakdown products crossing blood–brain barrier.

Grades of encephalopathy

- Stage I: personality/mood changes, anxiety, mild confusion, altered sleep/wake cycles, apathy, asterixis.
- Stage II: moderate confusion, disorientation, rigidity, asterixis.
- Stage III: severe confusion, somnolence, incontinence; Babinski's sign, asterixis.
- Stage IV: coma, decerebrate posturing.

Identify likely precipitants

- Sepsis, spontaneous bacterial peritonitis, fluid overload, albumin.
- Transjugular intrahepatic porto-systemic shunt, renal failure, CNS suppressants.
- Electrolyte abnormalities, diuretic overuse, GI bleeding.

Clinical

- Reversal of day/night sleeping, psychomotor dysfunction, impaired memory.
- Sensory abnormalities, poor concentration, disorientation, tremor, shuffling gait.
- Melena, haematemesis. Fetor hepaticus, flapping tremor, asterixis.

Investigations

- **FBC, U&E, and LFT**: raised WCC, AST/ALT, PT, blood ammonia level.
- **CT head** rules out acute bleeding.
- **Diagnostic ascitic tap** for spontaneous bacterial peritonitis.
- **EEG:** symmetrical slowing with characteristic (but nonspecific) triphasic waves.
- **Others**: exclude hypoxia, hypercarbia, uraemia, hypoglycaemia.
- **Ascitic tap**: exclude spontaneous bacterial peritonitis.

Management

- **Supportive**: manage dietary input including adequate protein. Avoid sedatives and other drugs.
- **Treat cause,** e.g. antibiotics, bleeding, fluids, alcohol, SBP.
- **Avoid constipation**: lactulose 20–50 ml BD and/or phosphate enemas to open bowels twice daily.
- **Rifaximin** (similar to rifampin) – a minimally absorbed broad spectrum antimicrobial which concentrates in GI tract and reduces ammonia-producing enteric bacteria. Rifaximin for 6 months maintained remission from hepatic encephalopathy more effectively than did placebo. Rifaximin treatment also significantly reduced hospitalisation. **Metronidazole** is also useful. Avoid neomycin.

- **Ornithine aspartase**: effective in treating hepatic encephalopathy in a number of European trials.

References:

Bass *et al*. (2010) Rifaximin treatment in hepatic encephalopathy. *N Engl J Med*, 362:1071.

Ginès & Schrier (2009) Renal failure in cirrhosis. *N Engl J Med*, 361:1279.

15.9 Acute fatty liver of pregnancy

About

- Serious complication of the end of pregnancy that needs recognition.
- 1 in 20 000, case fatality 1.8%. Mostly near term or early postpartum.

Pathophysiology

- Microvesicular steatosis in the liver due to impaired metabolism of fatty acids.
- Increased incidence in those with long-chain 3-hydroxyacyl-coenzyme A dehydrogenase (LCHAD) deficiency. The mother is heterozygote.
- Fetus may be homozygous and unable to oxidize fatty acids which are passed to the mother. This can lead to AFLP and so delivery is beneficial to mother.

Clinical

- Last trimester of pregnancy with jaundice, malaise, abdominal pain, nausea and upper GI bleed.
- AKI can develop with oliguria, uraemia, hypoglycaemic episodes.
- Fulminant liver failure – jaundice, encephalopathy, coagulopathy.
- Pancreatitis: abdominal pain into back can develop postpartum.

Differential

- HELLP syndrome, viral hepatitis, drug/toxin induced hepatitis.

Diagnostic criteria: in absence of other diagnosis – need >5 of:

- Vomiting, abdominal pain, encephalopathy, bilirubin >14, glucose <4 mmol/L.
- Urate >340, WCC >11, ascites / bright liver US, AST/ALT >42.
- Creatinine >150 µmol/L, PT >14 s, microvesicular steatosis on biopsy.

Investigations

- **FBC, U&E, LFT:** anaemia, AKI, raised urate.
- **LFT:** conjugated hyperbilirubinaemia, elevated AST and ALT, raised PT.
- **Clotting**: look for DIC: raised PT, low fibrinogen and antithrombin levels.
- **Amylase** increased if pancreas inflamed.
- **USS/CT abdomen**: USS may be normal or show increased echogenicity. Biopsy usually not done due to coagulopathy.
- **Hepatitis screen**: usual screen for hepatitis viral serology and other differentials.

Management

- Delivery of the fetus irrespective of gestational age within 24 h of diagnosis by induction or caesarean section. Ensure correction of coagulopathy.
- Patients may develop fulminant hepatic failure and management is detailed elsewhere.
- Plasma exchange seems to help. Prognosis for those who survive is usually excellent.

15.10 HELLP syndrome

About

- HELLP: **h**aemolysis, **e**levated **L**FTs, **l**ow **p**latelets. Part of the severe preeclampsia spectrum.
- Rarely can occur without hypertension and proteinuria.

> Unlike acute fatty liver of pregnancy liver function is normal.

Definition

- PET findings: BP >140/90 mmHg + proteinuria + 20+ weeks.
- Haemolysis, elevated LFTs, low platelets.

Clinical

- Patient is often well, hypertension may not be present.
- Epigastric pain, nausea, vomiting, jaundice. NO liver failure.
- Eclampsia can develop with seizures or coma.

Investigations

- **FBC:** low Hb, platelets <100 × 10^9/L, WCC normal. **LDH** >600 U/L (haemolysis).
- **LFT**: raised AST and GGT. **Liver USS** normal. **Urate** normal. **PT** normal.
- **Proteinuria** >300 mg/24 h. Urine dipstick >1+.

Management

- Vaginal delivery is indicated if >34th gestational week or the fetal and/or maternal conditions deteriorate.
- Higher maternal and perinatal morbidity and mortality rates.

15.11 Obstetric cholestasis

About

- Increased risk of spontaneous preterm birth, iatrogenic preterm birth and fetal death.
- Affects 1.5% of women of Asian (India and Pakistan) origin.

Pathophysiology

- Genetic and environmental factors, varies between populations worldwide.

Clinical

- Severe pruritus in the absence of a skin rash often worse at night.
- Pruritus that involves the palms and soles of the feet is particularly suggestive.
- Can lead to severe sleep deprivation.

Investigations

- **FBC, U&E, LFT: raised** AST, ALT, GGT 100–300, bilirubin and PT (occasionally).
- **ALP** × 4 (small rise normal in pregnancy – placental).
- **Liver ultrasound**: screen for other causes of liver disease.

Management

- Monitor LFTs every 1–2 weeks. If rapid escalation consider other diagnosis.
- Postnatal resolution of pruritus and abnormal LFTs should be confirmed.
- Consider induction of labour after 37 weeks of gestation.
- Skin – topical emollients are safe but their efficacy is unknown.
- Ursodeoxycholic acid (UDCA) improves pruritus and liver function.
- If PT prolonged then vitamin K (menadiol sodium phosphate) is indicated.

16 Haematological emergencies

16.1 Heparin-induced thrombocytopenia

About

- Heparin-induced thrombocytopenia (HIT) + thrombosis (HITT).
- Thrombocytopenia due to heparin which induces the formation of antibodies.
- Seen when a person on heparin develops a thrombosis with a fall in platelets.

Types

- Type I HIT is a relatively common, non-immune, clinically innocuous and benign reaction.
- Type II HIT is a rare, immune-mediated, potentially serious form of the disease.

Aetiology

- Propensity to form platelet-rich thrombosis 5–10 days after initiation of heparin therapy. The target antigen is a complex between **heparin and Platelet Factor 4**.
- HIT is commoner with unfractionated heparin (UFH) and very unusual with LMWH. HIT is caused by heparin-dependent IgG that activates platelets via their FcIIa receptors.

Clinical

- Arterial thrombosis: limb, stroke, MI, PE, renal artery, mesenteric arteries.
- Skin necrosis often at injection sites.
- Adrenal failure due to vein thrombosis and haemorrhagic necrosis.
- Combined DVT and HIT can cause venous limb gangrene. Seen day 10 post-UFH.

Consider HIT in any patient with a drop in platelets and heparin started within past 5–10 days.

Investigations

- **FBC and U&E**: platelet count <150 000 × 10^9/L or a decrease in the platelet count of 30–50% after the initiation of heparin therapy (the platelet count may still be within normal limits).
- **Peripheral blood smear:** examination shows frequent fragmented red blood cells.
- **Heparin-dependent platelet antibodies:** can be detected by platelet activation tests (platelet aggregation studies, serotonin release assay) or specific assays for antibodies to the heparin–PF4 complex (ELISA, flow cytometry).

Management

- All heparins (*UFH and LMWH and heparin line flushes*) must be discontinued immediately in patients strongly suspected to have HIT. Urgent haematology advice should be sought.
- Therapeutic doses of a non-heparin agent, e.g. fondaparinux or Hirudin can be considered but take expert haematology advice depending on what agents are available and suitable for the indication.
- Patient may be warfarinised but needs additional anticoagulation in interim whilst loading as it is a prothrombotic state (Protein C levels fall).

16.2 Disseminated intravascular coagulation

About

- Seen in 1% of inpatients. Uncontrolled microvascular clotting consumes platelets and clotting factors.
- Coagulopathy leads to massive haemorrhage, organ failure. Dreadful prognosis.

Aetiology

- Endothelial disruption and other initiators lead to a procoagulant state.
- Formation of microvascular thrombi consumes clotting factors, fibrinogen and platelets.
- Microthrombi can cause organ dysfunction. Bleeding due to coagulopathy.
- In malignancy DIC can be a more chronic process over weeks and months.

Clinical

- Severe spontaneous bleeding and bruising in an unwell patient.
- Haemorrhagic shock due to bleeding from lines, GI tract, genitourinary tract, epistaxis.
- Spontaneous intracerebral haemorrhage, post-operative wound bleed.
- Bleeding may be hidden, e.g. retroperitoneal, psoas.

Causes

- Trauma and tissue damage, sepsis and septicaemic shock (Gram negative).
- Malignancy, acute promyelocytic leukaemia / M3, massive transfusions.
- Obstetric emergencies (placental abruption, amniotic fluid embolism, eclampsia).
- Pancreatitis, vascular abnormalities, snake bites, recreational drugs.
- ABO transfusion incompatibility, transplant rejection, severe liver failure.

Differential

- Acute liver failure, HUS, HITT, thrombocytopenic purpura.

Investigations (*markers of severity)

- **FBC, blood film:** anaemia, low platelets, fragmented red cells.
- **U&E**: AKI, raised LDH and evidence of haemolysis.
- **Coagulation screen**: raised PT* (>+6 s) and APTT and TT all prolonged, low fibrinogen* (<1 g/L) and platelets* (50×10^9/L). Elevated FDPs* due to fibrinolysis (high).

Differential

- TTP and HUS, severe malignant hypertension.
- **Pregnancy**: pre-eclampsia, HELLP syndrome.
- Microangiopathic haemolytic anaemia.

Management

- **Supportive care**: admit ITU. Needs close observation, testing and management. IV fluids. Care with invasive monitoring as coagulopathy. Underlying condition is main focus. Find and treat the underlying cause. Early involvement of a haematologist.
- **Clotting factors**: give Vitamin K slow IV 10 mg stat. Replacement of clotting factors FFP, cryoprecipitate, platelets and red cell concentrates based on bleeding risk more than laboratory results. Give cryoprecipitate if fibrinogen is low. If there is a prolonged PT and APTT then consider FFP if high risk of bleed or procedure or active bleeding. If fibrinogen low (<1 g/L) despite FFP replacement consider fibrinogen concentrate or cryoprecipitate.

- **Platelets**: generally platelet half-life is short and platelets only given for acute bleeding when less than 50×10^9/L, or the need for a procedure and less than 50×10^9/L. If not bleeding and platelets low, consider transfusing when bleed risk high, e.g. platelets $10–20 \times 10^9$/L. Take advice if unsure.
- **Treatment targets**: platelets $>50 \times 10^9$/L, fibrinogen >1 g/L, Hb >80 g/L, PT and APTT $< \times 1.5$ normal.
- **IV HEPARIN**: may rarely be used to reduce the clotting. Indications include arterial or venous thromboembolism, severe purpura fulminans with acral ischaemia or vascular skin infarction. It should possibly not be stopped if patient already on it.
- **Avoid IV Tranexamic acid** except where there is severe bleeding and a hyperfibrinolytic state. One can augment mouth care with tranexamic acid solution as a mouthwash (1 g orally four times daily) which can help reduce oozing from friable oral mucosa.

Reference: British Committee for Standards in Haematology (2009) Guidelines for the diagnosis and management of disseminated intravascular coagulation. *Br J Haematol*, 145:24.

16.3 Sickle cell crisis

About

- Sickle cell disease causes a chronic haemolytic anaemia.
- Commonest in black patients but may also affect other groups.
- Homozygous inheritance of HbSS or HbSC.
- Most painful crises are managed at home.

Aetiology

- HbSS contains 2 defective β-globin chains due to a Valine to Glutamate substitution on the β6 position. Leads to a structural change and HbS polymerisation and sickling at low O_2 tensions.
- HbAS: no symptoms unless extreme hypoxia (sickle cell trait).

Acute crises seen with

- HbSS: (sickle cell anaemia) HbSS who only have HbS.
- HbSC: HbS from one parent and HbC from the other.
- HbS–β0: sickle cell + β-thalassaemia.

Clinical

- Crises triggered by infections and other illness or hypoxia.
- Usually severe chest/bone/back/limb/abdominal pain and anaemia.
- Anaemia from shortened RBC half-life needs transfusion but iron overload.

Complications

- Haemolytic anaemia, aplastic crises, lung fibrosis, stroke, hepatosplenomegaly.
- *Salmonella* osteomyelitis, sickling crisis, avascular necrosis of the hips, HiB infection.
- Renal failure, renal concentrating defects, renal papillary necrosis.
- Priapism – sequestration of red cells in corpus cavernosum.
- Acute chest syndrome due to pneumococcal pneumonia, lung infarction or fat embolism, bleeding in anterior chamber of eye (hyphaema).
- Osteoporosis – vertebral collapse, avascular necrosis of femoral head or dactylitis or swollen joints, skin ulcers, pigment gallstones, splenic infarction – autosplenectomy.

Investigations

- **FBC**: severe anaemia, low Hb, raised reticulocytes.
- **Blood films**: sickle cells, target cells, polychromasia.
- **Sickle solubility test**: positive in both sickle cell disease and trait.
- **Hb electrophoresis** confirms diagnosis.
- **CXR and ABG and ECG** and cardiac troponin if breathless or chest pain.
- **Cross-match** if symptoms severe and transfusion needed. Close matching of blood is needed beyond simple ABO and rhesus groups to reduce antibody formation.

Acute management

- **Supportive:** HR, BP, O_2 sats, respiratory rate, temperature. Most patients can drink freely but if any difficulties or nausea or vomiting then IV fluids will maintain hydration. Oxygen as per BTS guidelines.
- **Analgesia:** pain is almost always the dominating symptom and pain control the reason for admission. Mild pains try PARACETAMOL 1 g and IBUPROFEN 400 mg. If severe pains then add analgesia, usually **IV MORPHINE 5–10 mg (0.1 mg/kg) repeated until pain free**. Consider continuous infusion pump or patient controlled anaesthesia. Add LAXATIVE. Offer analgesia within 30 min of presentation with an acute painful sickle cell episode. Avoid pethidine.
- **Acute chest syndrome:** consider if chest pain, cough, fever, CXR infiltrates (may appear late), hypoxia. Due to fat embolism to lungs or infection. Give O_2 as per BTS guidance. Consider for ITU admission and ventilation if cannot keep PO_2 >8 kPa despite an FiO_2 of 0.6. Consider a trial of CPAP if hypoxic, but be prepared for intubation and ventilation. Take haematology and ITU help early.
- **Infection:** look for and treat any infection with IV/PO antibiotics as per local policy. 3rd generation cephalosporin/macrolide (cefotaxime/clarithromycin) combination. SALBUTAMOL nebuliser if wheeze.
- **Exchange blood transfusion** (6 units in and 6 units out) if remains hypoxic.
- **Priapism:** urgent urology referral.
- **LMWH:** VTE prophylaxis may reduce the length of stay of patients with an acute painful sickle cell episode.
- **Long-term:** haematology follow-up. Consider **Hydroxyurea:** raise HbF which decreases crises.
- **Bone marrow transplantation**. Screen at-risk patients before surgery/pregnancy.
- **Pregnancy**: acute management is the same and transfuse to reduce proportion of HbS and so sickling crises. Liaise with obstetric team.

Reference: NICE (2012) Sickle cell acute painful episode: management of an acute painful sickle cell episode in hospital. CG143.

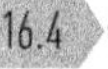

16.4 Haemolytic uraemic syndrome

About

- Seen in children with diarrhoeal illness and AKI but may be seen in adults.
- There is an intravascular haemolysis and a microangiopathic haemolytic anaemia.

Unlike DIC the coagulation tests are normal in those with HUS/TTP.

Aetiology

- Children: AKI due to verocytotoxin-producing *E. coli*, e.g. *E. coli* strain 0157: H7.60.
- Adults: drugs that damage endothelial cells.

- Familial (congenital) HUS – deficiency of factor H a plasma protein synthesised by the liver, which regulates the complement pathway.

Pathophysiology

- Toxin causes endothelial cell damage and renal microvascular thrombosis.
- Platelet aggregation results in a consumptive thrombocytopenia.
- Microangiopathic haemolytic anaemia – RBCs circulating through partially occluded microcirculation.

Classification of HAEMOLYTIC URAEMIC SYNDROME

	(D+) HUS involves diarrhoea	(D–) Atypical HUS form – no diarrhoea
Phenotype	Mainly children	All ages with significant co-morbidities
ADAMTS13 levels	Normal	Low
Causes	*E. coli* strain 0157: H7. Produces a verocytotoxin (shiga toxin) with A and B units. New strain *E. coli* 0104:H4 with high rate of complications. Toxins damage endothelium.	Usually due to a defect in complement levels. Mitomycin C, ticlopidine, cyclosporine, tacrolimus, QUININE, combination chemotherapy, radiotherapy, congenital, malignancies – prostate, gastric, pancreatic, scleroderma, antiphospholipid syndrome. *Strep. pneumoniae* can cause a rare form of atypical HUS.
	Infective cause as 95% of cases of HUS in children and infants.	Can be both familial and sporadic. Several genes have been associated. Seen at all ages.
Management	Paediatric renal service. Daily plasma exchange is sometimes tried but without evidence. Avoid antibiotics or antimotility agents. Complete recovery possible.	Plasmapheresis, supportive, renal replacement, **Eculizumab (Soliris).** Poorer prognosis. Liver transplantation for congenital anomalies in complement. In post *Strep. pneumoniae* avoid plasma infusion or plasmapheresis.

Clinical

- D+ patients: gastroenteritis and bloody diarrhoea usually in children.
- D– patients: underlying illness, drugs and co-morbidities.
- Red/brown urine, petechial rash, malaise, hypertension, uraemia.
- Jaundice, easy bruising and pallor from anaemia.

Investigation

- **FBC:** Hb <8 g/dL, low platelets. **U&E, LFT:** AKI, raised bilirubin (haemolysis).
- **Blood film**: schistocytes, fragmented, deformed, irregular, or helmet-shaped RBCs.
- Others: intravascular haemolysis, raised LDH and reticulocytes, low haptoglobin.
- **Coagulation:** normal PT, APTT, D-dimer and fibrinogen levels.
- **Coomb's test** results are negative.

- **Stool samples:** will be cultured for *E. coli* 0157: H7 and *E. coli* O104:H4.
- **Kidney biopsy** may be indicated to see degree and nature of kidney damage.
- **ADAMTS13** levels normal in D+ve disease.

Management
- Transfer to specialist (paediatric) nephrology unit or ITU. Avoid antibiotics or antimotility agents because they have been shown to worsen severity. Avoid platelet transfusions.
- Renal failure often requires dialysis in 50% of patients. However, 85% can go on to make a full recovery. Supportive management of hypertension, anaemia.
- **Daily plasma exchange** (plasmapheresis combined with FFP replacement) is treatment of choice. **Other agents:** unresponsive cases have been treated with **Vincristine or Ciclosporin A.** No role for steroids.
- **Appropriate supportive care**, affected children often recover completely. Irreversible renal damage and death can occur in more severe cases.

Prognosis in D− patients
- When seen in adults prognosis is usually poorer because there is an underlying cause, however, a new medication is available: **Eculizumab (Soliris)** binds to the terminal complement component 5, C5. It has been approved by the US FDA (September, 2011) for adults and children with **atypical haemolytic uremic syndrome (aHUS).** Approval was based on data from adults and children who were resistant or intolerant to, or receiving, long-term plasma exchange/infusion.
- **Eculizumab** demonstrated significant improvement in platelet count. Thrombotic microangiopathy events were reduced, and maintained or improved kidney function was also reported. Its use in the UK has been limited due to cost. See table above for more information.

Reference: Kavanagh & Goodship (2011) Atypical hemolytic uremic syndrome, genetic basis, and clinical manifestations. *ASH Education Book*, 2011:15.

16.5 Thrombotic thrombocytopenic purpura

About
- Activation and consumption of platelets, vessel occlusion, microangiopathic anaemia.

ADAMTS13 is a protease that breaks up large molecules of von Willebrand factor.

Aetiology
- Inhibition or lack of ADAMTS13 increases platelet adhesion to endothelium by vWF.
- This causes thrombosis and platelet consumption.

Causes
- Inherited deficiency, acquired secondary to antibodies to ADAMTS13.
- Ticlopidine, clopidogrel, ciclosporin, OCP, pregnancy, SLE, HIV, hepatitis.

Pathophysiology
- Platelet activation causes cerebral renal/gut microvascular thrombosis.
- Activation of coagulation cascade: increased platelet aggregation results in a consumptive thrombocytopenia. RBCs damaged passing through partially occluded microcirculation.

Differential

- DIC: there is a coagulopathy but not in TTP/HUS

Clinical

- Anaemia, fever. Thrombosis: phlebitis with superficial vein thrombosis.
- Thrombotic stroke, delirium, coma, cardiac/gut/renal ischaemia/infarction.
- Bleeding, e.g. mucosal, petechiae, purpura and bruising may be seen.

Investigation

- **FBC**: Hb <8 g/dL, low platelets.
- **Clotting screen**: normal PT, APTT, D-dimer, fibrinogen levels.
- **Blood film**: schistocytes. Fragmented, deformed, irregular, or helmet-shaped RBCs.
- **Intravascular haemolysis** elevated LDH, reticulocytes, bilirubin, and low haptoglobin.
- **U&E:** AKI. **Kidney biopsy** may be indicated to see degree and nature of kidney damage.
- **ADAMTS13 levels** low but wide variation of normal so unhelpful diagnostically.
- **Renal CT/MRI** may show areas of infarction.

Management

- **High volume total plasma exchange:** (plasmapheresis), which reduces 3 month mortality from 90% to almost 15%. This removes circulating antibody and increases ADAMTS13.
- Treat early even with moderate suspicion. Risks of treatment far outweighed by potential benefits. Replace total plasma volume daily (some replace 1.5 × plasma volume), e.g. 20–30 units of FFP given per session. Hypotension seen especially in those on ACE inhibitors.
- Platelets are generally contraindicated. Thrombosis is more a problem than bleeding so platelets generally not given and can even lead to thrombotic episodes. Take specialist haematological advice if active bleeding and low platelets.
- Supportive management and may need transfer to specialist centre. Watch daily bloods for response. Relapses may require steroids, rituximab or other immunosuppressive agents and splenectomy.
- Red cells given as needed for anaemia. Give folate 5 mg OD. Low dose aspirin 75 mg OD started once platelets $>50 \times 10^9$/L.

16.6 Severe thrombocytopenia

About

- Thrombocytopenia is platelet count $<150 \times 10^9$/L.
- Severe bleeding if count $<20–50 \times 10^9$/L, worsened by antiplatelets.

Pathophysiology

- Platelets survive 7–10 days. 35% of all platelets are found in the spleen.
- Reaction to vessel wall injury is rapid adhesion of platelets to the subendothelium and formation of a haemostatic plug, composed primarily of platelets.
- This is further stabilised by a fibrin mesh generated in secondary haemostasis.
- Significant quantitative or qualitative platelet dysfunction results in mucocutaneous bleeding.
- Platelet count $<20 \times 10^9$/L can be associated with severe bleeding.

Aetiology

- Platelets formed from developing megakaryocytes in the bone marrow.
- Low platelets can be due to a fall in production or raised consumption or sequestration.
- Platelet dysfunction with antiplatelets, drugs and diseases, e.g. uraemia.

Cause of thrombocytopenia	Notes
Sampling error	Platelet clumping can lead to a spuriously low platelet count. Repeat sample if any doubt. It is evident on a peripheral smear by the presence of platelet clumps.
Acute idiopathic thrombocytopenic purpura (ITP)	Seen in all ages. Immune mediated destruction of platelets usually to the platelet GP IIb/IIIa complex. May be postviral or drug induced. Rarely SLE or HIV. Treat with steroids (prednisolone 1 mg/kg) or other immunosuppression and IVIg and splenectomy if severe and persisting. Avoid giving platelets if possible. Note that ITP in pregnancy can lead to fetal thrombocytopenia with bleeding complications such as neonatal intracranial haemorrhage. Other newer agents include Danazol, Eltrombopag, Rituximab, Romiplostim.
Drug induced	Identify and stop drug. Pay great attention to drug history and simple over the counter medications. Quinine.
Chronic ITP	Adults with on-going thrombocytopenia. Insidious onset. Smear shows giant platelets.
Heparin induced thrombocytopenic purpura (HIT/T)	Patient is on UFH or LMWH and develops thrombocytopenia and thrombosis. Stop all heparins. See *Section 16.1*. Confirmed by *in vitro* testing to detect **heparin-dependent platelet antibodies.**
HUS/TTP	See *Sections 16.4* and *16.5*. Neurological involvement, renal failure and diarrhoea.
Pregnancy-related thrombocytopenia	Usually mild thrombocytopenia in an otherwise healthy pregnancy. May resemble a mild ITP. Infant does not develop thrombocytopenia.
Pre-eclampsia/ eclampsia syndrome	Causes increased platelet turnover, even when the platelet count is normal. Controlling BP and delivering the fetus leads to restoration of the platelet count.
HELLP syndrome	Sometimes thrombocytopenia is associated with haemolysis and raised liver enzymes and low platelet (HELLP) syndrome. Treat BP and deliver fetus.
Post-transfusion purpura	Typically occurs 10 days following a transfusion.
Disseminated intravascular coagulation	Pathological thrombin generation. There is consumption of platelets with thrombosis and bleeding. Seen in those with other overwhelming pathology.
Drug-induced thrombocytopenia	Drugs such as gold, ibuprofen, quinine, quinidine, methotrexate, amiodarone, valproate, cimetidine, captopril, carbamazepine, sulfonamides, glibenclamide, tamoxifen, ranitidine, phenytoin, vancomycin, piperacillin, cocaine.

Cause of thrombocytopenia	Notes
Bone marrow failure	Malignancy, infiltration, myelodysplasia, marrow failure.
Severe fever with thrombocytopenia syndrome	Serious infectious disease with a 12% case-fatality rate that has been documented in northeast and central China due to a novel bunyavirus.
Dengue fever, HIV	From endemic area or in risk groups. HIV test, CD4 count, viral load.
SLE	Check ANA dsDNA.
Hypersplenism	Thrombocytopenia rarely below 40×10^9/L.
Platelet dysfunction	Platelet numbers normal. Aspirin, clopidogrel, uraemia, etc. all prolong bleeding time.

Clinical

- Spontaneous petechiae, purpura, bleeding.
- Mouth may show evidence of bleeding. Check drug chart.
- Look for splenomegaly and lymph nodes, which may suggest a cause.
- Menorrhagia, epistaxis, haematuria.

Investigation

- **FBC:** Hb – anaemia, low platelets. If bleeding and platelets $>40 \times 10^9$/L look for exacerbating cause.
- **U&E:** AKI, check B12, folate, ferritin.
- **Blood film:** schistocytes, fragmented, deformed, irregular, or helmet-shaped RBCs suggests DIC.
- **Intravascular haemolysis:** raised LDH, reticulocytes, bilirubin, low haptoglobin, Coomb's test negative. Acute kidney injury (HUS/TTP or uraemic platelet dysfunction).
- **Coagulation:** normal PT, APTT, D-dimer and fibrinogen levels. Increased bleeding time.
- **Renal biopsy** if HUS may be indicated to see degree and nature of kidney damage.
- **ADAMTS13** levels of limited use.

Management

- **Treat cause**: look for underlying sepsis, drugs, other causes, and treat.
- **Bleeding:** direct pressure. If bleeding and count $<50 \times 10^9$/L then consider IV platelet transfusion and treat cause. Use local physical methods/surgery to stem bleeding.
- **Vitamin K** (10 mg IV or orally): if liver disease or vitamin K deficiency possible.
- **Avoid** NSAIDs, aspirin, clopidogrel, warfarin, heparins and NOACs.
- **Augment good mouth care** with tranexamic acid mouthwashes (1 g orally four times daily) added if there is bleeding from the oral mucosa.
- **Tranexamic acid 1 g PO tds**. Do not give if there is on-going haematuria and/or DIC.
- **Uraemia:** consider omitting antiplatelets. Manage uraemia.
- **Pre-eclampsia/ eclampsia/HELLP:** BP control and fetal delivery.

When to transfuse platelets

May replace at higher levels if patient has taken antiplatelets or has platelet dysfunction. Take haematological advice. Must determine cause before transfusion.

Platelets not usually indicated for TTP/HUS/HIT syndromes. In acute ITP only used for real risk of bleeding. The decision to transfuse should be supported by the need to prevent or treat bleeding. There may be a role for desmopressin in patients taking aspirin or uraemia.

A platelet count of >50 × 10^9/L is sufficient for most invasive procedures, including gastroscopy and biopsy, insertion of indwelling lines, transbronchial biopsy, liver biopsy, laparotomy, or similar procedures.

Platelets (× 10^9/L)	Advice when to transfuse platelets
<10	Prophylactic transfusion.
<20	Bleeding, fever, infection, platelet dysfunction, coagulopathy.
<50	Prior to minor procedures or in actively anticoagulated patients or in the presence of active bleeding.
<75	Prior to general surgery/childbirth.
<100	Prior to ophthalmic surgery or neurosurgery.

Reference: Lin & Foltz (2005) Proposed guidelines for platelet transfusion. *Brit Columbia Med J*, 47:245.

17 Acute infections

17.1 Returning pyrexial traveller

About

- The differential is all the home grown local infective causes plus exotic ones.
- In any infective presentation a travel history should be always be obtained.

Always be on the lookout for the patient with a fever and flu-like illness who has travelled to an endemic area who will die of complicated falciparum malaria unless you look for and diagnose the infection and treat it.

Geographical clues: first of all always consider malaria and actively exclude it (see below).

- **All:** HIV infection, bacterial sepsis, UTI, meningitis, HSV encephalitis, influenza, leptospirosis, rabies.
- **Africa, Asia, Caribbean, South America:** malaria, typhoid 'enteric' fever, viral hepatitis, dengue fever, poliomyelitis.
- **Africa:** rickettsial diseases, amoebic liver abscess, Katayama syndrome.
- **West Africa** (Nigeria, Niger, Mali, Senegal, etc.): viral haemorrhagic fever.
- **Horn of Africa:** visceral leishmaniasis.
- **South Asia:** enteric fever.
- **Others:** viral haemorrhagic fevers (Lassa fever), leptospirosis, trypanosomiasis.

Clinical

- History of where stayed, town or countryside, medications taken, night nets, unprotected intercourse with new person. Visiting game parks, farms, caves, health facilities, consumption of exotic foods, activities involving fresh or salt-water exposure, and sexual activity.
- Any bites, e.g. bats, dogs. Identify symptoms – malaise, photophobia, rash, dysuria, cough, phlegm, rash, eschar, hepatosplenomegaly, lymphadenopathy or jaundice.

Clues	Consider
Sexual contact	Acute HIV, disseminated gonorrhoea, syphilis, chlamydophila, chancroid, hepatitis B
IV drugs/blood borne	Hepatitis B and C, HIV
Mosquito bite	Malaria, dengue fever, chikungunya disease, tularaemia, filiariasis
Tsetse fly	African trypanosomiasis
Animals	Brucellosis, rabies, Q fever, plague, tularaemia
Faeco–oral	Hepatitis A and E, enteric fever
Fresh water	Leptospirosis, schistosomiasis (Katayama fever)
Incubation period <21 days	Malaria, typhoid fever, dengue fever, rickettsial diseases
Incubation period >21 days	TB, malaria, hepatitis

Clues	Consider
Tick bites	Rickettsial infections, Lyme disease, Rocky mountain spotted fever, ehrlichosis
Cold sores	*Herpes simplex* encephalitis
Teenager, adult <30	Infectious mononucleosis (EBV or CMV)
African safari	Rickettsial disease, African trypanosomiasis
Animal bite abroad	Immediate concern is always rabies – seek expert help
Africa	Malaria, dengue fever, rickettsial disease, enteric fever, viral haemorrhagic fevers, Ebola
Southeast Asia	Malaria, dengue fever, rickettsial disease, enteric fever, chikungunya disease
Eschar	Rickettsial disease, anthrax
Buboes	Bubonic plague, gonorrhoea, tuberculosis, chancroid or syphilis
Hotels and air conditioning	*Legionella*
IV drug users	*Staphylococcal aureus*, hepatitis B/C, HIV, anthrax, botulism

Historical clues

- **Infections: the usual illnesses:** although the patient may have returned from abroad, consider the usual familiar causes – influenza, UTI, chest infection, meningitis, endocarditis, TB or a lymphoma, Lyme disease.
- **Emergencies:** take advice early from infectious diseases specialist if the patient is particularly ill or has altered mental status. Although meningococcaemia, cerebral malaria and viral haemorrhagic fevers are highly uncommon, consider these diagnoses, because they are medical emergencies.
- **Pre-travel immunisations and chemoprophylaxis:** proper administration of vaccines against hepatitis A, hepatitis B, and yellow fever effectively rules out these infections (not malaria).
- **Travel itinerary:** the risk of acquiring a travel-related infection depends on the precise geographic location and the length of stay at each destination. Did they stay in a modern hotel or with locals or family. Infections can be acquired en route, so layovers and intermediate stops should be recorded. Mode of transport should be recorded.
- **Sex:** with whom, male/female, protected, prostitution, condom use, what type of sex. Risk of infection. Other STDs.

Management of pyrexia in a traveller (infective, inflammatory, malignancy)

- **Malaria**: if in endemic malarial area then assume falciparum malaria until you have a total of three negative smears which should be obtained 8–12 h apart over the course of 2 days. Discuss with infectious diseases specialist. If any signs of complications then consider starting treatment immediately (see *Section 17.2* below).
- **Bloods:** get FBC, blood film, U&E, LFT, HIV test, acute viral serology, blood cultures and CXR and CT head if any neurology. Consider lumbar puncture (check coagulation first). Serology and liver USS if liver abscess suspected. If bacterial meningitis or HSV encephalitis are a possibility, then treat appropriately.

- **Echocardiogram, cultures, CRP** if any cardiac signs. TFTs because thyrotoxic crisis could resemble infection. If still unclear then repeat history and examination to make sure all information extracted.
- **Get drug history:** is something non-infective going on: ?vasculitis, ?adult Still's disease. An eschar on the buttocks might be the clue needed to diagnose typhus and treat with doxycycline.

17.2 Tropical infections to recognise

Falciparum malaria

If suspected complicated disease start antimalarial immediately with whatever is available. Usually IV/PO quinine or Artesunate. If you are unsure, get help from local tropical diseases/infectious diseases unit.

About

- Falciparum malaria presents within 4 weeks but is seen up to 6 months post mosquito contact.
- Get urgent thick and thin films. Treat quickly. Falciparum malaria can kill within hours.
- Expert advice UK: London 0845 155 5000, Liverpool 0151 706 2000.
- Assume malaria as a possible cause and actively exclude if patient has been in endemic area.
- Be very cautious as fatal disease may present like 'flu'. Check films.

Appropriate prophylaxis with full adherence does not exclude potentially fatal malaria.

Endemic areas

- Africa, Asia, Papua New Guinea, South America, Western Pacific.

Aetiology

- Lethality with cytoadherance in which infected red cells adhere to the walls and block post-capillary venules by formation of *P. falciparum* erythrocyte membrane protein (PfEMP)-1.
- Rosetting is another finding where infected cells adhere to uninfected RBCs.

Clinical

- Flu-like malaise, fever >39°C (may be absent), headache, vomiting, malaise, myalgia.
- Severe cerebral malaria: coma, fits, paralysis – hemiparesis, blindness, brisk reflexes, extensor plantars and even decorticate or decerebrate posturing.
- Disease or treatment-induced hypoglycaemia can be misinterpreted as cerebral malaria.
- Diarrhoea, rigors, backache, drenching fevers, hepatosplenomegaly may be found.
- Acute renal failure needing dialysis in 10%, intravascular haemolysis, jaundice, haemoglobinuria.
- Malaria does not cause lymphadenopathy or rash (can have other infections/ illness).
- Record country and area of travel, stopovers, and date of return.
- Record what malaria prophylaxis was taken.

Complications

- Low GCS, seizures, oliguria <20 ml/h, ARDS/pulmonary oedema.
- Spontaneous bleeding/DIC, shock (algid malaria BP <90/60 mmHg).
- Haemoglobinuria (without G6PD deficiency).

Markers of severity

- Hb <8 g/dL, hypoglycaemia (<2.2 mmol/L), acidosis (pH <7.3, HCO_3 <15 mmol)
- Lactate >5 mmol/L, parasites >2%. Creatinine >265 µmol/L, increased bilirubin and jaundice.

Differential

- Malaria must first be excluded in any pyrexial illness from or in an endemic area.
- Typhoid, hepatitis, dengue, avian influenza, SARS, HIV.
- Meningitis/encephalitis and viral haemorrhagic fevers.

Investigations

- **FBC and U&E**: anaemia and haemolysis with raised urea and creatinine and LDH.
- **Thick and thin films**: (on same EDTA sample) to identify parasite infection. Thin Giemsa-stained blood films show the number of red cells infected and type. Need 3–4 thick/thin negative slides over 48–72 h to fully exclude malaria. Consider stopping antimalarial prophylaxis, because this may reduce parasitaemia, in order to get the films. Examination should identify the degree of parasitaemia.
- **Dipstick antigen detection tests**: some rapid tests are available. Treatment may give false negatives.
- **Chronic infection**: raised IgM and marked splenomegaly and anaemia.
- **Coagulation screen**: DIC seen, low fibrinogen raised, D-dimers low, platelets raised, FDPs elevated.
- **CXR**: non-cardiogenic pulmonary oedema, exclude pneumonia and other causes of fever.

Complications

- **Coma (cerebral malaria):** manage ABCs, exclude other treatable causes of coma (e.g. hypoglycaemia, bacterial meningitis); avoid harmful ancillary treatment such as corticosteroids, heparin and adrenaline; intubate and ventilate if necessary.
- **Hyperpyrexia**: administer tepid sponging, fanning, cooling blanket and antipyretic drugs.
- **Convulsions**: maintain airways; treat promptly with IV/PR DIAZEPAM if on-going.
- **Hypoglycaemia**: (check glucose <2.2 mmol/L), correct hypoglycaemia and maintain with glucose-containing infusion.
- **Severe anaemia**: (haemoglobin <5 g/100ml or packed cell volume <15%) transfuse with screened fresh whole blood.
- **Acute pulmonary oedema**: over-enthusiastic rehydration should be avoided so as to prevent pulmonary oedema. Prop patient up at an angle of 45°, give oxygen, give a diuretic, stop intravenous fluids, intubate and add PEEP/CPAP in life-threatening hypoxaemia.
- **Acute renal failure**: exclude pre-renal causes, check fluid balance and urinary sodium; if in established renal failure add haemofiltration or haemodialysis, or if unavailable, peritoneal dialysis. The benefits of diuretics/dopamine in acute renal failure are not proven.
- **Spontaneous bleeding and coagulopathy**: transfuse with screened fresh whole blood (cryoprecipitate, FFP and platelets if available); give vitamin K injection.

- **Metabolic acidosis**: exclude or treat hypoglycaemia, hypovolaemia and septicaemia. If severe, add haemofiltration or haemodialysis.
- **Shock**: suspect septicaemia, take blood for cultures; give parenteral antimicrobials, correct haemodynamic disturbances.
- **Hyperparasitaemia**: treat as below.

Management

- Oral/IV rehydration may be needed with fever, polyuria, poor intake. Give O_2 to achieve 94% saturation. Treat hypoglycaemia with IV glucose. Admit complicated malaria to the ITU and start treatment immediately. Use parenteral therapy if readily available and if not use oral quinine or artesunate until pharmacy can provide an IV preparation – which should be within a few hours.
- Do not delay antimalarials if patient has signs of complicated falciparum malaria. If the diagnosis unclear stop antmalarials to improve test accuracy. If unsure take expert help. Severe falciparum malaria is a medical emergency.

Antimalarial treatment

- **Non-falciparum malaria in adults**: Chloroquine 600 mg with Chloroquine 300 mg at 6, 24 and 48 h. If vivax/ovale then Primaquine 30 mg base/day for 14 days but check for G6PD deficiency first.
- **Uncomplicated falciparum malaria in adults**: one of the following:
    - Oral QUININE + DOXYCYCLINE/CLINDAMYCIN for 7 days
    - MALARONE 4 'standard' tablets daily for 3 days
    - Oral RIAMET (artemether and lumefantrine) 4 tablets then a further 4 tablets at 8/24/36/48 and 60 h.
- **Complicated or vomiting falciparum malaria in adults**: Artesunate is now the drug of choice for all patients with severe malaria. It has a rapid effect on parasite clearance. It reduces mortality compared to quinine. However, Artesunate is not yet licensed in the UK and most hospitals do not keep a supply. If not available give PO/IV quinine whilst waiting for Artesunate to arrive if it can be obtained.
    - **QUININE loading dose**: SLOW IV QUININE infusion unless already on quinine/melfloquine, followed by maintenance QUININE dose. Also give DOXYCYCLINE PO or CLINDAMYCIN for 7 days.
    - **IV ARTESUNATE** (unlicensed in EU) plus DOXYCYCLINE PO or CLINDAMYCIN for 7 days. When patient stable switch to oral QUININE for 7 days.

Pregnancy (take expert advice)

- Falciparum malaria in pregnancy may be more severe than suggested by the peripheral blood film due to marked placental sequestration. The fetus is usually unaffected but inadequate treatment may lead to placental insufficiency and stillbirth.
- Quinine is safe and effective in all stages of pregnancy and is used in standard doses. Artesunate is generally avoided in the first trimester of pregnancy but is probably safe and effective (ask expert).

Tropical infections

Infection	Notes
African tick typhus	**About:** tick bite inoculates patient with rickettsia. Rickettsia are obligate intracellular, Gram-negative bacteria. Game parks in southern Africa. Walking with exposed legs. **Clinical:** presents within 10 days with fever, headache, myalgia. Look for inoculation eschar at the site of tick bite, rash, lymphadenitis and reactive arthritis. **Complications:** pneumonitis, meningoencephalitis. Occasionally DIC or AKI with fatality rates up to nearly 20%. **Diagnosis:** exclude malaria. Confirmation of the diagnosis is retrospective and based on paired initial and convalescent-phase serum sample. **Management: DOXYCYCLINE 100 mg** BD PO/IV for least 7 days.
Katayama fever (acute schistosomiasis)	**Source:** endemic in parts of Africa. Swimming or bathing in fresh water lakes/ rivers allows cercariae released from snails to penetrate intact skin – 'swimmer's itch'. *Schistosoma mansoni, S. haematobium* and *S. japonicum*. **Clinical:** presents within 4–6 weeks. Fever, lethargy, myalgia, arthralgia, cough, headache. Urticarial rash, diarrhoea, hepatosplenomegaly and wheeze. **Diagnosis:** peripheral eosinophilia. Ova seen in urine. **Management: Praziquantel** will kill mature but not immature schistosomes. Treat at the time of diagnosis of Katayama fever and 3 months later. A short course of steroids may help alleviate acute symptoms.
Dengue	**Source:** endemic in Asia and S America and Caribbean; transmitted by day biting mosquito *Aedes aegypti*. Flavivirus. Presents within 4–8 days (range: 3–14 days) of mosquito bite. **Clinical: initial infection**: mild febrile, headache, retro-orbital pain, myalgia, arthralgia (back pain) and erythrodermic rash which may become petechial. **Dengue haemorrhagic fever** presents with haemorrhagic manifestations. **Dengue shock syndrome** (narrowing pulse pressure of <20 mmHg or a systolic BP of <90 mmHg). The last two (DHF and DSS) are rare in travellers but serious. Seen with a second or subsequent infection usually with a different serotype. Cause severe bleeding, capillary leak and hypotension. **Investigations:** platelets $<100 \times 10^9$/L and 20% increase in packed cell volume during course of illness due to plasma leak, hypoproteinaemia or clinical effusions. Raised LFTs. DIC. Confirm with a positive PCR or with a positive IgM-capture ELISA. Most managed with daily FBC and haematocrit and platelet count. **Management:** supportive. Avoid aspirin. Volume replacement. Transfusion.

Infection	Notes
Viral haemorrhagic fever *Urgent isolation and senior advice if contact with Ebola or from affected area*	**Source:** RNA viruses: arenaviruses, filoviruses, bunyaviruses and flaviviruses. Africa, S America and Asia. Very rare with a handful of cases per decade in the UK. Delayed diagnosis leads to further cases. Zoonosis. Usually from monkeys. As viruses depend on a host they are usually restricted to the geographical area inhabited by those animals. Humans are not the natural host for these viruses, which normally live in wild animals. **Types:** Lassa fever: visitors to Nigeria, Liberia, Sierra Leone. Ebola. Crimean–Congo haemorrhagic fever, Marburg and Ebola. Contact with dead. Sick animals. **Pathogenesis:** haemorrhage, severe capillary leak and shock. **Clinical:** some cause mild illnesses, others cause severe, life-threatening disease. Fever, fatigue, dizziness, muscle aches, loss of strength, and exhaustion. Petechiae, bruising, haemorrhage, mucosal bleeding, PR bleeding. Hypovolaemic shock, coma, delirium, and, seizures. AKI. **Investigations:** serology, FBC: fall in Hb and rise in haematocrit, U&E: AKI, coagulopathy, raised LFT. **Management:** exclude malaria. Contact local infection control unit and isolate patient, protective clothing, waste disposal. Largely supportive. *Person to person spread possible so strict precautions must be taken.* **IV Ribavirin**, an antiviral drug, has been effective in treating some individuals with Lassa fever or HRS. Convalescent-phase plasma has been used in some patients with Argentine haemorrhagic fever.
Ebola	**Source**: several viral types. Contact with bodily fluids of infected individuals (alive or dead) and some primates and bats. Humans only infectious when ill and symptomatic. IP 21 days. Endemic in parts of W. Africa. **Clinical**: myalgia, fever, vomiting, diarrhoea (infectious), haemorrhage. **Investigations**: serology, detectable RNA, coagulopathy. **Management**: immediately isolate (protect staff – mask, gown, goggles) and supportive. Dispose of corpse. **Prognosis**: fatality 60–90%. No vaccine.
Plague	**Source:** *Yersinia pestis*. sub-Saharan Africa. Reservoir is rodents. Plague is passed by bites from fleas. **Clinical:** classically causes swellings called buboes. Septicaemic and pneumonic forms as well as meningitis. **Investigations:** diagnosis by blood culture or from aspirate from bubo. **Management:** streptomycin IM for 7 days, gentamicin 5 mg/kg daily IV for 10 days.
Brucellosis	**Source:** *Brucella abortus*, *B. melitensis*, *B. suis*, *B. canis*. Gram-negative intracellular infection. Exposure to animals (goats, sheep, cattle, camels, pigs, dogs), unpasteurised milk, cheeses. Seen in Southern Europe, India. **Clinical acute:** infection phase 2–4 weeks. Undulant fever. Lymphadenopathy, hepatosplenomegaly, foul swelling sweat, arthritis, osteomyelitis, meningoencephalitis. Scrotal pain. **Investigations:** WCC and CRP can be normal so difficult diagnosis without serology. Culture is prolonged – blood, CSF, lymph nodes. Serology needed. **Management:** doxycycline 200 mg OD × 6 weeks. Rifampicin. Combined with streptomycin for 2 weeks.

Infection	Notes
Q fever	**Source:** *Coxiella burnettii.* From animals. Transmission is via dust, aerolised media, spores, and unpasteurised milk. **Clinical:** infectious phase 2–4 weeks with fever, headaches, myalgia, pneumonia, hepatitis, rarely endocarditis. **Investigations:** diagnosis by serology titres. **Management:** doxycycline 200 mg OD × 14 days.
Anthrax	**Source:** *Bacillis anthracis.* Gram-positive rods found naturally in soil as spores. May be used in bioterrorism. **Clinical:** *cutaneous*: handling infected material – blisters, itching and a black eschar. Lymphadenopathy. *Pulmonary*: inhalation of spores – breathlessness, haemoptysis, chest pain, cough, sweats, systemically unwell. *Gastrointestinal*: eating raw infected meat – fever, chills, neck lymphadenopathy, bloody diarrhoea. *Injectional*: a few cases of a heroin batch contaminated with spores – fever, skin abscess. **Investigations:** FBC, U&E, CRP: blood/sputum/CSF/skin swab for *B. anthracis* before antibiotics. *Serology* for *B. anthracis*. *CXR/chest CT*: enlarged mediastinum or pleural effusion. **Management:** no person to person spread except rarely with cutaneous form, however, until risks and source established full protection should be used and local guidance and isolate. Those at-risk without symptoms: anthrax vaccination can be considered. Ciprofloxacin or doxycycline can be given to exposed individuals before symptoms. *Cutaneous disease*: doxycycline for 7–14 days as outpatient. *Systemic anthrax*: hospitalisation, antibiotics (ciprofloxacin or doxycycline for 1–2 weeks) and antitoxin. **Raxibacumab**, a monoclonal antibody, may be useful against an anthrax bacterial antigen. Prognosis is very poor for those with inhaled or gastrointestinal or meningeal anthrax. Death is toxin-mediated and results in haemorrhagic/septicaemic shock.
Leptospirosis	**Source:** *Leptospira interrogan.* Found worldwide including in UK. Exposure to infected urine of rats, dogs, cattle and other domestic and wild animals. Acquire it from direct contact with urine or urine-contaminated water. Recreational water sports/occupations with animal/water exposure or flooding. Comes on 1–2 weeks following exposure. **Clinical:** varied from mild flu-like symptoms to a severe illness characterised by haemorrhage, jaundice and hepatorenal failure. Initial flu-like symptoms lasting 4–7 days, followed 1–3 days later by fever, myalgia (sore back and legs), HRS and haemorrhage. Conjunctival suffusion is suggestive. **Complications:** meningitis, renal failure, liver failure, myocarditis, pancreatitis and haemorrhage (purpura, ecchymosis, pulmonary and gastrointestinal haemorrhage). Most are self-limiting but occasionally severe and even fatal. Aseptic meningitis. Jaundice, hepatomegaly and bleeding, respiratory failure and lung infiltrates. ARDS. **Differential in tropics:** malaria, dengue, typhoid, scrub typhus, hantavirus. **Investigations:** *FBC*: raised neutrophils, low platelets, low Hb if haemorrhage. High CK. Raised LFTs. *Coagulation screen*: normal, usually PT may be a little prolonged but bleeding is due to capillary fragility and so tests of clotting are often normal. *U&E*: AKI, raised bilirubin and ALT. *Urinalysis*: may show proteinuria and haematuria. Organisms seen in 2nd week. *Serology:* cultures slow. Diagnosis

Infection	Notes
Leptospirosis – *cont'd*	needs serology with IgM titre >1 in 320. To confirm the diagnosis convalescent serology >10 days after symptom onset should be sent for IgM ELISA and microscopic agglutination test (MAT). *CSF and aerobic blood cultures*: (taken within the first 5 days of onset, before antibiotics) can be referred to the UK Leptospira Reference Unit. Keep blood cultures at room temperature prior to sending. *Urine* is not a suitable sample for the isolation of leptospira. **Management:** mainly symptomatic and supportive. AKI managed with dialysis if needed. Blood transfusion as needed. Treatment with **Benzylpenicillin IV 4 hourly or Ceftriaxone IV daily**. Evidence for antibiotic effectiveness is unproven. Those with jaundice can become very unwell despite therapy and may require renal or liver support. Severe disease is probably immunologically mediated.
Listeriosis *A cause of adult meningitis not covered by empirical treatment with ceftriaxone.*	**Source:** *Listeria monocytogenes*. Gram-positive. Found in environment. Contaminates food: salads, soft cheese, undercooked meat, chicken, pates. **At risk:** more severe infection in elderly, pregnant, immunocompromised. **Clinical:** acute gastroenteritis with nausea, vomiting, backache and diarrhoea. **Complications**: meningism, progressive coma, stroke-like episode, adult brainstem encephalitis (CSF may be normal), meningitis, stillbirth or premature labour, neonatal listeriosis causes sepsis or meningitis. **Investigations:** *FBC*: raised WCC. Elevated CRP, ESR. *MRI* changes for encephalitis or meningitis. *CSF* culture, raised WCC and normal glucose. **Management:** a prolonged course of IV AMPICILLIN + GENTAMICIN or CO-TRIMOXAZOLE.
Botulism	**Source:** toxin released by *Clostridium botulinum* in anaerobic conditions which is found as a spore in soil and is a large anaerobic Gram-positive spore-forming bacillus. Produces neurotoxins which block acetylcholine release with paralysis at motor nerve endings. Most powerful neurotoxin known to date. **Clinical:** food-borne, intestinal, wound infection. Neurological recovery can take months. Progressive blurred vision, bulbar and facial weakness, dysphagia, unable to speak. Progressive paralysis can lead to respiratory failure and death in 10%. Diarrhoea and vomiting, dry mouth, but some will be constipated. **Investigations:** *FBC, U&E, ABG*: hypoxia/hypercarbia, *FVC* measurements three times a day. **Management:** mostly supportive with active and passive physiotherapy for chest and paralysis. Antibiotics only for wound-based infection (**IV penicillin G or clindamycin or chloramphenicol**). NG/PEG feeding if no swallow. PPI or Ranitidine to prevent stress ulcer. Catheterisation for retention or incontinence. DVT prophylaxis. Wound infection: debridement and antitoxin and antibiotics. **Antitoxins**: essential for food-borne botulism and are equine derived and neutralise toxin. Severe cases (FVC <1 L) may need to be intubated/ventilated to avoid respiratory failure.

Infection	Notes
Clostridium perfringens	**Source:** *Clostridium perfringens* forms gas. Large Gram-positive anaerobic spore-forming rods. Five types (A–E) differentiated by surface antigens. A is commonest cause of human disease. Alpha toxin causes gas gangrene (lecithinase, haemolysis and necrosis). Found in soil, dust, faeces. **Pathogenicity:** gas gangrene – pain, massive tissue necrosis due to release of toxins, e.g. phospholipase C, lecithinase. Destroys polymorph. Local fermentation produces gas in the tissue. Potentially and rapidly fatal. **Clinical:** food poisoning – onset 12–24 h post-ingestion with diarrhoea which is usually self-limiting. Anaerobic cellulitis or infection of ischaemic limb. **Investigations:** G +ve spore-forming bacilli on Gram stain. Grows on anaerobic culture. Alpha toxin (lecithinase) production. Lipase production on egg yolk agar (Nagler plate). **Management:** debridement, hyperbaric oxygen chamber, benzylpenicillin 2.4 g IV 4–6 hourly + clindamycin 1.2 g IV 6 hourly.

Acute bacterial sepsis

Don't forget about common worldwide infections. Temperature, raised or low WCC, malaise, confusion. See *Section 17.1*. FBC, U&E, LFT. CRP. Screen urine, aerobic and anaerobic blood cultures, CXR, lumbar puncture, ascitic aspirate. Give broad spectrum antibiotics. See *Section 4.6*.

17.3 Common acute viral infections

Simple systemic viral infections can be potentially lethal in those with impaired immunity, e.g. malnutrition, malignancy, steroids, methotrexate, HIV, etc. Stop any immunosuppressive drugs. Patients may fail to volunteer this information so always check.

Infection	Notes
Measles *Take expert advice on stopping any immune suppression*	**Note:** severe in the immunocompromised patient. **Source:** caught from unvaccinated non-immune spread by respiratory droplets. Severe infection in older children/adults. Natural immunity lifelong. Infectious for 1–2 weeks. **Clinical:** prodrome of URT complaints, Koplik spots in buccal mucosa, generalised macular papular rash. Lymphadenopathy, diarrhoea. Otitis media and bacterial pneumonia. Viral encephalitis can occur acutely. Malnourished and immunocompromised get pneumonitis, encephalitis. Secondary bacterial pneumonia or severe diarrhoea or cancrum oris. Can be lethal particularly in developing countries. **Diagnosis:** clinical but IgM titres can be checked. **Complications:** pneumonitis, encephalitis; late: subacute sclerosing panencephalitis. **Management:** immunoglobulin reduces severity in immunocompromised if given within first 6 days. Vitamin A can help. Antibiotics for bacterial superinfections. MMR for unimmunised.

Infection	Notes
Chicken pox / varicella zoster *Take expert advice on stopping any immune suppression*	**About:** more severe in adults and immunosuppressed and pregnancy. Varicella pneumonia has a 10% mortality. Virus lives in dorsal root ganglion and can reactivate. Increased risk with pregnant, smokers, immunosuppressed. **Clinical:** causes crops of vesicles to pustules, which crust and dry on face, scalp and trunk. Can be feverish. Incubation period (IP) from contact to symptoms 2–3 weeks. Hypoxia, breathlessness and respiratory failure. Shingles much more severe in immunocompromised, e.g. HIV +ve. Can recur in later life as shingles with a dermatomal spread of vesicles. **Investigations:** serology if immunity unclear. Long-term calcification on CXR. **Management:** stop any immunosuppression and take expert guidance. HDU/ITU care to maintain respiratory support in severe varicella pneumonia. Childhood uncomplicated infection needs only supportive care. *Shingles*: oral Aciclovir 800 mg 5 times/day for 1 week. May need treatment for neuropathic pain. *Severe complicated infection*: IV Aciclovir 10 mg/kg tds. **Zoster immune globulin** (ZIG) for those without prior exposure and infection who are pregnant or immunocompromised.
Herpes simplex 1 and 2 *See Section 19.2 on HSV encephalitis*	**About:** usually benign but watch for HSV encephalitis. **Clinical:** severe mucocutaneous lesions – mouth, genitals, oesophagus. Often reactivation rather than new infection. Visceral involvement can be fatal, e.g. encephalitis. **Investigations:** LP for CSF. Stop immunosuppression. Expert consult. **Management:** oral Aciclovir 800 mg 5 times/day for 1 week. Severe complicated infection: IV Aciclovir 10 mg/kg tds; also consider Valaciclovir and Famciclovir. Look for and treat any bacterial superinfection.
Infectious mononucleosis	**About:** seen with EBV, CMV, HHV6 and HIV and toxoplasmosis. **Clinical:** syndromic presentation with severe sore throat and fever and malaise. Teenagers or young adults. Pharyngeal oedema/respiratory obstruction, rash with ampicillin, post viral fatigue. Hepatitis 80%, jaundice, myelitis, encephalitis. Guillain–Barré syndrome, low platelets, splenomegaly, nephritis, myopericarditis, splenic rupture. **Investigations:** positive monospot can be seen. Serology can be done for usual causes. Raised and atypical lymphocytes may be seen. **Management:** largely supportive. Avoid sports and trauma with splenomegaly. Manage complications as they arise.
Cytomegalovirus *Take expert advice on stopping any immune suppression*	**Source:** close contact human to human, saliva. Owl eye inclusion bodies and giant cells. **Clinical:** *immunocompetent*: get hepatitis and infectious mononucleosis, rarely Guillain–Barré syndrome. *Immunocompromised*: (solid organ and stem cell transplant) get a CMV pneumonitis mortality of 50%. *AIDS patients*: retinitis, CMV colitis and polyradiculopathy. *Pregnancy:* primary infection can affect fetus. With rash, hepatosplenomegaly and CNS complications. **Investigations:** swab and microscopy, serology and biopsy. Negative Paul–Bunnell test and no lymphadenopathy.

Infection	Notes
Cytomegalovirus – *cont'd*	**Management:** CMV infection is IV Valganciclovir (solid organ transplant patients) otherwise IV Ganciclovir. Needs expert help, particularly if pregnancy.
Epstein–Barr virus	**Source:** herpesvirus. Close contact human to human, saliva. **Clinical:** pharyngitis, severe pharyngeal oedema, cervical nodes, fever, splenomegaly. Macular/papular rash. **Investigations:** raised atypical lymphocytes, thrombocytopenia. Positive monospot. **Complications:** splenic rupture (avoid contact sport), encephalitis, airway obstruction. **Management:** rash with Ampicillin/Amoxil so avoid. Severe pharyngeal oedema treated with steroid. Antibiotics for bacterial superinfection, e.g. strep. throat. Antiviral not useful.
Influenza	**About:** caused by influenza A and B. Orthomyxoviruses. Most extensive and severe outbreaks are due to influenza A. **Virology:** virus has surface haemagglutinin (H) and neuraminidase (N) antigens. Haemagglutinin binds erythrocytes and initiates infection. Neuraminidase cleaves haemagglutinin and releases virus from cells. **Variants:** *avian influenza*: influenza A infection (H5N1) caused a more severe pneumonia. Seen mainly in SE Asia. Treat as for influenza with neuraminidase inhibitors. *Swine influenza*: seen in Mexico 2009. Influenza A infection (H1N1). Clinically more D&V symptoms. Increased risk with co-morbidities. Isolation. Neuraminidase inhibitors. **Clinical:** comes on within days of contact. Fever, headache, severe myalgia and malaise. Cough, sputum and respiratory tract symptoms. Diarrhoea. Secondary infection is common. *Staph. aureus* pneumonia. **Complications:** secondary pneumonia, myositis, Guillain–Barré syndrome, myocarditis, transverse myelitis, encephalitis, pericarditis. **Investigations:** PCR of nose swab. CXR cavitating secondary pneumonia. **Management:** supportive, hydration, analgesia, isolation, hand washing. Pandemic flu: needs special isolation and barrier nursing with staff wearing appropriate masks, goggles, gloves and protective gear. Patient wears a surgical mask. *Neuraminidase inhibitors*: **Oseltamavir 75 mg BD** or **inhaled Zanamivir** inhibit neuraminidase and work against influenza A and B, but must be given within 48 hours to reduce duration of illness.
Severe acute respiratory syndrome (SARS)	**About:** SARS is a coronavirus respiratory illness due to SARS-associated coronavirus (SARS-CoV). Since 2004, there have not been any known cases of SARS reported anywhere in the world. In cases prior to 2004, most patients had close contact with another infected person. **Clinical:** sore throat, rhinorrhoea, chills, rigors, myalgia, headache, diarrhoea. **Investigations:** raised WCC, CRP, ALT, CK, LDH. Get FBC, WCC, CXR. Blood cultures, test for viral respiratory pathogens, influenza A and B and respiratory syncytial virus. Legionella and pneumococcal urinary antigen testing if radiographic evidence of pneumonia (adults only). **Management:** supportive. Isolate, analgesia, oxygen.

Infection	Notes
Needlestick injury *Let it bleed and wash gently with soap and water. Urgent referral to occupational health or A&E.*	**About:** potential infection with HBV, HIV, HCV. Needle used to take blood or give IM/IV/SC injection pierces the skin of another. Infected fluids in eyes or ingested or on contact with mucocutaneous surfaces. Hepatitis C risk 3%, HIV risk 0.3%. All NHS staff should be immunised against hepatitis B. **Aetiology:** passage of blood-borne viruses. The risk of HIV infection is 1/300 if HIV +ve patient. HBV risk in HBV patient much higher but clinical staff should have been immunised. If there is a reasonable risk that the patient is HIV positive then treat as a medical emergency and injured person should either contact occupational health or go direct to the emergency department. **Management:** encourage wound to bleed freely and then wash with soap and water. Don't scrub such that further tissue damage occurs. Cover with waterproof dressing. If oral or eye contamination then wash and irrigate thoroughly with IV NS via giving set or tap water. Mouth contamination should rinse but don't swallow. *Report incident promptly to line manager and complete incident form when appropriate. In working hours contact occupational health, out of hours go to local emergency department (A&E). Do not try to manage this on the ward yourself or with your team.* Inform the patient and explore any particular risks for HIV/HBV/HCV, e.g. IV drug use, sexual history. Patient may allow a clotted sample for HBV/HCV/HIV. Patient should be aware that results will be divulged to the injured person. The consent should be recorded in their notes. All NHS clinical staff should be immunised against hepatitis B. Hepatitis B immunoglobulin may be given if required following expert assessment with emergency department or occupational health who may liaise with microbiology. The risk of hepatitis C is 3% and there is no post-exposure prophylaxis (PEP) but follow up should be carried out. For HIV the risk is 0.3% and depends on depth of wound, visible blood on device, needle from artery or vein and terminal HIV disease. **Risk of HIV transmission = risk that source is HIV positive × risk of exposure**. As part of risk assessment record size and volume of the inoculum, i.e. whether the needle was hollow, etc. Depth of injury. Visible blood on the device that caused the injury. Injury with a needle that had been placed in an artery or vein. If HIV possible, AZT reduces infection 5 fold. PEP is given which involves three antiretrovirals for 1 month and is started immediately. PEP should be taken following local expert risk assessment and guidance and policies; an exact protocol is not included here because local practice should be followed. **Reference:** Kuhar *et al*. (2013) Updated U.S. Public Health Service Guidelines for the management of occupational exposures to HIV and recommendations for post-exposure prophylaxis. *US PHS Guidelines for the Management of Occupational Exposures to HIV.*
Meticillin resistant *Staphylococcus aureus* (MRSA)	**About:** *Staphylococcus aureus* has acquired resistance to meticillin, flucloxacilln and oxacillin. This is by acquiring the *mec-A* gene. MRSA infections are falling. **Clinical:** line infections, soft tissue infections, pneumonias and septicaemia. MRSA is associated with a higher mortality than MSSA. Need good asepsis, hand washing and eradication policies.

Infection	Notes
Meticillin resistant *Staphylococcus aureus* (MRSA) – *cont'd*	**Investigations:** culture of blood, skin swabs, nasal and groin often screened. Lines. **Management:** MRSA septicaemia should receive **VANCOMYCIN or TEICOPLANIN. Others are** RIFAMPICIN and TETRACYCLINE. DOXYCYCLINE may be used for soft tissue infections.

Tuberculosis (*Mycobacterium tuberculosis*)

Pulmonary TB cavitation is synonymous with infectivity. Isolate patient.

About

- *Mycobacterium tuberculosis* is the typical and most common form in humans.
- *M. bovis* seen in developing countries from infected milk products (non-pasteurized).

Risks

- Increasing due to HIV/AIDS, homelessness, alcohol dependency.
- Immigrants from Sub-Saharan Africa, Bangladesh, India, Pakistan.
- Drug and multidrug resistant (rifampicin) TB is a problem.
- Age, malignancy, alcohol, immunodeficiency, malnutrition.
- Use of immunosuppression, anti-TNF-alpha drugs.

Pathology

- Classed as one of the granulomatous inflammatory conditions.
- Th1 reaction with epithelioid macrophages, Langhans giant cells, lymphocytes.
- Central caseous necrosis and production of interferon-gamma by T helper cells.
- The Ghon focus + local hilar lymphadenopathy is called a Ghon complex.

Clinical

- Weight loss, cervical or generalized lymphadenopathy, hepatosplenomegaly.
- Pyrexia of unknown origin, cervical lymph node (scrofula).
- TB of terminal ileum with a RIF mass, peritonitis, ascites, psoas abscess.
- Breathless, cough, sputum and consolidation and upper lobe scarring on CXR.
- Systemically unwell, miliary TB, fever, night sweats, weight loss.
- Renal TB: sterile pyuria with WCC in urine and normal cultures negative.
- CNS TB: TB meningitis – headache, cranial nerve palsies, etc.
- Vertebral disease: back pain – spinal infection, spinal cord compression.
- Skin: lupus vulgaris and erythema induratum.
- Cardiac: tuberculous pericardial effusion and constrictive pericarditis.
- Addison's disease with adrenal TB.

Investigations

- **FBC**: anaemia, raised WCC, raised ESR, CRP; LFTs: abnormal.
- **CXR:** pleural effusion, hilar lymphadenopathy, consolidation, fibrosis, upper and middle lobe infection, millet seed-like opacities on chest film <5 mm with miliary TB. Cavitatory disease suggests infectious, right mid zone collapse. Pneumothorax.
- **Sputum smear**: direct staining and microscopy of a smear from recently expectorated sputum. If bacilli seen it is classed as 'smear positive' and is infectious. Inducing sputum is said to be as effective as broncho-alveolar lavage.

Auramine O is an alternative to Ziehl–Neelson especially as the dye fluoresces under UV light and so the bacilli are easier to see.

- **Sputum cultures** are the gold standard but take 3–6 weeks to grow and then identify species.
- **Sputum analysis**: DNA analysis using PCR identifying serotype and drug sensitivity.
- **Serology**: HIV test and CD4 count.
- **Tuberculin test**: uses purified protein derivative (PPD) to elicit a delayed-type hypersensitivity response which is mediated by T lymphocytes. The reaction is maximal at 2–3 days after inoculation. Positive tuberculin testing does not always suggest active disease – it suggests a prior immune response, previous infection or BCG. So only a grade 3/4 (10 mm induration) or a negative test are useful in those with history of BCG. It is important to elicit a wheal to demonstrate that it is intradermal and not subcutaneous. Most with active TB will have a positive skin test (=10 mm). Must measure the induration, not erythema. Tuberculin skin tests are not contraindicated in BCG-vaccinated people and skin test reactivity should be interpreted and treated as for unvaccinated people. False negatives occur in immunosuppressed, steroids, malnourished, HIV, severe TB (e.g. miliary disease), early primary disease – becomes positive 2–12 weeks post primary infection.
- **Lumbar puncture**: CSF shows a raised lymphocyte count and protein levels but smears rarely positive in TB meningitis. Check CT to exclude any space occupying lesion.
- **Early morning urines** to culture for TB in suspected renal disease.
- **Renal imaging**. Image with CT or intravenous urogram.
- **Bronchoscopy and lavage**: may be useful to get samples in difficult cases when there is an unproductive cough and high clinical suspicion. It may help to exclude other causes such as tumours with a potential for biopsy of abnormal tissue.
- **Microbiological culture** from sputum analysis, gastric aspirate (used in children), urine for renal TB, bone marrow biopsy, CSF, liver biopsy, broncho-alveolar lavage.
- **Gamma interferon:** a high level of interferon-gamma production is presumed to be indicative of TB infection. There is current work on the use of such assays in the management of TB. There are two methods for detecting the interferon-gamma released by the T cell, an ELISA (e.g. QuantiFERON assay [QFT-TB]) and an enzyme-linked immunospot assay (ELISPOT, e.g. T SPOT-TB assay).

Management

- Needs to be a high level of suspicion in the high-risk groups identified and TB with widespread manifestations should always be considered. Those with smear-positive disease need to be isolated. It is a notifiable disease. Smear-negative patients are rarely infectious. Smear-positive patients can be considered not infectious after 2 weeks of treatment. Should be referred to specialist. Adequate tissue samples for diagnosis should be taken before treatment started.
- Patients should be treated with 4 drug regimen [RIPE] for 2 months and 2 drug regimen for 4 months. In those with a low chance of resistance then rifampicin, isoniazid and pyrazinamide only without ethambutol may be used [RIP]: RIPE 2 months and RI 4 months; RIP 2 months and RI 4 months – low chance of resistance. Exceptions: TB of CNS – treatment is for 12 months. Resistance to any of the drugs (isoniazid or rifampicin) means a 9 month course.

Acquired immunodeficiency syndrome (AIDS)

Episode	Notes
Acute HIV seroconversion **'Acute retroviral syndrome'**	**About**: HIV testing should be considered as routine in all who are sexually active or who use IV drugs. **Source**: worldwide. Symptoms within 2–6 weeks of infection. AIDS after years. **Risk groups**: men having sex with men. IV drug use and needle sharing. Casual unprotected sex with sex worker. Their sexual partners. Children of HIV-positive mothers. **Clinical (seroconversion):** fever, rash, joint pains, malaise, lymphadenopathy, headache, myalgia, pharyngitis. Lasts for days to 3 weeks. Medical attention often sought as severe. Highly infectious period. **Differential diagnosis of acute seroconversion**: exclude malaria in endemic area, glandular fever, influenza, and dengue. **Investigations:** HIV antibody not detected but there is HIV RNA or HIV p24 antigen in plasma. HIV test and repeat after 6 weeks and CD4 count and viral titres. CXR and ABG if suspected *Pneumocystis carinii* pneumonia (PCP). **Management**: patient highly infectious. Test also for syphilis and other sexually transmitted infections. Take expert advice as to need for post exposure prophylaxis. Refer to GUM for contact tracing and treatment with antiretroviral therapy. Over time the CD4 count falls. Those with a CD4 <200 cells/mm^3 are at high risk for opportunistic infections. If the CD4 <50 then high risk of CMV and atypical mycobacterial infections, e.g. disseminated *Mycobacterium avium intracellulare*. **ACQUIRED IMMUNODEFICIENCY SYNDROME** It is later with the clinical occurrence of infections and malignancies in the setting of a low CD4 count that AIDS is defined. All those with symptomatic disease should be offered antiretroviral treatment, usually as the count is <350 cells/mm^3. Those who are pregnant, need treatment of hepatitis B infection or have HIV nephropathy are treated regardless of CD4 count. The aim is to reduce the plama viral load (PVL) and improve the CD4 count. This typically requires 3 or more drugs. These drugs are potentially toxic.
Neurology	**Central nervous system** • **Stroke**: ischaemic stroke is seen. Exclude other causes. Look for usual causes. Easy to confuse subcortical lesions on CT with PML. Low threshold for MRI. • **Cryptococcal meningitis**: headache, neck stiffness, fever, photophobia, cranial nerve palsies and papilloedema. Chronic meningitis. CT: may be normal or cryptococcomas, hydrocephalus. Serum cryptococcal neoformans antigen in serum and CSF. CSF raised WCC and protein but occasionally normal. IV AMPHOTERICIN B. • **Cerebral toxoplasmosis**: host is cat. Ingestion of eggs. Infection before and held under check by immunity. Reactivates when CD4 <50 cells/mm^3. Progressive symptoms over days. Seizures, fever and reduced GCS. CT/MR shows multiple ring enhancing lesions in cortex and basal ganglia. Positive IgG serology useful. Take advice for treatment. Good response to treatment. Pyrimethamine, sulfadiazine and folinic acid. Repeat CT after 2 weeks shows improvement.

Episode	Notes
Neurology – *cont'd*	• **Progressive multifocal leucoencephalopathy**: onset can be over weeks. Usually CD4 <100 cells/mm^3. Can mimic white matter stroke disease due to JC virus. One or more focal non-enhancing lesions of gradual onset. Fever and headache uncommon and suggest toxoplasmosis. Can mimic stroke. CSF: PCR for JC virus. Optimise antiretroviral therapy. • **Tubercular meningitis**: cervical lymphadenopathy, headache, nausea, vomiting, pyrexia, meningism. IIIrd and VIth nerve palsies. CSF high opening pressure, raised protein and low sugar and raised lymphocytes. CD4 <200 cells/mm^3. Needs antiretroviral therapy and at least 12 months antitubercular therapy. • **Primary cerebral lymphoma**: progressive symptoms over weeks. Headache and focal neurology. No fever. More likely if toxoplasma serology negative or failure to respond to treatment for toxoplasmosis. Multiple periventricular lesions on imaging. Irregular and weakly enhancing. CD4 <100 cells/mm^3. • **AIDS dementia complex**: progressive cognitive and functional decline. CSF normal. CT shows atrophy. **Peripheral nervous system** • **Transverse myelitis**: sensory level with motor weakness, autonomic loss. • **Guillain–Barré syndrome**: see *Section 19.14*. • **Peripheral neuropathy**: typically a sensory neuropathy.
Cardio-pulmonary	• **Bacterial pneumonias**: see *Section 12.5*. Fever, breathless, productive cough. Will depend on degree of immunocompromise. 10 times commoner than in HIV negatives. Higher risks with IV drug abuse. Cover as well for PCP. Treat early. • **Pneumocystis pneumonia**: CD4 <200 cells/mm^3. High LDH. Breathless, dry cough, fever, for 2 weeks, desaturation. See *Section 12.6*. If the CD4 >200 cells/mm^3 or on prophylaxis and compliant then PCP much less likely. • **Tuberculosis**: test HIV in all those with evidence of TB. Assume infectious. Isolate and get sputum cultures and respiratory review once diagnosis confirmed. • **Cardiac**: may have a dilated cardiomyopathy and myocarditis. Needs Echo. Manage heart failure and arrhythmias.
Gastro-enterology	• **Oro-oesophageal candidiasis:** painful swallowing. Red painful bleeding mucosa. Can be candida. Treat with PO FLUCONAZOLE. Differential if ulcerated is CMV or HSV infection and OGD and swabs taken. If CMV consider IV GANCICLOVIR. If HSV then IV ACICLOVIR. • **Chronic diarrhoea:** some have an unknown cause. Others due to cryptosporidiosis infection. Also vulnerable to *Salmonella, Shigella, Campylobacter, Giardiasis* and some may be mixed pathogens. Leads to dehydration, weight loss due to malabsorption. Send stool cultures.
Dermatology	• **Multidermatomal herpes zoster**: can be seen with CD4 >500 cells/mm^3. Treat with ACICLOVIR 800 mg PO five times per day. Alternative is Famciclovir. Severe or ophthalmic involvement switch to IV ACICLOVIR. • **Herpes simplex**: oral, mucosal disease, hands, face. Crusted vesicles. Treat with ACICLOVIR 200 mg PO five times per day. Alternative is Famciclovir. • **Kaposi sarcoma**: purplish skin lesions. HHV6 infection.

Episode	Notes
Haematology	• Thrombocytopenia: see *Section 16.6*. • Neutropenia: see *Chapter 16*. • Lymphopenia: see *Chapter 16*.
Ophthalmic	• Any brain involvement involving optic nerve and tracts and occipital cortex can lead to hemianopia – see *Chapter 19*. • **CMV retinitis**: when CD4 count <50 cells/mm^3 or as part of IRIS (see below). Ophthalmology consult. Treat with GANCICLOVIR which may be given directly into the eye. • **Varicella zoster**: can affect ophthalmic branch of V and so the cornea. It can also cause an acute retinal necrosis simultaneously. Look for vesicular tingling and then painful rash over V1 distribution or may be multi-dermatomal. IV ACICLOVIR is given.
Antiretroviral drugs side effects	• **Lactic acidosis**: seen with nucleoside reverse transcriptase (NRTI). High mortality. Nausea, vomiting, raised lactate. • **Pancreatitis**: see with ddI, d4T and ddC drugs. • **Lipodystrophy**: d4T. • **Rhabdomyolysis**: protease inhibitors + statin. **Protease inhibitors are cytochrome p450 inhibitors**: enhanced toxicity of drugs metabolised on this pathway. Check *BNF* or equivalent. • **Toxic epidermal necrolysis/Stevens Johnson syndrome**: Nevirapine.
Immune reconstitution inflammatory syndrome (IRIS)	• Seen with introduction of antiretroviral therapy. Rapid fall in viral load and rise in CD4 count. More likely from a very low CD4 count. • There is a rise in T cells and enhanced immune response to infections that had been subclinical. Certain infections involved are: *Mycobacterium avium* complex, CMV retinitis, worsening pulmonary TB, worsening cryptococcal meningitis.

Relationship between CD4 count in cells/mm^3 and opportunistic infections	
CD4 – any	Kaposi sarcoma, pulmonary TB, herpes zoster, bacterial pneumonia, lymphoma
CD4 <250	*Pneumocystis* pneumonia, oesophageal candidiasis, PML, herpes simplex
CD4 <100	Cerebral toxoplasmosis, HIV encephalopathy, cryptococciosis, miliary TB
CD4 <50	CMV retinitis, atypical mycobacterial infection

17.4 Miscellaneous infections

Oropharyngeal infections

Organism	Notes
Glandular fever	Mentioned elsewhere – caused by CMV, EBV. Avoid amoxicillin.
Common viral	Measles, mumps, rubella, coryza and many of the common viral illnesses may cause some throat pain and associated pharyngitis.

Organism	Notes
Acute pharyngitis *Avoid ampicillin or amoxicillin*	Predominantly viral (adenovirus, rhinovirus, RSV). Management is supportive. Bacterial (*Streptococcus pyogenes* – Group A beta-haemolytic streptococci) more likely if fever and purulent tonsilar exudate and cervical lymphadenopathy without significant cough. Can confirm with rapid antigen detection test (RADT) and throat culture. Local complications include peritonsillar abscess. Treat with oral **PENICILLIN V (phenoxymethylpenicillin) 500 mg QDS** for 10 days or ERYTHROMYCIN. Complications: acute rheumatic fever, scarlet fever, post-streptococcal glomerulonephritis.
Acute epiglottitis	Acute onset of pain in throat and difficulty swallowing. Stridor and breathlessness. Usually seen in children. It may be a life-threatening compromise of the airway. *Haemophilus influenzae* type B (Hib), now less common. Now Group A beta-haemolytic streptococci has become more frequent. Drooling saliva, scared, stridor. Needs admission and rapid anaesthetic review. Treat with CEFOTAXIME or CEFTRIAXONE IV.
Diphtheria	**About:** *Corynebacterium diphtheria*, *C. ulcerans*. Fatality 5–10%. **Aetiology**: releases an exotoxin which blocks protein synthesis. Mild cases can go undiagnosed. Toxin acts as a RNA translational inhibitor. Local tissue necrosis. Toxaemia and paralysis due to demyelinating peripheral neuritis. Cardiac failure due to myocarditis. **Microbiology:** Gram-positive, aerobic, nonmotile, rod-shaped bacteria. Acquired from direct physical contact or breathing aerosolized secretion from infected person. **Clinical:** produces a grey thick membrane in pharynx. Nasal, laryngeal and pharyngeal mucosa affected. Can lead to airway obstruction and stridor. Sore throat, fever, malaise. Heart failure, heart block and arrhythmias. Cranial nerve palsies, diplopia, dysarthria, dysphagia. **Investigations**: *FBC, U&E, CRP. CXR. ECG*: heart block and arrhythmias. Culture of swabs from larynx/pharynx. Echocardiogram to assess LV function. **Management:** ABCs. Oxygen. Bed rest and telemetry initially. Isolation and treatment of the index case. Prevention with diphtheria toxoid immunisation and is also given with suspected diphtheria infection. Give BENZYLPENICILLIN IV or AMOXICILLIN IV or ERYTHROMYCIN if penicillin allergic. **Horse serum derived ANTITOXIN is given for acute infection.** Remove membrane by laryngoscopy or bronchoscopy to prevent airways obstruction. Two week course of penicillin or erythromycin. Also treat contacts. Seek expert help.
Lemierre's syndrome *First described by Lemierre in 1936 from a review of 20 cases. Mortality rate 5%.*	**About:** septic thrombosis of internal jugular vein (IJV). Smoking is a risk. **Microbiology:** *Fusobacterium necrophorum* produces a lipopolysaccharide endotoxin (leukocidin) and haemolysin which increases virulence. Also *Streptococcus* sp., *Bacteroides* sp., *Peptostreptococcus* sp., and *Eikenella corrodens*. **Aetiology:** disseminated abscesses. Septic thrombophlebitis of the internal jugular vein. Associated infection of the oropharynx due to Gram-negative anaerobic bacillus. Main sources of infection are tonsil, pharynx, and chest. **Clinical:** sore throat, painful swelling of the neck, fever, rigors. Haemoptysis and dyspnoea if lungs involved. Pustular exudates on tonsils. Thrombophlebitis of the internal jugular vein. Palsies of cranial nerves IX to XII. Septic emboli – joints, liver, spleen, osteomyelitis, meningitis.

Organism	Notes
Lemierre's syndrome – *cont'd*	**Investigation: FBC:** raised WCC, CRP, ESR. Blood cultures. **CXR**: cavitatory abscesses from septic emboli, pleural effusions. **CT thorax**: may find septic pulmonary emboli and internal jugular venous thrombosis and lung cavitation from abscesses. Pleural fluid/empyema. **Doppler USS** of neck veins shows occluded IJV. **Differential:** infectious endocarditis. Wegener's as lung lesions and ENT issues (check cANCA). **Management:** need HDU/ITU level care. Oxygen. Supportive. **Antibiotics:** take microbiological advice and consider prolonged high dose IV antibiotics, e.g. **TAZOCIN IV + METRONIDAZOLE IV**. Often sensitive to penicillin, clindamycin, chloramphenicol. Some beta-lactamase activity may be seen. **Anticoagulation with IV heparin/LMWH**: controversial and may speed recovery, though there may be worries about bleeding from septic emboli. Some reserve it only for evidence of clot progression towards cavernous sinuses, others for SVC thrombophlebitis. Those with uncontrolled sepsis and repeated septic emboli despite appropriate medical therapy, surgical ligation or excision of the internal jugular vein should be performed, although this treatment is rarely needed today. **Reference**: Golpe *et al.* (1999) Lemierre's syndrome. *Postgrad Med J*, 75:141.

17.5 Gastroenterology infections

Organism	Notes
***Clostridium difficile* colitis**	**About:** avoid use/duration of broad spectrum antibiotics as much as possible. Large Gram-positive anaerobic spore-forming bacterium. Found in the soil, bowel or environment as spores. **Aetiology:** broad spectrum antibiotics, especially cephalosporin, clindamycin and ampicillin. Rib type 027 causes a virulent form of infection with higher toxin production and quinolone resistance. **Risks:** elderly, broad spectrum antibiotics, PPI usage, antidepressants. Co-morbidities, inflammatory bowel disease. **Pathophysiology:** toxin A: enterotoxin inactivates Rho-GTPase; toxin B: cytotoxin. Toxins cause hypersecretion, disruption of tight junctions and death of colonic luminal cells. Together these cause ulceration and diarrhoea. **Clinical:** diarrhoea may begin within 4–10 days of antibiotic treatment but may be delayed up to 6 weeks. Asymptomatic to mild diarrhoea to pseudomembranous colitis with bloody diarrhoea. Copious liquid stool with fever, malaise, abdominal pain and distension and toxic megacolon. Acute abdomen, peritonitis and perforation and death. **Investigations:** FBC: raised WCC and CRP. U&E: AKI type picture. Prerenal failure. Stool culture, colonoscopy/sigmoidoscopy may show yellow adherent plaques. Anaerobic culture on cycloserine, cefoxitin and fructose (CCFA) media. EIA for detecting toxins A and B has sensitivity 80% and specificity 98%. AXR/CXR exclude perforation, ileus, megacolon. **Complications:** prerenal failure, toxic megacolon, colonic perforation. Severe disease: WCC >15, severe colitis, temp >38.5°C, raised creatinine.

Organism	Notes
***Clostridium difficile* colitis** – *cont'd*	**Management:** prevention: transmission can be reduced by good hand washing using alcohol hand gels in most infections, but not with *C. difficile* spores. Soap and water is advised. Patients should be isolated and receive either oral **METRONIDAZOLE PO** or **VANCOMYCIN PO 125 mg QDS (doses up to 500 mg QDS used when critically ill) NG or PO (capsules or give IV form orally)** until assays have proven or disproven diagnosis for up to 10 days. Loperamide and any drug which slows GI transit should be avoided. Involve gastroenterologists and surgeons in management if abdominal signs worsen (see below). Important to continue antibiotics even if nil orally. Acute surgical management especially with toxic megacolon or perforation requiring subtotal colectomy with ileostomy.

Advice	Indications to give vancomycin first line
Stop causative antibiotics. Stop antimotility agents (e.g. loperamide, opiates, etc). Stop PPIs if possible. Stop laxatives and review treatment chart for drugs that may exacerbate diarrhoea.	WCC $>15 \times 10^9$ cells/L Creatinine $>1.5 \times$ baseline Temperature >38.5°C Albumin ≤25 g/L Elevated lactate. Suspected or endoscopically confirmed pseudomembranous colitis or ileus. Major risk factors (e.g. ICU or immunosuppression). Colonic dilatation on CT scan / AXR >6cm.

Indications for surgery are age >65, WCC $>20 \times 10^9$/L, raised plasma lactate, peritonism, severe ileus, perforation or toxic megacolon. Prognosis is poor in elderly patients. About 25% can have a relapse.

Organism	Notes
Liver abscess	**Types: Pyogenic**: from appendicitis, cholecystitis. Older patients. Multiple lesions. **Amoebic**: *Entamoeba histolytica* from bowel infection. Found worldwide with highest prevalence in developing countries. Transmission is faeco-oral route. **Hydatid:** cysts usually asymptomatic and patients are well unless secondarily infected. **Clinical:** fever, abdominal pain, hepatomegaly, jaundice. Right pleural effusion, pleural rub. Occasionally abscesses are well tolerated and may present as PUO. Some will give a history of dysentery. Hydatid cyst rupture can lead to anaphylaxis. **Investigations:** *FBC*: anaemia, raised neutrophil, CRP, ALP, B_{12}. *Amoebic complement fixation text* has 90% sensitivity. *Hydatid disease* serology also useful. **CXR**: raised right hemidiaphragm. *Abdominal USS* and *CT diagnostic* for liver abscess. **Differential:** liver cyst, hepatoma, metastases.

Organism	Notes
Liver abscess – *cont'd*	**Management:** antibiotics are the first line in therapy and then some require open or radiologically guided percutaneous drainage depending on the response. • *Pyogenic*: IV antibiotics, e.g. **TAZOCIN IV tds.** Alternatives are **CEFOTAXIME IV BD**. Consider **METRONIDAZOLE** if causative organism unclear. • *Amoebic*: **METRONIDAZOLE 500 mg tds orally for 7–10 days** PO or IV if required and **diloxanide furoate** later to clear organism from bowel. Consider aspiration and drainage with radiological control. Left lobe abscesses are higher risk to rupturing into critical sites (e.g. the pericardium), which justifies more intervention. • *Hydatid cyst*: surgery remains the primary treatment and the only hope for complete cure. The puncture, aspiration, injection, and reaspiration (PAIR) technique is suggested with open surgery as a further option along with appropriate agents such as **albendazole or mebendazole**.
Gastroenteritis	**About:** usually a self-limiting bowel infection. Rarely can result in severe fluid/electrolyte loss. More severe in elderly, pregnant, immunocompromised, co-morbidities who may need admission. **Causes:** viral: norovirus, rotavirus, adenovirus, etc. Bacterial: non-typhoidal *Salmonella*, *Campylobacter*, *Shigella* (blood dysentery stools), cholera (*Vibrio cholera*, rice water stool). **Clinical:** colicky abdominal pain, diarrhoea and dehydration are main symptoms, with hypotension. Oliguria, syncope. Can be bloody diarrhoea. **Investigations:** FBC, U&E, stools for microscopy and culture. **Prevention is key:** avoid contact for 24–48 h after symptoms have stopped. Side room or home if can manage and hydrated. Hand washing soap and water. Wear glove and aprons where advised. **Management:** isolation and good hand washing and infection control. Oral rehydration therapy for mild cases. More severe need IV fluids. Most resolve without antibiotics. Severe cases consider antibiotics as below. **Antibiotics**: treat if >6 type unformed stools per day, fever, blood or significant co-morbidities beware that antibiotics should be restricted to most severe cases and most will resolve naturally. **CIPROFLOXACIN PO** is the antibiotic of choice in most infections. However, antibiotics best avoided if you suspect *E. coli* 0157 as increases risk of HUS. **METRONIDAZOLE** for giardiasis and amoebiasis. Oral **METRONIDAZOLE or VANCOMYCIN** for *C. difficile*. **CIPROFLOXACIN** or cotrimoxazole for *Shigella*. For *Campylobacter* use **ERYTHROMYCIN** PO for 5 days. Non-typhoidal *Salmonella* **CIPROFLOXACIN** for 5–7 days or **CEFTRIAXONE**. For cholera try **DOXYCYCLINE** 300 mg single dose.
Escherichia coli **infection**	**About:** disease depends on previous exposure and pathogenicity. From animal contact and foods. **Microbiology:** *clinical correlates of different forms*: • *Enteropathogenic* (EPEC) mild to severe disease with bloody diarrhoea. • *Enterotoxigenic* (ETEC) causes marked diarrhoea and vomiting. • *Enteroinvasive* (EIEC) damages colonic cells with watery (bloody) diarrhoea but no toxin, usually mild and self-limiting.

Organism	Notes
***Escherichia coli* infection** – *cont'd*	• *Enterohaemorrhagic* (EHEC) with verocytoxin (VTEC) such as 0157:H7 and others. Usually from poorly cooked food. Milk and meat. The enterotoxins can affect kidneys, heart and brain and cause HUS. Made worse by antibiotics. **Clinical:** water or bloody diarrhoea, dehydration, AKI. **Management:** self-limiting so usually supportive and oral or IV rehydration as needed. Avoid antibiotics, especially if 0157:H7 suspected.
***Staphylococcal* food poisoning**	**About:** infection from handling cheese, meats. Poor hygiene and storage. **Clinical:** sickness within 3–6 h. Mostly severe vomiting rather than diarrhoea. Toxins may act as superantigens. Severe dehydration can occur. **Management:** needs oral/IV rehydration and anti-emetics.
Shigella	**About:** *Shigella dysenteriae, Sh. flexneri, Sh. boydii, Sh. sonnei.* **Source:** contaminated food, flies, men having sex with men. Institutions. Gram-negative. Invade colonic mucosa. **Clinical:** diarrhoea, colic, abdominal pain. Bloody purulent stools. Fever and dehydration. Later Reiter's syndrome (red eye, arthritis). **Complications:** rectal prolapse, megacolon, Reiter's syndrome, HUS. **Management:** supportive. Consider **CIPROFLOXACIN**.
Enteric fever (typhoid paratyphoid)	**About:** *Salmonella typhi* causes typhoid fever (TF) and *Salmonella paratyphi* causes paratyphoid fever. Can be life-threatening unless treated promptly. **Aetiology:** infects terminal ileum and Peyer's patches and spreads via thoracic duct to lymph nodes and reticuloendothelial system. **Clinical:** usually 2–3 weeks of progressive symptoms. Dry cough. Contact to symptoms 5–21 days. Fever, headache, bradycardia (TF). Constipation or diarrhoea. Rose spots (easily missed), meningism, encephalopathy. Apathy, hypo- and hyperactive delirium is frequent (TF), hepatosplenomegaly (TF). Worsening over 2–3 week period leading to intestinal haemorrhage, bowel perforation, and death. **Investigations: blood and stool cultures** positive in first 2 weeks (stools positive in chronic carriers). **FBC**: fall in WCC and platelets. **U&E**: AKI, raised LFTs. **Serology** is possible. **Management: CIPROFLOXACIN** less effective with increasing resistance. First line is **CEFTRIAXONE IV for 10–14 days** for severe cases or where resistance suspected (acquired in Asia). Supportive care is required. Surgery for any bowel perforation. **Reference:** Fiddian–Green (2009) Treatment of enteric fever. *BMJ*, 338:b1159.
Bacillus cereus	**Source:** seen classically from fresh rice. Heat stable exotoxin. **Clinical:** severe vomiting. If toxin-producing organisms ingested may be more of a watery diarrhoea presentation. Usually self-limiting within a day. **Management:** needs oral rehydration if possible. IV if severe and dehydrated.
Cholera	**About:** infected diarrhoea or vomitus. Water-borne as survives in fresh and salt water. **Aetiology:** *Vibrio cholera* serotype 01. Toxin activates acetylate cyclase in intestinal mucosa. Causes active secretion of water and chloride. **Clinical:** acute watery diarrhoea. Significant volume loss and hypovolaemic shock.

Organism	Notes
Cholera – *cont'd*	**Investigations:** U&E: raised urea, creatinine. AKI. **Diagnosis**: dark field microscopy. **Management:** needs salt and water replacement. Oral rehydration but usually needs IV replacement. Use IV Ringer-lactate. Can lose 10 L/day which needs to be matched. Give **TETRACYCLINE or DOXYCYCLINE** or **CIPROFLOXACIN.**
Amoebic dysentery	**About:** *Entamoeba histolytica.* **Clinical:** diarrhoea. **Management:** give metronidazole PO 800 mg tds for 5 days and then **DILOXANIDE FUROATE PO 500 mg tds** to eradicate cysts.
Giardiasis	**About:** *Giardia intestinalis.* **Clinical:** acute watery diarrhoea. **Management: METRONIDAZOLE** PO 2 g OD for 3 days or PO 400 mg tds for 5 days.

17.6 Bone and joint and skin infections

Organism	Notes
Osteomyelitis *Infection of bone which can lead to pain, deformity and chronic disease if untreated*	**Aetiology:** differing picture in adults and children. Association with sickle cell disease and salmonella infection. Infection either haematogenous or direct from local wound sepsis. **Adult disease:** 60% are due to *Staphylococcus aureus*, *Enterobacter* or *Streptococcus*. In older adults the vertebral bodies are more likely to be infected, due to changes in blood flow with spinal osteomyelitis. TB still remains prevalent in certain groups. **Risks:** open fractures, prostheses, diabetes, diabetic foot, alcoholism, AIDS, immunosuppression. Sickle cell, IV drug abuse – blood spread to vertebrae, chronic steroids. **Clinical:** toxic, febrile and rigors, localised bone pain, tenderness, warmth and swelling. Children can have just vague symptoms for weeks. **Investigations:** *plain X-ray*: unreliable (will take 2–4 weeks for demineralization of bone). *CT or MRI or USS* or three-phase bone scan. *Blood cultures* are positive in 50% of cases of acute osteomyelitis. *FBC, CRP and ESR*: ESR and WCC are typically raised. *Obtain pus* by open surgery or needle aspiration. *Bone biopsy* for culture and histology. **Differential:** synovitis, trauma and fracture, bone cancer, sickle cell crisis. **Management:** rapid diagnosis and orthopaedic and microbiology liaison to choose optimal antimicrobial therapy. *Acute osteomyelitis*: **FLUCLOXACILLIN IV** +/– **SODIUM FUSIDATE** PO. *Penicillin allergy*: **VANCOMYCIN IV + SODIUM FUSIDATE PO**. Duration of therapy: usually 4–6 weeks (minimum 2 weeks IV). Discuss with microbiology. **Surgical:** debridement and removal of necrotic tissue and drainage of any abscess or collections. Replacement of dead space with tissue flaps or bone grafts. Internal/external fixation. Amputation may be needed. **Sickle cell disease:** *Staph. aureus* and salmonella often involved organisms.

Organism	Notes
Septic arthritis *An infected joint needs urgent assessment and treatment so discuss immediately with orthopaedics to enable aspiration and treatment*	**About:** infected joint can become a permanently painful and destroyed joint. Involve orthopaedic team and microbiology immediately. **Aetiology:** destruction of cartilage begins within 48 h due to pressure, proteases and cytokines from macrophages, bacteria and inflammatory cells. **Microbiology:** *Staph. aureus*, *Streptococci*, *Gonococci*, Gram-negatives, Lyme disease, salmonella (sickle cell). Viral – hepatitis B, parvovirus B19, and lymphocytic choriomeningitis viruses. **Risks:** immunosuppressed (those with RA particularly) and elderly people. Prosthetic joints are at increased risk. Recent joint injections, e.g. steroids, diabetes. Sickle cell, IV drug user, disseminated gonococcal infection. **Clinical:** new joint pain/swelling or increase in usual pain, erythema. Immobility (held in maximal position of comfort), systemic fever. Knee 50%, hip 22% and shoulder. Also ankles, wrists, elbow, and PIPs and DIPs. Also sternoclavicular and sacroiliac joints in generally decreasing frequency. Note that concurrent immunosuppression can dampen clinical findings. **Differential:** gout, pseudogout, fracture, reactive arthritis, osteoarthritis. RA itself does not give this presentation but it can have secondary infection. Crystal deposition uncommon in RA affected joints. **Investigations:** *FBC*: raised WCC, ESR, CRP, U&E, LFT, bone, urate, glucose, blood culture, CXR. *Joint aspiration*: turbid pus with raised WBC, predominantly neutrophils. Send aspirate for Gram stain, microscopy for crystals and culture. Consider *urethral culture* for gonococcus or skin lesion if STD likely. *Plain X-rays* to look for bony changes. *Ultrasonography:* can detect effusions and synovial changes. *MRI* can show bone and joint destruction and osteomyelitis. *Radionuclide leucocyte scans* can detect inflammation. **Management:** urgent consult with orthopaedics as requires joint aspiration. This will relieve pressure and pain and provide microbiological information. **FLUCLOXACILLIN IV**. Add **GENTAMICIN IV** if coliforms are likely. If *N. gonorrhoea* likely give **CEFTRIAXONE IV**. For penicillin allergy consider **VANCOMYCIN IV** (adjusted to renal function) + **SODIUM FUSIDATE PO** (not to be used IV). Contact consultant microbiologist if risk factors for, or evidence of, MRSA colonisation or infection or HIV positive patient. Orthopaedic review as arthroscopy or open surgery may be required. **Prosthetic joint infections:** all cases of prosthetic joint infection should be discussed with the microbiologist and should be seen by orthopaedics team. Empirical therapy is usually not indicated unless patient is septic. Later physiotherapy and rehabilitation may be required.

17.7 CNS infections

Organism	Notes
Bacterial meningitis	See *Section 19.3*.
Viral encephalitis	See *Section 19.2*.
Brain abscess	See *Section 19.3*.

Organism	Notes
Neuro-cysticercosis	See *Section 19.3*.
Rabies *Uniformly fatal*	**About:** found worldwide. Lyssavirus of *Rhabdovirus* family. Zoonosis. Encephalomyelitis. Acquired via dog or other animal bite. Infectious phase 1–3 months. Less if wound is head and neck. **Clinical:** hydrophobia, agitation, tremor, muscle spasms, ascending flaccid paralysis. **Investigations:** saliva, CSF PCR. Negri bodies within cytoplasm. Brain biopsy of dog. **Management:** there is no effective treatment. ITU care. Supportive. Post-exposure prophylaxis with antirabies immunoglobulin and vaccination can be tried.
Tetanus *Clostridium tetanus seen mostly in Western world in older non-immunised adults*	**About:** prevention is the key. **Aetiology:** obligate anaerobe Gram-positive bacillus with a drumstick spore produces tetanospasmin which causes clinical signs and lethality. Damage to interneurons inhibiting motor nerves. Travels from distal lesion in reverse axonal transport to the cord. Toxins: tetanolysin and tetanospasmin. **Clinical:** symptoms seen weeks after stepping on nail with spores, wounds. Hypertonic muscles with rigidity, spasms, clonus and ophisthotonus. Contraction of masseter gives trismus, cranial nerve palsies (cephalic tetanus). **Investigations:** FBC, U&E, LFT, check FVC, ABG, ECG. **Prognosis:** adverse findings: short IP, rapid onset, acquired from burns, wound, umbilical stump, septic abortion, delayed treatment, head or neck lesion. **Management:** supportive. Admit to ITU. Give HUMAN TETANUS IMMUNOGLOBULIN or IMMUNE EQUINE TETANUS IMMUNOGLOBULIN. Antibiotics: IV METRONIDAZOLE may be preferable to IV PENICILLIN. Intubation and ventilation if needed, nutrition, skin care, physiotherapy, sedation. Manage any seizures as indicated – diazepam or lorazepam. Spasms: diazepam, baclofen, muscle relaxants, magnesium. Monitor for autonomic complications. Survival usually results in a full recovery.

Renal emergencies

18.1 Haematuria

Taking referral / answering bleep

- When did it start? Quantity? Clots? Is patient passing urine or in retention?
- Pyrexial, pain – cystitis/pyelonephritis? Recent catheterisation? Prostate disease? Pregnant? Known bladder malignancy? On any anticoagulants?
- 30% of patients with painless haematuria have a malignancy.

Investigations

- FBC, U&E, CRP, urinalysis. Cystoscopy, intravenous urogram, renal USS. β-hCG.
- PSA and formal microscopy, culture and sensitivities.
- CRP/echocardiogram/blood cultures if endocarditis considered.
- False positive dipstick for blood may be seen with menstruation or trauma (which includes vigorous exercise or sexual activity within 24 hours or local lesions – ulcers, warts.

On arrival

- Indications for admission include clot retention, cardiovascular instability, uncontrolled pain, sepsis, acute renal failure, coagulopathy, severe co-morbidity, heavy haematuria or social restrictions.
- Those not needing admission should drink plenty of clear fluids and return for further medical attention if the following occur: clot retention or worsening haematuria despite adequate fluid intake, uncontrolled pain or fever, or inability to cope at home.
- Repeat observations and review medications and consider stopping anticoagulants depending on their need. Hypotension or tachycardia may suggest sepsis or haemorrhage.
- Follow-up by a urological team should be arranged promptly, ideally within the 2-week cancer referral target. Consider bladder and prostate cancer in those males over 40. In those under 40, cystoscopy may not be mandatory if another cause found.
- **Significant macroscopic (visible) bleeding** can cause clot retention resulting in outflow obstruction and often a three-way catheter irrigation system should be used. In bleeding of this severity, reverse all anticoagulation and get urological advice. Ensure check Hb and replace blood. **Will need urgent cystoscopy** if persists and imaging of whole renal tract.
- **Microscopic haematuria** (not visible but positive dipstick) and protein consider as UTI. Lack of protein in dipstick could suggest tumour or stones.
- **Microscopic haematuria and proteinuria** consider nephrology and a more medical cause, e.g. glomerulonephritis.

Causes	Notes
Urinary tract infection (cystitis and pyelonephritis)	Commonest cause. Pain, dysuria, blood, protein, leucocytes in urine. Positive cultures. Confusion, suprapubic discomfort. Usually elevated WCC and CRP. May present as acute confusion or 'off legs' in the elderly.

Causes	Notes
Traumatic bladder catheterisation	Often seen post-catheter or any form of instrumentation. Exacerbated by any antithrombotics. Bleed should settle, but if it persists investigate.
Bladder cancer	Common in older population and needs cystoscopy for diagnosis, staging and treatment.
Renal cell cancer	Look for a renal mass, fever, USS or CT abdomen. Bladder cancer: persisting haematuria. Cystoscopy.
Prostate cancer	Elevated PSA, bony metastases, prostatism, hard craggy prostate on PR. Urology referral.
Prostatitis	Pain and UTI like symptoms.
Renal stones	Pain loin to groin. Passing grit in the urine.
Thrombocytopenia	Check FBC and causes.
Antithrombotics and anticoagulants	Warfarin, dabigatran and other NOAC, aspirin and clopidogrel and heparin can worsen bleeding and are not uncommon causes. Need risk assessed on temporary stopping or reduction of dose.
Infective endocarditis	Murmur, raised CRP, stigmata of endocarditis, needs echo.
Acute glomerulonephritis	Haematuria and proteinuria. May be RBC casts and dysmorphic RBCs. Check anti GBM, ANCA, ASO titres and usual renal work up.
IgA nephropathy	Glomerulonephritis: younger patients than other causes.
Tuberculosis	Weight loss, overseas, CXR, sterile pyuria classically.
Sickle cell	Usually known sickle cell anaemia.
Schistosomiasis	Overseas exposure due to *Schistosoma haematobium*. Also called bilharzia. Chronic bladder inflammation. Risk factor for bladder cancer.
False positive dipstick	Myoglobinuria, e.g. rhabdomyolysis.

18.2 Reduced urinary output (oliguria)

Taking referral / answering bleep

- If patient catheterised, assess amount of urine produced in last few hours. Quantify input oral and IV and losses in the past few days. Oliguria: <500 ml/day urine output which is about 20 ml/h. Anuria usually suggests obstruction.
- If the patient has poor intake and is not in heart failure then speed up fluids over next 30–60 min and review. Oliguria might suggest hypoperfusion and sepsis or other causes of shock. Attend quickly if low BP, raised temp, raised HR, raised Early Warning Score.
- If anuric think obstruction first. Has patient any suprapubic pain or is catheter blocked or is it acute retention. Reasonable to ask staff to flush or change the catheter if one is in place. Bladder scan will tell you if bladder full or empty and then catheterise. If obstruction still considered then a renal USS is usually diagnostic.
- If low BP assess as for hypotension. If renal cause suspected ask about new drugs or IV contrast for an X-ray or angiogram that could precipitate or cause AKI. Is there rhabdomyolysis or severe infection?

On arrival

- What's the BP, HR, temp? In most cases the cause is pre-renal and the patient just needs careful fluid replacement. Ensure accurate fluid balance chart. If low BP then treat and manage as pre-renal AKI. Get IV access. Look and treat individual causes. Omit antihypertensive on drug chart. Correct any volume loss.
- If BP normal then look for renal and post-renal causes. Catheterise if unsure of output. Is there a residual volume? If so leave catheter in for now and monitor.
- Check bloods – if high urea and creatinine and you have given volume replacement and excluded pre- or post-renal causes then this suggests AKI – manage supportively and discuss with renal team. You may have to refer for dialysis to manage hyperkalaemia, pulmonary oedema. Make sure there are no pre- or post-renal problems.
- If the patient is euvolaemic and still remains oliguric then it may be useful to try diuretics to get some renal flow. Discuss with renal team. Those with post-renal causes need to be discussed with urology for surgical or radiologically placed drainage before definitive management. See *Section 18.3* for more information.

Differential

- Recording error – fluid balance underestimates urine output.
- Pre-renal failure – oliguria and recent hypotension. Cardiogenic, haemorrhagic shock, sepsis, obstructive shock. Excessive antihypertensives.
- AKI – ischaemic, nephrotoxic drugs, nephritis.
- Post-renal – obstruction at renal pelvis, ureters, bladder, urethra. Stones, tumour, prostate.

18.3 Acute kidney injury

About

- AKI has replaced the term 'acute renal failure' to emphasis potential reversibility.
- Sudden rapid reduction in GFR and there may be oliguria and anuria.
- Mortality varies from 10 to 80% depending on population studied. Increased length of stay and mortality.
- Prevalence of AKI is about 5% in hospital patients. A minority need a nephrologist. Most managed by generalists. Only 1% need dialysis.

RIFLE and AKIN classification for AKI in adults

Stage	Creatinine (μmol/L)	Urinary output
1: Risk	Creatinine >120, increased by >26 within 48 h Creatinine >×1.5–1.99 baseline value <7 days	<0.5 ml/kg/h for 6 consecutive hours
2: Injury	Creatinine × 2 (creatinine >240) Creatinine >× 2.0–2.99 baseline value <7 days	<0.5 ml/kg/h for 12 consecutive hours
3: Failure	Creatinine increased ×3 or >354 mmol/L or dialysis needed	<0.3 ml/kg/h for 24 consecutive hours or anuria for 12 h
Loss	Complete loss of function needing RRT >4 weeks	
End	End stage renal disease needing RRT >3 months	

Risk factors for AKI

- Age >75, CKD (eGFR <60 ml/min/1.73m^2) cardiac failure, liver disease, DM.
- Peripheral vascular disease, nephrotoxic medication, hypovolaemia, sepsis.

In a nutshell

- Simple questions – pre-renal? Clues are low BP and oliguria. Requires fluid replacement. Is it post-renal with oliguria/anuria, e.g. obstructed kidney, ureter, bladder, urethra seen on renal USS which needs surgical urostomy?
- Lastly that leaves renal where the management may involve immunosuppression or simply cessation of toxic medications and time and supportive measures for acute tubular necrosis (ATN) to resolve.

In rapidly progressive glomerulonephritis early management may save nephrons. If you suspect vasculitis, e.g. systemically unwell, rash, fever, raised CRP, pulmonary haemorrhage, seek nephrology help immediately.

- If Wegener's/Goodpasture's syndrome suspected then get an urgent cANCA/anti-GBM and refer to nephrology team immediately.

Reduced renal function

- Impaired control of water and electrolytes. Impaired excretion of drugs and other metabolites. Impaired acid–base control – need to excrete acid load.
- Impaired BP control, impaired EPO synthesis, impaired vitamin D hydroxylation.

Causes	Notes
Acute tubular necrosis (45%)	Acute fall in GFR: tubule cell damage and cell death. Ischaemia or toxin driven. Ischaemia usually due to prolonged prerenal failure. There can be recovery over 1–2 weeks with diuresis. May also be due to nephrotoxic drugs or DIC or myoglobinuria, radiocontrast.
Prerenal failure (21%)	E.g. shock, hypovolaemia, sepsis, heart failure, cirrhosis.
Acute or chronic renal failure (13%)	Mostly due to ATN and pre-renal disease.
Urinary tract obstruction (10%)	Stones, tumour, papillary necrosis, surgical.
Glomerulonephritis	Neoplasia, autoimmune, drugs, genetic abnormalities and infections.
Rapidly progressive glomerulonephritis	Vascular/vasculitis (4%) – Wegener's granulomatosis, HUS, TTP, hypertension, scleroderma, renal artery stenosis.
Acute interstitial nephritis	Hereditary, systemic, toxic and drug-induced.
Atherosclerosis / emboli	Atherosclerosis/emboli.

Clinical

- Malaise, lethargy, delirium, nausea, vomiting, generalised anorexia. Volume depletion suggesting pre-renal with postural hypotension and tachycardia.
- Oliguria helps define AKI but is non-specific. Anuria suggests post-renal obstruction. Polyuria: CKD with impaired renal concentrating ability or hypercalcaemia or an osmotic load (glucose) or diabetes insipidus.
- Breathless and haemoptysis – pulmonary oedema, consolidation, alveolar haemorrhage with vasculitis (Wegener's granulomatosis or Goodpasture's syndrome). Pericardial rub due to uraemic pericarditis. A pericardial effusion may be seen on echo or CXR. Occasionally this may progress to tamponade.

- Skin: palpable purpura, neuropathy might suggest vasculitis. Skin pigmentation, pallor and itch are common with evident scratch marks. Impaired platelet function and bruising is seen.

State		Investigations
Acute pre-renal (60%)	Hypotensive, shocked, tachycardia. Acute setting. Burns, gastrointestinal losses, sepsis. **Uraemia**: drowsiness, poor appetite, itch, encephalopathy, pericardial rub. Late: seizures and coma.	Low urine Na <20 mmol/L. Low urine specific gravity. USS: normal kidneys. Old tests show normal creatinine.
Acute renal (25%)	Uraemic symptoms. Nephrotoxic drugs, vasculitis, pulmonary renal syndromes (Wegener's, anti-GBM disease). Acute tubular necrosis. Acute interstitial nephritis.	Normal urine Na >40 mmol/L. Intrinsic renal disease: proteinuria and haematuria and red cell casts. Normal urine specific gravity. USS: normal kidneys. Old tests show normal creatinine.
Acute post-renal (15%) *'clot, calculus, compression, cancer'*	Uraemic symptoms + anuria or oliguria. Prostatic symptoms, Cervical carcinoma or other gynaecological tumours, retroperitoneal fibrosis, tumour, clot.	USS: normal kidneys but evidence of obstruction with dilated system. Old tests show normal creatinine.
Chronic	Absence of signs or symptoms of an acute illness. Progressive uraemic symptoms. Diabetes, hypertension. Chronic fatigue. Multiple co-morbidities. Polyuria and nocturia if concentrating defect.	USS: small kidneys (not amyloid or diabetes of polycystic kidney disease). Normocytic normochromic anaemia, low calcium. Raised phosphate. Old tests show raised creatinine.

Investigations

- **FBC and film**: anaemia not typical with ARF, look for an alternative cause. Raised WCC, platelets? Haemolysis? Microangiopathic anaemia – check blood films.
- **Urinalysis** shows blood, protein and red cell casts on microscopy. Positive protein values of 3+ and 4+ on reagent strip testing of the urine suggest intrinsic glomerular disease and this is reinforced if there are a high number of red cells. Increased white cells (>5 per high power field) are non-specific but are found more commonly with acute interstitial nephritis, renal or urinary tract infection and glomerulonephritis.
- **U&E:** raised urea and creatinine. May be raised potassium.
- **Calcium:** hypocalcaemia – CKD, hypercalcaemia – malignancy, myeloma, primary hyperparathyroidism.
- **LFTs:** albumin is low with nephrotic syndrome. **Blood glucose:** elevated with diabetes.
- **ABG:** to assess the severity of acidaemia associated with AKI and any respiratory compromise. Metabolic acidosis with failure of the kidneys to remove organic acids and regenerate bicarbonate.
- **Coagulation tests** can be abnormal if DIC associated with sepsis.
- **Blood cultures:** if sepsis is suspected.

- **Creatine kinase:** rise suggests rhabdomyolysis or acute MI.
- **CXR:** pulmonary oedema or alveolar haemorrhage. Cavitating lesions suggesting a pulmonary/renal syndrome.
- **ECG:** look for cardiac disease (LVH, STEMI/non-STEMI) or hyperkalaemia.
- **CT renal tracts:** exclude structural lesion or retroperitoneal fibrosis.
- **Renal USS:** perform within 24 h if obstruction suspected. Assess renal size and exclude obstruction.
- **Renal biopsy:** shows a crescentic type picture in rapidly progressive glomerulonephritis. Biopsy if suspected glomerulonephritis / rapidly progressive glomerulonephritis / tubulointerstitial nephritis or vasculitis. Raised ESR – myeloma or infection. Raised CRP if infection/vasculitis/autoimmune disorder.
- **PPE and urine Bence-Jones:** always do both when looking for multiple myeloma.
- **Autoantibodies:** ANCA (MPO and PR3), anti-GBM Goodpasture's syndrome. Check ANA, dsDNA.
- **Complement** C3 and C4 and cryoglobulins. **HIV test**: where risk factors exist.
- **Magnetic resonance angiography** (MRA) if suspicion of renal artery stenosis.

Prevention

- Some causes are predictable and preventable. Those at risk of contrast-induced AKI (CI-AKI) should have pre-procedure volume expansion with NS or isotonic sodium bicarbonate if clinically indicated. Currently there is no compelling evidence for the routine use of *N*-acetylcysteine to prevent CI-AKI. Those at risk of developing AKI secondary to rhabdomyolysis should receive IV volume expansion with NS and sodium bicarbonate.
- In those at risk of AKI, nephrotoxic drugs should be stopped or used sparingly and doses adjusted to match for renal clearance and to avoid nephrotoxicity.

Management

- **Hyperkalaemia:** refractory hyperkalaemia related to AKI needs dialysis so urgently contact the renal team.
- **Exclude POST-RENAL cause with renal tract obstruction:** if obstruction is possible, then get a renal USS <24 h to exclude an obstructive cause and if so liaise with urology. A catheter placed in the bladder will relieve any possible prostatic or urethral obstruction. If a per-urethral catheter cannot be placed due to an enlarged prostate or urethral stricture then a suprapubic catheter is needed. The finding of a dilated ureter and hydronephrosis will require percutaneous nephrostomy. Inserting a urinary catheter in a patient with AKI (indeed in any patient) introduces the risk of a UTI and should be made on an individual basis and is dependent upon the cause of the AKI, e.g. bladder outflow obstruction, the clinical context, and severity of illness. If a urinary catheter is required it is important not to routinely administer gentamicin as antibiotic cover, because it is nephrotoxic. Remove catheter as soon as it is not adding value as risk of iatrogenic urosepsis.
- **Medical management:** if non-obstructive liaise closely with renal physicians. The cause may be obvious, such as volume depletion or intravascular loss or renal toxic drugs, and management is by cautiously correcting fluid balance and stopping or adjusting doses of all drugs to take into account the current renal function, or lack of. In mild cases renal function will improve over several days with cautious fluid management. In those with impaired cardiac function small challenges with 250 ml fluid aliquots and then reassessment of urine output and fluid balance and pulse and postural BP is reasonable. In selected severe

cases central vein catheterisation may help to estimate CVP and arterial lines can help measure BP. Once fluid balance is normal, then watch for an improvement in urine output suggesting pre-renal cause. If a hydrated patient is oliguric and non-obstructed then a diuretic stimulus with FUROSEMIDE 100–120 mg may be given slowly IV over 10–20 min. A failure to respond suggests that things have progressed beyond simple pre-renal failure and we may be dealing with ATN. There is no evidence for furosemide or dopamine in the management of AKI.

- Manage euvolaemia with **fluid replacement = output + 500 ml per day**. Frequent assessment of BP/HR/skin turgor. Daily weights and other clinical assessments of volume should be done. Normal enteral nutrition should be maintained as much as possible. Stop/avoid drugs such as ACE inhibitors, NSAIDs, AT2 blockers and reduce the dose of other drugs that are renally cleared.
- Always refer to the *BNF* for specific prescribing advice. Further investigations such as renal biopsy are for the nephrologists to deal with. There may well be a return of function in the short term over the first few weeks, but in some patients cortical scarring means a progressive course into chronic renal failure and a need for lifelong renal replacement strategies. AKI following the administration of radiological contrast tends to occur within 72 h and often resolves after around 5 days.
- **Specialist management:** where rapidly progressive glomerulonephritis is suspected then quick card test for cANCA and anti-GBM and, once confirmed, then rapid transfer to renal team to consider immunosuppressives.
- **Post-renal failure:** once post-renal causes are treated there may be a marked diuresis which needs to be compensated for in the fluid management plan. Frequent monitoring of U&E is required.
- **Renal replacement management:** it may be that conservative measures are insufficient and urgent renal replacement therapy is indicated. Usual indications are listed below. The patient will need either ITU for haemofiltration or renal unit transfer. Haemofiltration is most commonly used acutely as volume shifts are less and can be provided in an ITU set up. Be sure to talk to your intensivists and renal physicians early before this situation arises if at all possible.
- **Urgent renal replacement:** AKI plus refractory hyperkalaemia, AKI plus pulmonary oedema, AKI plus severe acidosis (pH <7.2), AKI plus encephalopathy, AKI plus bleeding due to uraemia and pericarditis. Ethylene glycol poisoning.

References:

www.renal.org/clinical/guidelinessection/AcuteKidneyInjury.aspx

KDIGO Group (2012) Clinical practice guideline for acute kidney injury. *Kidney Int Suppl*, 2:1.

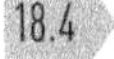

18.4 Urinary tract infections

About

- UTI usually symptomatic bacterial infection of the urinary tract.
- Kidney (acute pyelonephritis) – young females.
- Bladder (acute cystitis) – young females.
- Prostate (prostatitis) – older males, due to urinary infection, in younger often an STI.

Note

- Asymptomatic bacteriuria (ABU) does not itself require treating in uncomplicated patients. UTI denotes symptomatic disease. However, ABU during pregnancy is associated with complications such as preterm birth and perinatal mortality for the fetus and with pyelonephritis for the mother.
- Treatment of ABU in pregnant women decreases the risk of pyelonephritis by 75%. Uncomplicated UTI refers to acute cystitis or pyelonephritis in non-pregnant outpatient women with a normal anatomy and no instrumentation of the urinary tract.

Risks

- Catheterisation or instrumentation of urinary tract, pregnancy.
- Post-coital: void afterwards because organisms milked into bladder.
- Diabetes mellitus (women only), incontinence, lack of circumcision in men.

Microbiology

- *E. coli* accounts for 85%. *Staphylococcus saprophyticus* for 10%.
- Others include *Klebsiella, Proteus, Citrobacter, Pseudomonas aeruginosa*.
- Gram-positive enterococci and *Staphylococcus aureus* and even yeasts.

Clinical

- General malaise, fever, nausea and vomiting, most often female.
- Pyelonephritis: classically unilateral loin pain, rarely bilateral, fever, rigors.
- Cystitis: suprapubic discomfort, frequency, dysuria.
- Prostatitis: dysuria, perineal pain, frequency.

Investigations

- **FBC, U&E, CRP:** raised WCC and CRP. U&E typically normal unless underlying renal issues.
- **Urine dipstick: test for nitrites.** Not all bacteria convert nitrate to nitrite, and a sufficient concentration must be present to be detectable. Test for **leukocyte esterase**: enzyme found in polymorphs in the urine. Either is a positive test when the clinical picture is suggestive. A negative dipstick test is not good enough to exclude bacteriuria in pregnant women – send a sample for culture.
- **Urine microscopy**: a WCC can be a useful indicator as per the table of infection before a culture result is available at 24 h. As can be seen, a lower threshold is used in women than men.
- **Urine culture**: gold standard but contamination from poor sampling can complicate matters.
- **USS renal** can be considered in recurrent UTI to exclude anatomical issue.

Diagnostic criteria for UTI

Level of coliforms/WCC to call it a UTI	Patient group
$\geq$100 coliforms/mm^3 + 2 samples WCC $\geq$10/mm^3	Symptomatic young females
$\geq$100 coliforms/mm^3	Symptomatic young females
$\geq$1000 coliforms/mm^3	Symptomatic male
$\geq$100 000 coliforms/mm^3 on two occasions	Asymptomatic young females/males

Complications

- Bacteraemia and urosepsis.

- **Diabetic:** obstructive uropathy associated with acute papillary necrosis causing AKI if bilateral.
- Staghorn calculi if chronic infection develops, renal/perinephric abscess formation.
- Emphysematous pyelonephritis where gas-forming bacteria proliferate.

Management

- If vomiting ensure adequate hydration, analgesia and nutrition and IV fluids. Look for and treat any causes. Once urine has been sent for culture (in some patients, e.g. confused incontinent older female – sampling is very difficult and in these cases it can be prudent and pragmatic to treat empirically rather than wait for a sample that can never be obtained).

Infection	Management
Cystitis/lower UTI (simple cystitis without fever or loin pain)	Take advice if urosepsis or there has been a multi-resistant pattern in antibiotic sensitivity seen in previous isolates. **NITROFURANTOIN 50–100 mg QDS PO** (avoid if creatinine clearance is less than 60 ml/min, G6PD deficiency, porphyria) OR **TRIMETHOPRIM 200 mg BD PO** (if creatinine clearance is less than 60 ml/min or if nitrofurantoin is not tolerated). Duration of treatment: 3 days in non-pregnant women, 7 days in men.
Cystitis/lower UTI: (simple cystitis without fever or loin pain) and PREGNANT	Approximately 2–10% of pregnancies are accompanied by ABU and of these 40% develop infection. Most due to *E. coli*. Screening at 12–16 weeks. Send a sample for culture and sensitivities. **AMOXICILLIN** and **CEPHALOSPORINS** for 1 week are safe and effective. Avoid trimethoprim where pregnancy possible.
Acute pyelonephritis	**CO-AMOXICLAV (Augmentin) 1.2 g tds IV**. Switch to oral CO-AMOXICLAV 625 mg tds PO when apyrexial >48 h. If pyrexial after 48 h, consider renal USS to exclude renal abscess. Review with results of culture. Treat for 2 weeks. **IV ERTAPENEM 1 g OD** or **IV GENTAMICIN 5 mg/kg OD**. Take advice if pregnant.
Indwelling urinary catheters	Antibiotic treatment is not required unless patient is systemically unwell. Treatment should follow antibiotic sensitivity test result with changing/removal of the catheter. For empirical management: discuss with consultant microbiologist.

18.5 Renal colic

About

- Calculi in kidney and/or ureters. Care in those with single kidney or CKD.
- Renal stones seen in 10% of adults at some time. Admit under Urology.

Stones

- Calcium oxalate and calcium phosphate in 80% (radio-opaque).
- Urate stones in 10% (radio-lucent). Cystine in 1% (radio-opaque).
- Struvite (magnesium ammonium phosphate) in 5% (radio-opaque).

Causes

- Distal renal tubular acidosis, idiopathic hypercalcaemia and hyperparathyroidism.

- Cystinuria, polycystic kidneys, dietary or internal hyperoxaluria. Hyperuricosuria.
- Stone formation exacerbated by hot climates with resultant oliguria.

Clinical

- Excruciating back or abdominal or flank pain: 'loin to groin/labia'.
- Patient writhing around in agony, **unlike** peritonitis who lie still.
- The pain can last minutes or hours and there can be intervals of no pain.
- Chronic distension is painless.
- Can be associated nausea, vomiting, frequency, dysuria, oliguria, and haematuria.

Investigation

- **FBC: raised** WCC and CRP can suggest infection (urinalysis positive too).
- **Urinalysis:** nitrites suggest UTI. Red cells compatible with stone disease.
- **AXR (kidneys–ureter–bladder):** sensitivity for stones 45–60%.
- **U&E calcium and urate**: ensure no stone-forming causes and renal function.
- **β-hCG:** if pregnancy possible.
- **Non-contrast helical CT abdomen:** accuracy > 95%. Detects radio-opaque and radio-lucent stones. No need for intravenous contrast medium.
- **Intravenous urography (IVU):** shows level of ureteric obstruction and defines pelvicaliceal anatomy. It can miss some radio-lucent ureteric or renal stones (10–20% of stones). It is about 70–90% accurate.
- **USS renal tracts:** use in pregnancy, in children, and in febrile people. A low 50% diagnostic accuracy for stone detection, but main use is to diagnose hydronephrosis in people with complicated renal colic.

> Special care must be taken with those with renal stones and pre-existing renal disease, single kidney, kidney transplant, bilateral renal obstruction, pregnancy.

Differentials

- Appendicitis (pain is right-sided), diverticulitis (pain is left-sided).
- Ectopic pregnancy, pyelonephritis, salpingitis in women, ruptured AAA.

Management

- **Conservative:** try to sieve all urine to catch stone which can be sent for biochemical analysis. Encourage oral fluids as needed and maintain hydration and urine flow. In general, patients whose stones are 5 mm or less in diameter have a good chance of spontaneous passage, whereas the chance of spontaneous passage for larger stones diminishes considerably. 80–85% of stones pass spontaneously and so management is conservative and mainly pain control and in uncomplicated cases care may be at home. Advise the person left at home to seek urgent medical assistance if fevers or rigors, pain worsens or abrupt recurrence of severe pain.
- **Caution:** admit under Urology those with signs of infection, single or transplanted kidney, pre-existing renal impairment, bilateral obstructing stones are suspected, significant analgesic need, dehydration and unable to maintain oral intake, pregnancy, patient preference, diagnosis uncertain in older patient or ectopic pregnancy in younger female. Choices for analgesia include DICLOFENAC 100 mg PR or 75 mg IM which may be repeated up to 150 mg per day. DIAMORPHINE or MORPHINE. Antiemetic: consider CYCLIZINE 50 mg IV or METOCLOPRAMIDE 10 mg IM (avoid in those <20 years old). Reduce the dose by 25–50% in moderate or severe renal impairment.

- **Medical expulsive therapy:** α1-adrenergic blockers are indicated for those with adequate renal function reserve with a newly diagnosed distal ureteric stone (less than 10 mm), whose symptoms are controlled, and who have no clinical evidence of sepsis. TAMSULOSIN OD is the drug of choice and has been shown to reduce time to expulsion and need for intervention. NIFEDIPINE XL 30 mg daily can also increase stone expulsion rate from 35% to 79% when combined with a steroid. PREDNISOLONE 10 mg BD in a 5 day burst can be added to both. This may be helpful by reducing the intense inflammatory reaction. Tamsulosin preferred over nifedipine as it has fewer side effects.
- **Surgical removal:** consider if stone does not pass with basket extraction, surgical removal or lithotripsy.
- **ESWL:** (lithotripsy) focused sound waves fracture stone. Non-invasive and can be done as outpatient.
- **Percutaneous nephrolithotomy:** used for larger stones and staghorn calculi. A nephroscope is inserted into renal pelvis and collecting system and stone broken up and extracted.
- **Ureteroscopy** can be done with a laser to break up the stone. Ureteric injury low in experienced hands.
- **Open surgery**: done with large stones, multiple stones, etc.
- **Discharge:** if pain settles and there is no stone or the stone is 5 mm or less on KUB X-ray, the patient may be discharged with an NSAID orally, e.g. Voltarol 50 mg tds. An urgent IVU should be requested and referral to urology. If the pain does not settle admit. Higher risk patients are those with a solitary or transplanted kidney, pre-existing renal impairment or where bilateral obstructing stones are suspected.

Complications

- Urinary tract obstruction and upper UTI. Pyelonephritis, pyonephrosis, urosepsis can ensue. AKI.

18.6 Renal obstruction

About

- Cause of post-renal failure. Complete obstruction causes anuria.
- Early treatment (usually surgical/radiological) can restore renal function.
- Can occur at any level from renal calyces to the distal urethra. Admit under Urology if diagnosis suspected.

Aetiology

- Normal sites of narrowing are junctions between renal pelvis and ureter, ureter and bladder, bladder and urethra (bladder neck) and urethral meatus.
- Acquired causes and congenital cases seen in children.

Causes

- Congenital narrowing usual at sites mentioned above; posterior urethral valves.
- Phimosis and meatal stenosis. Infection with oedema and scarring.
- Tumour – cervix, uterus, colorectal, bladder, prostate.
- Debris: blood clots, sloughed papillae, benign prostatic hypertrophy.
- Pregnant uterus pressure, retroperitoneal fibrosis.
- Malignancy extrinsic compression – cervical, ovarian, bowel.
- Abdominal aortic aneurysm. Trauma at any level.
- Neurological – diabetic neuropathy, spinal cord disease.
- Accidental ligation at abdominal surgery.

Aetiology

- Depends on whether obstruction is slow and progressive.
- Depends if it affects both or a single kidney.
- Is there underlying renal disease?

Clinical

- Acute obstruction: pain due to build up of hydrostatic pressure in kidney.
- Bilateral acute obstruction: anuria and AKI.
- Partial obstruction: polyuria and nocturia as concentrating ability impaired.
- Chronic picture: hypertension and polycythaemia.
- Look for phimosis or meatal stricture, full bladder, flank pain or abdominal masses.
- PR examination for prostate enlargement and rectal tumour.
- Gynaecological exam: uterine or cervical or ovarian disease.

Investigations

- **Bloods:** FBC, U&E, CRP: check anaemia, infection, WCC, AKI, Ca, CRP.
- **Urinalysis**: protein, leucocytes, glucose.
- **Bladder scan**: urine in bladder, post-voiding volume.
- **Non-contrast CT** is modality of choice. **IVU**: can delineate level of stenosis.
- **USS renal tracts**: useful to see obstruction and a dilated system with hydronephrosis or hydroureter.
- **Voiding cystourethrography**. Antegrade/retrograde urography for renal pelvis and ureter.

Management

- Urgent relief of obstruction is needed to restore function and reduce risk of urosepsis. Drainage by nephrostomy/ureterostomy/urethral or suprapubic catheter as is appropriate.
- **Supportive**: manage hydration, electrolytes and acid–base balance. Treatment of any infection. Individualised treatment of particular cause. There is often a post-obstruction diuresis following treatment requiring fluid replacement to avoid pre-renal problems.

Neurology emergencies

19.1 Acute delirium / confusion

Taking referral / answering bleep

- What is patient doing and how long for? How were they yesterday? Is it new?
- Why is patient in hospital? Check set of observations.

On arrival

- See notes, review observations and medication. Confusion in new admissions with poor cognitive reserve is common and may suggest some serious issues and poorer prognosis. Is this confusion, psychosis or dysphagia?
- Determine if this is confusion on a background of milder confusion or normality.

The Confusion Assessment Method

(A) Acute onset and fluctuating course	Is there evidence of an acute change in mental status from baseline? Does abnormal behaviour come and go? Fluctuate during the day? Increase/decrease in severity?
(B) Inattention	Does the patient have difficulty focusing attention? Are they easily distracted? Do they have difficulty keeping track of what is said?
(C) Disorganized thinking	Is the patient's thinking disorganized, incoherent? Does the patient have rambling speech/irrelevant conversation? Unpredictable switching of subjects? Unclear or illogical flow of ideas?
(D) Altered level of consciousness	Alert, vigilant, lethargic, stuporous, comatose.

Confusion assessment method: delirium = A + B + either or both C and D (Inouye)

Assessment

- A comprehensive clinical assessment from top to toe needed as well as drug history and try to get as much corroborating history as possible. Work through common causes, e.g. infection (chest / urine), metabolic (low Na), malignancy (high calcium), drugs, e.g. codeine.
- Establish baseline. Use and record answers to the mental test score (MTS) or some standard questions in terms of cognition, orientation to time and place, speech, comprehension and attention span.
- The abbreviated MTS can be done or the more complex mini mental state examination. Any recording of cognition is useful.

Abbreviated mental test score (AMTS)

- What is your age? (1 point)
- What is the time to the nearest hour? (1 point)
- Memory test, e.g. an address which should be told and then tested at end (1 point)
- What is the year? (1 point)
- What is the name of the hospital or number of the residence where the patient is situated? (1 point)
- Can the patient recognise two people (the doctor, nurse, home help, etc.)? (1 point)
- What is your date of birth? (day and month sufficient) (1 point)
- In what year did World War 1 begin? (1 point)
- Name the present monarch/dictator/prime minister/president (1 point)
- Count backwards from 20 down to 1 (1 point)

Causes	
Hypoglycaemia	Check capillary blood glucose.
Occult head injury	Was there head trauma which has been missed by emergency department? Is a CT needed? Look for bumps and abrasions and cuts. Blood in ear canal.
Sepsis	Chest: pneumonia. UTI, meningitis (a very common cause in elderly). Assess temp, WCC, CRP. CXR. Check urine and treat empirically. Consider LP.
Delirium tremens	Hyperactive with long alcohol history and withdrawal (give Pabrinex IV/ Thiamine before glucose IV).
Wernicke's encephalopathy	Eye signs, delirium, ataxia, B1 deficiency.
Acute stroke	Dysphasia often misinterpreted as confusion.
Acute pain	Elderly person and acute urinary retention, or fractured neck of femur, or acute abdomen, or MI. Agitated. Incoherent.
Cardiac	ACS/silent MI, elderly, diabetes.
Hypoxia and hypercarbia	Check ABG, CXR, COPD, carbon monoxide.
Drugs	Illicit drugs: cocaine, heroin, amphetamines; codeine, opiates (may be a patch), tramadol, morphine, L-dopa, alcohol, large dose steroids, anticholinergics.
Acute psychosis	Schizophrenia or other mental health disorder.
Metabolic	Hyponatraemia, liver failure, renal failure, myxoedema madness, thyrotoxicosis, hypercalcaemia, Addison's disease, pituitary failure, SIADH.
Vitamin	Thiamine deficiency, B12 deficiency.
Malaria	Travel or endemic area send thick/thin films. Treat if real possibility.
Structural brain pathology	Abscess, stroke, SAH, encephalitis, meningitis, tumour, hydrocephalus; CT scan helpful. Consider LP.
Seizure or non-convulsive status	EEG, CT/MRI/ LP. Treat and see if resolves.
Malignancy	Hypercalcaemia, liver metastases, brain metastases.
Inflammatory disease	Any acute inflammatory illness or flare up.
Encephalitis	Infectious, autoimmune.
Creutzfeldt–Jakob	Can quickly deteriorate over weeks. Myoclonus is a helpful clue. CSF elevated protein 14-3-3.

Investigations

- Blood glucose, FBC, ESR, U&E. Calcium, B12 and folate. TFTs. Urinalysis.
- CXR, ECG – silent MI. ABG – hypoxia, hypercarbia.
- CT head: can be difficult but looking for major pathology, e.g. SDH, haemorrhage, tumour, oedema, etc.

- Lumbar puncture: meningitis/encephalitis/SAH.
- In some cases EEG. Malaria thin and thick films.

Management

- **Supportive**: manage anxiety. Low dose Haloperidol acutely if in danger or very unsettled, keep lights on, calm, friendly reassurance, involve family members. Work through potential causes as listed above. May need mild sedation or even full sedation and airway management for a CT brain.
- **Sedation:** go slow. **LORAZEPAM 1–4 mg PO/IM/IV** can be tried or **HALOPERIDOL 1–5 mg PO/IV/IM/SC (low doses 0.5–2 mg in elderly)** are useful. Get help if risk of over-sedation and airway management. Very low threshold for a CT head is needed.
- **Antibiotics/Aciclovir:** if suspicion for bacterial meningitis and HSV encephalitis treat both. Get LP.
- **Thiamine IV** as PABRINEX prior to dextrose IV. Look and treat hypoglycaemia quickly.
- **Stop opiates.** Remove any transdermal opiate pain patch and give naloxone.
- **Give phenytoin** if non-convulsive status. Measure ammonia: ?encephalopathy.

Reference: Inouye *et al*. (1990) Clarifying confusion: the confusion assessment method. A new method for detection of delirium. *Ann Intern Med,* 113:941.

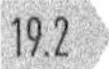

19.2 Viral encephalitis

For HSV encephalitis aciclovir IV greatly improves mortality and morbidity.

About

- Serious form of encephalitis due to *Herpes simplex* and West Nile virus.

Aetiology

- Acute inflammation of brain parenchyma +/– spinal cord in adults due to **HSV-1**.
- Favours temporal lobes, frontal and limbic system. Haemorrhagic necrosis.

Clinical and viral causes

- **General:** headache, fever, pyrexia, reduced GCS, hemiparesis, altered speech, psychosis/delirium, brainstem signs. Enquire about recent exposure to ticks or travel to areas with endemic viral encephalitides.
- **HSV:** "general" + cold sores, high fever, temporal lobe involvement. Younger.
- **VZV:** "general" + widespread vesicular rash. All ages.
- **West Nile virus** (WNV): (arbovirus mosquito). Erythematous rash. Age >50. 10% fatality.
- **Japanese encephalitis:** (arbovirus) "general" + movement disorder.
- **Enterovirus:** Coxsackie/Echo virus. Seen in summer/autumn. General symptoms.
- **Others:** measles, mumps, rubella, rabies, EBV, HIV JC virus.

Investigations

- **FBC:** raised WCC, CRP. U&E: may see hyponatraemia.
- **CT:** to exclude abscess and to show lesions in the temporal lobes. May be necrosis and haemorrhage.
- **MRI:** temporal lobe oedema/necrosis with HSV. Thalamic changes with WNV.
- **Lumbar puncture:** if no C/I. CSF raised lymphocytes and protein. PCR for HSV / WNV (West Nile virus) if suspected. Bloody CSF can result in a falsely negative PCR.
- **EEG:** slowing and periodic discharges.

- **Brain biopsy**: HSV encephalitis shows neuronal inclusion bodies called Cowdry Type A, found in the neuronal nucleus.

Poor prognostic indicators for HSV

- Age >30. Coma at presentation. Bilateral EEG abnormalities.
- High CNS viral load, treatment delayed (4 days), abnormal CT.

Management

- **ABC**, O_2 as per BTS guidelines. Arrange imaging, **LP** and **CSF** to confirm diagnosis. Monitor renal function. ITU involvement if low GCS. Specialist advice.
- Any suspicion of the diagnosis must give **ACICLOVIR IV × 21 days**. Untreated HSV is a tragedy with disability and death. Treatment reduces mortality from 54% to 28%. Check CSF is free of HSV before ending treatment. Suspected CMV infection Ganciclovir IV.
- Ensure hydration and NG feeding as required. Often initially managed in HDU setting. Of those who survive there is a high risk of on-going neurological deficits. There is no evidence base for steroids.

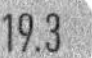

19.3 Acute bacterial meningitis

> Typical empirical therapy does not cover *Listeria* species which should be considered in older, diabetic or immunocompromised patients.

About

- Bacterial infection in the subarachnoid space. Notifiable disease.
- Delayed treatment increases mortality and morbidity.
- Difficulty is those with an atypical presentation. Treat on clinical suspicion alone.

Aetiology

- Pneumococcus/meningococcus/HiB all capsulated.
- They colonise nasopharynx and secrete IgA protease.

Pathology

- Purulent exudate in the subarachnoid space. Loss of cerebral autoregulation.
- Localised thrombophlebitis and vasogenic oedema.
- Arterial/venous thrombosis and infarction. Protein levels rise.

Infection	Notes
***Streptococcus* pneumonia**	Main adult cause. Related to pneumococcal pneumonia, sinusitis, otitis media. Commoner in alcoholics. Diabetes, post-splenectomy, complement deficiency, basal skull fractures and CSF rhinorrhoea. Give BENZYLPENICILLIN if sensitive. **CEFTRIAXONE IV or CEFOTAXIME IV.** VANCOMYCIN IV may be added. 2 week course.
Neisseria meningitidis	Epidemics type A and C. Affects children and adolescents. Petechial (non-blanching) rashes or purpura are vital to early diagnosis. Complement deficiencies, e.g. properdin, increase risk. Septicaemia – Waterhouse–Friederichsen syndrome with adrenal haemorrhage causing shock. DIC. Haemorrhagic rash. **BENZYLPENICILLIN** if sensitive. **CEFTRIAXONE IV or CEFOTAXIME IV.**
Haemophilus influenzae	Reduced due to HiB vaccination. **CEFTRIAXONE IV or CEFOTAXIME IV.**

Infection	Notes
Gram negatives	Seen in debilitated, diabetics and cirrhotics. Post-craniotomy. **CEFTRIAXONE IV or CEFOTAXIME IV**. 3 week course.
Group B streptococci	Traditionally a neonatal infection. Now being seen in all ages including elderly. **BENZYLPENICILLIN or AMPICILLIN**.
Listeria monocytogenes	Elderly, pregnant and immunocompromised. Food-borne – soft cheese, coleslaw and undercooked meats. **AMPICILLIN IV 3 week course**. GENTAMICIN IV daily may also be given. Listeria is resistant to cephalosporins and so not covered by empirical treatment. May cause brainstem signs.
Staphylococcus aureus	VANCOMYCIN is drug of choice.
Viral meningitis	Usually benign. Suspected HSV meningitis consider Aciclovir if severe. Any neurology beyond headache and meningism consider encephalitis.
Cryptococcal (fungal)	Seen in immunosuppression, e.g. AIDS (see *Section 17.3*), lymphoma. **AMPHOTERICIN B IV**.

Clinical

- Neck stiffness, meningeal irritation, resists passive neck flexion; Kernig's sign: patient supine with thigh flexed back to abdomen and knee flexed.
- Pain elicited on straightening the knee; Brudzinski's sign: supine and flexing neck causes flexion of hips and knees. Signs may be muted in the young and elderly or immunocompromised.
- Chest infection, craniotomy, rhinorrhoea, petechiae (non-blanching), hands and feet and conjunctiva.
- Atypical presentation with delirium, stroke-like episodes, falls.
- Unexplained fever, nausea, vomiting, photophobia, seizures, with progression – VI nerve palsy, papilloedema. Reduced level of consciousness, decerebrate posturing, falling heart rate, raised BP.

Complications

- Seizures, stroke from arterial/venous thrombosis, hyponatraemia.
- Raised ICP, hydrocephalus, cerebral abscess/empyema, and cerebral herniation.

Investigations

- **FBC, U&E, CRP, blood cultures** should be taken immediately and antibiotics commenced.
- **CT/MRI scan** if any suggestion of raised ICP or focal signs or reduced level of consciousness, or papilloedema, or immunocompromised, or elderly, or recent seizure. Family physicians may treat on suspicion prior to cultures being done. Take as soon as possible after.
- **LP and CSF analysis** if possible, but not if there is coagulopathy (petechiae) or CT suggests an imminent herniation syndrome.
- **CSF: raised WCC** (neutrophils) >1000/mm^3, raised protein, low glucose and raised CSF pressure. PCR for bacterial DNA. Latex agglutination to pneumococcus, meningococcus, influenzae, *E. coli* and Group B streptococci. Very high protein and low glucose are bad prognostic predictors. Cryptococcal antigen in CSF or blood.
- Biopsy of petechial skin lesions can reveal organisms.

Differential

- Viral meningitis, HSV encephalitis, Rocky Mountain spotted fever in USA, SAH.
- Acute disseminated encephalomyelitis. Cerebral abscess.
- For those with HIV/AIDS see *Section 17.3*.

Management

- **Supportive**: ABCs, O_2 as per BTS guidance. Manage care in an HDU or ITU setting.
- **Antibiotic choice:** treat on suspicion then follow up with investigations, but endeavour to get LP and CSF before antibiotics. However, if delayed start CEFTRIAXONE IV or CEFOTAXIME IV as initial blind therapy. CSF will guide therapy as will patient's age. This does not cover *Listeria* so if considered (age >55, pregnant, immunocompromised) then add AMPICILLIN for 14 days). Meningitis post-head injury/neurosurgery/brain abscess: MEROPENEM IV. If you suspect penicillin-resistant pneumococcus then add VANCOMYCIN IV. Suspect pseudomonas then add VANCOMYCIN + CEFTRIAXONE. Cryptococcal meningitis needs AMPHOTERICIN B IV.
- **Close contacts receive:** RIFAMPICIN. Take microbiological advice if unsure. Staff do not need prophylaxis unless they gave mouth to mouth resuscitation.
- **Steroids:** adults with proven or suspected pneumococcal meningitis should receive Dexamethasone 10 mg IV QDS for 4 days. Reduces mortality, improves functional outcome. Start with first dose of antibiotics.

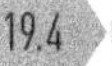

19.4 Brain abscess

Risk factors

- Alcoholism, immunodeficiency, skull fracture, associated mastoiditis or localised infection. Dental abscess, bronchiectasis, TB, AIDS, endocarditis.

Microbiology

- *Staphylococcus aureus* from penetrating skull trauma.
- Pseudomonas from ears, anaerobes and streptococci from oral cavity.
- Mixed infections. Immunocompromised – toxoplasma and nocardia.

Clinical

- General malaise, drowsiness, symptoms of space-occupying lesion. Headache, focal seizure. Delirium.
- Neurological signs, poor dentition. Evidence of neglect/alcoholism.

Investigations

- **Bloods**: elevated CRP, WCC. Blood cultures, HIV serology.
- **Echocardiogram**: endocarditis. **CXR**: bronchiectasis, exclude lung tumour.
- **CT brain with contrast /MRI brain with gadolinium**: shows ring-enhancing lesions. Look for hydrocephalus and signs of raised ICP. Look for any radiological signs of local sepsis, e.g. sinusitis, mastoiditis.
- **LP** avoided due to risk of coning and herniation syndrome.

Management

- Stereotactic biopsy and culture to confirm diagnosis and identify organism.
- Antibiotics (given IV and accompanied by surgical aspiration or excision): *oropharyngeal/dental source*: Cefuroxime + Metronidazole. *Middle ear infection*: Ampicillin + Metronidazole. *Mastoiditis/sinusitis*: consider adding Ceftazidime or Gentamicin. *Penetrating trauma*: Flucloxacillin. Take Microbiology advice.
- Anticonvulsants may be needed. Neurorehabilitation.

Neurocysticercosis

About

- Tapeworm (*Taenia solium)* infection ingested from infected food or water.
- Widespread outside Europe. Cysts form in the CNS.

Clinical

- Epilepsy, cerebellar and brainstem signs, dementia. May be asymptomatic.

Investigations

- **Bloods:** leukocytosis, eosinophilia, and raised ESR.
- **CT/MRI:** lesions in different stages: vesicular, colloidal and nodular–granular stage.
- **CSF:** raised protein, oligoclonal bands, eosinophilia.

Management

- May develop hydrocephalus needing external ventricular drainage.
- Needs **PRAZIQUANTEL** or **ALBENDAZOLE** combined with steroids.
- Management of seizures. Biopsy rarely needed.

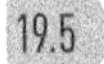

19.5 Seizures and status epilepticus

About

- Epilepsy is a tendency to have seizures so need at least 2 to diagnose.
- Status diagnosed if a seizure persists 5+ minutes without regaining consciousness or seizures quickly recur.
- Few single seizures will last more than several minutes.
- Status epilepticus (SE) is a medical emergency. Mortality for SE is 17–26% (by older definition). 10–23% of patients who survive are left with new or disabling neurological deficits.

Causes

- Primary epilepsy, pre-eclampsia (pregnant >20 weeks, BP >140/90, proteinuria).
- Hypoglycaemia, encephalitis, meningitis, space occupying lesion.
- Brain tumour, brain abscess, haematoma, stroke – bleed or ischaemia.
- Cerebral vasculitis, severe hyponatraemia, severe hypocalcaemia, head trauma.
- Low anticonvulsant levels – compliance, dosing, interactions. Sepsis, acute alcohol or alcohol withdrawal.
- Cocaine, opiates, overdose of tricyclics or phenothiazines. Idiopathic, pseudoseizures, cerebral malaria.

Advice: things to check

- Is there suspicion of a structural lesion needing CT brain and/or LP?
- Consider causes of coma and treating for such.
- Drugs that lower fit threshold: alcohol commonest, cocaine, TCAs, theophylline.
- Drug withdrawal, e.g. alcohol and sedatives. Exclude hypoglycaemia.
- Infection, particular HSV encephalitis, chest and urine. Brain tumour/abscess.

Clinical

- Usually generalised cry and then fall, and patient then has rhythmic contraction of limbs and is unresponsive. In SE the fit-like movement and unresponsiveness remains or recurs.
- A witnessed history of the fit is vital to making the diagnosis.
- Some will recall have a preceding aura: smells, tastes, especially with a temporal lobe focus.

- Tongue biting and urinary incontinence all suggest a generalised seizure as a differential. Most seizures are followed by a post-ictal phase of several hours for complete recovery which is useful in differentiating from other causes of collapse which recover quickly, e.g. vasovagal and Stokes–Adams attacks.
- Nocturnal seizures – wake up with headache, wet bed, bruises, confused.

Seizure classification

- **Generalised:** involve cerebral hemispheres. There is loss of consciousness. Different forms are absence, atonic, tonic-clonic, tonic, myoclonic.
- **Simple partial**: these can be simple partial in which awareness and consciousness are unaffected, for example, motor (e.g. jerking and movements), sensory, transient weakness or loss of sensation, autonomic and even psychic. No LOC and patient can give clear history. Differential is TIA and migrainous aura. Usually self terminate without treatment.
- **Complex partial**: consciousness or memory impaired automatisms (such as lip smacking, picking at clothes, fumbling), unaware of environment, may wander, amnesia for seizure events, mild to moderate confusion during, sleepy afterwards.
- **Partial seizures that evolve to generalised seizures:** can be an initial simple or partial seizure.

Differential of seizures

- **Generalised convulsive movements**: syncope with jerking movements, severe rigors in obtunded patient, cardiorespiratory compromise with anoxic seizures, non-epileptic attack disorder.
- **Drop attacks**: cardiac disorders, cataplexy, metabolic disorders, vertebrobasilar ischaemia.
- **Transient motor attacks**: tics, TIA, spasms, movement disorders.
- **Confusion or fugue states**: transient global amnesia, hysteria, intermittent psychosis, encephalopathy.

Investigations

- **Bloods:** FBC, U&E (hyponatraemia), Ca and Mg. **LFTs:** alcohol withdrawal.
- **Glucose:** hypoglycaemia.
- **CRP:** infection or inflammation, vasculitis, malignancy. **ECG** should be done.
- **Brain imaging**: low threshold to CT acutely and then later MRI when stable if needed. MRI is the imaging modality of choice, but acutely CT is more available, quicker and allows monitoring.
- **EEG** is useful but not usually immediately available, but very useful in diagnosing non-epileptic attack disorders.
- **Lumbar puncture** post-seizure if encephalitis/meningitis or SAH or HIV suspected.
- **Toxicology screen** for cocaine or other drugs if suspected. Anticonvulsant levels should be taken for later assessment.
- **Prolactin level (PRL)** goes up with generalised and some focal seizures but not with pseudoseizures. Take within 30 min of post-ictal period. If elevated may be useful at a later date to determine baseline PRL level as mild hyperprolactinaemia is not uncommon in the general population for various reasons.

Management

Time	Actions
0–10 min	ABC and start O_2 as per BTS guidelines. Monitor with 10 min temp, BP, pulse, GCS and pupils. Note time of onset to know duration. Place in safe recovery position. Protect airway and head. Get IV access (send bloods: U&E, glucose, Ca, Mg, anticonvulsant level, toxicology if needed). Manage in an area with appropriate monitoring and staff ratios. Do not insert anything in the mouth. Fit usually terminates in 2–5 min. No need to give any medications if this is the case. IV access, fluids and monitor. If at any time seizure has self-terminated and not recurred after several minutes, then manage supportively and allow to wake up after post-ictal period. Continue to monitor for further seizures and look for precipitant.
0–30 mins	On-going seizure. Close monitoring. Glucose: 50 ml of 50% solution +/– thiamine 250 mg IV or as Pabrinex if any suggestion of alcohol abuse or impaired nutrition. Start Phenytoin or Fosphenytoin infusion unless already on oral phenytoin. See alternatives below. If seizures continue or airway management needed get anaesthetic help and consider for ITU. Start fluids, e.g. 1 L NS over 4 h.
0–60 mins	Get anaesthetic help if airway unsafe or GCS <8 and not quickly improving. If the fit has terminated and the patient is simply post-ictal there is no need to give anything. Establish aetiology if possible. Identify and treat complications.
30–90 mins	If fit continuing then need to transfer to ITU. EEG monitoring. Consider monitoring intracranial pressure. Revision of AED therapy.
EEG monitoring	Necessary for refractory status. Consider the possibility of non-epileptic status. In refractory convulsive SE, the primary end-point is suppression of epileptic activity on the EEG, with a secondary end-point of burst-suppression pattern (that is, short intervals of up to 1 second between bursts of background rhythm).

Phenytoin loading dose should be given slowly (over 30–60 minutes) with cardiac monitoring at no more than 50 mg/min.

Acute AED therapy

- **Prehospital**: diazepam 10–20 mg given rectally, repeated once 15 minutes later if SE continues to threaten, or midazolam 10 mg given buccally. If seizures continue, treat as below.
- **Lorazepam** (IV) 0.1 mg/kg (usually a 4 mg bolus, repeated once after 10–20 min; rate not critical). Give usual AED medication if already on treatment. For sustained control or if seizures continue, treat as below. Should be given within first 10 min if seizure on-going or quickly recurs. Alternatives are diazepam (Diazemuls) 5–10 mg slow IV up to 20 mg. Midazolam 5 mg slow IV up to 10 mg IV. With all these drugs watch for respiratory depression.
- **Phenytoin**: consider IV loading dose of PHENYTOIN or FOSPHENYTOIN with cardiac monitoring. If the patient on phenytoin then send level and consider maintenance phenytoin IV dose only or consider another agents. DO NOT give phenytoin IM. *Never mix phenytoin with a 5% dextrose solution*. Phenytoin has zero order kinetics, resulting in a large exponential rise in serum concentration as the

dose increases. Watch levels (therapeutic range 10–20 mg/L or 40–80 μmol/L). Oral dose is 300 mg per day. Switch to preferred oral agent later.

- **Refractory seizures**: general anaesthesia. Choose one of **Propofol** OR **Midazolam** or **thiopental sodium** titrated to effect (the dose regimen is beyond this text and the patient will be under ITU care); after 2–3 days infusion rate needs reduction as fat stores are saturated. Anaesthetic continued for 12–24 h after the last clinical or electrographic seizure, then dose tapered.

Simple uncomplicated seizure

- **Discharge**: consider discharge if known epilepsy, full recovery to baseline, well, self-caring independent patient, seizure was short lasting and terminated without sedation. Prefer patient to be under supervision or a responsible adult to check-up on patient and on normal adequate anticonvulsant therapy. Arrange neurological follow-up if needed.

Other considerations

- **Hypoglycaemia**: check blood glucose and give 25–50 ml 50% dextrose if hypoglycaemic or once sample taken and suspicion. Excess opiates: consider naloxone (0.4–2.0 mg slow IV) if opiate toxicity possible or suspected.
- **Ask why**. Exclude encephalitis (consider Aciclovir IV if possible), drug toxicity, metabolic causes, sepsis (check WCC, lactate). Look for head injury, alcohol withdrawal. Have a low threshold to neuroimaging and LP. If there are additional signs suggestive of HSV encephalitis or meningitis then treat empirically. Try to obtain collateral history and context so as to determine cause. Is there head injury, drugs, history of epilepsy and medications taken? If the patient is pregnant then always consider eclampsia.
- **Complications:** aspiration pneumonia, rhabdomyolysis, AKI, trauma, dislocated shoulders.
- **Malnourished or alcoholic**: consider Pabrinex IV or THIAMINE IV (see Investigations section above). This is really to prevent precipitating Wernicke's encephalopathy before you give lots of glucose IV.
- **Pregnancy and eclampsia**: give **Magnesium IV** in addition to lorazepam and get obstetric help. If seizures continue then load with anticonvulsant. Choice will depend if patient already taking AED. Choice of phenytoin, fosphenytoin or valproate IV is available (see below).
- **Recovery:** patients who present with generalised seizures are expected to awaken gradually. If the level of consciousness does not improve by 20 min after cessation of movements, or the mental status remains abnormal 30–60 min after the convulsions cease, non-convulsive SE (NCSE) must be considered or some other explanation should be sought.
- **Pseudoseizures** (non-epileptic attack disorder)**:** difficult diagnosis because many are incredibly convincing and a patient with enough drive can end up intubated and ventilated. EEG and neurology input should help. Some do also have genuine seizures and some have never had seizures but have convinced neurologists they do and are on several agents and it can be near impossible to untangle.

Starting anticonvulsants

- For first seizure the need for on-going AEDs depends upon the presence of an on-going precipitant and the ability to avoid precipitants. In most cases medication is not commenced after a single seizure. Where there is an active on-going precipitant, e.g. a tumour or a structural abnormality, then sodium valproate 300 mg BD which can be titrated upwards is reasonable, as is phenytoin, carbamazepine or newer agents such as lamotrigine. Efficacy varies little between drugs and choice is more limited by side-effects and interactions and pregnancy. All patients with first seizure should have a specialist neurology review. Pregnant patients require neurological consult before starting any agent. **Agents:** PHENYTOIN 300–450 mg per day, VALPROATE 800–2000 mg per day, carbamazepine 400–1000 mg per day. For a second generalised tonic–clonic seizure try sodium valproate and second line is lamotrigine. Lamotrigine can worsen myoclonic seizures in those with juvenile myoclonic epilepsy. For focal seizures carbamazepine is first line and lamotrigine second line. For absence seizures then consider valproate or ethosuximide or lamotrigine. Specialist input recommended.

- **General advice**: further refinement should be left to the neurologist. In the meantime advice regarding no driving, avoiding machinery or situations where unexpected loss of consciousness would cause harm, e.g. using hazardous machinery, cycling in traffic, climbing ladders or swimming unaccompanied (this list is not comprehensive), then advice to curtail the activity should be given until more specialist assessment. DOCUMENT DRIVING ADVICE GIVEN IN NOTES.
- **Sudden unexpected death in epilepsy** (SUDEP). Rare. May occur after a generalised tonic–clonic seizure. Commoner in those with over 3 GTCS per year, those not on AEDs or sub-therapeutic levels, early adulthood and epilepsy of long duration and mental retardation. May be related to suffocation exacerbated by central apnoea. Related to nocturnal seizures.
- **SE in pregnancy:** establish the ABCs, and check vital signs, including oxygenation. Maternal airway and oxygenation should be maintained at all times. Get obstetric team – assess the fetal heart rate or fetal status. Rule out eclampsia – BP, urine, platelets, LFTs (see above). IO or venous access should be in SVC distribution. **If seizures associated with eclampsia then use magnesium sulphate**. If seizure persists give **LORAZEPAM or DIAZEPAM** as per usual protocol**. Consider PHENYTOIN IV**. Check laboratory findings, including electrolytes, AED levels, glucose, and toxicology screen. If signs of fetal distress consider urgent delivery. Delivery should be expedited following a seizure during labour, and neonatal expertise should be available. Liberally use CT to exclude intracranial pathology if fits are atypical or symptoms or signs suggest new pathology or worsening baseline pathology, e.g. enlarging meningioma. Women with epilepsy should be delivered in a consultant-led maternity unit and one to one midwifery care given during labour. Low threshold for epidural anaesthesia. AED medication should be continued during labour and post-natally in women unable to tolerate oral medication. An elective Caesarean section should be considered if there have been frequent tonic–clonic or prolonged complex partial seizures towards the end of pregnancy.
- **Possible causes of first fit in pregnancy:** idiopathic, eclampsia, sagittal vein thrombosis, anti-phospholipid syndrome, infarction, intracerebral haemorrhage, thrombotic thrombocytopenic purpura, amniotic fluid embolism, gestational epilepsy, alcohol withdrawal, brain tumour, SAH, vasculitis and other causes.

References:

Arif *et al*. (2008) Treatment of status epilepticus. *Semin Neurol,* 28:342.
NICE (2013) CG137: Epilepsy.

19.6 Non-convulsive status epilepticus

About

- Patient is comatose due to ongoing seizures. A cause of delirium in the elderly.
- Possibly under-diagnosed condition. Consider treatment with benzodiazepine.

Aetiology

- All age groups – infants to elderly. May follow benzodiazepine withdrawal.
- May follow a generalised seizure in a patient who fails to recover quickly.
- Less metabolic derangement. Risk of sustaining focal damage.

Clinical

- Anorexia, aphasia, mutism, amnesia, catatonia, coma, confusion, delirium, lethargy, agitation/aggression, automatisms, blinking, crying, delusions, echolalia, staring, facial twitching, laughter, 'stroke-like' state. Mislabelled as TIA or acute delirium.
- Nausea/vomiting, nystagmus/eye deviation, perseveration, psychosis tremulousness.

Investigations

- FBC, U&E, CRP: as for SE.
- **CT brain scan**: may show underlying pathology, e.g. tumour, stroke, haemorrhage, abscess, encephalitis.
- **EEG**: diagnostic generalised spike and slow wave discharges.

Management

- Minimal evidence of lasting neurologic deficits due to NCSE.
- Try midazolam at 1 mg/dose, and assessing clinically for a definite clinical or EEG improvement. Stop if any respiratory depression, hypotension, or other adverse effect.
- Additional treatment is to start PHENYTOIN IV or FOSPHENYTOIN or other AED and assess clinical response. Investigations and management are much the same as SE (see *Section 19.4* above).

Reference: NICE (2013) CG137: Epilepsy.

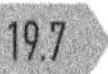

19.7 Neuroleptic malignant syndrome

About

- Seen in 1 in 200 individuals taking antipsychotic drugs. Mortality 10%.

Causes

- Neuroleptics, e.g. HALOPERIDOL (Haldol), METOCLOPRAMIDE.
- Withdrawal of L-DOPA and DOPAMINE agonists. Restart medication.

Clinical

- Exhaustion, dehydration, hyponatraemia, catatonic, pyrexia even >41°C.
- Impaired consciousness and even catatonic.
- Tachycardia, autonomic instability, severe muscle rigidity.

Investigations

- FBC, U&E: elevated WCC/CRP. AKI, elevated urea and creatinine.
- CK >1000 mmol/L. Check Ca^{2+}, Mg^{2+}, TFTs.

Management

- **ABC. High FiO_2** as per BTS guidelines. Consider ITU.
- Intensive care may be needed if GCS <8. Ensure cooling and adequate hydration.
- Dantrolene sodium and Bromocriptine and also levodopa, pergolide, benzodiazepines.

19.8 Transient ischaemic attacks

Definition

- Focal transient ischaemia of the brain or retina lasting <24 h (in reality often <20 min). TIA and small strokes are risk factors for large disabling strokes. Risk is greatest in the days following TIA.
- TIA patients should be seen urgently in a stroke prevention (TIA) clinic in order to confirm diagnosis, rapid screening and manage risks factors.

TIA differentials

Causes	Notes
Migraine with aura	Usually the aura part is confused with TIA. May be positive flashing lights, fortification spectra, a moving scotoma with a bright margin, word-finding difficulties, stuttering expressive dysphasia like episode (never receptive in my experience) tingling and paraesthesia. The headache usually comes on later. Common in young and females but may commence in later years. Migraine aura and no headache is acephalic migraine. Stereotypical repeated episodes likely migraine.
Hypoglycaemia	Always exclude. Usually diabetics on hypoglycaemic agents. Acute alcohol. Quinine. Insulinoma.
Hypocalcaemia anxiety attack	Especially with hyperventilation with tingling and generalised weakness.
Partial motor/ sensory seizures	Sensory symptoms, tingling, slow progression over a minute moving over face and arm. Unwanted movements in face, hand or leg have been reported with TIA. Needs EEG and MRI to exclude irritative focus. Ask about other seizure-like activity. See *Section 19.4*. Difficulty with speech associated with focal seizure 'speech arrest'.
Pre/syncope	Often easy as there is a global deficit. TIA does not cause presyncope or syncope, though a vasovagal may be associated with tingling and transient neurology.
Transient global amnesia	A historical diagnosis and if the history is compatible then no further action needed. Not TIA. Aetiology unclear. Benign.
Optic neuritis	A visual loss from optic neuritis. Sensory or motor symptoms. Usually coming on over hours rather than seconds.
Pressure neuropathy	A radial, common peroneal nerve, median nerve, ulnar nerve. Usually in setting where nerve compressed.
Others	Anything can be referred to a TIA clinic from dizziness caused by a PE, to subdural haematoma (SDH), to known brain metastases and anxiety states. Even a large SDH with shift can give transient focal neurology.

Aetiology

- Thrombotic: localised plaque stenosis causing typical episodes as flow drops.
- Embolic: from cardiac or aorta. Unlikely to cause identical events as embolus can go anywhere in brain circulation. Left/right and anterior/post circulation symptoms/signs.
- Difficult: are they microscopic bleeds, seizures, functional, anxiety?

Clinical

- Unilateral weakness of face/arm/leg. Variable hemisensory loss – face/arm/leg.
- Transient dysphasia, transient ataxia, transient hemianopia, or transient monocular blindness.
- Ask about headache – can suggest haemorrhage/stroke/migraine/temporal arteritis.
- Look for AF, residual neurology, and temporal artery tenderness. Residual weakness, mild or subtle dysphasia, ataxia. Look for pronator drift. Difficulty heel/toe walking. Look for hemisensory loss.
- Listening for bruits is useful but the decision for carotid imaging depends on symptoms of ipsilateral carotid territory ischaemia.

Clinical TIA less likely with:

- +ve phenomena, e.g. flashing lights, fortification spectra.
- Isolated vertigo without other brainstem symptoms. Bilateral symptoms.
- Syncope or presyncope or altered consciousness. Memory loss.
- Repeated stereotypical episodes for weeks/months would seem to be unusual for TIA – ?focal seizure.
- Unlikely to be cardioembolic if same neurological deficit each time.

$ABCD_2$ score (risk score) – non diagnostic and assumes correct diagnosis	
Age: >60 (+ 1)	**Blood pressure**: **SBP** >140 and/or **DBP** >90 mmHg (+ 1)
Clinical: unilateral weakness (+2) or dysphasia/dysarthria no weakness (+1)	
Duration: 10–59 mins (+1), >60 mins (+2)	**Diabetes** (+1)
Repeated episodes in 1 week gives an automatic score of 4 (high risk) **Risks:** score of 6–7 gives 2 day stroke risk of 8% and 7 day risk of 12%. Score of <4 gives 2 day risk of 1% and 7 day risk of 1% (Lancet, 2007;369:283). Others consider those with repeated episode, a carotid bruit or AF as a high risk priority.	

Investigations

- **FBC, U&E, ESR** (giant cell arteritis) with headache or amaurosis fugax, age >50. Fasting blood glucose and lipids.
- **CXR:** especially in smokers (lung cancer + brain metastases).
- **ECG, echocardiogram** (age <50, abnormal ECG, murmur, recent MI).
- **Carotid doppler** scan in those with TIA and potential candidate for endarterectomy.
- **CT brain:** can help exclude TIA mimics or infarction/haemorrhage.
- **MRI with diffusion weighted imaging**: modality of choice (the more prolonged the episode the more likely to see changes).

Comments

- TIA can be a soft diagnosis – by definition there are no residual signs or symptoms and imaging may be entirely normal. With stroke and imaging the diagnosis is far more solid.

- The stroke physician must weigh up the history in the context of *a priori* risk and the likely probability of a TIA that could suggest imminent stroke. Avoid labelling unexplained 'odd spells' as TIA.

Management

- **ASPIRIN 300 mg OD (or loading dose CLOPIDOGREL 300 mg then 75 mg OD)** immediately without CT scan (transient neurology is very rarely haemorrhagic). Start simvastatin 40 mg OD.
- We do not generally admit high risk TIA referrals unless very concerned (most are not TIAs) but see them immediately in TIA clinic same day with **doppler/CT/MRI** or next morning if they have someone to stay with them overnight with strict instructions to call 999/911 if any change because the emergency department is set up for urgent thrombolysis if needed.
- **Driving:** not to drive for 28 days (UK-DVLA). There is usually no need to involve DVLA if complete resolution, but should inform motor insurance. The exception is if the patient drives a lorry, bus, coach or taxi when DVLA need to be involved and needs their approval before can drive.
- Adhere to local policies. There are some questions over the validity of $ABCD_2$ and stroke risk. Ideal is to see all urgently. See and MRI (CT if MRI not possible) and doppler scan within 24 h. If TIA confirmed then consider carotid endarterectomy within 48 h if symptomatic stenosis >70%.
- **CLOPIDOGREL 300 mg stat and then 75 mg** long term. Alternative is combined **ASPIRIN 75 mg OD + Dipyridamole MR 200 mg BD** but headache remains a problem as well as compliance.
- If AF, then consider rapid **warfarin** or **new oral anticoagulant,** e.g. dabigatran/similar agent. Smoking cessation and hypertension management. Depending on age and strength of diagnosis other tests such as echo/trans-oesophageal echo and thrombophilia screens may be undertaken. Many of our high-risk TIA referrals are migraine, focal seizures, syncope and some remain unexplained symptomatology.

19.9 Stroke

Introduction

- Third commonest cause of death. 80% are ischaemic and the remaining 15% haemorrhagic with 5% subarachnoid haemorrhage. Similar pathologies can cause both – venous infarction famously can cause haemorrhage, dissections can lead to SAH, SAH can lead to delayed cerebral ischaemia, septic emboli from endocarditis can cause obstruction and bleeding. In the vast majority the cause is simple. In selected cases (beyond the scope of this book) one needs to think beyond the obvious.
- Any atypical or young stroke, consider asking yourself the **VIVID list**: is this **vasculitis, infective, venous, inflammatory or dissection.** If you never consider an unusual aetiology you will never diagnose it.

19.10 Ischaemic stroke

About

- Sudden onset of focal neurological symptoms and signs. Related to reduced blood flow supplying an area of the brain. Focal brain ischaemia and infarction. 80% of strokes are ischaemic.

Aetiology

- Thrombotic, embolic (artery to artery, cardiac to artery) or low flow or venous infarction.

Definitions

- WHO definition of stroke: neurological deficit of cerebrovascular cause that persists beyond 24 h or is interrupted by death within 24 h. It includes brain, retinal and spinal ischaemia.
- There is tissue damage but this may not be seen on initial early imaging.

Causes

Causes	
Large artery disease	Atherosclerosis within aortic arch and its branches, ICA especially at its bifurcation within carotid siphon and within large intracranial vessels. Same is seen in the vertebral artery and basilar artery. Disease is caused by progressive increase in plaque size and obstruction. Plaque rupture and thrombosis or even distal embolisation of thrombus and debris (artery to artery stroke). If stenosis comes on gradually over time there is a chance of development of collaterals making subsequent occlusion less severe. Atherosclerosis common within the aortic arch or its branches and can lead to obstruction or embolisation of thrombus. Arterial dissection of carotid or vertebral can cause local acute occlusion or thromboembolism into its area of perfusion.
Cardio-embolism (30%)	Commonest cause is AF particularly when associated with valvular heart disease. Other causes include endocarditis, MI and apical thrombus, atrial myxoma and paradoxical emboli across a patent foramen ovale (PFO)/atrial septal aneurysm. There is an increased incidence of PFO in young cryptogenic strokes, but association does not prove causality. Echocardiography (transthoracic and transoesophageal) is indicated. 24 h tape may pick up paroxysmal AF.
Small artery disease (40%)	There is localised stenosis and thrombosis usually of deep perforating arteries of the cerebral hemisphere and brainstem. The driver behind this is diabetes and hypertension. These are end arteries with little collateralisation. The result is lacunar infarction. These are small deep lesions usually less than 1.5 cm in diameter. Over time the cumulative effect of multiple lacunar infarcts is a subcortical vascular encephalopathy.
Venous thrombosis	Can cause haemorrhagic infarction. Atypical, crosses arterial boundaries. Suggests local infection or thrombophilia
Low flow	Causing watershed infarction between ACA and MCA and MCA and PCA.

List of general causes that predispose to ischaemic stroke

- Atherosclerosis – age, hypertension, DM, hyperlipidaemia, smoking.
- Arterial dissection – hypertension, trauma.
- Connective tissue disease, fibromuscular dysplasia. Vasculitis – temporal arteritis.
- Polyarteritis nodosa, Behcet's, arterial spasm – migraine, SAH.
- Embolic – AF, endocarditis, valve disease, atrial myxoma, PFO, LV dysfunction, mural thrombus.
- Thrombophilia – prothrombin, Factor V Leiden, protein C and S deficiency, malignancy. Oestrogens, antiphospholipid syndrome, hyperviscosity.

Differentials

- **Focal/generalised seizure**: motor or sensory. Todd's paresis. Usually as part of a generalised seizure which may not be witnessed or nocturnal. Weakness resolves. Patient obtunded. May be an epilepsy history. Nocturnal seizure: suspect if patient wakes up with sore head, incontinent, tongue bitten, feels unwell. Post-stroke seizures tend to be seen months after the stroke with a focus in the territory of the previous stroke.
- **Migraine**: younger patient with known history of stroke-like symptoms as part of migraine with aura. If this is first ever presentation then treat as stroke. Positive symptoms: flashing lights, speech disturbance, headache. Care needed as some strokes seem to be accompanied by migraine-like episodes. Take specialist advice if within thrombolysis window.
- **Old stroke systemic illness** (I call these 'Ozzies'): CT shows old stroke, history of a stroke with a sudden worsening of symptomatology on same side and same weakness. Usually precipitated by fatigue, infection or metabolic cause. Once treated neurology resolves.
- **Functional:** younger patient, challenging life, often smokers and risk factors but atypical signs. Arms drift down, no pronation. Give way weakness. Excessive effort. Power stronger when limbs tested separately. Incongruent abilities with therapists. Bizarre gaits. Normal imaging. Need positive stroke team support with full expectation of recovery.

Clinical syndromes (ischaemic stroke)

Artery	Clinical – think what is the culprit vessel?
Middle cerebral artery	C/L hemiplegia affecting face and arm with relative sparing of the leg. C/L hemisensory loss and a homonymous hemianopia. Aphasia if dominant side affected. Anosognosia/neglect if non-dominant.
Anterior cerebral artery	C/L hemiplegia affecting leg more than face and arm. Gait disturbance. Urinary incontinence. Primitive reflexes. Abulia.
Posterior cerebral artery	C/L homonymous hemianopia with macular sparing. Memory loss, somnolescence, cognitive changes.
Vertebral and posterior inferior cerebellar artery	Lateral medullary syndrome, Horner's syndrome, ipsilateral cerebellar signs, spinothalamic loss.
Lacunar strokes	**Pontine perforators**: C/L lacunar-type motor/ataxic syndromes. Cranial nerve palsies. **Medial and lateral lenticulostriate**: C/L lacunar syndromes. Pure motor, pure sensory, dysarthria + clumsy hand, ataxic hemiplegia.
Basilar artery occlusion	Diplopia, hemianopia, vertigo, progressive coma, ophthalmoplegia.

Initial investigations

- **Bloods:** FBC, CRP, ESR, U&E, LFT, glucose, lipids.
- **ECG:** primarily to find AF or recent MI/LVH/cardiomyopathy.
- **CXR:** cardiomegaly, tumours with brain metastases mimicking stroke.
- **Non-contrast CT head** may initially be normal and may take 6–12 h for hypodensity to show. Earlier signs include subtle signs such as loss of grey/white matter,

cortical differentiation, thrombus in MCA or basilar arteries, sulcal effacement, loss of insular ribbon. Cortical and subcortical atrophy and small vessel disease may be seen.

- **1–7 day tape**: done in most patients where paroxysmal AF suspected, e.g. cardioembolic strokes in different sides and both anterior and posterior circulations.
- **MRI**: DWI for infarction, gradient echo for haemorrhage.

Additional tests in selected patients

- **Carotid doppler**: mild non-disabling stroke/TIA and fit and willing enough for a carotid endarterectomy if a symptomatic stenosis is found.
- **Echocardiogram:** age <50, significant murmur, ECG changes, cardiac symptoms.
- **CT angiogram:** can show up Circle of Willis demonstrating acute occlusion of a major branch, e.g. MCA. It can also show neck vessel stenosis of occlusion (carotid and vertebrals). However, only done as initial work up in selected centres. It needs to be considered if there is a plan to refer for vascular intervention. May be done as option to look for AVM or dissection but most centres use MRA.
- **CT + contrast:** when a tumour is suspected. Looking for enhancement.
- **MRI + DWI T1/T2 :** where stroke location or diagnosis is in doubt.
- **MRV** if venous thrombosis suspected. **MRA** if aneurysm or dissection or vascular anomaly considered.
- **Troponin**: ACS suspected. **BNP** if heart failure suspected.
- **Vasculitis screen:** raised CRP. Younger, seizure, headache, multiple infarcts/bleed.
- **Sickle test:** if sickle cell anaemia suspected.
- **Thrombophilia** screen in those <45 with history of venous/arterial thrombosis or family history of VTE or venous thrombosis in unusual site, e.g. cerebral/portal/ hepatic vein. Other than cardiolipin there is a very poor correlation with arterial strokes and these thrombophilias. Most useful for venous infarcts.

Hyperacute management

- **Thrombolysis**: screen and see thrombolysis protocol below if indicated.
- **Stroke unit:** regular neurological observations – temperature, pulse, BP, GCS, pupillary responses. Stroke unit admission is fundamental and key for improving outcomes and reduces mortality.
- **General care:** IV hydration and swallowing assessment before eating, skin care, nutrition. Consider NG tube if unsafe swallow after 12 h.
- **VTE prevention:** pneumatic calf compression preferred as well as early mobilisation. Some give VTE prophylaxis LMWH after a few days. Follow local guidance.
- **Decompressive hemicraniectomy:** for those with malignant MCA syndromes with any fall in level of consciousness on NIH stroke scale in those under 60 years. Take urgent neurosurgical advice. It is possible to have both thrombolysis and hemicraniectomy.
- **Medical:** if not for thrombolysis and non-haemorrhagic, start **ASPIRIN 300 mg stat PO/PR** for 2 weeks.
- **Hypertension** not treated acutely unless SBP persistently over 200 mmHg for ischaemic stroke and 180 mmHg for haemorrhage. Reductions in BP should be very gradual or can severely reduce cerebral perfusion.

Acute medical care

- **Antiplatelet: ASPIRIN 300 mg PO/PR × 2 weeks.** Add a PPI if history of dyspepsia. Then convert **ASPIRIN 300 mg to CLOPIDOGREL 75 mg OD** (1st line therapy). Use combined **ASPIRIN 75 mg + dipyridamole 200 mg BD** if unable to take clopidogrel.

- **Hypertension:** it is usual to delay treatment up to 1 week unless severe, i.e. BP >200/100 mmHg and if so then consider thiazide + ACE inhibitor, e.g. Bendroflumethiazide 2.5 mg OD / Ramipril 1.25 mg OD or amlodipine 5 mg via NG or PO may be given. Lower BP slowly over hours and days.
- **Cholesterol:** simvastatin 40 mg OD start after 48 h if new, or continue if already on statin.
- **Anticoagulant:** warfarin for those with AF or PAF with no C/I, after patient consent commence low dose 3–4 mg per day around day 10. Aim for INR of 2–3 by day 14. Use CHA_2DS_2VaSc and HAS-BLED score to assess relative risks of anticoagulation. Those with a stroke or TIA with AF should be anticoagulated.
- **Diabetes:** blood glucose: maintain between 7 and 11.0 mmol/L. Use a VRIII and convert to regular insulin ASAP. Avoid hypoglycaemia in comatose patients.
- **Oxygen:** give sufficient O_2 as per BTS guidelines.
- **Fluids/nutrition**: bedside swallow assessment ('SIP test') and if normal then allow normal intake but keep under review. Get speech and language therapy review if unsure. If nil orally start IV fluids, preferably NS 2–3 L/day initially. If swallow remains poor then start NG feeding if indicated after assessment at 24–48 h. Do not place NG immediately unless vital oral meds required, e.g. sinemet, etc.
- **Carotid stenosis**: doppler or CTA to screen for symptomatic carotid stenosis in those who would be candidates for urgent carotid endarterectomy, i.e. **TIA and mild non-disabling strokes.**

CHA_2DS_2VaSc score

Assess stroke risk in those with AF who would benefit from anticoagulation:

- CCF history (+1)
- Hypertension history (+1)
- Age: 65–74 (+1), >75 (+2)
- Diabetes mellitus (+1)
- Stroke/TIA or thromboembolism (+2)
- Sex: female (+1)
- Vascular disease or coronary artery disease (CAD), MI (heart attack), peripheral artery disease (PAD), or aortic plaque (+1)

Adjusted annual stroke risk by score:
0: 0%, **1**: 1.3%, **2**: 2.2%, **3**: 3.3%, **4**: 4.0%, **5**: 6.7%, **6**: 9.8%, **7**: 9.6%, **8**: 6.7%, **9**: 15.2%

HAS-BLED score

Assess potential bleeding risk in those to be started on oral anticoagulants in atrial fibrillation:

- Hypertension (SBP >160 mmHg) (+1)
- Abnormal renal (+1) and/or liver function (+1)
- Stroke in past (+1)
- Bleeding (+1)
- Labile INR (+1)
- Elderly age >65 (+1)
- Drugs (+1) or alcohol abuse (+1)

A score of 3 or more indicates increased 1 year bleed risk on anticoagulation sufficient to justify caution or more regular review. Risk is for intracranial bleed, bleed requiring hospitalisation or a haemoglobin drop >2 g/L or that needs transfusion.

Stroke thrombolysis assessment

Should only be done by those formally trained in stroke thrombolysis.

RCP Thrombolysis Guidance 2012 based on current evidence:

- Aged ≤80 up to 4.5 h from stroke onset and aged >80 up to 3 h from stroke onset. Stroke onset is from when patient last known stroke free.

Thrombolysis criteria

Clinical exclusion criteria	Imaging / laboratory exclusion criteria
• GCS <9, rapidly resolving symptoms. • Pathology other than stroke likely. • SBP >185 mmHg or DBP >110 mmHg despite treatment. • NIH score <4 or >25 (caution >22). • Fixed head or eye deviation. • Seizure at stroke onset and residual deficit is post-ictal weakness. • Thunderclap headache suggestive of SAH.	• CT hypodensity or sulcal effacement in >1/3 of MCA territory. • CT shows bleeding, tumour, abscess, or developed stroke, AVM or aneurysm. • Blood glucose <3 mmol/L or >22 mmol/L. • Platelet count $<100 \times 10^9$/L. • Hb <10 g/dL or haematocrit <25%. • APTT > upper limit of normal for laboratory. • Abnormal INR >1.7 or APTT >36 sec. • Heparin within previous 48 h.

If there is no clinical reason whatsoever to suspect an abnormal lab result, thrombolysis should not be delayed to wait for the results. Results should be obtained as quickly as possible nevertheless and acted upon.

Exclusion criteria for stroke thrombolysis

- **Trauma**: recent puncture of non-compressible blood vessel, LP in past 7 days or traumatic CPR less than 10 days, surgery or visceral biopsy in past 4 weeks, major surgery within 3 months, recent head injury, significant trauma (fracture or internal injuries) in past 3 months.
- **Bleeding**: history of recent bleeding (PR/PO/PU/gynae/epistaxis), severe anaemia Hb <10 g/dL, any neoplasm with increased bleeding risk including intracranial neoplasm, endocarditis, pericarditis, arterial aneurysm, arteriovenous malformations: aortic aneurysm or ventricular aneurysm. Any known bleeding problem or blood disorder. Haemorrhagic retinopathy (untreated proliferative diabetic retinopathy).
- **Pregnancy**: pregnant (discuss) or childbirth <4 weeks ago, desire to breast-feed after treatment.
- **Stroke**: ischaemic stroke in past 3 months, haemorrhagic stroke any time in the past, arteriovenous malformation or aneurysm.
- **Gastrointestinal**: ulcerative GI disease in past 3 months, oesophageal varices, active peptic ulcer disease, severe liver disease, coagulopathy or suspected varices.

Management pre and post treatment

- Monitor BP every 15 min to ensure <185/110 mmHg.
- BP >185/110 mmHg and within pre-treatment thrombolysis window, then treat with 10–20 mg doses of LABETALOL given IV push within 1 h unless contraindicated. Second line is GTN IV. If, despite this, BP >185/110 mmHg then do not give ALTEPLASE.
- If not confident that you can maintain BP <185/110 mmHg for the next 12–24 h then do not treat.

ALTEPLASE: give **0.9 mg/kg body weight** (maximum 90 mg) infused IV over 60 min. Give 10% of the total dose administered as an initial IV bolus.

PATIENTS MUST BE CLOSELY MONITORED BEFORE, DURING AND AFTER DRUG ADMINISTRATION, and for at least 24 h following administration for potential side effects and complications. Should be prescribed by and administration supervised by a doctor (Registrar or above) once the approval has been obtained from the stroke/neurology consultant.

- In the first 24 h immediately after stroke thrombolysis try to avoid NG tube and urinary catheter unless in retention. Avoid IM injection. Discuss with stroke team.
- Do not give aspirin, persantin, asasantin, dipyridamole, warfarin, phenindone, acenocoumaral, plavix, clopidogrel, heparin, enoxaparin, ibuprofen, diclofenac, naproxen or other NSAIDs. Paracetamol IV/oral/PR is safe for analgesia or pyrexia.

If suspected intracranial (fall in GCS, seizure, worsening headache) bleed then alteplase should be stopped immediately and an emergency CT scan should be obtained.

Difficult cases

- **Top of the basilar occlusion**: acute comatose, eye signs, extensor plantars. Bright basilar dot on CT. If suspected then consider CTA to confirm thrombus. If no good other explanation and no other contraindications, then may consider off-licence alteplase. Prognosis usually grim so worth attempting. Get consent. Specialist decision. Alternatively consider referral for intravascular intervention.
- **Artery of Percheron occlusion**: subtle coma and eye signs out of proportion to stroke size. Bilateral thalamic infarction. Might consider alteplase off-licence. May need urgent DWI to confirm. Specialist decision.

Complications

- **Anaphylaxis/angioedema**: manage as for anaphylaxis.
- **Malignant MCA syndrome**: analysis of studies of hemicraniectomy for malignant MCA infarction has shown that mortality is reduced from 70 to 30%; survival with good functional outcome is doubled from 20 to 40%. One-third survive with substantial disability. **Consider** if: age <60, imaging evidence of >50% MCA infarction (involving deep and superficial MCA territory), >2/3 MCA infarction (if only superficial territory involved), >145 cm^3 volume of infarction (if local imaging allows quantification), within 48 h of stroke onset. Patients will usually have an NIHSS >15, particularly if dominant hemisphere infarct. Patients with dominant as well as non-dominant hemisphere infarcts are suitable for decompression. **The following may not be suitable:** age >60, significant medical or neurological co-morbidity that would hinder survival or rehabilitation, bilateral fixed dilated pupils, time >48 h after stroke onset, 3 vascular territories involved (e.g. bilateral ACA and MCA; combined ACA, MCA and PCA) at any age, 2 vascular territories involved >45 y (e.g. ACA and MCA, MCA and PCA).
- **Suspect ICH:** sudden fall in GCS. Headache. Seizure. Raised NIH score at 2 h. Acute hypertension. Nausea and vomiting. See bleeding advice below. Arrange a CT scan. Inform family and discuss prognosis which is usually very poor depending on the extent of bleeding.
- **Extracranial haemorrhage**: suspect extracranial haemorrhage if there is a fall in BP, rise in HR, shock, epistaxis, melaena, haematuria, haematemesis, abdominal pain and bruising or pain in flanks or thighs. Appropriate referral, e.g. ENT for persisting epistaxis, gastroenterology for melaena, haematemesis, etc. *Immediately stop infusion of ALTEPLASE*. Use direct pressure if possible to control bleeding from arterial or venous puncture sites. Check fibrinogen, PT, APTT, full blood count and arrange appropriate cross-match and urgent transfusion to match blood losses. Support circulation with fluids and blood transfusion as appropriate. If bleeding has been confirmed by imaging, that blood should be taken for group and save, FBC and coagulation screen. Fibrinolysis causes a low

fibrinogen which can be replaced by cryoprecipitate with a target fibrinogen level of 1 g/L.

- If the patient has received antiplatelet therapy such as ASPIRIN then a platelet transfusion should also be considered. Liaise with haematology. Consider transfusion of FFP and/or cryoprecipitate depending upon the results of a coagulation screen. Most patients who have bleeding can be managed by interruption of thrombolytic and anticoagulant therapy volume replacement and manual pressure applied to an incompetent vessel.
- Protamine should be considered if heparin has been administered within 4 h of the onset of bleeding. In the few patients who fail to respond to these conservative measures, judicious use of transfusion products may be indicated. Transfusion of cryoprecipitate, FFP, and platelets should be considered with clinical and laboratory reassessment after each administration.

19.11 Haemorrhagic stroke

About

- Many different causes and patterns. Up to 15–20% of strokes are haemorrhagic.

Types

- Lobar cortical haemorrhages, deep subcortical bleeds.
- Putaminal, thalamic, brainstem bleeds. Subarachnoid haemorrhage.

Causes

- **Hypertension:** causes lobar and deep bleeds in the basal ganglia, thalamus, cerebellum, pons.
- **Arteriovenous malformations:** tends to cause lobar haemorrhages.
- **Cavernoma (cavernous angioma):** seizures, bleeds in younger patients.
- **Cerebral amyloid angiopathy** causes lobar haemorrhages in those over 70 usually without hypertension.
- **Warfarin/haemophilia/thrombolysis/DIC**: warfarin or any coagulopathy.
- **Embolic stroke:** higher rate of haemorrhagic transformation seen with embolic strokes and any large stroke especially if hypertensive.
- **Cerebral venous thrombosis**: haemorrhagic stroke can be seen.
- **Endocarditis:** mycotic aneurysms from septic emboli bleed.
- **Sickle cell disease:** both ischaemic and haemorrhagic stroke.
- **Malignancy:** primary or metastatic stroke.
- **Vasculitis:** polyartertis nodosa, SLE, Wegener's granulomatosis, Takayasu's, temporal arteritis.
- **Systemic:** sarcoid, Behcet's disease.
- **Trauma:** history should be suggestive. Signs of head injury. Not stroke.

Haemorrhagic stroke mimics

- Head trauma – look for soft tissue injury. Did patient fall and hit head and bled or did the bleed come first.
- Tumours, e.g. melanoma.
- Infarct with haemorrhagic transformation.
- Endocarditis with haemorrhage from septic emboli.
- Cortical vein thrombosis and secondary haemorrhage.

Pathology

- Haematoma formation usually splits white fibre bundles.

- Secondary oedema exacerbates increased ICP and coma/coning.
- Progressive bleeding not uncommon, especially if anticoagulated.
- Older atrophied brain may allow more room for expansion.
- Some bleeds may be low pressure, e.g. cavernomas from venous side.
- Bleeding into ventricular system. Obstructive hydrocephalus.

Prognosis

- 15% of strokes are due to intracerebral haemorrhage.
- 5% are due to SAH. 30–50% death within 30 days.

Investigations

- **Bloods:** FBC: low platelets, raised INR if warfarin/liver disease, CRP, ESR, glucose. U&E: (low Na with SAH). LFTs.
- **CT imaging:** CT very sensitive for blood and shows haematoma in brain substance +/− oedema, +/− extension into ventricles, +/− hydrocephalus and signs of raised ICP. Presence of intraventricular blood is a poor prognostic indicator.
- **MRI imaging:** almost as good as CT initially but most helpful later when the haematoma has resolved. Old bleeds show a slit-like appearance with signs of haemosiderin. Repeat interval scan at 6 weeks can help exclude an underlying vascular lesion e.g. tumour, AVM, cavernoma
- **MRA imaging:** shows the circle of Willis and can identify aneurysms and AVM.
- **CTA:** allows imaging of aneurysms and dissections and vascular malformations.
- **CT with contrast:** if suspicion of tumour.
- **MRV imaging:** consider if any suspicion of venous thrombosis with haemorrhage.
- **Digitial subtraction cerebral angiography:** reserved for selected cases in tertiary centres for those with SAH or AVM. 1% stroke risk associated with the procedure. Involves selective catheterisation of carotids and subclavian arteries.
- **Echocardiography:** CRP and work up if endocarditis suspected. Septic emboli can bleed.
- **Lumbar puncture** for red cells and xanthochromia if SAH suspected.

Management

- **Supportive**: ABC, IV fluids, ITU if GCS <9 and high early warning scores.
- **Admit to stroke unit**. Monitor temperature, pulse, BP, GCS, pupillary responses.
- **Neurosurgery**: younger patients, cerebellar bleeds, superficial lobar bleeds.
- **End of life care**: the decision may be for palliation, though some patients should not be written off too soon in the first 24 hours and may make some recovery. Take experienced advice.
- **Coagulopathy**: if on warfarin and INR >1.4 give **VITAMIN K 10 mg IV** stat and prothrombin complex concentrates, e.g. **OCTAPLEX/BERIPLEX**. Discuss with haematologists. Warfarin must be stopped and reversed in the short term even with metal prosthetic valves.
- **Surgery:** consult with neurosurgeons, especially if cerebellar haematoma >3 cm diameter and/or developing hydrocephalus for **external ventricular drainage (EVD)** or evacuation of the lesion and shunting. Little evidence to suggest neurosurgical benefit in supratentorial bleeds, the exception being young patient with a superficial bleed close to the cortex and easily accessed. Infratentorial bleeds benefit from clot evacuation or shunt insertion for hydrocephalus, especially if there are signs of developing coma.
- **IV steroids** have no evidence base and may raise BP and glucose.
- **Stop drugs:** statins and all anticoagulants and antiplatelets must be stopped.

- **VTE prevention**: early mobility, some give LMWH after several weeks if high VTE risk and bleed risk has diminished.
- NG tube and PEG if normal feeding delayed.
- **Blood pressure:** manage BP but 'hands off' approach first week unless BP consistently 185/100 mmHg. Lower high BP cautiously by 10–20% over hours and days.
- **Manage diabetes:** (blood glucose 4–11 mmol/L).
- Multidisciplinary approach to rehabilitation.
- **Anticonvulsants:** for seizures.

19.12 Subdural haematoma

About

- Acceleration–deceleration injury. May cause vague neurology. If any concern then CT head.

Aetiology

- Rupture/tearing of bridging veins crossing subdural space.
- Mild to severe trauma. Worsened by concomitant coagulopathy.
- Risk are falls and trauma, anticoagulants, elderly patients, alcohol abuse.

Clinical

- Reduced GCS, IIIrd nerve palsy, coning, delirium, seizure, headache, unsteadiness.
- C/L hemiparesis or hemisensory loss, Cheyne–Stokes respiration.

Investigation

- **FBC, U&E:** ensure normal – hyponatraemia.
- **Coagulation**: check INR, platelets or coagulation screen if on warfarin or liver disease.
- **Non-contrast CT:** rim of hyperdense crescent-shaped extraxial blood which over time gradually has density of brain and then CSF. Look for midline shift and signs of raised ICP.
- **MRI scan** can be helpful if suspected that subdural isodense with brain on CT.

Management

- **Supportive:** ABC oxygen as per BTS guidelines, IV fluids if swallow unsafe.
- **Neurosurgery:** small subdurals managed conservatively. Larger haematomas need surgical removal and craniectomy. Evacuate all with a rim >10 mm or midline shift >5 mm. Over time, acute SDH can become chronic with recurring bleeding and it may take 3 months or so for things to settle. Chronic SDH managed with burr holes as the usually jelly-like clot has liquefied into a 'motor oil' consistency which can be aspirated by burr-hole craniostomy without craniectomy.
- **Clinical criteria:** fall in GCS by 2 points. Fixed dilated pupils or an increase in intracranial pressure >20 mmHg.
- **Post surgical complications:** seizures, subdural empyema, aspiration, sepsis, haemorrhagic stroke, SIADH, pneumonia.

19.13 Epidural haematoma

About

- Usually seen by trauma and orthopaedics rather than physicians because head injury related.
- Rarely non-traumatic with bleeding disorders.

Aetiology

- Usually a tear of middle meningeal artery with bleeding. May be associated skull fracture. Can also be bleeding from veins and from fractured bone.
- May have rapid expansion and seen often in young where there is little room for any increase in intracranial volume. ICP rises quickly with devastating results.

Clinical

- Classically a head injury (perhaps with LOC) followed by lucid period and then sudden decline.
- Signs of raised ICP. Reduced GCS, IIIrd nerve palsy, coning, delirium, seizure, headache, unsteadiness.
- C/L hemiparesis or hemisensory loss, Cheyne–Stokes respiration.

Investigation

- **Non-contrast CT:** there is a hyperdense lens-shaped convexity of blood on the inner surface of the skull restricted by the suture lines of the skull. Look for midline shift and signs of raised ICP. May be contrecoup injuries seen and subarachnoid and intraparenchymal haemorrhage.
- **X-ray C-spine** and full trauma assessment.

Management

- **Discuss with neurosurgeons.** Needs rapid transfer and surgical drainage combined with drugs, hypothermia and ventilation to lower ICP and neurocritical care. Recommended to evacuate all epidural haematomas with volume >30 cm^2 irrespective of GCS (www.braintrauma.org). Pupillary abnormalities and GCS <9 should be evacuated as quickly as possible.
- Smaller bleeds may be managed conservatively following a period of monitoring with immediate access to intervention. Bleeding and haematoma expansion can occur. Ensure any other injuries are managed, e.g. long bone fractures, C-spine injuries, abdominal injuries, etc. In those rare cases of bleeding disorder being involved this needs urgent correction.

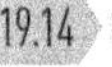

19.14 Subarachnoid haemorrhage

About

- Berry aneurysms are found in 2% of population, but SAH much less common. Identifying symptomatic aneurysms is important, so do all to prove that a SAH has occurred when CT normal.
- Non-traumatic bleeding from blood vessels on the surface of the brain into the subarachnoid space and occasionally direct into the parenchyma. Blood tends to track into sulci and ventricles and basal cisterns.
- Main early risks are rebleeding, vasospasm, arrhythmias, hydrocephalus, seizures.

Causes

- Berry aneurysms cause the majority (80%); arteriovenous malformations (10%).
- Vasculitis (rare), intracranial arterial dissections (rare).
- Perimesenchephalic: unknown cause but good prognosis.
- Non-aneurysmal SAH: amyloid in older patients.

Risks

- Smoking, binge drinking, illicit drugs, no real evidence for role for hypertension.
- Adult polycystic kidney disease (10% have aneurysms). SLE.

- Marfan's and Ehlers–Danlos syndromes, pseudoxanthoma elasticum and sickle cell disease.
- **Berry aneurysms:** aneurysms <7 mm diameter in the anterior circulation have the lowest risk of rupture, whereas risk is higher for aneurysms in the posterior circulation and increases with size. In contrast to sporadic aneurysms, familial aneurysms often larger (>10 mm) and multiple. Berry aneurysms develop with increasing age and usually arise at areas of vessel branching. Rupture rate increases with size. Small aneurysms are commoner and so bleeds are seen more in smaller aneurysms. Related to hypertension, smoking and excessive alcohol.
- **Arteriovenous malformations**: these are vascular anomalies which consist of a plexiform network of abnormal arteries and veins linked by one or more fistulae. They lack the typical capillary bed interposed between the arteriole and venule and have arterioles with a thinner than normal muscularis. Annual rate of bleeding is about 2% amongst patients with no history of bleeding. Annual rate of repeat haemorrhage is 18%. Can present initially as bleeding or seizures.
- **Peri-mesencephalic**: SAH on CT and LP but no aneurysm or AVM seen. Tend to do well. Possibly venous blood. Blood around brainstem.
- **Trauma**: SAH can be seen with head injury.

Clinical

- Worst ever headache comes on very acutely – 'hit round back of head'. Some cases less acute and consider any with maximal headache onset <4 min.
- Be careful with differential as triptans can help all headaches.
- Comes on at rest or exertion, during sleep, coitus and straining. Enquire after associated collapse/syncope and then recovery. Headache may be occipital or cervical, photophobia and neck stiffness, vomiting, diplopia. Beware the sore stiff neck with meningeal irritation.
- Progressive bleeding leads to coma, coning and sudden death. Some claim warning headaches over preceding weeks 'herald bleeds'. Headache and IIIrd nerve palsy suggests an ipsilateral posterior communicating aneurysm.
- Arrhythmias and myocardial dysfunction and even pulmonary oedema.

Differential of thunderclap headache

- Primary thunderclap headache: when all tests are negative this is the presumed diagnosis. Cerebral venous thrombosis, benign orgasmic cephalgia.
- Migraine or cluster headache, reversible cerebral vasoconstriction syndrome.
- Primary parenchymal haemorrhage, tumour with bleed, carotid/vertebral dissection.

Grading of subarachnoid bleeds : World Federation of Neurological Surgery

I. GCS 15 no focal deficits.
II. GCS 13–14 no focal deficits.
III. GCS 13–14 focal deficits present.
IV. GCS 7–12 irrespective of deficits.
V. GCS 3–6 irrespective of deficits.

Investigations

- **Bloods:** FBC, U&E: hyponatraemia (naturiesis or SIADH) slightly more difficult to see a small SAH on CT if severely anaemic.
- **ECG and CXR**: arrhythmias and pulmonary oedema possible. Dynamic T wave and ST changes may be seen but don't necessarily suggest ACS. Measure troponin and cardiology review if concerns. Obviously do not anticoagulate.

- **CT head with thin cuts through base of brain:** shows high signal attenuation in the basal cisterns. MCA aneurysm blood in the sylvian fissure. ACA or anterior communicating artery blood in intrahemispheric fissure. CT showing higher concentrations of blood over the convexities or within the superficial parenchyma of the brain is more consistent with the rupture of an AVM or a mycotic aneurysm. Blood also seen around the brainstem in prepontine, premedullary and interpeduncular cisterns as well as within ventricles. CT is 98% sensitive in the first 12 h. Blood on CT less clear if severe anaemia/low Hct.
- **Lumbar puncture (if CT negative):** normal CT with SAH presentation needs LP done at earliest 12 h after onset (NOT BEFORE): SAH causes uniformly bloody CSF on LP with xanthochromia from haemoglobin breakdown which is present for up to 3 weeks. Interpretation is variable. A traumatic tap may be suggested by a fall in red cell numbers in successive bottles, however, caution must be taken and this is not an absolute rule. The absolute level of RBCs must be taken and a high baseline level should still raise some suspicion of SAH. A count of <10 RBCs/mm^3 constitutes a negative tap, RBC >100/mm^3 in all tubes should be considered positive, especially if xanthochromia (bilirubin) is present. Opening pressure should be measured routinely in all lumbar punctures.
- **CSF xanthochromia** (breakdown product of haem) suggests recent bleed with haemolysis and so not a bloody tap. In some centres there is restricted access as samples now go to reference laboratories. Xanthochromia can be determined visually or by spectrophotometry which is not available in some hospitals. CSF, especially if bloody, should be spun down immediately and if the supernatant is yellow (compared with water against a white background), the diagnosis of SAH is practically certain. The specimen should be stored in darkness, preferably wrapped in tinfoil because the ultraviolet components of daylight can break down bilirubin. Spectrophotometry can not only confirm the presence of bilirubin but also exclude it.
- **CT/MR angiography:** may be used as an alternative. Not as good as catheter angiography.
- **Catheter cerebral angiography:** gold standard and has the best resolution to identify the bleeding source and is usually only done following admission to a tertiary neuroscience centre.
- **Transcranial doppler:** can detect vasospasm in the MCA.
- **MRA and CTA** can pick up aneurysms but will miss the smaller ones.

Early complications

- **Rebleeding**: needs intervention at neurosurgical centre.
- **Delayed cerebral ischaemia/vasospasm**: causes ischaemic stroke which may be distant to bleeding aneurysm even on opposite side. Seen in about 30% with further resultant brain injury.
- **Obstructive hydrocephalus**: detected by CT. Refer for EVD.
- **Arrhythmias and myocardial dysfunction**: telemetry.
- **Hyponatraemia** can be due to renal sodium loss or SIADH**.** Determine which using serum/urine osmolality as management differential.
- **Seizures**: manage as below.
- **Death**: from raised ICP and coning due to massive haematoma or coning. 10–15% of patients die before hospital: 40% within the first week, and about 50% die in the first 6 months.

Management

- **Prehospital care** with ABCs and rapid triage and transport to hospital and urgent CT. An early CT within 6 h is more sensitive than delayed imaging and is a reason to justify earlier diagnostic imaging in patients.
- **Bed rest.** Codeine and laxative/stool softener. Hydration and slight hypervolaemia is suggested with 3 L/day. Hyponatraemia may well be due to renal sodium loss rather than SIADH and, unless SIADH proven, fluid restriction should be avoided.
- **Rebleeding:** early intervention and management of aneurysm. 19% will rebleed, of whom approximately 70% will die. Rebleeding is commonest within the first 2 weeks of the SAH. A bimodal peak of the first 24–48 h and between days 7 and 10. Prevent with early angiography and then treatment of aneurysm either by coiling or clipping. Transfer to neurosurgeons for early CT/cerebral angiography, or to place small soft titanium coils within the aneurysm to induce thrombosis, or microsurgical clipping of aneurysm, or management of AVM in order to prevent rebleeding. Note 10–15% of patients have more than one aneurysm. If brain injury sustained then will need later neuro-rehabilitation depending on the extent of the brain injury. Post surgery or coiling is usually transferred to neuro-rehabilitation setting if there is a brain injury for ongoing assessment and rehabilitation.
- **Delayed cerebral ischaemia/vasospasm** of branches of the Circle of Willis can lead to ischaemic stroke which may be distant to the aneurysm. Start **Nimodipine 60 mg PO/NG every 4 h for 21 days to reduce vasospasm**. Evidence for Mg usage to prevent vasospasm is controversial. May need ITU if comatose and needs airway protection. Orotracheal intubation and mechanical ventilation if falling GCS <9 or progressive neurology.
- **Intracranial hypertension**: hyperventilate to maintain $PaCO_2$ of 30–35 mmHg to reduce elevated ICP. Mannitol reduces ICP 50% in 30 min which peaks in effect after 90 min, and lasts 4 h. Used in ITU setting with ICP monitoring. If acute hydrocephalus on CT due to ventricular blood then EVD and maintain ICP at <20 mmHg and CPP >60 mmHg.
- **Seizures**: if occur (anticonvulsants may be given as prophylaxis) then start PHENYTOIN infusion.
- **Telemetry**: risk of cardiac arrhythmias/myocardial dysfunction.
- **Hypertension:** manage BP with **LABETALOL IV** if BP >180/110 mmHg. Target SBP <140 mmHg.
- Long term prevention of further SAH is helped by **BP control and smoking cessation.**
- Rehabilitation for any resultant disability due to bleed or subsequent ischaemic injury and take advice on screening family members.

References:

Greenberg (2010) *Handbook of Neurosurgery*, 7th Edition. Thieme.

SIGN (2008) 107: Diagnosis and management of headache in adults. A national clinical guideline.

Tofteland & Salyers (2007) Subarachnoid haemorrhage. *Hospital Physician*, 31.

19.15 Guillain–Barré syndrome

In suspected respiratory muscle weakness measure FVC qds (caution if FVC <1.5 L and intubate when FVC <1 L). Check ABG to look for a rise in $PaCO_2$ which occurs before any hypoxia.

About

- Acute onset over days of weakness with areflexia. Neuromuscular weakness with respiratory failure in some cases. Early diagnosis and management is important.

Aetiology

- Possible cross-reacting autoimmune reactive T cells mediate response instigated by infectious antigen, e.g. *Campylobacter jejuni* infection, CMV, HIV, EBV, *Mycoplasma*, Lyme disease.
- AIDP (acute inflammatory demyelinating polyneuropathy) commonest in West.
- AMAN (acute motor axonal neuropathy) seen in Asian populations (?*C. jejuni*).

Pathology

- Most are multifocal demyelination and raised CSF protein. Slowed conduction.
- Axonal variants have axonal disruption and Wallerian degeneration.

Different forms (most are demyelinating)

- **Acute inflammatory demyelinating polyneuropathy** (AIDP) (90%): various antibodies.
- **Acute motor (+/– sensory) axonal neuropathy** (AMAN and AMSAN 5%): anti-GD1a/GM1 antibodies.
- **Miller–Fisher syndrome (5%)**: ophthalmoplegia, ataxia, areflexia: anti-GQ1b and anti-GT1a.
- Acute motor (+/– sensory) autonomic axonal neuropathy (1%): acute sensory / autonomic neuropathy.

Clinical

- Proximal weakness comes on over hours/days, usually at worst by 14 days.
- Weakness moves from legs to trunk to chest and arms and head. Tingling hands/feet. Difficulty rising from a chair. Severe back pain, respiratory and swallowing weakness.
- Distal sensory loss. Loss of distal reflexes. Papilloedema due to high CSF protein.
- Hypertension, arrhythmias, bilateral facial weakness, ptosis, ophthalmoplegia.
- Assess power of neck flexion/extension/shoulder abduction – correlates with diaphragmatic weakness.

Hughes functional grading scale

Grade 0: healthy
Grade 1: able to run
Grade 2: can walk 5 m independently
Grade 3: can walk 5 m with help
Grade 4: chair/bed bound
Grade 5: ventilated
Grade 6: death

Differentials (exclude cord or cauda equina syndrome)

- **Poliomyelitis** (and similar viral illness): will give LMN weakness. Most immunised.
- **Botulism:** flaccid paralysis, ophthalmoplegia, bulbar weakness, dry mouth, hypotension, constipation.
- **Tick paralysis**: toxin within the tick. Seen more in children. Removal of the tick is associated with improvement within hours in some cases and progression in others. Consider if recent tick exposure.
- **Acute spinal cord compression**: when signs still remain flaccid before tone increases.
- **Chronic inflammatory demyelinating polyneuropathy**: slowly progressive.
- **Acute myelopathy**: HIV, paraneoplastic. May be flaccid weakness early. MRI useful.
- **Cauda equina lesion**: flaccid weakness. Consider MRI.
- **Acute neuropathy**: porphyria, arsenic, thallium, organophosphates, lead.

Investigations

- **Bloods:** FBC, U&E to check K^+. Low Na due to SIADH can be seen.
- **ECG**: autonomic neuropathy so arrhythmias and ST/T wave changes.
- **CSF:** protein >1 g by 2nd week, WCC <10/mm^3. Glucose normal.
- **MRI spine**: if any diagnostic doubt exclude a cord/cauda equina lesion. Will depend on pattern of weakness. GBS can cause spinal nerve root enhancement with gadolinium but this is nonspecific.
- **Nerve conduction studies:** most show demyelination with slowed nerve conduction velocities and prolonged F wave. May show axonal degeneration in AMAN.
- **Antibody measurements** rarely useful except prognostically, e.g. anti-GD1a or anti-GQ1b found in Miller–Fisher variant.

Management

- **ABC and O_2** as per BTS guidelines. Respiratory support where required. Tracheal suction can cause hypotension due to autonomic instability and so ongoing telemetry and BP monitoring, for autonomic difficulties which can lead to dysrhythmia, are required.
- **Monitor low FVC (not PEFR)** at least 6 hourly for respiratory muscle weakness. HDU monitoring if FVC <1.5 L. Consider intubation FVC <1.2 L for a 65 kg person.
- **Neurology consult:** recommended before treatment. Close liaison with ITU and outreach teams should be maintained. Treatment is either IV immunoglobulin (IVIg) or plasmapharesis. Steroids not effective. In cases where response is poor a second course may be considered or plasma exchange tried.
- **Immune modulation: high dose IVIg at a dose of 0.4g/kg/day for 5 days given within first 2 weeks.** As with any blood-derived product there are issues of allergy. Can give headache, malaise. C/I with renal failure and IgA deficiency. Check IgA level first. **Plasmapheresis:** is equally effective as IVIg. Give four alternate-day exchanges over 7–10 days for a total of 200–250 ml/kg. Steroids have no benefit.
- **VTE prophylaxis**: prevent VTE with LMWH and early mobilsation
- **Ongoing rehabilitation** over weeks and months.
- **Speech and language therapy** to assess swallow safety and speech.
- **NG feeding** in the interim and PEG if delayed return of bulbar function.
- **Neuropathic pain**: carbamazepine and gabapentin and opiates as required. Amitriptyline should be avoided acutely because it can theoretically cause arrhythmias.
- **Laxatives** to avoid constipation from opiates and immobility.
- **Outcome:** 85% may have a good recovery, others are left with a degree of disability, usually monophasic but can recur and may even become progressive resembling chronic inflammatory demyelinating polyneuropathy. Worse outcome post-diarrhoea, older patient, rapid onset, muscle wasting.

Reference:

Winer JB (2002) Treatment of Guillain-Barré syndrome. *Q J Med*, 95:717–721

Zhong & Cai (2007) Current perspectives on Guillain–Barré syndrome. *World J Pediatr*, 3:187.

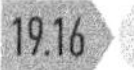

19.16 Myasthenia gravis

Check all drugs in *BNF* before prescribing for patients with MG – common medications can worsen condition.

About

- Myasthenic crisis can cause severe respiratory compromise.
- It can be brought on by medications and any acute illness.

Aetiology

- Autoantibodies to the nicotinic acetylcholine receptor or muscle specific protein kinase (musk) protein.
- Complement-mediated damage with a reduction of receptors and post-synaptic response to acetylcholine.

Clinical associations

- Rheumatoid arthritis, pernicious anaemia, systemic lupus erythematosus, sarcoidosis. Sjogren's disease, polymyositis, ulcerative colitis, pemphigus.

Clinical

- Fatigable weakness of skeletal, ocular and respiratory and bulbar musculature.
- Fluctuating proximal weakness worsens with exercise – fatigability.
- Sustained upward gaze causes diplopia and symmetrical ptosis. Eyelid twitch response (Cogan's lid twitch) is characteristic. Normal pupils.
- Respiratory muscle weakness and usually matches with neck flexion weakness.
- Difficulty in chewing, abnormal smile, dysarthria, and dysphagia are also common. Bulbar nasal quality speech, dysphagia and risk of aspiration.
- Pregnancy: MG worsens in 1st trimester of pregnancy and then improves.
- Myasthenic crises: profound weakness leads to respiratory failure.

Drugs and events exacerbating weakness

- **Common**: penicillamine, aminoglycosides, tetracycline, phenytoin can all exacerbate weakness.
- **Antibiotics:** aminoglycosides, fluoroquinolones, tetracyclines, macrolides, clindamycin.
- **Anaesthetic agents/neuromuscular blockers:** care must be taken before any anaesthesia (check *BNF*).
- **Cardiac:** beta blockers, calcium channel blockers, some antiarrhythmics, statins.
- **Other:** narcotics, steroids, anticholinergic, anticonvulsants, antipsychotics, lithium.
- **Events**: acute illness, surgery or infections can worsen symptoms.

Differential

- Lambert–Eaton syndrome: paraneoplastic, non-fatiguable.
- Botulism: bacterial toxin, tinned foods, mydriasis.
- Drug-induced myasthenia (penicillamine, aminoglycosides).
- Chronic progressive external ophthalmoplegia.
- Cholinergic crisis: excessive acetylcholinesterase inhibitors, salivation, miosis.
- Guillain–Barré syndrome: protein and WCC LP findings.
- Motor neuron disease and myopathies.

In myasthenia 10% are negative for autoantibodies.

Investigations

- **Bloods: FBC, U&E, ESR, TFTs:** check potassium/calcium/magnesium levels.
- **Autoantibodies:** acetylcholine receptor (90%), muscle specific receptor tyrosine kinase. Thymoma patients: antibody to muscle proteins ryanodine and titin. However, 1 in 10 is antibody negative.

- **Tensilon test**: edrophonium chloride (Tensilon). Cardiac monitor and resuscitation equipment in case of bradycardia/asystole needing ATROPINE. Edrophonium chloride 1 mg IV test dose given and if no problems then 2 mg IV given with determination of clinical improvement in motor power. Further edrophonium up to 10 mg IV in total may be given. Particularly useful in MG patients with ocular symptoms. Onset <1 min and lasts for 5 min. Also give placebo.
- **Ice cube test:** placed over eyelid with ptosis for 1–2 minutes and improves ptosis. Cold reduces activity of cholinesterase.
- **Repetitive nerve stimulation and single fibre electromyography** is the most sensitive test (>95%) for diagnosing MG. When a motor unit is activated, the action potentials reaching muscle fibres are not all synchronous. It is highly accurate in confirming MG by detecting 'jitter'.
- **MRI/CT thorax**: detect anterior mediastinum thymoma (found in 12% of patients with MG). All should be considered for thymectomy.

Acute management

- **Myasthenic crisis:** monitor respiration: fall in FVC, a rise in CO_2 or weak neck flexion suggests respiratory muscle weakness. A fall in PO_2 may be late. May be exacerbated by bulbar weakness. Needs immediate access to **intubation and ventilation** so liaise closely with ITU. Steroids may worsen clinical state acutely. Stop any drug that may have exacerbated the condition and manage any other acute illness. Anticholinesterases may need to be stopped as they can cause excess secretions
- **Prednisolone 40–80 mg/day** as a single slow reducing dose may be used but can cause initial worsening so some start at smaller but less effective dose, e.g. Prednisolone 20 mg OD. Usually started under inpatient supervision.
- **Immunomodulating:** acute crisis use **plasmapheresis** or **IVIg**. **Plasmapheresis**: five sessions spread over 1–2 weeks. A reduction in acetylcholine receptor antibody levels correlates to clinical response. **IVIg therapy** is typically given at a dose of 2 g/kg *divided over 5 days*. Check for IgA deficiency. Close liaison with neurologists. Later other agents include Azathioprine, Mycophenolate and Ciclosporin.
- **Pyridostigmine 30–60 mg orally 4 hourly** initially has an onset of effect in 30 min and a duration of 4 h. Long acting formulations are available for overnight. S/E include miosis, sweating, and hypersalivation, severe weakness, bradycardia, and hypotension.

19.17 Acute spinal syndrome

About

- Identify acute spinal cord or cauda equina pathology early and act quickly to prevent long term consequences. Surgical causes might be missed despite trauma assessment in the emergency department and the patient may be admitted medically.
- Bilateral leg weakness can be flaccid with reduced reflexes and loss of sphincters early in both spinal and cauda equina lesion. MRI of the whole spine in those with malignant disease as other subclinical lesions may be present.

Anatomy

- Spinal cord starts at foramen magnum and descends within the spinal canal to lower border of L1.

- Nerve roots exit cord carrying efferent motor and afferent sensory and autonomic fibres to sweat glands and sphincters run down in spinal canal to pass out via corresponding vertebral foramina.
- Cord compression will give UMN motor and sensory level signs. Cord lesions below T1 will result in weak legs, between C5 and T1 will give leg and arm weakness. Above C5 will give quadriparesis.
- Below L1 the spinal canal contains the remaining nerve roots which form the cauda equina. This ends with the conus medullaris at the lower border of S2. These are peripheral nerves but compression can be permanent with severe neurological damage so rapid diagnosis and treatment needed.
- Cauda equina damage is LMN and lowermost sensory fibres come from perianal region, saddle area and backs of legs so there will be saddle distribution anaesthesia.
- Some medical and compressive lesions can give a partial cord lesion with dissociated sensory loss and asymmetrical signs. Weakness, however, is very rarely completely unilateral.

Skeletal level	Spinal cord level
C1–C4	C1–C5 roots exiting cord and passing down to their formina
C5–C7	C6–T2 roots exiting cord and passing down to their formina
T1–T6	T3–T8 roots exiting cord and passing down to their formina
T5–T10	T8–T12 roots exiting cord and passing down to their formina
T10–T12	Lumbar roots merge
T12–L1	Sacral roots emerge
Below L1 to S2	Conus medullaris and cauda equina roots remaining

Note, for example, at L2 vertebra the canal contains the exiting L2 root and all the other nerve roots below that level.

Different clinical syndromes

Cause	Notes
Trauma to spinal cord/ cauda equina	RTA: 50%, especially if thrown from vehicle. Falls: 25% even from standing in elderly, especially at C2. Violence (especially gunshot wounds): 15%. Sports accidents: 10%, e.g. diving, rugby. Others: 5%. **Increased risk:** ankylosing spondylitis, cervical spondylosis, narrow spinal canal.
Inflammatory demyelinating	Transverse myelitis, multiple sclerosis, neuromyelitis optica.
Vascular	Cord infarction or haemorrhage 'spinal stroke', e.g. related to aortic aneurysm surgery or embolism/thrombosis, cavernomas and AVM or coagulopathies.
Chronic weak legs	Syringomyelia, MND, hereditary spastic paraparesis. B12 deficiency – posterior column and corticospinal loss. Tabes dorsalis – dorsal column loss.
Epidural haematoma	Can cause sudden acute cord injury (on anticoagulants/bleed from AV malformation, post lumbar puncture/epidural). Epidural abscess, e.g. spinal tuberculosis or other infection. Reverse anticoagulants.

Cause	Notes
Cancer	Spinal metastases can impinge the vascular supply to the cord as well as cause direct pressure. Most are epidural arising from the vertebrae such as lung (CXR), breast (breast mass) or prostate (raised PSA and ALP), thyroid, renal, myeloma. Most commonly thoracic then lumbar then cervical. Image whole cord as 2nd lesions may coexist. Primary tumours: ependymomas, astrocytomas, haemangioblastomas. Most have pain and bone destruction on plain films.
Acute porphyria	May cause a generalised muscle weakness even quadriparesis. Clues may be abdominal pain, psychiatric symptoms. See *Section 13.14.*
Disc prolapse	Soft central part of the disc, the nucleus pulposus, may rupture through the outer layers of the disc (annulus fibrosus). Most commonly posterolateral. If fragment of nucleus compresses nerve root patient experiences pain, e.g. sciatica. Also numbness and weakness in dermatome/myotome. Commonest discs to prolapse are the L4/5 on L5 root and the L5/S1 discs on S1 root. Causes pain with straight leg raise as nerve stretched. Others are possible including L3/4. A central disc protrusion can compress the central part of the canal. Effects depend on size and position of herniated disc and canal size. Central disc prolapses below L1 can cause the rare cauda equina syndrome. Discs can also rarely herniate at cervical level with nerve root pain into arm and LMN signs in the region of the compressed root. A central cervical disc lesion may cause progressive spasticity and abnormal gait below.
Neuromyelitis optica	**Transverse myelitis + optic neuritis.** Transverse myelitis may benefit from steroids. Over hours can be cancer or MS or infectious.
Anterior cord syndrome	Spastic bilateral weakness and spinothalamic loss. Preserved posterior columns (seen with anterior spinal artery infarction). Central cord syndrome: cervical level hyperextension can cause ischaemic central cord damage. Weakness and loss of sensation in both arms, intact motor and sensation in legs.
Conus medullaris	This is an intermediate level between cord and cauda equina at L1/2. Mixed UMN and LMN signs as both present at this level. Urinary retention, constipation, sacral anaesthesia, back pain, erectile dysfunction.

Clinical presentations

Cause	Notes
Bilateral leg weakness +/– arm weakness and/or sensory weakness	Should immediately suggest cord disease. If both arms and legs are weak then the problem is likely cervical or more than one lesion. Detect localised back pain and spinal tenderness, which could suggest mechanical cause. Check reflexes, brisk below lesion, absent at lesion level, but normal above. Check bladder and bowels. Immediate imaging.
Parasagittal lesion	Causes bladder dysfunction and lower leg weakness and possibly upper limb weakness which is UMN. Any facial weakness in addition to arm/leg is very useful as it means the lesion is above the pontine nuclei of VIIth nerve and not spinal.
Spinal cord dysfunction	Acute trauma to cord (UMN) can cause spinal shock – loss of reflexes below lesion, flaccid limbs below, atonic bladder, loss of vasomotor control, atonic bowel. Can last 2 weeks. Heightened activity – after 1–2 weeks with spasticity

Cause	Notes
Spinal cord dysfunction – *cont'd*	of limbs, increased reflexes, upgoing plantars, spastic bladder, increased autonomic function with sweating and vasomotor responses. Midline pain especially on any movement and local tenderness and sensory level below which sensation is lost. Log roll to examine back – assess perianal sensation and anal tone. Diaphragmatic breathing as intercostal damaged and only C3–5 intact. Acute paraplegia and quadriplegia if damage above T1. Priapism due to lost sympathetic tone as well as hypotension and bradycardia.
Hemisection of cord (Brown–Sequard syndrome)	Loss of ipsilateral posterior columns (vibration and proprioception) and corticospinal (UMN weakness) and C/I spinothalamic (pain and temperature).
Cord (acute myelopathy	Motor arms are C5 to T1. Motor to legs L2 to S3. Dermatomes same so sensory level too: a UMN cord lesion may be associated acutely with weakness, hyporeflexia and reduced tone. UMN signs may develop later. Lesions above T1 gives arm and hand symptoms. Lesions above C5 can affect breathing and diaphragmatic weakness. Back pain usually cervical or thoracic.
Cauda equina	Weak areflexic legs. Signs may be asymmetrical. Root pain down one or both legs. Also lower roots to S1–S5 affected which supplies cutaneous sensation from soles of feet, backs of legs centering on S5 in the perianal region with weak reduced tone anal sphincter, urinary retention, erectile issues. Can be devastating with paralysis from the waist down with inability to walk, no sensation to the backs of legs and loss of bladder and bowel control.

Investigations

- **Trauma:** simple radiology is vital but in non-traumatic cases or where possible go straight to MRI when cord/cauda equina pathology suspected. The whole of the spine should be visualised and symptoms and signs correlated with findings. Lateral/anteroposterior and odontoid peg views of spine. Lateral view must show C7/T1 junction. CT scan head and cervical spine (especially C1/2 lesions) and may be done instead of plain films. Fractures may exist at multiple levels. MRI is better for showing bone and ligamentous injury.
- **Medical/oncological:** urgent MRI is required to diagnose and assess or exclude a mechanical cause. Infarction of the cord may show up as may inflammatory lesions and different levels of cancer involvement. Also consider FBC, ESR/CRP, ALP, myeloma screen, U&E, LFTs, HIV test, ECG (AF with vascular lesion), INR (warfarin), CXR (lung cancer/metastases/TB), B12/folate, syphilis serology, lumbar puncture.

Management

- **General:** ABCs. Manage BP and O_2, IV fluids. Skin care with 2 hourly turns to prevent pressure or neuropathic ulcers, intermittent or temporary urinary catheterisation to prevent over distension of bladder and infection. If trauma and spine may be unstable, then spine must be immobilised using a hard collar initially and additional with sandbags. High cord lesions (above C5) with respiratory compromise may necessitate rapid sequence induction protecting C-spine.
- **MRI shows cord compression:** discuss with surgeons and give dexamethasone 10 mg IV and then 8 mg bd PO. Transfer to surgical centre for decompression. Surgery may be needed for spinal instability and to prevent further damage and to allow early mobilisation and rehabilitation. Coexisting other trauma must be looked for and managed. If possible then transfer to a spinal unit within 24 h which improves outcome.

- **Extradural haematoma:** compresses the cord. Requires drainage and reversal of anticoagulation or treatment of any coagulopathy.
- **Extradural abscess:** compresses the cord. Needs orthopaedic review and surgical drainage and IV antibiotics.
- **Oncological:** dexamethasone 4 mg IV 6 hourly. Get imaging. Take urgent advice as may need radiotherapy, chemotherapy or surgery.
- **Criteria for spinal surgery in malignancy:** single compressive lesion, unknown primary or other areas to biopsy, radio-resistant tumour, progressions despite radiotherapy, bone compression or vertebral collapse in patient with good performance status. If there are none of these but there are spinal metastases then radiation without surgery should be considered. Discuss immediately.
- **If the MRI is normal then look for a medical cause:** needs LP to look for cells and protein and consider neurology referral. Consider MRI brain if MS suspected to look for additional evidence of disseminated lesions.
- **Cauda equina lesion:** is also a surgical decompression emergency often due to a central disc prolapse below L1. Low back pain, weak legs and reduced reflexes. Saddle anaesthesia. Urgent MRI of lumbar spine and referral for surgical review. Oncology also if malignant.

19.18 Acute dystonic reactions

About

- Can be quite dramatic/bizarre and occurs even after innocuous drugs.
- Often seen in those on antipsychotics. Stop the causative drug.
- Commoner in males, recent cocaine, family history of dystonia, young.

Take a detailed drug history as innocuous drugs can cause dystonia including erythromycin, haloperidol, metoclopramide, prochlorperazine, SSRIs, cocaine, sumatriptan, ranitidine, carbamazepine.

Aetiology

- Nigrostriatal D2 receptor blockade with excess striatal cholinergic output.
- Starts within 7 days of commencing. Alcohol and cocaine use increases the risk.

Clinical

- Oculogyric crises – sustained upward gaze, torticollis, tongue protrusion, trismus.
- Sustained contractions of facial muscles, neck, trunk, pelvis, extremities, larynx.
- Everything else is normal, e.g. cognition, consciousness, vital signs.
- Can very rarely compromise airway with laryngeal/pharyngeal dystonia.

Differential

- Tetanus and strychnine poisoning, hyperventilation (carpopedal spasm).
- Hypocalcaemia and hypomagnesaemia, Wilson's disease.

Management

- Identify and stop causative drug. Give an antimuscarinic or diazepam.
- Consider PROCYCLIDINE 5–10 mg IM/IV or BENZTROPINE 1–2 mg by slow IV.
- A small dose of **DIAZEPAM 1–5 mg IV** has been used in those who fail to respond.

Reference: Campbell (2001) The management of acute dystonic reactions. *Aust Prescr*, 24:19.

20 Toxicology emergencies

See suicide and assessment (*Section 26.19*) for those with an episode of deliberate self harm.

General principles

- The following includes some general principles on overdose management. It is not comprehensive and so **Toxbase** (www.toxbase.org) should be consulted on all drugs taken. Poisons information can also be found in the *BNF* with contact numbers.
- *Check salicylate and paracetamol levels on all deliberate overdoses as common treatable posionings.* In most overdose cases the first 12 h are the most critical with maximal clinical deterioration, the notable exception being *paracetamol and iron poisoning and paraquat* where death often occurs on day 3–5. Not all appreciate the toxicity of some substances, e.g. iron tablets in children.
- Death following overdose is thankfully rare but can be further reduced with simple observation and supportive management with access to ITU as needed.
- A table of drugs with antidotes is included below. In most cases management is supportive and directed at particular problems, e.g. airway protection, ventilatory support, arrhythmias, seizure and psychosis management, etc.
- All deliberate overdoses require psychiatric evaluation when medically well.
- In the UK, online support is available at **Toxbase** which can be accessed from NHS computers. The UK National Poisons Agency is at 0870 600 6266 and will redirect calls to one of four regional centres. Consult local guidelines for expert help.

Clinical signs	Possible cause
Pink rosy colour	Cyanide, carbon monoxide.
Nausea, vomiting	Paracetamol overdose, opiates, NSAIDs, iron toxicity, salicylates.
Small pupils	Opiates, gamma hydroxybutyrate, pontine bleed, cholinergic syndrome (insecticides).
Large pupils	Cocaine, tricyclic antidepressants, amphetamines, anticholinergic syndrome – ATROPINE, 'belladonna'.
Severe hypertension	Cocaine, amphetamines.
Bradycardia	DIGOXIN, β-blockers, CCBs, opioids.
Hypoglycaemia	Insulin, sulphonylurea, meglitinides, alcohol, QUININE, salicylates.
Hyperglycaemia	Organophosphates, Theophyllines, MAOIs.
Hyperventilation	Salicylates.
Renal failure	Renal failure, salicylates, paraquat, ethylene glycol.
Hyperthermia	Serotonin syndrome, cocaine, ecstasy, MAOIs, theophylline.
Hypothermia	Exposure due to sedation/alcohol, phenothiazines, barbiturates.

Clinical signs	Possible cause
RUQ pain/jaundice	Paracetamol poisoning, organic solvents, iron toxicity.
Abdominal pain	Iron poisoning, lead toxicity, NSAIDs.
Seizures	Mefenamic acid, TCAs, opioids, theophylline, cocaine, alcohol.
Rhabdomyolysis	Amphetamines, neuroleptics.
Chest pain	Cocaine, carbon monoxide.
Oral ulcers	Corrosives, paraquat.
Elevated osmolar gap	Acetone, mannitol, methanol, acetone, ethanol, ethylene glycol.
Anion gap metabolic acidosis	Methanol, metformin, renal failure, diabetic/alcoholic ketoacidosis, iron, isoniazid.
Lactic acidosis	Ethylene glycol, cyanide, carbon monoxide, toluene, salicylates.

20.1 Drugs with specific antidotes

Drug	Antidote
Arsenic	Dimercaptosuccinic acid (Succimer), dimercaprol
Benzodiazepines	Flumazenil 200 mcg over 15 sec then 100 mcg at minute intervals. Use only with severe respiratory depression. It may provoke seizures. Most benzodiazepine overdoses are 'slept off' with simple observation of ABCs.
Beta-blockers	Severe bradycardia consider ATROPINE 1–3 mg IV and/or GLUCAGON 2–10 mg IV bolus
Caesium/thallium poisoning	Prussian blue
Calcium channel blockers	CALCIUM CHLORIDE/gluconate
Carbon monoxide	100% O_2 or hyperbaric oxygen
Cyanide	High flow O_2 and cyanide kit – amyl nitrate, sodium nitrate, sodium thiosulphate, hydroxycobalamin
DIGOXIN	DIGOXIN-specific Fab antibodies (Digibind)
Ethanol	Supportive and haemodialysis
Ethylene glycol	Alcohol or Fomepizole and haemodialysis
Heparin	Protamine
Insulin/oral hypoglycaemics	Oral or IV dextrose and IM glucagon
Iron salts	Desferrioxamine 15 mg/kg/h IV
Drugs causing **met-haemoglobinaemia**	Methylene blue

Drug	Antidote
Methanol	Alcohol or Fomepizole and folinic acid
Methotrexate and trimethoprim	Leucovorin/folinic acid
Nerve agents	ATROPINE 2 mg IV (every 2 min until pulse >70/min) and Pralidoxime 30 mg/kg
Opioids	NALOXONE 0.4–2.0 mg IV/IM may need to be repeated depending on half life of opiate; NALOXONE has a short half life
Organophosphate	ATROPINE 2 mg IV (every 2 min until pulse >70/min) and Pralidoxime 30 mg/kg
Paracetamol	Oral methionine or IV *N*-acetyl cysteine
Phenothiazine dystonic reactions	Benzatropine 1–2 mg IV
Salicylates	Sodium bicarbonate IV
Sulphonylureas	Glucose, Octreotide
Tricyclic antidepressant	Sodium bicarbonate IV
Warfarin	Vitamin K 5 mg slow IV and prothrombin complex concentrates (PCC) or FFP if PCC not available

20.2 Methods to reduce absorption

- As with all drugs the risk of the methods to reduce absorption need to be considered in light of the potential toxicity of the ingested substance. In some cases gastric lavage is attempted and in others not.
- **Gastric lavage:** now used much less than before. Airway protection against aspiration is fundamental to avoid aspiration. Only done if serious and difficult to manage overdose taken within last hour. Ideally patient intubated with anaesthetist at hand. Ensure O_2 and suction at hand. Place patient in left lateral head down position. Raise foot of bed. **Not if corrosive agents or petroleum products** which can cause a chemical pneumonitis and ARDS if aspirated. A lubricated size 36–40 FG stomach tube inserted and attached to a funnel. Listen over stomach for injected air or aspirate gastric juices. If intubated then concerns about being in the trachea are unwarranted. Pour in 300 ml aliquots and then allow aspirate to come out. Massage over stomach to help tablets out. Finish with 50 g of activated charcoal.
- **Ipecac:** was once used to induce vomiting in poisoned patients for whom there was a chance to get the toxin out of the body. Now rarely used. Many believe that ipecac and gastric lavage are essentially worthless, potentially harmful, and unlikely to alter morbidity and mortality in the real world.
- **Activated charcoal:** high degree of microporosity; 1 g has a surface area in excess of 500 m^2. Consider when less than 1 h since tablets taken. Binds materials by van der Waal's forces or London dispersion force. **Does not bind alcohols, glycols, strong acids and bases, metals and most inorganics, such as lithium, sodium, iron, lead, arsenic, fluorine, and boric acid very well, or hydrocarbons.** Activated charcoal is estimated

to reduce absorption of some substances by up to 60%. It remains within the GI tract and eliminates the toxin in faeces. Large amounts require laxative to ensure passage. Best taken by cooperative patient or if not then consider administration via NG tube. For drug overdose or poisoning: 50–100 g of activated charcoal is given at first. Unless a patient has an intact or protected airway, the administration of charcoal is contraindicated.

- **Multi-dose activated charcoal:** for drug overdose or poisoning: 50–100 g of activated charcoal is given at first, followed by charcoal every 2–4 h at a dose equal to 12.5 g/h. Used to interrupt enteroenteric, enterogastric, and enterohepatic circulation of absorbed drugs. Used for **carbamazepine, dapsone, phenobarbital, QUININE, or theophylline toxicity.** Unless a patient has an intact or protected airway, the administration of charcoal is contraindicated.
- **Total bowel irrigation:** polyethylene glycol is given via NG tube into bowel. About 2 L/h given. Useful for body packers, sustained release formulations. This does not cause fluid shifts. Administer until clear effluent from bowels.
- **Dialysis:** useful for substances not heavily protein bound: alcohol, DABIGATRAN, salicylates, lithium and ethylene glycol, valproate, methanol, theophylline, carbamazepine.

20.3 Drug toxic syndromes

Anti-cholinergic syndrome	**About:** 3 Ds (dry/dilated pupils/delirium): blockade of the neurotransmitter acetylcholine in the central and the peripheral nervous system at muscarinic receptors. **Clinical:** dry flushed skin and mouth, mydriasis, delirium, fever, sinus tachycardia, decreased bowel sounds, functional ileus, urinary retention, hypertension, tremulousness, and myoclonic jerking. Centrally these cause ataxia, confusion and disorientation, short-term memory loss, hallucinations (visual, auditory), psychosis, seizures (rare), coma, respiratory failure, and cardiovascular collapse. **Causes:** antihistamines, antipsychotics, antidepressants, atropine-like drugs, belladonna and other plant-derived agents. **Management:** generally supportive, IV DIAZEPAM/LORAZEPAM for seizures. IV fluids, ECG monitoring. β-blockers for tachycardia. Catheterisation for urinary retention.
Opioid syndrome	**Clinical:** small pinpoint pupils, comatose, bradycardia and hypotension, constipation, itch. Respiratory depression. See opioid overdose in *Section 20.4*. **Management:** O_2 as per BTS guidelines. Give **NALOXONE 0.4–1.2 mg**. Watch ABG. May need intubation and repeated Naloxone.
Serotonin syndrome	**Aetiology:** excess serotonin. **Clinical:** tachycardia, shivering, sweating, mydriasis, diarrhoea, myoclonic jerks, hyperreflexia, clonus, hyperthermia. Increased vigilance and agitation, metabolic acidosis, rhabdomyolysis. DIC, AKI, seizures. **Cause:** some antidepressants (SSRIs and SNRIs) and opioids, TCAs, MAOIs, lithium. **Management:** DIAZEPAM IV for seizures and agitation and can reduce muscle tone. IV fluids. Supportive. β-blockage for arrhythmias. Should settle once causative drug stopped. Give O_2 as per BTS guidelines.

Cholinergic syndrome	**About:** overstimulation of central and peripheral acetylcholine-based nicotinic acid receptors at the neuromuscular junction and at muscarinic receptors due to an excess of acetylcholine. May be due to reduced breakdown of acetylcholine by acetylcholinesterase. Seen with sarin/organophosphate poisoning and carbamate pesticides. Excess medications for myasthenia or dementia. **Clinical:** flaccid paralysis, respiratory failure, increased sweating, hypertension, urination, diarrhoea, salivation, bradycardia, copious bronchial secretions, miosis, seizures. **DUMPSS:** diarrhoea, urination, miosis, paralysis, seizure, secretion. **Management:** ABCs. O_2 as per BTS guidelines. Cholinergic crisis can be treated with antimuscarinic drugs like atropine given IV and Pralidoxime. Intubation and ventilation if not improving. Atropine blocks muscarinic sites. Pralidoxime blocks muscarinic and nicotinic sites. Supportive management.

Generic issues

Problems	Management
Respiratory depression	Naloxone as indicated. May need airways management and intubation and ventilation. Enlist help of anaesthetists.
Hyperthermia	Fans, IV fluids, iced baths, dantrolene.
Ongoing seizures	Lorazepam, phenytoin/fosphenytoin.
Acute anxiety	Diazepam, lorazepam, haloperidol (not if seizure).
Bradycardia	ATROPINE IV, ISOPRENALINE, ventricular pacing, calcium/hyperinsulin normoglycaemic therapy for CCBs, GLUCAGON. Digibind for DIGOXIN OD.
Nausea/vomiting	METOCLOPRAMIDE, ondansentron.

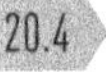

20.4 Specific drug overdoses

Amphetamines

About

- Various types: methamphetamine ('crystal meth') and ecstasy.

Clinical

- Euphoria, hallucinations, agitation, tachycardia, hypertension.
- Bruxism, dilated pupils, sweating, psychosis, seizures, cerebral oedema.

Complications

- Can cause DIC, fulminant liver failure, AKI and rhabdomyolysis.

Investigations

- **Bloods:** FBC, U&E, Mg, Ca, ECG, glucose.
- **CT head/LP**: if fever, coma, confusion to exclude other causes.

Management

- **Supportive**: give O_2 as per BTS guidelines and reassess after ABG. ECG monitoring. Give IV crystalloid if normonatraemic and euvolaemic or hypovolaemic. If ingestion very recent then activated charcoal may be used. For huge amounts, e.g. body packing for drug trafficking, then whole bowel irrigation may be considered. May require ITU.

- **Seizures:** as per status epilepticus (*Section 19.4*). *Agitation/psychosis*: DIAZEPAM or HALOPERIDOL (may lower seizure threshold so combined with benzodiazepines) for agitation/seizures. Effects may last up to 12 h.
- Manage complications as discussed elsewhere. Watch temperature. Cooling may be needed for hyperthermia, e.g. ice baths.

Beta-blockers

About

- Competitively blocks β1 and β2 adrenoreceptors.

Clinical

- Bradycardia-related hypotension. Bronchospasm. Worsening cardiac failure.

Investigations

- FBC, U&E, Mg, Ca, glucose. ECG: heart blocks and bradycardia, QT changes.

Management

- **Supportive**: ABC, physiological monitoring, IV crystalloid, telemetry. Consider gastric lavage if very early presentation. Bronchospasm managed with **SALBUTAMOL** nebulisers.

Severe bradycardia and circulatory failure

- **ATROPINE** up to 3 mg IV and/or temporary pacing may be needed. **DOBUTAMINE** may be used.
- **GLUCAGON** 2–10 mg IV may be used as a bolus and infusion. If helps then followed by a continuous IV infusion at a rate of 2–5 mg/h (maximum: 10 mg/h) in 5% dextrose injection.
- **INSULIN: hyperinsulinaemic euglycaemic (HIE) therapy** where high dose insulin is given along with IV dextrose to prevent hypoglycaemia. Infusion doses starting at 0.5 U/kg and increasing to 1.0–10 U/kg/h have been given with 10–20% dextrose, being careful to avoid hypoglycaemia and hypokalaemia.
- **Intra-aortic balloon pumping** has been used for circulatory support.

References:

Engebretsen *et al*. (2011) High-dose insulin therapy in beta-blocker and calcium channel-blocker poisoning. *Clin Toxicol*, 49:277.

Shepherd (2006) Treatment of poisoning caused by beta-adrenergic and calcium-channel blockers. *Am J Health Pharmacy*, 63:1828.

Benzodiazepines

About

- Diazepam, Clonazepam, Temazepam. Generally used as sedatives.

Clinical

- Drowsiness and coma. If coma (GCS <10) look for other drugs or pathology.
- Pupils may be partially dilated, ataxia, dysarthria.
- Higher risk where combined with alcohol or underlying chest disease and elderly.

Investigations

- FBC, U&E, Mg, Ca, ECG, glucose. ABG if comatose or low saturations or breathless.

Management

- **Supportive**: ABCs. Within 1 h activated charcoal may be given. Most overdoses are slept off. Give O_2 as per BTS guidelines. Recovery position and nasopharyngeal airway if needed. IV fluids.

- **Severe respiratory depression** and GCS <9 and concerns about the airway flumazenil 200 mcg (0.2 mg) over 15 sec and then 100–300 mcg (0.1–0.3 mg) might be given up to a maximum dose of 3 mg, but there is a risk of lowering seizure threshold, especially in a mixed overdose with other drugs that also lower seizure threshold, e.g. alcohol, TCAs.
- Lone overdoses will rarely need ITU. Most are stable <24 h depending on severity of overdose.

Calcium channel blockers

Occasionally lethal so do not underestimate seriousness, admit CCU/ITU and give IV calcium.

About

- Amlodipine/Felodipine and Nifedipine act peripherally and may cause hypotension. Verapamil and Diltiazem act on the heart.

Aetiology

- Block influx of calcium into myocardial and vascular tissues via L-type channels.

Clinical

- Severe bradycardia and hypotension, circulatory collapse, cardiac arrest, cardiogenic shock.

Investigations

- **Bloods**: FBC, U&E, Mg, Ca, ECG.

Management

- **Supportive**: ABC, O_2, ECG monitoring. Best on CCU or ITU/HDU. Give 500–1000 ml IV crystalloids and treat bradycardia with IV ATROPINE 0.6–1.2 mg.
- Whole-bowel irrigation with polyethylene glycol and activated charcoal can treat overdose with sustained-release VERAPAMIL.
- **CALCIUM: give 10–20 ml 10% CALCIUM GLUCONATE/CHLORIDE IV** and an infusion may improve cardiac contractile function. Aim for mild hypercalcaemia. Maintain monitoring for at least 12 h especially with modified release preparations.
- **ADRENALINE** IV with close monitoring in a HDU/ITU with senior advice if hypotensive/bradycardia at a rate of 1 mcg/min (as the hydrochloride) and increased as necessary. Watch ECQ and for ST changes.
- **INSULIN: hyperinsulinaemic euglycaemic (HIE) therapy** where high dose insulin is given along with IV dextrose to prevent hypoglycaemia. Infusion doses starting at 0.5 U/kg and increasing to 1.0–10 U/kg/h have been given with 10–20% dextrose, being careful to avoid hypoglycaemia and hypokalaemia.
- **GLUCAGON** for hypotensive patients: give IV bolus 3 mg (0.05 mg/kg) and then an infusion.
- **DOPAMINE** at 5–20 mcg/kg/min can reduce systemic vasodilation, but may also need noradrenaline.
- **Cardiac pacing** may be considered for persisting significant bradycardia-induced hypotension.

References:

Engebretsen *et al*. (2011) High-dose insulin therapy in beta-blocker and calcium channel-blocker poisoning. *Clin Toxicol*, 49:277.

Shepherd (2006) Treatment of poisoning caused by beta-adrenergic and calcium-channel blockers. *Am J Health Pharmacy*, 63:1828.

Cannabis (marijuana)

About

- Cannabis is derived from parts of the plant *Cannabis sativa*.
- Can be smoked (effects within 10–20 min) or ingested (effects 1–2 h).

Clinical

- Low doses cause acute euphoria and altered reality, relaxation.
- Hallucinations, drowsiness, visual distortions, hypertension, tachycardia.
- High doses: acute delirium, anxiety attacks, depersonalisation.
- IV usage of cannabis can cause renal failure, pulmonary oedema and DIC.

Investigations

- FBC, U&E, Mg, Ca, ECG, CXR and/or coagulation screen as indicated.
- Urine toxicology: can be detected in urine for several days.

Management

- If sedation for acute anxiety then **DIAZEPAM IV** or **HALOPERIDOL IV/IM**.
- IV crystalloid for hypotension. Serious poisoning rare. Most resolve quickly.
- Those with IV use need particular care and admission for ongoing observation.

Carbon monoxide

> O_2 sats by pulse oximetry can be falsely normal. If you suspect CO you must check ABG and COHb and ECG.

About

- Odourless, colourless gas, from the incomplete combustion of fossil fuels.

Clues

- Deliberate overdose, e.g. exhaust fumes or accidental from poorly ventilated faulty home heating.
- Low dose toxicity may be subtler in its presentation, e.g. 'flu' like illness.
- A new cold period where gas/solid fuel home/water heating used, changes to home heating or ventilation.

Aetiology

- CO binds avidly to Hb with 240 times greater affinity than oxygen and inhibits cytochrome oxidase A3.
- Saturation probes treat COHb as O_2Hb giving a false normal SaO_2.
- Normal COHb is 3–5% with levels up to 10% in smokers. Result is tissue hypoxia and metabolic acidosis.
- The result is leftward shift in O_2 haemoglobin dissociation curve.
- Causes myocardial and cerebral hypoxia and cerebral oedema.

Clinical

- Drowsiness, headache, fatigue, breathlessness, coma and death.
- Pink rosy colouration.

Investigations

- **Bloods**: FBC, U&E, lactate, ABG. Troponin.
- **Measure COHb** specifically if diagnosis considered. Patients get O_2 en route and so hospital COHb may not represent prior levels or the extent and severity of any hypoxia. **Severe when** COHb >10%.

Differential

- Excess opiates, sedatives, and excess alcohol. Stroke.
- Subdural or other intracranial lesion.

Management

- **Remove source**: open windows, switch off heating/car engine.
- **Supportive**: O_2 sat probe unreliable. Check ABG. Give **oxygen therapy**: give 100% O_2 unless COPD and Type 2 RF and if so consider ventilation. 100% O_2 will reduce half-life of CO from 4 h to 40 min. Give O_2 12 L/min via CPAP mask for at least 6 h until COHb is less than 5%; may be needed for 12–24 h.
- **Severe cases:** (when COHb >10% or ECG shows ischaemia or signs of cerebral oedema) cause fitting and cardiorespiratory arrest. Prone to cerebral oedema so do neurological observations. Patients may need IV mannitol. Risk of long term neuropsychiatric damage, Parkinsonism and cerebellar symptoms.
- **Indications for hyperbaric O_2 which reduces CO half-life to 20 min are**: COHb >40%, coma, neurological or psychiatric problems, ECG changes, e.g. ST depression, T wave changes, arrhythmias, pregnancy (fetal COHb is to the left of mother's). Transporting patients to a distant hyperbaric chamber can be hazardous and difficult and the role of hyperbaric O_2 is controversial. Take expert advice.

Cocaine

About

- Always ask about usage with anxiety, BP, chest pain, stroke.

Aetiology

- Cocaine is a CNS stimulant derived from the leaves of the coca plant.
- Blocks reuptake of dopamine, serotonin and noradrenaline.
- Chronic usage may actually accelerate atherosclerosis.
- Pleasurable effects from raising dopamine levels in the mesolimbic reward centres.

Administration

- Snorted and absorbed via well vascularised tissues (that normally heat and humidify air) lining the nose – causes localised vasoconstriction and eventual damage to the nasal mucosa.
- Smoked or taken IV – these give a rapid response but a shorter high than snorting. Rubbed on the gums or small amounts taken orally, or taken as a suppository.
- Cocaine-induced chest pain usually due to spasm and generally not treated with thrombolysis. Users often have coexisting atherosclerotic disease which are actually more prone to spasm.

Clinical

- Chest pain, neurological signs from ischaemic/haemorrhagic stroke, aortic dissection, hypertension.
- Tachycardia, hyperthermia, euphoria, psychotic, dilated pupils, long term myocarditis, atherosclerosis.

Investigations

- **Bloods**: FBC, U&E, troponin at baseline and 12 h. CXR cardiomegaly.
- **ECG**: ischaemia or look for STEMI, LVH. **CT head** if any neurology.

Management

- **Supportive**: O_2 as per BTS guidance. IV fluids. Suspected ACS with ST elevation necessitates primary PCI. Thrombolysis is generally avoided especially where markedly hypertensive. Give **GTN** sublingually and then **IV GTN** as a prelude to PCI. Caution with β-blockade, which will cause HTN due to unopposed α effects.
- **Hyperthermia** is a side effect of cocaine and should be treated with fluids, cooling and dantrolene.
- **Agitation**: DIAZEPAM PO/IV. Avoid HALOPERIDOL, phenothiazines which lower fit threshold.

Cyanide

About

- Accidental exposure may be seen in the chemical industry.
- Suicide or homicide attempt.

Aetiology

- Burning of plastics/foam with smoke inhalation.
- Excess **sodium nitroprusside** infusion.
- Inhibits cytochrome a3, blocking mitochondrial oxidative phosphorylation.

Clinical

- In lethal overdoses death is usually pre-hospital. Survival to hospital bodes well.
- Evidence of smoke inhalation, **cherry-red skin colour,** smell of bitter almonds on the breath. Chest pain and dyspnoea, seizures, coma.

Investigation

- FBC, U&E, LFT, CXR, ECG.
- **ABG**: metabolic acidosis, increased lactate suggests significant overdose.

Management

- **Supportive:** ABC and respiratory support with high flow O_2. ITU if high early warning scores.
- **Dicobalt edetate 300 mg IV over 1 min** followed by 50 ml of 50% dextrose, but only if severe toxicity confirmed because it is itself very toxic. Otherwise, **Hydroxycobalamin 5 g** over 15 min, which combines to form cyanocobalamin. Alternatively, **Sodium thiosulphate** (25 ml of 50% solution), which enhances the conversion of cyanide to thiocyanate, which is renally excreted. Take expert advice.

Digoxin

About

- Commonly available and occasionally overdosed accidentally.
- Lethal dose = 10 mg (adult) and 4 mg (child). Well absorbed orally.
- Half-life 30–40 h, with peak toxicity at 6 h and death at 6–12 h post ingestion.

K^+ >5.5 mmol/L suggests severe potentially fatal DIGOXIN toxicity.

Aetiology

- Blocks Na/K ATPase pump: raises intracellular Ca^{2+} and reduces AV conduction.
- Causes bradycardia, raised vagal tone, automaticity, and hyperkalaemia.

Clinical

- Nausea and vomiting, yellow vision, abdominal pain.
- Bradycardia, AV block, SVT (with AV block), AF, VT and even VF.

Investigations

- **Bloods**: FBC, U&E, calcium, DIGOXIN level.
- **Serial ECGs**: CCU monitoring for arrhythmias.

Management

- **Supportive: DO NOT GIVE CALCIUM in any form.** Admit for CCU monitoring: can lead to low BP, arrhythmias, cardiac arrest. ATROPINE 0.6 mg IV for AV block.
- **Gastric lavage** if seen within 1 h. Give activated charcoal if within 1 h of ingestion in cooperative patient. Repeated dosing may be helpful. Manage hyperkalaemia with sodium bicarbonate and/or insulin/dextrose. Give **MAGNESIUM IV** and consider **LIDOCAINE 50–100 mg IV** for refractory VT/VF.
- **DIGOXIN immune Fab:** given where adult dose >10 mg ingested, serious life-threatening arrhythmias, DIGOXIN level >15 nmol/ml (12 ng/ml), K^+ >5 mmol/L. **Note**: each Digibind vial will bind approximately 0.5 mg of DIGOXIN (or digitoxin), so multiple vials will need to be given in a significant overdose, e.g. 10 mg DIGOXIN taken. You will have to summon as much as possible, e.g. 20 vials. It is expensive and not always stocked. Contact poisons advisory service for nearest stores. If renal failure, then plasmapheresis may be needed to clear DIGOXIN–Fab complexes. In a cardiac arrest continue to give multiple vials of this for up to 30 min as resuscitation continues.

Ethanol (C_2H_5OH)

About

- Metabolised to acetaldehyde by alcohol dehydrogenase which is metabolised to acetate by acetaldehyde dehydrogenase found in liver mitochondria.
- Significant toxicity in overdose and mixed with other sedatives.
- Seen in mouthwashes, hand-washes, antiseptics. Ingested alcohol is almost totally absorbed within 1 h.

Clinical

- Small amounts cause mild incoordination, euphoria and reduced reaction time.
- Moderate amounts lead to a cerebellar-type ataxia, dysarthria and even diplopia, sweating and tachycardia. Disinhibition, aggression and resulting violence and accidents.
- Severe overdose: coma, respiratory depression and aspiration and death.

Investigations

- **Bloods**: FBC, U&E, LFTs. Chronic usage – elevated GGT and macrocytosis.
- **ABG:** acute intake can cause a metabolic acidosis.
- **Ethanol levels**: mild: <150 mg/dL, moderate: 150–300 mg/dL, severe: 300–500 mg/dL.

Complications

- Coma, aspiration, head injury (low threshold for CT if concerns), hypoglycaemia.
- Alcoholic ketoacidosis, lactic acidosis, AKI, rhabdomyolysis.

Management

- **Supportive**: ABC, give sufficient O_2 as per BTS guidance. ITU if high early warning scores. Rapid gastric uptake renders lavage and charcoal unhelpful. Neuro-observations and physiological monitoring (O_2 sat, BP, HR, blood glucose). Most are slept off in recovery position with close monitoring, but some require intubation and ventilation for severe respiratory depression. **IV NS** to ensure hydration.

- **IV thiamine 50–100 mg or Pabrinex IV** should be given in chronic alcoholics.
- **Hypoglycaemia** may be seen and should be treated with 10% dextrose IV.
- **Benzodiazepines**: LORAZEPAM/DIAZEPAM for seizures.
- **Haemodialysis** with blood ethanol levels >4 g/L (400 mg/dL) or severe metabolic acidosis pH <7.0–7.1. Most patients have stabilised by 12 h.

Ethylene glycol

About

- Sweet taste; it is harmless until metabolised by alcohol dehydrogenase.
- Used as antifreeze and has been added to alcohol drinks. Alcohol is an antidote.

Clinical

- Coma, Kussmaul's breathing, aspiration, seizures, cerebral oedema, ARDS, AKI.

Investigations

- **U&E, LFT, ABG**: AKI, severe raised anion gap metabolic acidosis.
- **Calcium/urinalysis**: hypocalcaemia and calcium oxalate crystalluria.
- **Ethylene glycol:** >20 mg/dL, osmolar gap >10 mOsm/L, pH <7.3.

Management

- **Supportive**: ABC, give O_2 as per BTS guidelines. IV fluids. Airways management if comatose. Consider ITU if high early warning scores.
- Treat if there is clear evidence of ethylene glycol/methanol ingestion or suspicion and evidence of metabolic disturbance – osmolar gap >10 mmol/dL, arterial pH <7.3, raised anion gap metabolic acidosis.
  - 1st line: **FOMEPIZOLE IV** to block alcohol dehydrogenase.
  - 2nd line: **ETHANOL IV or PO/NG** if fomepizole unavailable.
- Acidosis should be corrected with IV sodium bicarbonate.
- Haemodialysis and fomepizole if pH <7.25, AKI, EG levels >50 mg/dL.
- Seizures as per standard treatment.

Reference: Brent (2009) Fomepizole for ethylene glycol and methanol poisoning. *New Engl J Med*, 360:2216.

Gamma hydroxybutyrate (GHB)

About

- White powder, dissolved in water forms an odourless, colourless liquid.
- Mild euphoric effects. Abused as a date rape drug or sleep aid or by bodybuilders.

Aetiology

- It stimulates release of growth hormone. It is a GABA agonist.
- Gamma butyrolactone (GBL) is a similar drug with similar effects.

Clinical

- Excitement, miosis, agitation, amnesia, bradycardia, myoclonic jerks.
- Hypotension, respiratory depression and coma.

Investigations

- **Bloods**: FBC, U&E, ABG as needed. Toxicology if other drugs taken.

Management

- **Supportive**: ABC and O_2 as per BTS guidelines and airways protections; ITU if high early warning scores.

- IV fluids, and watch for expected improvement which can be rapid when it occurs. Effects enhanced with alcohol/other drugs. Effects unpredictable even in same individual.

Insulin

About

- Commonly available and potentially lethal. May be deliberate or accidental.
- Long acting insulins more difficult to manage.

Pathophysiology

- Insulin excess results in hypoglycaemia. Long acting insulins active >24 h.

Clinical

- Hypoglycaemic: confusion, tremor, hunger, panic, altered behaviour, confusion, coma, violence.

Investigations

- Check blood sugar every 30–60 min and when there are symptoms.
- Check FBC, U&E and LFTs (liver injury).
- Check C peptide (not elevated if exogenous insulin).

Management

- **Supportive**: ITU if high early warning scores. Regular observation and blood glucose testing every 30–60 min. Use IV glucose 10% infusion to maintain blood glucose at >4 mmol/L by peripheral or central line.
- New long acting insulins with significant overdose need IV glucose.
- Surgical removal of insulin injection site has been used for overdose of long acting insulin.

Reference: Eldred *et al*. (2013) The patient who has taken an overdose of long-acting insulin analogue. *Acute Med*, 12:167.

Iron (ferrous sulphate)

About

- Often taken accidentally. Highly toxic, particularly for children.

Clinical

- Minor overdoses: nausea, vomiting, dyspepsia to haematemesis and melaena.
- Large overdoses: cardiovascular collapse, Kussmaul's breathing, hepatorenal failure.
- After 48 h: liver failure can occur. Later liver fibrosis and scarring.

Investigations

- Iron level at 4 h, lactate, ECG, U&E, LFTs.
- KUB film: radio-opaque iron tablets seen suggest **whole-bowel irrigation.**
- Metabolic acidosis (raised anion gap), AKI.
- Liver injury: raised LFTs and prothrombin time and hypoglycaemia.

Management

- **Supportive:** ABCs, resuscitate, IV crystalloids. ITU if high early warning scores.
- **Assess risk:** ingested dose 20–60 mg/kg will give GI effects, and 60–120 mg/kg systemic toxicity. A dose >120 mg/kg is potentially lethal. In children, 1–2 g can be fatal. Act quickly.

- **Perform whole-bowel irrigation:** those with radio-opacities on KUB until the opacities clear or for amounts taken >60 mg/kg. Surgical or endoscopic removal for significant overdoses.
- **IV DESFERRIOXAMINE infusion chelation therapy:** for toxic levels >90 µmol/L at 4–6 h post ingestion. Metabolic acidosis or altered mental state can be life saving. **DESFERRIOXAMINE IM** administration is preferred and should be used for PATIENTS NOT IN SHOCK.

Lithium

About

- Alkali metal widely used for bipolar affective disorders. Rapid GI absorption. No protein binding. Toxicity with dehydration or use of diuretics.

Clinical

- Acute toxicity causes tremor, dysarthria, confusion, delirium, seizures, coma.
- Thirst, and polyuria due to an induced nephrogenic diabetes insipidus (NDI).
- Chronic toxicity: encephalopathy with neuropathy and cerebellar dysfunction.

Investigations

- **U&E**: hypernatraemia due to NDI. **ECG:** T wave flattening.
- **Lithium levels:** therapeutic range 0.6–1.2 mmol/L. Symptoms increase when levels >2.0 mmol/L, coma occurs at >3.0 mmol/L, with massive overdose at >5.0 mmol/L.

Complications

- Truncal and gait ataxia, nystagmus, short-term memory loss and dementia.
- SILENT – syndrome of irreversible lithium-effectuated neurotoxicity.

Management

- **Supportive:** rehydration with IV NS and 5% dextrose to match urine losses. Polyuria due to nephrogenic diabetes insipidus can take weeks to recover.
- **Whole bowel irrigation:** GI decontamination method of choice. Lithium is not protein bound so **haemodialysis** effective in removing lithium.

Methanol (CH_3CHO)

About

- Slightly sweeter than ethanol and is metabolised to toxic formic acid.

Aetiology

- Rapid absorption orally. Peak methanol concentrations within 60 min.
- 10 ml can be severely toxic with blindness within the first day post ingestion.

Clinical

- Nausea, vomiting, abdominal pain, tachypnoea, tachycardia, coma and death.
- Dilated pupils, hyperaemia of the optic disc, retinal oedema and blindness due to optic nerve toxicity.
- Metabolic acidosis with Kussmaul's respiration.
- Later polyneuropathy, tremors, rigidity, spasticity and hypokinesis.
- Later a Parkinsonian-like extrapyramidal syndrome with mild dementia.

Investigations

- **Methanol level**: lethal dose range of 300–1000 mg/kg. Serum level >500 mg/L confirms severe poisoning. Methanol is measured in usual toxicology screen, but treatment should start empirically.

- **ABG**: increasing severe metabolic acidosis with an increased anion gap (formic acid). Elevated osmolar gap. Lactate and ketones minimally elevated.

Management

- **Supportive**: ABC, give O_2 as per BTS guidance. IV fluids. HDU management if comatose.
- **Treatment indicated:** clear evidence of ethylene glycol/methanol ingestion or suspicion and metabolic disturbance – osmolar gap >10 mmol/dL, arterial pH <7.3, raised anion gap metabolic acidosis.
    - 1st line: **FOMEPIZOLE IV** to block alcohol dehydrogenase.
    - 2nd line: **ETHANOL IV or ORAL** if fomepizole unavailable.
- **Acidosis:** should be corrected with IV sodium bicarbonate.
- **Haemodialysis** can be used to remove methanol and correct metabolites.
- **Seizures:** as per standard treatment.
- **FOLINIC ACID** may help prevent ocular toxicity.

Reference: Brent (2009) Fomepizole for ethylene glycol and methanol poisoning. *New Engl J Med*, 360:2216.

3,4 Methylenedioxymethamphetamine (Ecstasy)

About

- Increasing need to take higher doses for same effect.

Clinical

- Euphoria, agitation, tachycardia, dilated pupils, sweating, trismus.
- Thirst and excess fluid intake + SIADH can cause severe hyponatraemia.
- Seizures, cerebral oedema, DIC and fulminant liver failure, AKI and rhabdomyolysis.

Investigations

- U&E: low Na, AKI, raised CK, FBC, blood glucose, LFTs.

Management

- **Supportive:** may require ITU if GCS <9 or high early warning score. Give IV NS if normonatraemic and euvolaemic or hypovolaemic. ECG monitoring.
- **Hyponatraemia**: management is dependent on fluid balance and sodium level and clinical status.
- **IV DIAZEPAM** or **HALOPERIDOL** for agitation. Cooling and Dantrolene for hyperthermia.
- **Manage seizures** as per status epilepticus (*Section 19.4*). Manage complications as discussed elsewhere.
- Fatalities rare due to liver failure and cerebral oedema.

Novel / new oral anticoagulants (NOACs)

About

- Thrombin inhibitor (TI) and factor Xa inhibitors (XAI).
- Used in stroke prevention in non-valvular AF and VTE prophylaxis and treatment.
- Dabigatran (TI) has a half-life of about 12–14 h.
- Others: Apixaban, Rivaroxaban (both XAI).

Properties

- 80% renally excreted. Enhanced toxicity in renal disease.
- In haemorrhage find out when last dose taken.

Clinical

- Haemorrhage: intracranial, extracranial, GI, urine.
- Retroperitoneal bleed, psoas, intramuscular, intradermal blood.

Management

- Apply direct pressure. Surgical input as needed. Transfuse and supportive.
- Half-life short and wears off after 24 h but bleed risk may continue for several days especially if impaired renal function. Renal dialysis is suggested to remove drug.
- Discuss other options, e.g. Octaplex/Beriplex and discuss FFP with haematologist.
- Currently there is no actual antidote and this is likely to be an increasing future problem.
- Guidelines changing so take expert advice.

Non-steroidal anti-inflammatory drugs (NSAIDs)

About

- Commonly seen in overdose. Patients may take excess to manage pain.
- Commonest are ibuprofen and mefenamic acid (Ponstan).

Clinical

- Gastric irritation and mild abdominal pain.
- Mefenamic acid can famously cause seizures.
- Overdose may also cause AKI and metabolic acidosis.
- Low GCS, drowsiness, nystagmus and tachycardia rarely seen.

Investigations

- FBC: iron deficiency anaemia with gastritis, U&E: AKI. ABG: low HCO_3.

Management

- Give activated charcoal 50 g if more than 10 tablets in past 1–2 h.
- **Seizures**: ABC, O_2. Recovery position. Manage as per status epilepticus (*Section 19.4*).
- **Gastritis**: oral PPI if symptoms. Manage upper GI haemorrhage.
- **Discharge**: most medically fit for discharge by 12 h if stable. Psychiatric evaluation in all overdoses.

Opioids

About

- May be seen as accidental overdose in a drug addict, or deliberate or accidental overdose.
- Include drugs from codeine, coproxamol to DIAMORPHINE and MORPHINE.

Aetiology

- Opiates bind to kappa and mu CNS opioid receptors.
- Opioid withdrawal is unpleasant but not life threatening.

Clinical

- Coma and respiratory depression. Pinpoint constricted pupils.
- Signs of opiate abuse, e.g. needle marks. May be taken with alcohol.
- May be cardiac effects, e.g. QRS widening, arrhythmias and heart block with dextropropoxyphene.
- Look for skin patches of opiate medications.

Investigations

- If deliberate overdose check paracetamol/salicylate levels, toxicology screen.
- U&E, FBC, ABG, LFTs, CXR. CT head if coma diagnosis unclear.

Management

- **Supportive:** ABC, O_2 as per BTS guidance. High dependency area. Recovery position. If airway unsafe consider intubation and ventilation especially if GCS <8 and not rapidly responsive to naloxone. If any doubt look for other causes of coma and consider CT head.
- **Remove transdermal opiate patches:** opiate usage can be easily missed in those with fentanyl and other patches. Can lead to opiate toxicity but the patch can be easily overlooked.
- **NALOXONE 0.4–1.2 mg IV in 10 ml syringe** diluted with NS. Give 1–2 ml every 2 min. Consider infusion if helps. Give 2/3rds of the dose needed to wake the patient as an infusion. IM naloxone has been used. Drug abusers may become agitated with naloxone-induced withdrawal. If no response is observed after 10 mg of NALOXONE then search for an alternative diagnosis. Signs of reversal – enlarging pupils, improving respiratory rate and GCS.
- **Opiate reversal when used in terminal care:** the aim is to reduce opiate induced respiratory depression without removing beneficial effects. Give small doses of naloxone 20 mcg repeated as needed. Make up 200 mcg (0.2 mg) in 10 ml NS and give as repeated 1 ml bolus.
- **Note: tramadol and naloxone:** overdoses of tramadol can cause serious potential consequences of respiratory depression and seizure. Naloxone will reverse some, but not all symptoms caused by overdosage.

Organophosphates

About

- Accidental, deliberate usage. Similar to action of the nerve agent Sarin.

Aetiology

- Organophosphates (OPs) phosphorylate the enzyme acetylcholinesterase making it inactive.
- Leads to increased acetylcholine causing autonomic symptoms and muscle weakness.
- Excess bronchial secretions and respiratory muscle weakness causes respiratory failure.

Clinical

- Nausea, vomiting, colic, diarrhoea, sweating, rhinorrhoea, bronchorrhoea, miosis.
- **Nicotinic receptors** (muscle): weakness, fasciculation, flaccid paralysis, weak respiratory muscles and respiratory compromise. Intermediate syndrome occurs 48–96 h later with muscle weakness and respiratory distress and failure requiring ventilation and respiratory support; usually make a full recovery within 3 weeks.
- **OP-induced delayed polyneuropathy** (OPIDN): develop a distal symmetrical flaccid weakness involving limbs and hands and later can develop some UMN signs with increased tone and spasticity.

Investigations

- **Erythrocyte cholinesterase activity** is low (better guide than serum cholinesterase activity).
- FBC, U&E, CXR: oedema, consolidation. ABG: Type I RF.

Management

- **Supportive: ABC,** give O_2 as per BTS guidelines. High dependency area. Intubation and ventilation if GCS <8. Ensure you do not get contaminated with OPs. You must carefully remove and discard contaminated clothes: needs skin wash with soap and water to avoid further transcutaneous absorption and toxicity. OPs are hydrolysed in aqueous solutions with a high pH. Staff must take special care in handling the patient and wear protective clothing. OPs can penetrate latex – use locally advised kit. Treat contaminated clothing as hazardous waste.
- **ATROPINE:** immediate aggressive use of atropine may avoid need for intubation. If toxicity suspected give a test dose of **ATROPINE 1 mg IV** (a rapid increase in HR and skin flushing eliminates the possibility of significant cholinergic syndrome if that was a concern). Patient should be given adequate **ATROPINE 2–3 mg IV** as soon as diagnosis made to ensure complete and early atropinisation. Tachycardia and mydriasis should not stop or delay subsequent doses of atropine. OP toxicity is primarily respiratory failure from excessive airway secretions. Goal is to dry pulmonary secretions and oxygenate.
- **Torsades de pointes** should be treated as discussed in *Section 11.5*.
- **IV magnesium sulphate** may be beneficial for OP toxicity.
- **Pralidoxime (2-PAM) 1–2 g slow IV** is given for nicotinic (weakness) symptoms.
- **Seizures:** manage as per seizure section (*Section 19.4*). Use Lorazepam.

Paracetamol (acetaminophen)

About

- Liver failure and death in those who present late or are inadequately treated.
- Hepatotoxicity very unlikely if *N*-acetylcysteine (NAC) started <8–10 h after the ingestion.
- Toxicity with doses of 150 mg/kg taken in less than 1 hour or 75–150 mg/kg in any 24-hour period.

Pathophysiology

- Paracetamol converted to highly reactive toxic metabolite (*N*-acetyl-*p*-benzoquinone imine (NAPQI)) by hepatic cytochrome P450 2E1 (CYP2E1). Causes liver failure and renal failure. NAPQI usually inactivated by glutathione but this is rapidly consumed in overdose.
- **Those at increased risk for liver failure**: chronic alcoholic, starvation/fasting depletes glutathione. Taking enzyme-inducing drugs (e.g. carbamazepine, phenytoin, barbiturates, isoniazid, and rifampicin), AIDS, cystic fibrosis, and other liver disease. Low BMI, urinalysis positive for ketones, low serum urea concentration. These factors no longer play a part in dosing algorithm.

Natural clinical history

- **1–24 h**: nausea and vomiting.
- **24–72 h**: nausea and vomiting and RUQ pain/discomfort. Raised LFT and PT.
- **72–96 h**: hepatic necrosis and fulminant liver failure, progressive jaundice, coagulopathy, delirium, encephalopathy, death. Consideration for transplantation.
- **4 days – 2 weeks**: resolution or death. Post-transplant recovery if performed.

Investigations

- **Paracetamol (and salicylate) level**: 4 h or later post ingestion.
- **Bloods:** FBC, U&E, LFTs and baseline prothrombin time at baseline and then at least daily. ALT >1000 IU/L indicates severe liver damage.

- **Lactate**: may then be elevated. Prothrombin time (PTT) very useful prognostically. Watch for AKI.

Management

- **Activated charcoal** if a dose of paracetamol >150 mg/kg was taken in the previous hour.

Patients come to harm when non-immunological adverse reactions to NAC are interpreted as anaphylaxis and NAC is withheld.

- **Unable to establish position on treatment graph**: if overdose timing uncertain or unknown or staggered overdose or history unclear, then start NAC immediately in all patients at potential risk. The threshold for treatment is low. Check levels but it may be difficult to correlate with any timings. There would be even more of an incentive to treat if patient is high risk for hepatic failure.
- **Able to establish position on the treatment graph:** if overdose timing clear then check paracetamol levels at 4 h post ingestion or later and assess level using nomogram (see below). Determine if patient is above or below the treatment line. Treat those on or above the treatment line with NAC.
- **Presenting 8+ hours following ingestion or with symptoms of toxicity**: treat any late presenters with evident liver disease or symptoms immediately with NAC. *Do not wait for levels but give NAC prior to results*. Assess paracetamol level and time post overdose on the graph and use to guide treatment. Take specialist advice. Have a low threshold for considering paracetamol toxicity and giving NAC in all with acute unexplained liver failure.
- **Give the antidote IV *N*-ACETYLCYSTEINE (NAC) if any doubts**. NAC can cause a reaction with rash, angioedema, wheeze and hypotension, but should be continued where needed. Give chlorphenamine IV. If cannot take NAC then consider oral methionine but this can be hard to obtain out of hours and may not be in stock. If for some reason NAC or methionine cannot be given, then **haemodialysis** may be considered.

_N_-Acetylcysteine dose and administration – run bags immediately after each other

- **First infusion** (150 mg/kg) – add acetylcysteine concentrate for IV infusion to 200 ml glucose IV infusion 5%; infuse over 1 h.
- **Second infusion** (50 mg/kg) – add acetylcysteine concentrate for IV infusion to 500 ml glucose IV infusion 5%; infuse over 4 h.
- **Third infusion** (100 mg/kg) – add acetylcysteine concentrate for IV infusion to 1 L glucose IV infusion 5%; infuse over 16 h.

- **Fulminant hepatic failure**: discuss patient with evident sign of liver failure as early as possible with the regional liver centres. Supportive treatment and transfer. **Orthotopic liver transplant:** may be the only hope of survival with fulminant liver failure following paracetamol. Criteria below are used in UK. Do not wait for criteria to be met before picking up telephone. Some are transferred and may settle.
- **Post recovery:** for those who recover they must be seen by psychiatry prior to discharge.
- **Pregnancy:** pregnant patients should be treated same as non-pregnant.

Kings College criteria for liver transplant

- **Paracetamol-induced liver failure:** an arterial pH <7.3 at 24 h after ingestion OR a prothrombin time >100 sec. Creatinine >300 μmol/L. Grade III or IV hepatic encephalopathy.
- **Non paracetamol-induced liver failure.** Prothrombin time >100 sec OR 3 of the following: (1) drug induced, (2) age <10 or >40, (3) more than 1 week between jaundice and encephalopathy, (4) prothrombin time >50 sec, (5) bilirubin >300 μmol/L.

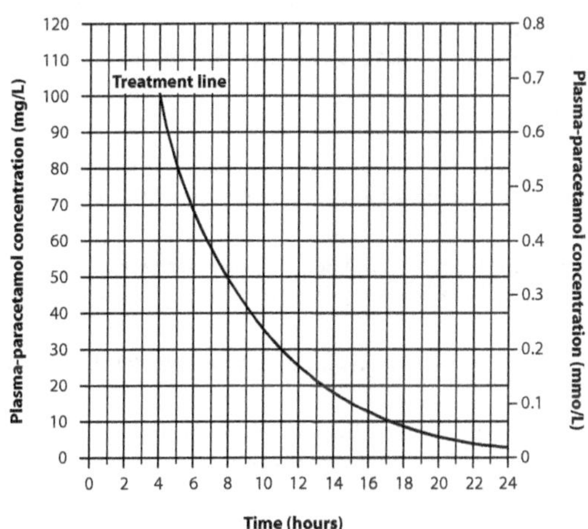

Nomogram for paracetamol overdose. Treat above line.
Reproduced from the MHRA with permission.

Reference: Bateman (2011) Management of paracetamol poisoning. *BMJ*, 342:d2218.

Paraquat

About

- Herbicide. A mouthful of 20% Gramoxone is almost certainly fatal.

Pathophysiology

- Causes a pulmonary–renal syndrome. Mechanism unknown.
- Possibly formation of superoxides and free radicals.

Clinical

- Mucosal ulceration, vomiting, diarrhoea. Alveolitis, AKI. Oesophageal perforation and mediastinitis.
- Cardiac failure, renal failure, respiratory failure.

Investigations

- **U&E**: AKI. **CXR:** ARDS with oedema and progressive pulmonary fibrosis.
- **ABG**: Type 1 RF and metabolic acidosis. **Check paraquat levels.**

Management

- ABC, give sufficient O_2 to deliver sats of 94–98% or 88–92% if severe COPD and reassess after ABG. Some advocate even less to avoid any oxygen toxicity to match a saturation of 92%. Eventually Type 1 RF occurs and increased FiO_2 will be needed.
- Remove any contaminated clothing and wash from skin or mucous membranes. Give activated charcoal up to 50 g orally/NG and get early expert advice.
- Extracorporeal removal by prolonged haemodialysis or haemoperfusion have been used until paraquat levels are undetected. IV fluids to force diuresis.
- Consider cyclophosphamide and steroids. Salicylates may also be of benefit. Lung transplantation has failed whenever used.
- **Prognosis:** dose >6 g is fatal, 1.5–6 g mortality is 60–70%, and <1.5 g is rarely fatal.

Quinine toxicity

About

- Quinine is used to treat chloroquine-resistant malaria and nocturnal cramps. Toxic on retinal photoreceptor cells with localised spasm/vasoconstriction.

Clinical

- Partial or complete blindness, nausea, vomiting, headache, fatigue.
- Tremor, ataxia, coma. Respiratory depression, arrhythmias, hypotension.

Investigation

- **ECG**: widened QRS and prolonged QTc, risk of VT, Torsades de pointes and VF.

Management

- Activated charcoal and gastric lavage if early presentation.
- Bradycardia: ATROPINE 0.6 mg IV or transvenous pacing.
- **Give IV $NaHCO_3$** if QRS >120 msec aiming for a pH of 7.45–7.55.

Salicylates / aspirin

About

- Weak acids uncouple oxidative phosphorylation leading to hyperthermia.

Aetiology

- Initial hyperventilation as stimulates respiratory centre with respiratory alkalosis.

Clinical

- Dehydration, hypokalaemia and a progressive metabolic acidosis occur late.
- Nausea, vomiting and tinnitus, vertigo, hyperventilation, tachycardia.
- Agitation, delirium, hallucinations, convulsions, lethargy, and stupor may occur.
- Hyperthermia is an indication of severe toxicity, especially in young children.

Investigations

- **U&E, FBC, glucose**: hypoglycaemia is seen. Raised lactate.
- **Salicylate**: normal salicylate levels 15–30 mg/dL. Symptoms if >40–50 mg/dL, with severe toxicity if >100 mg/dL. Always check paracetamol levels and treat accordingly.
- **ABG** should be checked regularly.

Management

- Gastric lavage is suggested in this situation as gastric emptying may be delayed. Repeated doses of activated charcoal are possibly useful for early presentation. Consider whole bowel irrigation with **polyethylene glycol** with a significant overdose. Promote diuresis with IV fluids.
- **Urinary alkalinisation**: $NaHCO_3$ (e.g. 1500 ml of 1.26% with 40 mmol KCl over 3 h).

- **Haemodialysis** with toxicity levels >700 mg/L or renal/cardiac failure or seizures or severe acidosis.

Selective serotonin reuptake inhibitors

About

- Commonly used drugs which raise CNS serotonin. Less toxic than TCAs.
- SSRIs includes fluoxetine, citalopram and venlafaxine.

Clinical

- Drowsiness, seizures and coma in severe overdose.
- Nausea, vomiting, diarrhoea, tremor, agitation. Hypertension, tachycardia.

Investigations

- U&E, ECG, paracetamol and salicylate levels. Consider CT head if seizure/coma.

Management

- Activated charcoal if <1 h from overdose and 10+ tablets taken.
- Supportive management. Usually medically stable by 12 h.

Tricyclic antidepressant

About

- Significant toxicity due to the wide pharmacological effects of TCAs.
- Include amitriptyline, imipramine, dothiepin.
- Avoid or controlled access in those at high risk of suicide.

Aetiology

- Anticholinergic effects, adrenergic blockade. Inhibition of noradrenaline and serotonin reuptake.
- Blockade of fast Na channels in myocardial cells (quinidine-like membrane-stabilising effects).
- Block HERG potassium channels. Histamine receptor blockers.

Clinical

- Seizures, coma, hypotension, drowsiness, dilated pupils. Urinary retention.
- Arrhythmias, respiratory depression, hyperthermia. Hyperreflexia.

Investigations

- FBC, U&E, ABG where necessary. ECG. Paracetamol, salicylate levels.
- CT head if seizure/coma to exclude other brain pathology.

Management

- **Supportive:** ABCs. O_2 as per BTS guidelines and IV fluids and CCU/ITU monitoring. Give activated charcoal if >10 tablets ingested in past 1–2 h.
- **Monitor ECG**: QRS >140 msec suggests (sodium channel blockade) serious risk of fits/arrhythmias. Antiarrhythmics avoided generally.
- **Serum alkalinisation** (sodium bicarbonate 50 ml of 8.4% IV) where QRS prolonged or hypotension or arrhythmia and is useful therapy in overdose. Aim for alkalinisation of the serum to a pH level of 7.45–7.55 which increases protein binding, decreases the QRS interval, stabilises arrhythmias, and increases blood pressure in patients with TCA poisoning.
- **Ventricular arrhythmias** may be managed with overdrive pacing and **MAGNESIUM SULPHATE**. Also consider sodium bicarbonate IV and **LIDOCAINE 100 mg IV**.
- **Tricyclics** are highly protein bound so haemodialysis not indicated. Risk of further complications uncommon after 24 h. Once medically stable involve psychiatry liaison for all overdoses.

Theophylline

About

- Used to treat asthma/COPD. Narrow therapeutic window.
- Inhibits phosphodiesterase with elevated cAMP and adrenergic stimulation.

Clinical

- Nausea, severe vomiting, abdominal pain, tachycardia, seizures.

Investigations

- **ABG:** metabolic acidosis. Low K^+, PO_4, Mg^+. Hypo/hypercalcaemia. Hyperglycaemia.
- **Check levels**: therapeutic range 10–20 mcg/ml, toxic levels >20 mcg/ml.
- **ECG and telemetry**: all arrhythmias, AF / atrial flutter / SVT / VT / VF.

Management

- **Limit absorption: multidose activated charcoal (MDAC)** enhances elimination of theophylline and is vital. Control nausea and vomiting (e.g. ondansentron) in order to perform MDAC treatment.
- **Gastric lavage if recently (<1 h) ingested** a significant amount or sustained-release preparation of theophylline. It should only be considered in intubated patients.
- **Whole bowel irrigation** in patients with exposure to sustained-release theophylline preparations.
- **Stop any oral or IV theophyllines**. ABC, give O_2 as per BTS guidelines.
- **Seizures: manage as per status epilepticus** (*Section 19.4*)**.** (Coexisting respiratory compromise may require intubation and ventilation.)
- **Hypokalaemia**: cautious correction of hypokalaemia.
- **β-blockers** (except with asthma) for arrhythmias or **Disopyramide** suggested for ventricular arrhythmias.

Warfarin

About

- Causes excessive bleeding. Reverse with vitamin K and prothrombin complex concentrates.

Pathophysiology

- Antagonises vitamin K-dependent clotting factor synthesis.

Clinical

- Bleeding: GI, urinary, retroperitoneal, intramuscular, and intracranial.
- Any signs of shock on anticoagulants should raise the issue of bleeding.

Investigations

- Check INR and FBC. Group and hold/cross-match if bleeding.
- Urgent CT head if any neurology.
- Endoscopy if upper GI bleed.
- CT abdomen/pelvis or USS if retroperitoneal or psoas or pelvic bleed suspected.

Management

- Direct pressure, surgical review and usual bleed management where possible.
- Reverse with **vitamin K 5–10 mg PO/slow IV** depending on urgency.
- Consider prothrombin complex concentrates (Octaplex/Beriplex) or FFP.
- Transfuse as needed. Manage as haemorrhagic shock if hypotensive.

21 Miscellaneous emergencies

21.1 Amniotic fluid embolism

About

- Amniotic fluid (fetal cells, hair, or other debris) enters maternal circulation with cardiac arrest/shock. Suspect if sudden unexpected death in labour/caesarean or within 30 min post-partum.

Aetiology

- Usually during labour but also abortion and trauma. Resembles anaphylaxis.
- Fetal squamous cells found in the maternal pulmonary circulation.
- These are also found in well patients. Possibly complement activation.

Clinical

- Acutely dyspnoeic with hypotension and hypoxia, cough, seizures, cardiac arrest.
- Coagulopathy or severe haemorrhage.

Investigations

- **ABG**: Type 1 RF. **CXR**: pulmonary oedema. **ECG**: non-specific.
- **Coagulation screen**: coagulopathy.

Management

- As per cardiac arrest (see *Section 1.2*). CPR, ABCs, intubate and ventilate.
- Manage with IV fluids for hypotension.
- Invasive monitoring and exclude alternative diagnoses.
- Manage any coagulopathy. Haemodialysis with plasmapheresis for AKI.
- Steroids if immune-mediated mechanism suspected.

21.2 Fat embolism

About

- Consider with any recent fracture with sudden dyspnoea (may not be a PE).
- A skin rash or new neurology. Consider in sickling crisis chest syndrome.

Aetiology

- Fat enters the venous circulation and passes into the systemic circulation.
- Results in vascular occlusion and release of inflammatory mediators.
- Fat from marrow from long bone (femur usually) or pelvis fractures.
- Also lipid infusions, recent steroid administration.

Causes

- Blunt trauma, acute pancreatitis, and sickle cell crisis.
- Decompression sickness. Parenteral lipid infusion.

Clinical

- Breathlessness, tachycardia, febrile. Type 1 RF, petechiae, confusion, delirium.
- Coma, retinal haemorrhages with fatty lesions.

Investigations

- **FBC**: low platelets, Hb and fibrinogen.
- **Urinalysis**: fat globules in the urine are common after trauma.

- **CXR:** infiltrates. **ABG:** hypoxia and Type 1 RF. **U&E:** AKI.
- **CT chest:** ARDS picture, infiltrates.
- **CT head:** diffuse white-matter petechial haemorrhages.

Management

- ABC and give O_2 as per BTS guidelines. Supportive, oxygenation, circulatory support.

21.3 Air embolism

About

- Air within the circulation results in obstructive shock.

Aetiology

- Air sucked into negative pressure venous circulation above right atrium passes into the heart and leads to loss of pumping effectiveness, with vascular occlusion and sudden death. Risk in any operative procedure where the exposed site is >5 cm above the right atrium.

Causes

- Surgical procedures, e.g. neurosurgery or ENT where patients sit upright.
- Back street abortion – air accidentally injected into pelvic venous plexuses.
- Penetrating chest injuries with bronchopulmonary venous fistulae.
- Central venous catheterisation can provide entry point, especially with loss of connections.

Clinical

- Most episodes are clinically silent or result in mild, transient hypotension.
- Acute dyspnoea, chest pain, agitation or disorientation.

Investigations

- **ABG:** hypoxia, hypo/hypercarbia, respiratory and/or metabolic acidosis.
- **ECG**: tachycardia ST/T changes of ischaemia. CXR: oligaemia.

Management

- Give 100% O_2. Fluid resuscitation and inotropes. Clamp or remove any central line that is entry point.
- Put patient head down and left lateral decubitus (on left side with head down) to trap the air in ventricle and not in right ventricular outflow tract.

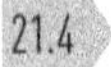

21.4 Falls

Wards often have policies to reduce falls – make sure these are in place and being adhered to.

Taking referral / answering bleep

- How is the patient now? Observations? Why did the fall happen?
- Any head injury? If so, what is GCS? Any bony pain – hip, back pain, wrist, etc.?
- What were the events of fall – hypotension, chest pain, breathless, confusion.

On arrival

- See notes, review observations and medication. Mechanical fall, i.e. simple trip with clear consciousness.

- Medical fall – patient unwell or presyncopal or faint or hypoglycaemia or confused prior? Assess any obvious injury: fracture or head injury and arrange imaging as needed. Analgesia and orthopaedic review for fracture. CT head if any persisting neurology.
- General examination especially for low BP. Neurological observations if head injury or seizure occurred. Document findings – take advice if on warfarin. ECG and telemetry and regular observations best on CCU if any suggestion of arrhythmia or vascular cause.
- **Secondary trauma**: exclude subdural and ruptured spleen and fractures. Non-displaced hip fracture may be missed and not all have classical leg shortening and external rotation. Repeated examination may be needed. Pain may not be noted until attempts to mobilise. Initial trauma surveys can miss things so have a low threshold to repeat examination and imaging if there is evidence or suspicion of possible problems. Do not get distracted by the secondary trauma and so forget about the primary cause of syncope.

21.5 Hypothermia

About

- Unintentional drop in core body temp below 35°C. Elderly and babies are at highest risk.
- Core temperature below 32°C is moderate and below 28°C is severe.

Note

- With cardiac arrest do not stop resuscitation until patients are warm and 'dead'.

Aetiology

- Body heat generated by basal metabolic rate and muscle activity.
- Heat lost to environment by conduction, convection and evaporation.
- Hypothalamus manages temperature. Core temperature set at 37°C +/− 0.5°C.
- Peripheral vasoconstriction and shivering are normal response.

Risks

- Falls, stroke, sepsis, confusion, patient with dementia and wandering, e.g. going outside in cold.
- Alcohol, phenothiazines, immersion in cold water. Is this part of a suicide attempt?

Clinical

- In extremes it may resemble death. Mild hypothermia causes reflex shivering and the desire to put on warm clothes and turn up heating. Mild ataxia, confusion and dehydration. Bradycardia, hypotension.
- Confusion and lack of awareness so no attempt is made to reduce heat loss.
- Severe (less than 28°C) coma, absent pupillary responses, absent corneal reflex, cardiac standstill. Seen with stroke or falls patients incapacitated in a cold environment.

Investigation

- **FBC:** raised haematocrit and urea/creatinine from dehydration.
- **U&E:** raised K^+ as a consequence of rhabdomyolysis.
- **Cardiac troponin** if any signs of ACS/MI.
- **ECG:** arrhythmias are possible. May show classic J or Osborne waves and rhythm disturbances such as AF. The height of the Osborne wave is roughly proportional to the degree of hypothermia.

- **Arterial/venous blood gases**: metabolic acidosis, lactate.
- **TFT**: raised TSH as hypothyroidism can cause hypothermia.
- **Cortisol/short synacthen**: low threshold for suspecting hypoadrenalism.
- **Amylase:** raised in pancreatitis which may be subclinical.
- **Toxicology screen:** overdose may have been taken, e.g. opiate, benzodiazepine, paracetamol, aspirin.
- **Carboxyhaemoglobin**: carbon monoxide poisoning.
- **CT head:** if comatose or focal neurology.

Management

- **ABCs and give O_2 as per BTS guidelines.** Consider urinary catheter to detect oliguria/anuria. Always use a low reading rectal thermometer. Axillary, tympanic and oral temperatures can all be misleading. Full monitoring and resuscitation facilities must be available as patient may develop VF and need defibrillation.
- **Get IV access** and correct dehydration cautiously with warmed fluids if possible. Use warm blankets and warm drinks if able and not severe – beware excess vasodilation which can drop BP. Cardiac monitoring and repeated bloods in severe cases.
- Always consider rare possibility of **hypopituitary, hypoadrenalism and/or hypothyroidism**. Consider IV hydrocortisone as well as need for IV dextrose/thiamine/naloxone.
- Warmed IV fluids (without potassium) or warmed fluids via NG tube. Warming strategies: in extreme cases peritoneal warmed fluids or even cardiac bypass can be used. Hot baths are useful but run the risk of haemodynamic compromise with vasodilation and impossible to defibrillate, but are indicated for immersion victims. Keep a close watch on blood gases and potassium. Hypothermic patients in cardiac arrest should be resuscitated until they have a normal core temperature.

Differential

- Stroke or any brain injury – consider urgent CT. Drug overdose – alcohol, opiates, benzodiazepines, etc. Myxoedema coma, hypoglycaemia (see *Chapter 6* on coma).

21.6 Malignant hyperpyrexia

About

- Previous uneventful anaesthesia with triggering agents does not preclude MH.
- Usually precipitated by drugs in those genetically susceptible.

Aetiology

- Autosomal dominant, 1 in 20 000. Genetic defect, e.g. Ryanodine receptor on 19q13.
- Acute rises in cell calcium causes rigidity and rhabdomyolysis.

Drug causes

- All inhalational agents except nitrous oxide: Halothane, Methoxyflurane, Suxamethonium.

Clinical

- Onset within 1 h of drug administration. Masseter muscle spasm an early sign.
- Hyperpyrexia >40°C, tachycardia, muscle stiffness.
- Monitoring: elevation of end-tidal CO_2 is early, sensitive and specific sign of MH.

Investigation

- **FBC:** raised WCC. **Glucose:** may be raised. **Coagulation**: monitor for DIC.
- **U&E** : raised K^+. AKI from dehydration or myoglobinuria, **raised CK, phosphate.**
- **ABG:** lactic acidosis.
- Watch for complications: AKI due to rhabdomyolysis, arrhythmias, raised K^+, DIC.

Management

- **ABC, high FiO_2** initially and then O_2 as per BTS guidelines and reassess after ABG. Telemetry for raised K^+. Try cooling and allow heat loss. Tepid sponging, fans, avoid paracetamol/salicylates. Later counsel family members as is genetic predisposition.
- **Acute anaesthetic management**: stop causative drug immediately and stop surgery if possible. Do not waste time securing another anaesthetic machine, use an Ambu bag and an O_2 cylinder initially. Hyperventilate the patient with 100% O_2 at 10 L/min via a clean breathing circuit. Otherwise maintain anaesthesia with IV agents such as Propofol until surgery is completed.
- **Cooling management** – cool IV fluids and ice packs.
- **Dantrolene 2 mg/kg** as a bolus and then repeat doses of 1 mg/kg (up to a maximum of 10 mg/kg) should be given until the tachycardia, rise in CO_2 production and pyrexia start to subside.

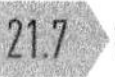

21.7 Acute rhabdomyolysis

About

- Muscle damage can lead to AKI.

About

- Damage to striated muscle can lead to myoglobinuria. Plasma myoglobin levels exceed protein binding. Precipitates in the tubules can lead to AKI, renal vasoconstriction and direct nephrotoxicity.

Causes

- Trauma and crush injuries, high voltage electrical injury, near drowning.
- Falls and lying on floor for prolonged periods, severe exercise.
- Neuroleptic malignant syndrome (NMS), malignant hyperthermia.
- Cocaine and heroin use, amphetamines, ketamine, LSD.
- Generalised seizures, alcohol, methanol, ethylene glycol, carbon monoxide.
- Ischaemic limb with muscle necrosis, polymyositis, viral myositis – influenza.
- HIV, Coxsackie, echovirus, statins +/– fibrates, hypothyroidism, hyperthyroidism.
- Snake bites with action of phospholipases, compartment syndrome.
- Muscle genetic disorders – carnitine deficiency, caffeine, aspirin.
- Hypokalaemia, hypophosphatemia, diabetic ketoacidosis and HHS.
- Sepsis with bacterial infections, MI or myocarditis can raise CKMB.

Clinical

- Muscle pain and weakness. Muscles hard and tender especially when crush injury.
- Dark urine – burgundy coloured or dark tea. Cause may be apparent, e.g. trauma.
- Evidence of trauma or falls or prolonged immobility.
- Family history might suggest genetic cause.
- Drug history – neuroleptics.
- Fever, increased tone, neuroleptic malignant syndrome.

Investigations

- **FBC**: raised WCC. **U&E**: raised urea, creatinine.
- **Tissue damage**: raised K^+, CK, urate, myoglobin, phosphate, myoglobinuria.
- **ABG**: metabolic acidosis. **Coagulation screen**: DIC. **MRI** can be useful to identify muscle damage.
- **ECG** and **cardiac troponin** if myocardial injury suspected.

Complications

- Raised K^+, hypovolaemic shock, AKI. DIC, sepsis, death.

Management

- **Supportive**, ABCs, IV fluids, watch and treat high K^+. Risk of AKI low if CK <15 000–20 000 units/L. CK >60 000 units/L is predictive of AKI and death.
- **Early hydration** (even prior to hospitalisation) with NS. Goal is a good diuresis (200–300 ml/h). Carefully monitor for fluid overload, particularly in elderly/CCF. Furosemide can enhance diuresis if overloaded.
- **Alkalinisation of urine**: enhances myoglobin solubility. Target urine pH >6.5 with IV $NaHCO_3$ where CK >6000. Consider **dialysis** in AKI or refractory hyperkalaemia or fluid overload.
- **Mannitol** can be added to enhance diuresis, renal vasodilator and free radical scavenger.
- **Bromocriptine or Dantrolene** in the case of neuroleptic malignant syndrome.
- **Fasciotomy** for any compartment syndrome. Revascularisation for limb ischaemia.
- **Treat DIC** with FFP, cryoprecipitate, and platelet transfusions.

21.8 Acute limb ischaemia

About

- Early action may preserve limb, either thrombotic occlusion or embolic.
- Rarely severe venous thrombosis can lead to ischaemia.

Clinical

- Limb is pale, painful, pulseless, paraesthesia, perishing with cold.

Aetiology

- AF is a common cause. On heparin? HITT must not be missed – check platelets.
- LV thrombus from MI, cardiac murmurs, aortic aneurysm.

Investigation

- **FBC:** WCC, platelets (low platelets with HITT). **Coagulation screen.**
- **U&E**: AKI, hyperkalaemia, glucose, troponin. **CXR**: cardiomegaly. **ECG**: AF, MI.
- **Doppler ultrasound:** can give evidence of flow and flow rates.
- **Angiography:** evidence of thrombus.

Management

- **Vascular surgical emergency**. Refer quickly and meantime **ABC,** give O_2 as per BTS guidelines and reassess after ABG. Get IV access and start 1 L NS. **Analgesia**: MORPHINE 5–10 mg IV + CYCLIZINE 50 mg IV. Watch for respiratory depression.
- **Senior vascular surgical review**: mottled white leg with skin petechiae with hard painful muscles is beyond salvage and may consider amputation or palliation. Consider co-morbidities. Conservative management may be recommended. With an acute white cold leg without more chronic changes then a quick decision

must be made as to active treatment which can be angiography initially with plan for thrombolysis, embolectomy or angioplasty, or even arterial bypass.

- **Heparinisation/thrombolysis/embolectomy**: consider heparin 5000 units IV bolus and then 1000 units/h with APTT 2–2.5. Embolectomy can be done under local anaesthesia. Compartment syndrome may require fasciotomies to be done. Warfarin should be considered post-operatively.
- **Amputation** finally is indicated if all options are futile. In some cases consider percutaneous lumbar sympathectomy which requires CT guidance.
- Rare cases of leg ischaemia due to **severe venous thrombosis** can be treated by elevation, starting heparin and providing analgesia.

Complications

- Death in 20%, limb loss, ARDS, pneumonia, sepsis, rhabdomyolysis, hyperkalaemia, AKI.

21.9 Painful leg

Taking referral / answering bleep

- Painful since when? Was there trauma or fall? Is patient mobile on it? Any redness, shortened and externally rotated?
- Pyrexia? Normal observations? Why is patient in hospital? Anticoagulants – ?haematoma.

Differentials

- **Trauma – soft tissue injury – bruising and swelling.** Rest, ice, elevate. Severe trauma can cause rhabdomyolysis and compartment syndrome. Follow appropriate criteria, e.g. Ottawa guidance for ankle pain. Bony tenderness should warrant suspicion if fracture. Experience in older patient is to reasonably assume any patient with leg pain warrants exclusion of pelvic/hip fracture or long bone fracture as clinical signs can be reduced and difficult in confused/dementia patients.
- **Deep vein thrombosis:** warm, dilated veins, swollen, calf tender, raised D-dimers. Important differential as can rapidly kill if missed and untreated. If suspected begin treatment immediately.
- **Compartment syndrome**: post trauma or fracture or ischaemic limb needs fasciotomy. Distal ischaemia and reduced pulses. Surgical emergency.
- **Haematoma:** trauma +/– excessive anticoagulants and muscle haematoma. Check clotting. Reverse warfarin or stop heparin or manage bleeding disorder.
- **Inflammation:** acute gout or pseudogout or septic arthritis: red-hot joint with effusion. Aspirate joint.
- **Osteomyelitis**: acute or chronic bony pain, sickle cell. May be associated soft tissue infection, e.g. diabetic foot. Sciatica – pain radiating down leg corresponding to disc lesion. Limited straight leg raising.
- **Cellulitis**: usually a newly warm red tender leg starting distally and moving proximally. Bilateral cellulitis should make one question diagnosis. Florid red legs may be chronic and cool to the touch. Check for diabetes and skin infection entry points. Emollients for dry skin. Antibiotics for confirmed cellulitis.
- **Rheumatoid arthritis:** can affect the knee as a tender warm joint with synovial thickening and may have an effusion. Rarely acutely inflamed. Patient has clinical features of rheumatoid arthritis. Check ESR/CRP and serology. Must aspirate knee if joint sepsis suspected.

- **Lymphoedema**: unilateral swollen leg maybe painful. Look for evidence of malignancy if new. Check nodes at groin. Pyoderma gangrenosum – may be seen with bowel disease and presents as a painful non-healing violaceous rash with ulceration. Needs management of underlying condition. Dermatological referral.
- **Necrotising fasciitis**: hard woody feeling, intense pain, gas bubbles below skin, margin which is moving. Needs urgent surgery.
- **Acute ischaemic limb:** mottled, pale, painful, pulseless, perishing with cold. A vascular emergency.

On arrival

- Check general observations and review notes. Examine legs: front and back for tenderness, red – possible cellulitis. Tender muscles: suspect rhabdomyolysis – check CK and statin usage or other causes.
- Recent trauma/ischaemia and pain – compartment syndrome which will need urgent surgical decompression. Recent fall – even something trivial can cause a fracture. Fractured neck of femurs have few signs if undisplaced. Check for pubic bone fracture. **Any doubts X-ray**.
- Acute gout can cause a painful large toe – check urate. Tender erythematous. Calf – always consider DVT and D-dimer may help but may need USS leg veins. Start LMWH treatment whilst you get doppler if DVT suspected.

22 Oncological emergencies

22.1 Neutropenic sepsis

About

- Temp >38°C or other signs or symptoms of sepsis and neutrophil count $<0.5 \times 10^9$/L. High mortality once neutrophil count $<0.5–1.0 \times 10^9$/L.

Microbiology

- Gram-positive infections via indwelling lines. Invasive *Aspergillus* and candidal infections. Gram-negative sepsis from enteric organisms as well.

Common causes

- Bone marrow suppression 1–2 weeks post chemotherapy would be commonest.
- Carbimazole/propylthiouracil cause agranulocytosis, infection.
- Idiosyncratic drug reaction (check all new drugs): azathioprine and allopurinol.
- Malignant bone marrow infiltration, SLE, RA, splenic sequestration.

Clinical

- Care as may be septic but no fever. Usually temp >37.5°C, diarrhoea, malaise.
- Sore throat, cough, sputum, dysuria, hypotension, tachycardia, oliguria, rigors after flushing a central line. Inspect mouth, skin and perineum for infection. Defer PR examination until antibiotics given.
- Look for other infections, e.g. herpes zoster. Look for tenderness or erythema around cannula/central line sites.
- Chronic neutropenia causes chronic sinusitis and mouth ulcers.

Investigations

- **FBC and WCC** and platelets, U&Es, LFTs and ESR/CRP.
- Lactate. Urine dipstick and culture.
- Culture Hickman lines, blood. CXR if any pulmonary signs or symptoms.
- Additional: serum folate, vitamin B12, iron and ferritin, serum liver enzymes, serum proteins, ANA and anti-dsDNA antibodies and rheumatoid factor and TFTs.

Management

- **Emergency first line:** unwell and compromised then ABC and high flow O_2 if shocked and resuscitate as for sepsis. Take blood as above. Start IV fluids. Isolate and reverse barrier nursing. If patient completely well then observe and take blood cultures. Manage sepsis as detailed in *Section 4.6*. Do not remove central venous access devices as part of the initial empiric management of suspected neutropenic sepsis.
- Give O_2 as per BTS guidelines and reassess after ABG. Adhere to local policies. Liaise with microbiologist/haematologist/oncologist. Different groups to consider in terms of risk. Guidance here refers to highest risk group who are immunocompromised, neutropenic and possibly septic. Temperature control with tepid sponging and paracetamol (0.5–1 g orally or rectally qds) or NSAIDs can be used.
- **First line is TAZOCIN IV (Piperacillin and Tazobactam).** Continue empiric antibiotic therapy in all patients who have unresponsive fever unless an alternative cause of fever is likely. Do not switch antibiotics in patients with unresponsive fever

unless there is clinical deterioration or a microbiological indication. Discontinue empiric antibiotic therapy in patients whose neutropenic sepsis has responded to treatment, irrespective of neutrophil count.

- If fever persists then **GENTAMICIN IV** (or dose as per local guidance) normally given as a single daily dose unless advised otherwise. Levels should be checked 16–20 h after the first dose (and satisfactory clearance annotated) and then at least every 3–4 days (more frequently if there is evidence of renal impairment) according to local protocols. If fever persists and central line *in situ* add **VANCOMYCIN IV** for suspected line sepsis to cover meticillin resistant or coagulase-negative staphylococcal sepsis.
- For penicillin allergy take advice because it will depend on agents available locally, e.g. **MEROPENEM**. Take microbiological advice.
- Persisting symptoms may lead to consideration of **AMPHOTERICIN IV** if fungal infection suspected but this should be based on microbiological advice.
- **Colony stimulating growth factors** (G-CSF, GM-CSF) may be considered in cytotoxic therapy induced neutropenia. **Autoimmune neutropenia** may require steroids and colony stimulating growth factors may be considered. This is determined following senior haematological assessment.

Reference: NICE (2012) CG151: Neutropenic sepsis.

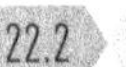

22.2 Malignancy-related hypercalcaemia

About

- Causes polyuria and dehydration and delirium.
- Seen in 10–20% of all adults with cancer.

Causes

- Solid tumours, such as lung or breast cancer tumours.
- Multiple myeloma and other haematological malignancies.

Aetiology

- **PTH-related peptide** increases renal calcium reabsorption.
- Humoral hypercalcaemia due to circulating tumour secreted factors.
- Osteolytic hypercalcaemia due to primary or secondary bone lesions.

Clinical

- Severe dehydration, bone pain, anorexia, nausea, and vomiting.
- Signs of underlying malignancy.

Investigations

- FBC, U&Es, PTH, PTH-related peptide, CXR.
- Serum immunoglobulins, Bence-Jones protein, skeletal survey.

Management

- Management may be palliative in selected patients.
- If severe, then rehydrate with 3–6 L NS over 24 h.
- Close watch on renal function and level of calcium and cardiac status.
- Once rehydrated repeat calcium and consider renal function before IV pamidronate or a Zoledronate 4 mg infusion.
- Also see hypercalcaemia section (*Section 13.5*) for further detail.

22.3 Tumour lysis syndrome

About

- Seen with treatment of chemosensitive malignancies.
- Rapid tumour cell death leads to metabolic derangements.

Aetiology

- Seen with tumours with high tumour bulk, high turnover, chemosensitive.
- Marked rise in LDH with raised uric acid pre-chemotherapy or impaired renal function.

Chemotherapy for malignancies

- Acute leukaemias (ALL, AML, APML, CLL/CML with blast crisis).
- High-grade non-Hodgkin lymphomas, Burkitt's lymphoma.
- Breast cancer, small cell lung cancer, sarcomas.

Investigations

- **FBC:** watch Hb, WCC and platelets.
- **U&E**: AKI with raised urea and creatinine.
- **Urate:** raised uric acid, phosphate, K^+ and low Ca.
- **CRP**: raised can suggest infection/inflammation/malignancy.
- **ECG:** and telemetry to detect effects of high K^+.
- **Raised lactate, ABG**: high anion gap metabolic acidosis.
- **Coagulation screen**: rarely a coagulopathy can develop such as DIC.

Management

- Prevent with IV fluids and ensure optimal hydration. Central line if needed (4–5 L per day). Cardiac monitoring for raised K^+. Standard replacement for K/Ca/Mg.
- Monitoring bloods 2–3 times daily for 48–72 h after chemotherapy initiation.
- Hyperuricaemia: ALLOPURINOL 300 mg PO tds started prior to treatment or RASBURICASE.
- Some patients with renal impairment may need to be on dialysis prior to the initiation of therapy.
- Urinary alkalinisation with $NaHCO_3$ to maintain a urine pH >7.0 can help clearance of uric acid.

22.4 Malignant cord compression

About

- Malignant compression of the spinal cord or cauda equina.
- Any new back pain in a patient with known malignancy warrants urgent investigation.
- 5% of lethal malignancies show signs of spinal cord compression.

Aetiology

- Malignant usually extradural cord compression.
- Tumour, usually within the vertebral body, enlarges.
- Compression causes ischaemic damage to the cord.
- Cord ends at lower edge of L1 vertebra.
- Cord is UMN, cauda is LMN.
- 60–70% is thoracic, 20% lumbosacral and 10% cervical.

Cancers

- Lung, prostate, breast, renal cell, myeloma, colorectal, lymphoma.

Clinical

- May have a known malignancy or this may be the presentation.
- Worsening back pain and tenderness can help localise lesion, radicular pain.
- Tone flaccid initially but then increased + spasticity, extensor plantars and sensory level.
- Up-going plantar reflex suggests significant cord compression.
- Cauda equina damage: saddle anaesthesia, loss of sphincters and LMN signs with bilateral leg weakness.
- Electric shock sensation (Lhermitte's sign) with flexion suggests cord involvement.

Investigation

- **Bloods:** FBC, U&Es, ESR, Ca, PSA, CRP, CXR, myeloma screen.
- **Abdominal CT**: to help find primary if unknown.
- **Plain films** may show bony changes, e.g. 'erosion of pedicle', 'bone lesions'.
- **MRI scan +/– gadolinium** to detail extent of spinal cord compression. 25% have multiple lesions. If MRI not available then **CT or CT myelogram** may be considered.
- **Bladder scan**: retention >150 ml suggests neurological damage.

Management

- Pain control is key – often needing opiates. Median survival is now 6 months.
- If compression found then speak to neurosurgeons and consider use of high dose steroids such as **Dexamethasone** 10 mg IV then 8 mg bd PO.
- Try to preserve remaining neurology through surgical consult for resection/ decompression of any lesions or radiation therapy. Systemic chemotherapy can help certain patients. Urgent oncological advice is key. Surgery where possible has better outcomes. It may allow a tissue diagnosis and spinal stabilisation.

Cerebral tumour

About

- Can be a primary or secondary.

Causes

- Primary: usually single (primary CNS lymphoma often multifocal).
- Metastatic: single or multiple.

Risk

- **Primary brain**: radiation, HIV (see AIDS, *Section 17.3*), genetics – von Hippel–Lindau disease, tuberous sclerosis, Li–Fraumeni syndrome, and neurofibromatosis.
- **Secondary**: smoker and lung cancer.

Clinical

- Seizures, morning headache, vomiting, raised ICP, papilloedema, cognitive, behavioural changes.
- Focal neurology dependent on site, e.g. weakness, cerebellar signs, hemianopia, personality change.
- May present as stroke, e.g. with subcortical hypodensity or with a haemorrhage.

Signs of an extracranial primary malignancy

- Lung: weight loss, cough, hoarseness, Horner's syndrome.

- Breast lump, Paget's disease of nipple, localised nodes.
- Testicular mass.
- Haematuria, renal mass: renal cell tumour.
- Anaemia: gastrointestinal primary.
- Skin pigmentation: look for melanoma.

Investigations

- **Bloods:** FBC: anaemia from gut malignancy, U&E, LFT, Ca, ALP: liver metastases.
- **CT + contrast**: usually a well demarcated ring-enhancing lesion often sited at grey–white matter border or even within the dura, with associated vasogenic oedema. In adults most are in the cerebral hemispheres with a minority in the posterior fossa. Look for hydrocephalus. Melanomas, renal cell carcinomas, lung tumours and choriocarcinomas and anticoagulated tend to bleed.
- **MRI head with gadolinium**: FLAIR, T1 and T2 with contrast can confirm lesion.
- **PET scan**: specialist use only.
- **CXR**: lung tumour or lung metastases.
- **CT chest abdomen pelvis** for primary malignancy.
- **Brain biopsy:** to confirm histology at open craniotomy or CT-guided stereotactic techniques.
- **LP:** generally avoided especially with a large space occupying lesion and oedema and risk of brain herniation.

Differential: cerebral abscess, stroke, encephalitis.

Metastatic tumours (64 per 100 000 per year)

- Lung cancer, renal cell cancer, colonic tumour.
- Melanoma, breast cancer, testicular tumours/choriocarcinoma.

Primary tumours (10 per 100 000 per year)

Gliomas

- Grade IV: glioblastoma multiforme is particularly aggressive (high grade)
- Grade III: anaplastic astrocytomas (high grade)
- Grade II: astrocytoma
- Grade I: pilocytic

Oligodendrogliomas

- Anaplastic oligodendroglioma (high grade)

Ependymal: lining of ventricles:

- Anaplastic ependymoma (high grade)

Others

- Medulloblastomas (posterior fossa in children)
- Meningiomas (Falx, sphenoid, base of skull, complete resection usual)
- Pituitary tumours (see *Section 13.9*)
- Craniopharyngiomas
- Vestibular schwannomas
- CNS lymphoma: immunocompromised, deep in brain, cause seizures, multiple

Acute management

- Will depend on age, morbidities and underlying health status as well as the nature of the tumour, its size and its responsiveness to surgery or radiotherapy and patient choice. Determine primary if possible – for some metastatic tumours the primary is elusive.
- **Steroids**: symptoms of raised ICP and oedema – usually Dexamethasone 10 mg stat PO and 6 mg BD PO increasing to 24 mg per day in divided dose. Don't give doses after 5 pm as will cause insomnia. The only exception is where primary brain lymphoma is suspected when it is preferable to do a brain biopsy first. If falling GCS – see *Section 2.6* and consider IV Mannitol.

- External ventricular drainage if acute hydrocephalus. Consider starting Phenytoin if there has been any seizure-like activity.

Ongoing management

- Referral to a neuro-oncology MDT: oncology, neuro-radiologists, neurosurgeons, palliative care.
- Some tumours can be removed and cured, e.g. meningioma, pituitary, solitary lesions. More difficult if brainstem or language or sensorimotor areas or basal ganglia.
- Palliative surgical resection or debulking of the primary or secondary tumour.
- Radiotherapy: whole brain radiotherapy or stereotactic radiosurgery.
- Chemotherapy rarely useful except for primary cerebral lymphoma.
- Median prognosis is 6 months and depends on primary.

22.5 Hyperviscosity syndrome

About

- Increased plasma viscosity.

Causes

- Waldenstrom's macroglobulinaemia, multiple myeloma causing high levels of serum immunoglobulins (usually IgM, then IgA and IgG), immunoglobulin M (IgM) paraproteins.
- Leukaemias (WCC >100), myeloproliferative diseases, polycythaemia and thrombocytosis.

Clinical

- Visual disturbances, bleeding (GI bleeds, mucous membranes, epistaxis).
- Neurological manifestations, e.g. stroke/TIA, vertigo and hearing loss.

Investigations

- **FBC, U&Es, ESR, Ca, PPE**: monoclonal band, urinary Bence–Jones protein.
- **CT brain:** if stroke/TIA, **CXR:** if breathless.

Management

- ABC, IV access, hydration, treat infection.
- Plasma exchange via plasmapheresis is the gold standard of treatment.

22.6 Malignant superior vena caval obstruction

Malignant causes	Non-malignant causes
• Lung cancer (non-small cell lung cancer / small cell lung cancer) • Metastases, lymphoma, testicular • Breast or thrombosis from malignancy	• Mediastinal fibrosis: histoplasmosis, TB, sarcoid • Thrombosis: central line/pacemaker/ ICD leads • Compression from thoracic aortic aneurysms • Behcet's syndrome, fibrosis from radiation

Clinical

- Breathless, oedema of face and neck, headache and sensation of fullness.
- Cough, haemoptysis, weight loss, dilated veins in upper chest and neck.
- Horner's syndrome, effusion, clubbing, hoarseness.

- Lymphadenopathy, testicular mass, hepatosplenomegaly.
- Cerebral or laryngeal oedema suggests a poor prognosis.
- Raised SVC pressure can even lead to oesophageal varices and bleeding.

Investigations

- **FBC, U&Es, ESR, Ca.**
- **CXR/CT**: tumour mass, BHL, fibrosis, TB. **CT-guided biopsy**: primary lung tumour.
- **MRI brain with gadolinium**, bronchoscopy, sputum cytology, staging and biopsies.

Management

- ABC, O_2 as per BTS guidelines. Airways management, remove central venous lines. Steroids: malignancy consider DEXAMETHASONE 4 mg PO qds.
- **Diuretics:** have been given for malignant causes unresponsive to other options.
- **Endovascular stenting** indicated for an extrinsic compressive cause and this also helps non-malignant/fibrotic causes. The rare downside of stenting is that the sudden improved venous return can lead to pulmonary oedema.
- **Anticoagulation**: may need anticoagulation at least for VTE prophylaxis. Full anticoagulation if the obstruction is thrombotic.
- **Chemotherapy**: consider treatment where tumours are chemosensitive, e.g. small cell lung cancer or lymphoma.

23 Dermatological emergencies

23.1 Cellulitis, bites, surgery

About

- Beware overtreating chronic bilateral warm legs.
- It's possible, but unusual, for cellulitis to be symmetrical.

Organism

- These are usually sensitive to flucloxacillin.
- Cellulitis mostly due to beta-haemolytic streptococci.
- Less common *Staph. aureus* and MRSA.

Clinical

- Subcutaneous skin infection. Red, painful swelling often of a limb. Pyrexia and malaise.
- Look for the point of entry – dry cracked skin between toes or insect bite or trauma. Look at heels.

Management

- **Mild–moderate cellulitis:** non-severe – afebrile and systemically well and no osteomyelitis. Give **FLUCLOXACILLIN** PO for 7–14 days. If penicillin allergic then **CLARITHROMYCIN** for 7–14 days. **MRSA positive** consider **VANCOMYCIN or TEICOPLANIN** IV OD.
- **Severe cellulitis: FLUCLOXACILLIN IV/PO** until patient shows clinical improvement, no sepsis and tolerating oral intake then switch to oral therapy.
- **Orbital cellulitis (serious infection):** has various causes and may be associated with serious complications including visual loss. Prompt diagnosis and proper management are essential for curing the patient with orbital cellulitis. Needs admission and CT + contrast and monitor function and IV antibiotic therapy (**CEFTRIAXONE IV and METRONIDAZOLE IV**) should be continued for 1–2 weeks and then followed by oral antibiotics for an additional 2–3 weeks. Fungal infection requires IV antifungal therapy along with surgical debridement.
- **Leg ulcers, pressure sores:** treat with antibiotics only if demarcated cellulitis or systemic infection observed. Refer to the cellulitis guidelines above. Wound cleaning and skin management. Discuss with tissue viability specialist.
- **Animal bites/human bites. CO-AMOXICLAV PO (IV** for severe infection). For penicillin allergy **DOXYCYCLINE PO + METRONIDAZOLE PO**. Severe human bites, take advice. Duration: 7 days.
- **Following clean surgery**: *mild/moderate*: FLUCLOXACILLIN PO/IV. *Severe*: BENZYLPENICILLIN IV + FLUCLOXACILLIN IV. *MRSA colonised/infected*: TEICOPLANIN IV.

23.2 Toxic epidermal necrolysis

About

- Involves skin as well as mucous membranes – mouth, genitals, vagina, eyes.
- TEN is a more severe form of Stevens Johnson syndrome (SJS).
- Ask about drugs within the preceding 2 months as a reaction may be delayed.

Aetiology

- Idiopathic – worse prognosis than drug-induced.
- Drug-induced – sulphonamides, cephalosporins, antibiotics, anticonvulsants.
- Commoner with HIV and in slow drug acetylators.

Clinical

- Preceding flu-like illness with myalgia, fever in recent days.
- Milder: erythema, target lesions, blistering on skin and oral/genital mucosa.
- Spreading tender erythema and confluent blistering rash followed by loss of sheets of epidermis. Pain may be severe. Involves skin and oral/genital mucosa.
- Detachment of the skin and mucosal epidermis. Progressive exfoliation.
- Recovery may lead to scarring, altered pigmentation and loss of sweating.
- Positive Nikolsky sign when slight lateral pressure to the epidermal surface.

Differential

- *Staphylococcal* scalded skin syndrome (seen in children and mucosa spared).
- Toxic shock syndrome, phototoxic skin reactions. Drug reaction with eosinophilia.

Prognostic severity factors for toxic epidermal necrolysis	
(1) Age >40 years or HR >120	(4) Urea >10 mmol/L
(2) Cancer or haematological malignancy	(5) HCO_3 <20 mmol/L
(3) Involved body surface area >10%	(6) Blood glucose level >14 mmol/L

Mortality rates: based on the number of positive criteria are as follows: 0–1 factor = 3%, 2 factors = 12%, 3 factors = 35%, 4 factors = 58%, 5 or more factors = 90%.

Investigation

- **Bloods**: FBC, U&Es, LFT, CRP. Blood cultures, urine culture, CXR if febrile.
- **Skin biopsy**: necrotic keratinocytes with full thickness epithelial necrosis and sheets of epidermal detachment helps differentiate from *Staphylococcal* scalded skin syndrome.

Management (speak with dermatologist)

- Stop all possible drug causes, early detection and management of any sepsis.
- Transfer to burns unit. Supportive – fluid balance and nutrition, avoid hypothermia. Some may consider IVIG but steroids/immune suppression not indicated.
- Appropriate bedding – Clinitron mattress, avoid IV lines to reduce sepsis.
- Fluid/nutrition orally or via NG tube. Eye care to avoid scarring. VTE prophylaxis.

23.3 Necrotising fasciitis

About

- A surgical emergency – minutes matter because infection proceeds rapidly and lethally.
- Always consider if extremely painful cellulitis with a hard woody feel.

Aetiology

- Infections with group A β-haemolytic streptococci.
- Diabetics, arterial and venous vascular disease. Can follow mild trauma.

Clinical

- Severe localised pain, myalgia, malaise, fever. Localised defined erythema.
- Crepitus and surgical emphysema from gas-forming bacteria in the soft tissue.
- Blistering and hardening. Mark out limits of erythema.

Differential

- Cellulitis, *Pyoderma gangrenosum*.

Investigation

- **FBC**: raised WCC, ESR and CRP. **U&Es**: AKI, hyperkalaemia.
- **Plain X-ray** of affected area may show gas in soft tissues.
- **MRI/CT:** may be used to detect soft tissue infection, however, surgery should not be delayed for confirmatory radiology if clinical suspicion high.
- **Needle aspirate:** at edge of lesion and Gram stain can help.

Management

- **ABC, high flow O_2** to get saturation 100% unless severe COPD. Resuscitation. IV fluids and antibodies and immediate surgical consult.
- **Immediate surgery can decrease mortality**: once diagnosed patient requires burns unit or trauma unit transfer to those with experience in extensive debridement and reconstructive surgery. Hyperbaric O_2 where facilities available.
- **IV CLINDAMYCIN** – as well as antimicrobial effect it is a potent suppressor of bacterial toxin synthesis. May be combined with **IV BENZYLPENICILLIN and GENTAMICIN IV**. Liaise closely with microbiology.

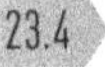

23.4 Erythroderma (exfoliative dermatitis)

About

- Erythroderma is the presence of erythema >90% of the skin. Several causes.
- Determine underlying cause but 25% are idiopathic. Commoner in males.

Aetiology

- Dermatitis (atopic, contact and seborrhoeic types).
- Psoriasis. Drug eruptions. Cutaneous T-cell lymphoma, idiopathic.

Clinical

- Scaling erythematous dermatitis with erythroderma and heat/fluid loss.
- Risks of hypothermia, heart failure, fluid/electrolyte imbalance.
- Erythrodermic psoriasis, there may be an additional feature of pustulation.

Differential

- Cellulitis, cutaneous T-cell lymphoma.

Investigation

- **FBC**: raised WCC. U&Es: AKI, raised CRP, ESR. LFTs: low albumin.
- **Skin biopsy** may be required. Increased serum IgE in some cases.

Management

- Detect and treat any underlying cause. Bed rest, bland emollients. Fluid and electrolyte management.
- Erythrodermic pustular psoriasis is one of the few indications for systemic steroids in psoriasis, but care is required because withdrawal of systemic steroids is a trigger for erythrodermic pustular psoriasis.

24 Ophthalmological emergencies

24.1 Acute visual loss

Consider high dose steroids if GCA is suspected as cause of arteritic AION.

Cause	About
Arteritic anterior ischaemic optic neuropathy	Arteritic AION usually due to giant cell arteritis. Oclusion of posterior ciliary artery which supplies optic nerve. Usually painless. Raised ESR/CRP. Aged >50. Temporal artery tenderness. Usually unilateral but may proceed to complete visual loss in both eyes. Afferent pupillary defect. Start steroids if suspected. See giant cell arteritis (*Section 24.2* below).
Non-arteritic anterior ischaemic optic neuropathy	Atherosclerotic or thromboembolic occlusion of posterior ciliary artery which supplies optic nerve. Usually painless, associated with arteriosclerotic vascular disease, older males. Usually unilateral but may proceed to complete visual loss in both eyes. Atrial fibrillation. Main issue is differential from GCA. Afferent pupillary defect. Treat as for stroke disease. Carotid doppler may show plaques or stenosis on affected side; assess and manage vascular risk factors.
Central retinal artery occlusion	Sudden severe visual loss in seconds. Afferent pupillary defect. May be complete or affect branches. Retina is pale and white with a cherry-coloured spot at macula. Associated with vascular risk factors. If seen within first hour sudden pressure and release to the globe may dislodge embolism or propel it peripherally. Should have carotid dopplers and ESR/CRP to exclude GCA. Give steroids immediately if GCA suspected.
Retinal detachment	Painless progressive visual loss depending on retinal area detached. If macuar affected then central vision is lost. May see floaters and describe flashes of light.
Central retinal vein occlusion	Sudden severe visual loss in seconds. Afferent pupillary defect. May be complete or affect branches. Retina is red with haemorrhage with bloody venous infarction and engorged dilated retinal veins. Associated with vascular risk factors. If seen within first hour sudden pressure and release to the globe may dislodge embolism or propel it peripherally.
Corneal ulcer	See red eye section below (PAIN + RED EYE + VISUAL LOSS).
Acute angle closure glaucoma	See red eye section below (PAIN + RED EYE + VISUAL LOSS).
Occipital stroke	May give only clinical finding as visual loss. Haemorrhagic or infarction. May give homonymous hemianopia but bilateral strokes may occur depending on aetiology. See acute stroke management (*Section 19.8*).
Occipital tumour	Visual loss and hemianopia progressive +/– headache.

Cause	About
Optic neuritis	Eye movements may be painful. May be seen as a first presentation of later multiple sclerosis. Often young and more commonly female. Monocular blindness comes on over hours so more subacute than acute. Afferent pupillary defect. Altered colour perception initially. Optic disc may be normal or swollen. Some recovery over 2–6 weeks with residual temporal pallor. Discuss high dose methylprednisolone with neurology.
Vitreous haemorrhage	May be due to proliferative retinopathy. Blood may obscure retina and loss of red reflex and afferent pupillary defect.
Pituitary apoplexy	Sudden headache and visual loss and IIIrd nerve palsy. Needs steroids for acute pituitary insufficiency and urgent neurosurgical decompression (see *Section 13.9*).

Red eye

Consider urgent ophthalmic referral for severe ocular pain, photophobia, sudden reduction in vision, coloured halos around point of light, proptosis or smaller pupil in affected eye.

Cause	About
Conjunctivitis	Viral infection usually but also bacterial (more purulent discharge) or allergic (history and other features of atopy). Conjunctiva is red and infected and there may be a discharge and anything from tingling to pain. Vision is normal. Cornea normal. Treat with chloramphenicol eye drops. If viral ensure good hand hygiene as easily transmitted. Occasionally due to gonorrhoea where it is very severe with discharge and chemosis and preauricular node enlargement. Needs topical penicillin. Can also be due to chlamydia.
Anterior uveitis (iritis): red eye + pain + visual loss	Both redness and ocular pain on palpation over the sclera and involvement of the anterior chamber which can blur vision. Vessels dilated around the cornea. Pupil constricted, keratic precipitates and hypopyon in anterior chamber. Ophthalmic referral. Check CRP/ESR, ANA, RF, etc. Associated with ankylosing spondylitis (HLA-B27), inflammatory bowel disease, sarcoid, tuberculosis, syphilis, toxoplasmosis, Behçet's syndrome, etc. Management for inflammatory causes is topical steroids with cyclopentolate 1%.
Corneal ulcer: red eye + pain + visual loss	Inflammation of the cornea. May be due to HSV. Pain, foreign body sensation and photophobia and lacrimation. HSV ulcer shows up with fluorescein. Needs Aciclovir ointment 5/day for 2 weeks.
Acute angle closure glaucoma: red eye + pain + visual loss	Angle close (narrow angle) glaucoma is an emergency and patients have an acute elevation in intraocular pressure. Mid dilated pupil. IOP >45 mmHg. Aged >50. May have systemic symptoms of nausea, vomiting even abdominal symptoms. Seen later in day / evening as pupils dilate. Exam shows narrow anterior chamber and needs urgent ophthalmic referral. Give IV acetazolamide 500 mg (check for contraindications) and pilocarpine 4% drops to constrict pupil.

Cause	About
Subconjunctival haemorrhage	Common, painless, may be associated with trauma or simple coughing and exacerbated by anticoagulants (check INR if on warfarin). Conservative management.
Orbital cellulitis	See *Section 23.1*.

24.2 Giant cell (temporal) arteritis

About

- Inflammation of small and mid-sized arteries with occlusion/infarction.
- Occluded posterior ciliary arteries causing an anterior ischaemic optic neuropathy.
- Atypical cases occur. Treat first and get TAB and expert opinion later.

Aetiology

- Inflammatory vasculitis may affect any artery. Commoner in females.
- Superficial temporal, posterior ciliary and ophthalmic arteries.
- Immune attack may be to the internal elastic lamina of the vessel wall.
- Large vessel disease can show aortic inflammation on PET scanning.

Clinical

- Headache, jaw and tongue claudication (pain when chewing). Temporal artery tender and pulseless. Transient or permanent monocular visual loss.
- Systemic symptoms, e.g. weight loss, malaise, fever.
- Can have symptoms of PMR – pain over shoulders, proximal weakness.
- Fundoscopy: white optic disc oedema with splinter haemorrhages at disc margin.

Differential

- Migraine, TIA, non-arteritic AION.
- Optic neuritis, causes of sudden monocular blindness.

Investigation

- **FBC**: normocytic normochromic anaemia. **B12 folate ferritin**: normal.
- **ESR**: elevated >50 mm/h (classically >100 mm/h). **CRP:** elevated. **ALP:** elevated.
- **Temporal artery biopsy** (TAB): needed within 7–14 days of starting steroids.
- **American College of Rheumatology classification criteria:** three of the following five criteria were required to meet the diagnosis for giant cell arteritis: sensitivity of 93.5% and a reported specificity of 91.2% for the classification of giant cell arteritis compared with other vasculitides:
  (1) Age 50 years or older.
  (2) New onset localised headache.
  (3) Temporal artery tenderness or decreased temporal artery pulse.
  (4) ESR >50 mm/h.
  (5) TAB characterised by mononuclear infiltration or granulomatous inflammation.

Management

- **High dose steroids** started immediately to avoid potential visual loss where there is significant suspicion of the diagnosis: **Prednisolone 1 mg/kg usually**. Higher doses may sometimes be used.

- **TAB organised urgently**. Steroids: reduce slowly over 18 months titrated to clinical response and ESR/CRP. Steroid-sparing agents may be used. Start osteoporotic bone protection.
- Consider **ASPIRIN 75 mg OD** and PPI as well as good BP and vascular risk factor management. TIA/stroke seen in these patients.

25 Medical problems in pregnancy

About

- The call to the obstetric unit for medical issues can be intimidating to even the most accomplished doctor. This is a collection of a few basic facts and principles to help you. As ever, if unsure of what you are doing then get help. This is to deal mainly with acute and on-call questions. Pregnancy is covered within resuscitation, asthma and DVT/pulmonary embolism and headache sections.

General principles

- Most women in pregnancy are healthy. Those with known or anticipated medical disorders require expert care which is really the preserve of the obstetric team liaising with medical specialists as needed. Communication is key.
- Medical disorders can be considered in terms of disorders caused by the pregnancy and pre-existing disorders exacerbated by the effects of the pregnancy, e.g. heart disease, asthma, immune disorders, clotting disorders, epilepsy.
- It is important to involve senior members of the obstetric team when making any significant management plans that can affect the pregnancy.

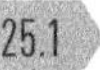

25.1 Acute medical advice in pregnant patients

Medical advice on managing pregnant patients

- There are two (or sometimes more) patients.
- Give folate prior to conception and in the first trimester.
- Investigations and treatments can affect mothers and/or fetus.
- Normal BP can be misleading (BP may not fall until 1500 ml blood loss).
- Tachypnoea or tachycardia must not be ignored.
- A pink venflon is useless in a sick pregnant patient.
- Ectopic pregnancy can be atypical, e.g. 'fainting, D&V'.
- ALP (placental) rises in 3rd trimester so beware overdiagnosis of liver disease.
- CXR safe (3 days background radiation exposure) and fetus can be screened.
- Most X-ray concerns are outweighed by need for accurate diagnosis.
- Avoid prescribing in 1st trimester unless proven safety.
- Avoid NSAIDs, ACE inhibitors, ARBs, trimethoprim, warfarin.
- For anticoagulation use LMWH or IV heparin.
- Consider managing PE by diagnosing a DVT first.
- Untreated hyperemesis can lead to severe thiamine deficiency (give Pabrinex).
- Salbutamol and steroids and magnesium can be given for asthma.
- Magnesium is drug of choice for preventing eclamptic seizures.
- Magnesium toxicity causes cardiac arrests. Treatment with IV calcium.
- Maximum cardiac physiological stress is at 14 weeks and just following delivery.

25.2 Hypertension in pregnancy

- Hypertension during pregnancy carries risks of increased perinatal mortality, preterm birth and low birth weight.

- Pre-eclampsia and gestational hypertension come on later in pregnancy.
- Pre-existing hypertension can be discovered at initial contact.
- ACE inhibitors and ARB drugs are teratogenic and contraindicated in pregnancy.

Degrees of HTN	Values
Mild	DBP 90–99 mmHg and SBP 140–149 mmHg
Moderate	DBP 100–109 mmHg and SBP 150–159 mmHg
Severe	DBP > 110 mmHg and SBP >160 mmHg

Causes of HTN in pregnancy (BP >140/90 mmHg, 2 readings seated 6 h apart)

- Gestational (pregnancy-induced) HTN (new onset but minimal proteinuria).
- Pre-eclampsia and eclampsia (new hypertension with proteinuria).
- Chronic hypertension (renal disease, primary/essential hypertension).
- Pre-eclampsia superimposed on chronic hypertension.

25.3 Eclampsia and pre-eclampsia

Low-dose aspirin is beneficial in the prevention of pre-eclampsia in selected high-risk women.

About

- Reported frequencies from 2 to 7% of all pregnancies after 20 weeks.
- Only 1 in 2000 pregnancies have hypertensive proteinuria before fit.
- **Pre-eclampsia (PET):** after 20 weeks + BP >140/90 mmHg + proteinuria >300 mg/24 h.
- **Severe** = pre-eclampsia (PET) + end organ damage.

Moderate risk factors	High risk factors (give aspirin 75 mg OD from 12 weeks)
• First pregnancy, age >40 years	• HTN during previous pregnancy
• Pregnancy interval >10 years	• Chronic kidney disease
• BMI >35 kg/m^2 at first visit	• Antiphospholipid syndrome
• Family history of pre-eclampsia	• Type 1 or type 2 diabetes
• Multiple pregnancy	• Chronic hypertension

Clinical

- **Pre-eclampsia:** severe headache, severe pain just below ribs, epigastric or hypochondrial (hepatic congestion/liver capsule stretching). Is baby moving normally (fetal wellbeing)? Visual problems such as blurring or vomiting, flashing before eyes, sudden swelling of face, hands or feet. Disorientated, hyperreflexia, clonus, stroke and cerebral oedema.
- **Severe pre-eclampsia:** severe headache, visual problems, papilloedema, clonus >3 beats. Liver tenderness.
- **Eclampsia:** grand-mal seizures last 60+ sec preceded by facial twitching. There is generalised muscle contraction. May be coma and period of hyperventilation.

Complications

- **Stroke:** ischaemic or haemorrhagic get CT head, manage BP, aspirin where indicated. Exclude cerebral venous thrombosis and SAH.
- **HELLP**: platelets <100×10^9/L, haemolysis (raised LDH), elevated LFTs. Fatal in 2%.
- **AKI** (acute cortical or tubular necrosis): fall in GFR, elevated creatinine, urea. Oliguria, proteinuria >5 g/24 h.
- **Others:** fetal growth retardation, fetal death, placental abruption, ARDS, hepatic infarction, DIC.

Investigations

- **FBC**: low platelet count (HELLP syndrome). Anaemia due to microangiopathic haemolysis (peripheral smear – schistocytes, burr cells, echinocytes) or physiologic haemodilution of pregnancy.
- **U&E**: AKI: renal dysfunction (late), raised urate in eclampsia.
- **LFTs**: raised AST/ALT, mild: increase LDH or bilirubin. Low haptoglobin levels with haemolysis.
- **Clotting**: (not routinely if platelets >100×10^9/L). MSU to exclude UTI as cause of protein.
- **Fetal assessment**: fetal HR, USS for growth, CTGs. Maternal: cervical assessment (depending on gestation).
- **CT head**: arrange post seizure to exclude haemorrhage or other pathology.
- **Prevention:** aspirin 75 mg started at 12 weeks treatment to reduce risk of PET. Moderate but consistent reductions in PET, preterm delivery and serious outcomes. Start in those at high risk – hypertensive disease during a previous pregnancy, chronic kidney disease, systemic lupus erythematosus or antiphospholipid syndrome, type 1 or type 2 diabetes, chronic hypertension.

Management

- **Antihypertensives in pregnancy**: the following are acceptable: methyldopa, labetalol, clonidine, prazosin, doxazosin, nifedipine.
- **HTN**: mild consider **LABETALOL** PO and monitor closely to keep BP <150/80–100 mmHg. In more severe cases consider **labetalol IV/oral**, **hydralazine** (IV) and nifedipine (oral).
- **Eclamptic seizures:** IV magnesium is recommended and is better than phenytoin or diazepam for preventing eclampsia in severe PET. Regimen for **MAGNESIUM SULPHATE**: loading dose of 4 g given intravenously over 5 min, followed by infusion of 1 g/h for 24 h. Further dose of 2–4 g given over 5 min if recurrent seizures. Monitor urine output, reflexes and respiratory rate. Ongoing seizures managed as per status epilepticus (see *Section 19.4*).
- **Delivery**: recommended but timing depends on gestational age and fetal maturity and risk to mother of continuing the pregnancy. Obstetrician may give steroids to improve lung maturity if delivery planned within 1 week.
- **Gestational hypertension:** avoid ACE inhibitors, ARBs. Give aspirin from 12 weeks. Consider α-methyldopa, hydralazine, labetalol and nifedipine. Diuretics avoided.
- **Chronic hypertension**. Stop ACE inhibitors, ARBs. Switch to safer drugs in pregnancy. Give aspirin from 12 weeks. Ensure underlying causes excluded, Consider α-methyldopa, hydralazine, labetalol and nifedipine (avoid sublingual as it can cause sudden hypotension). Diuretics avoided.
- Warfarin, ACE inhibitors and AT2 blockers are absolutely contraindicated in pregnancy. Diuretics are not contraindicated but are generally avoided.

Reference: NICE (2010) CG107: Hypertension in pregnancy.

25.4 Pharmacology in pregnancy

Sources of prescribing advice in UK

- *BNF* or your local equivalent. National Teratology Information Service (NTIS) in Newcastle – call 0191 2321525 (5944 urgent monday to friday 17.00–20.00); 08448920111 – emergency 24 h advice line for poisoning/chemical exposure in pregnancy.
- Websites: http://toxbase.org; http://toxnet.nlm.nih.gov; http://ukmicentral.nhs.uk. Also consult with local obstetric medicine team. The safety of any drug used in pregnancy must be checked with manufacturer's data sheet or *BNF*.
- **Known or potential teratogens to stop/avoid:** ACE inhibitors, AT2 blockers, cigarette smoking, cocaine, warfarin, fluconazole, isotretinoin (Accutane), lithium, misoprostol, penicillamine, tetracyclines, doxycycline, thalidomide, valproic acid.
- **Some possible teratogens:** alcohol binge drinking, carbamazepine, colchicine, disulfiram, ergotamine, glucocorticoids (benefits often outweigh risks), lead, metronidazole, primidone, quinine (suicidal doses), streptomycin, vitamin A (high doses), zidovudine (AZT).
- **Drugs to avoid when breastfeeding:** chloramphenicol, metronidazole, nitrofurantoin and sulphonamides (haemolysis with G6PD deficiency), tetracycline (stains teeth and bones), lithium, antineoplastics and immunosuppressants, psychotropic drugs (relative).
- **Drugs which can be used in pregnancy:** heparin and LMWH, ampicillin, cephalosporins, clindamycin, erythromycin, gentamicin, paracetamol (acetaminophen), folate, pyridoxine, thyroxine, steroids, salbutamol, aspirin, magnesium, anticholinergic inhalers, theophyllines, lorazepam, diazepam, phenytoin. Give usual doses of GTN, IV nitrates, furosemide, morphine, calcium blocker, mechanical support, e.g. IABP, LVAD, digoxin, β-blockers.

26 General management issues

26.1 Assessing fluid balance

Situation	Dehydration	Overhydration	Euvolaemic
General exam	Sunken eyes, dry mouth and reduced skin turgor, complains of thirst. With time becomes obtunded	Raised JVP, usually gravitational dependent oedema, ascites, anasarca, breathless if CCF	Warm, well filled
Observations	Low BP, postural hypotension, weak low volume pulse, tachycardia	Normal BP or hypertension, tachycardia if in CCF	BP and HR normal
Body weight	Reduced	Increased	Normal
Urine	Anuria/oliguria with low urinary Na	Normal or increased urine output and urine Na	Normal output
Bloods	Raised Hb, increased urea more so than creatinine, hypernatraemia if free water loss	Normal unless pre-existing disease. Hyponatraemia possible	Normal
Evidence	Vomiting, diarrhoea, obstructed fluid-filled bowel, polyuria, sweating, fistulae	Excess intake, liver/ cardiac/renal failure	N/A
CVP	Reduced	Increased	Normal
Fluid balance chart	Net fluid loss	Net fluid gain	Normal balance
Management	Appropriate fluid replacement. Is it just water depletion or salt too and other electrolytes?	Fluid restriction, diuretics	Match losses + 500 ml orally if possible

Assessment

- Examine for hypovolaemia (low BP, postural hypotension, tachycardia, reduced skin turgor). Seek help if still unsure (it can be difficult) about volume status especially when complex, e.g. where there is ongoing organ failure (e.g. cardiac/ renal/liver) or sepsis, pyrexia and drains losing fluids.
- Examine the notes – cause of admission, past history, procedures? Examine the chart – drugs, observations, pyrexia, BP, HR, urine output, output of drains all of which should be stored within the fluid balance chart. What has preceded the assessment? Surgery, new drugs given?
- Do not hang your diagnosis on one sign – the fluid balance chart may be badly completed, a raised JVP might suggest RV infarction or a PE and a need for filling rather than overload, a CVP line may be blocked or erroneously measured, a BP might be recorded in an arm with atherosclerotic arteries and be misleadingly low so check other side. Healthy scepticism is always wise especially when appearance of patient and signs don't match.

- Fluid losses may be hidden unless looked for, e.g. ascites and intestinal luminal or generalised oedema can contain significant fluid losses. During sepsis and inflammation increased fluid can be found in the interstitium and depletes the circulating volume.
- Finally body weight, if recorded, is a simple and usually hard piece of data. A litre of water weighs 1 kg and recent fluctuations in body weight are likely to be due to fluid losses or gains. It is an important point to always try to get a baseline weight on any new admissions.
- Other ways to assess fluid balance is measuring urine output, which is a crude measure of renal perfusion. Oliguria/anuria where there is no evidence of post renal obstruction suggests renal water and sodium retention and even incipient AKI. Many resort to using the JVP but this is not without its limitations and potential complications and should be reserved for the patient on HDU/ITU.
- The physiological response to volume loss is the release of ADH and free water retention as well as increased sodium retention through the renin–angiotensin–aldosterone mechanism. Stress/surgery and pain also cause cortisol release and ADH release. If there is impaired renal function this mechanism may be impaired. The hypovolaemic patient is typically vasoconstricted with cold peripheries and a mild tachycardia and dry mucous membranes. The patient is also typically oliguric with a low urinary sodium.
- **Other losses**: the values here are very rough with wide variation and generally all prescriptions of IV fluids must take into account renal/cardiac function, latest blood results, fluid balance status, drugs prescribed.

26.2 Gastrointestinal losses

Fluid	Vol (L/day)	Na (mmol/L)	K (mmol/L)	Cl (mmol/L)	HCO_3 (mmol/L)
Saliva	1–1.5	50	15	30	90
Gastric aspirate	1–2.5	60	10	140	0
Bile	0.5–1.0	200	10	50	40
Pancreatic juice	1–2	120	10	40	100
Small bowel secretions	2–3	140	10**	variable	variable

**Raised in inflammatory conditions.

26.3 Replacing losses

Situation	Choice of replacement (NS = 0.9% normal saline)
General GI losses	Replace with equivalent volumes of NS
Significant diarrhoeal losses	These tend to contain significant amounts of K (e.g. 40 mmol/L) and so hypokalaemia can occur which may well worsen any ileus and other problems. Potassium should be monitored and replaced with NS + added K

Situation	Choice of replacement (NS = 0.9% normal saline)
Fistulae and overactive ileostomies	Loss of chloride and bicarbonate – replace with NSI and treat cause
Systemic sepsis with 3rd space losses	Replace with NS
Pyrexia/sweating Insensible losses	Replace with NS

Normal oral intake is best. Involve dietician if calorific or other needs identified. Ensure adequate access and able to hold beaker or use straw or other handheld devices. Good nursing/health care assistance if unable to swallow. Short term consider NG tube and longer term consider PEG tube placement. IV fluids only when above routes are unsatisfactory. If enteral replacement is not possible then IV fluids to consider are described below.

26.4 Choices of fluids

Fluid	Comments
5% dextrose	Glucose-containing solution that uses glucose (sugar) as the solute make it isotonic. It becomes hypotonic once glucose (solute) metabolised by the body's cells. Used mainly when there is free water loss, e.g. severe hypernatraemia secondary to diabetes insipidus.
(0.9% NaCl) NS	Crystalloid high in sodium content. *First line for hypovolaemic shock*. Can cause a hyperchloraemic metabolic acidosis. It has a short half-life and remains in the vascular space for only 15 min. In the UK the favoured choice of most physicians.
Dextrose–saline	A hybrid containing 0.18% NaCl (only one-fifth of the concentration of NS) and 4% dextrose. Again it has a short half-life and remains in the vascular space for only minutes.
Hartmann's (lactated Ringer's)	Isotonic crystalloid solution containing NaCl, KCl, $CaCl_2$ and sodium lactate all dissolved in sterile water. *Indicated for shock.* Distributed equally throughout the extracellular space and is rapidly lost from the intravascular space. Favoured choice of anaesthetists. Contains a high level of Na (at 131 mmol/L) and little K (at 5 mmol/L), and there is a small amount of calcium (2 mmol/L). The 29 mmol/L of lactate may be helpful for buffering acidosis. It does have a lower Cl concentration than normal saline (111 mmol/L rather than 154 mmol/L).
Plasmalyte (PL148)	Similar to Hartmann's and is a 'balanced' crystalloid solution. It mimics human plasma in its content of electrolytes, osmolality, and pH. Has buffer capacity with anions such as acetate, gluconate, and even lactate that are converted to bicarbonate, CO_2, and water. It can manage volume and electrolyte deficit and acidosis. Excess leads to fluid overload. It contains magnesium. Few studies on its use in trauma or hypovolaemic shock. No evidence that it is superior to other crystalloids for the prehospital management of traumatic hypovolaemia.
Gelofusine	Colloid formed from gelatin. Remains for longer within intravascular compartment. May cause histamine release and rash and bronchospasm. No evidence superior to crystalloids.

Crystalloids versus colloids

- There has been much discussion about the relative merits of crystalloids versus colloids in critically ill patients. The use of 4% albumin appears to increase mortality especially in trauma. There is no evidence that crystalloids are better or worse than colloids. Crystalloids should be used first line.
- **Crystalloid:** e.g. NS which is 0.9% NaCl or Hartmann's. First line in volume replacement.
- **Colloid:** which contains starch-like substances, e.g. Dextran or Gelofusine.
- **Blood and blood products** which remain in the vascular space for longer; red cells have O_2 carrying capacity, platelets and white cells have additional important functions.

Fluid	Na mmol/L	K mmol/L	Cl mmol/L	Mg mmol/L	Ca mmol/L	Lactate mmol/L	Osmolality mOsm/L
0.9% Saline (NS)	154	0	154	0	0	0	308
0.18% Saline 4% dextrose	30	0	30	0	0	0	284
0.45% Saline 5% dextrose	77	0	77	0	0	0	405
Gelofusion	154	0	154	0	0	0	274
Hartmann's	131	5	111	0	2	29	278
Plasmalyte 148	140	5	98	1.5	0	Acetate 27	297
5% Dextrose	0	0	0	0	0	190 kcal/L	278

Osmosis

- Water moves to dilute any solvent. If the interstitium and blood is hypertonic then water moves out of cells into the vascular space.
- If the blood is hypotonic it moves into cells and can cause cellular oedema and more worrying cerebral oedema (see *Section 13.10* on hyponatraemia).

26.5 Fluid replacement regimens

- These are for those having no oral or feeding intake usually, such as those who are post-operative or comatose, e.g. stroke patients. They should only be used transiently and feeding issues should be contemplated, because there is no significant calorific intake here.
- When patients are perioperative and on IV fluids then electrolytes should be checked at least every 24–48 h, or more often if there is any abnormality or any additional factors or deterioration. Avoid excessive fluid replacement in those with cardiac failure or renal failure and take expert advice if unsure.

In uncomplicated average patient requiring fluid replacement consider

Traditional regimen: (one salt + two sweet)

- 1 L Saline 0.9% + 20 mmol KCl (over 8 h) +
- 1 L Dextrose 5% + 20 mmol KCL (over 8 h) +
- 1 L Dextrose 5% + 20 mmol KCL (over 8 h)

= 3 L H_2O + 154 mmol Na + 154 mmol Cl + 60 mmol K + small amount of glucose.

Other regimens are acceptable as long as they replace similar amounts of water (3 L), sodium (150 mmol/day) and potassium (60 mmol/day) without upsetting serum osmolality.

Potassium replacement

- Normal needs are 60–100 mmol/day. May be omitted or reduced in the first 1–2 days post-surgery or where there is significant trauma/burns/blood transfusions as tissue damage will release potassium.
- Frequently check levels (e.g. twice daily). Maintain between 3.5 and 5 mmol/L, usually 4–5 mmol/L on the CCU. Take advice if unsure. See *Section 13.3* on management of hyperkalaemia if situation arises.
- Most potassium-containing fluids come prepared, e.g. with NS or 5% dextrose. Concentrated potassium should never be given directly IV but only given slowly and diluted, usually 20–40 mmol/L.
- The most concentrated infusion one would use outside a typical HDU/ITU/CCU setting would be 40 mmol/L in 500 ml given at 20 mmol/h. Rapid IV potassium infusion could lead to cardiac arrest. Any infusion must be closely controlled and given by an infusion pump.

26.6 Blood products

Product	Details	Indication
Red cell transfusions (packed red cells)	Red blood cells that have been separated from whole blood for transfusion purposes and stored at 4°C. Consider if Hb <10 g/dL, though the exact threshold for transfusion depends on the context. In the setting of haemorrhage then blood is needed and the Hb may indeed be normal acutely. It is thought that transfusion in non-haemorrhagic anaemia may not be needed until Hb <7–8 g/dL. Risks of infection, fluid overload, transfusion reactions, etc. Laboratory need to ensure ABO and rhesus compatibility. A bag of packed cells lasts 35 days and is kept refrigerated at 4°C. Volume is between 220 and 320 ml and should raise Hb by 10 g/L.	Acute haemorrhage, bone marrow failure, haemolytic anaemia (thalassemia/sickle cell), myelofibrosis, myelodysplasia, anaemia where Hb <7–8 g/dL and symptoms.
Platelet transfusions	Rhesus compatibility more important than ABO compatibility, but ABO compatible platelets are more effective. Platelet function is also important and platelets needed in those with bleeding on drugs such as clopidogrel. If there is more substantial bleeding then a target of 75–100 × 10^9/L should be aimed for. Platelet count can be a poor estimate of platelet functional activity. Each bag contains 300 × 10^9/L platelets in 300 ml and raises count by 20–30 × 10^9/L. Reactions can include all those seen with a blood transfusion.	Any cause of severe thrombocytopenia, avoid in HITT and TTP. Usually avoided in ITP. Used once platelet count <10 × 10^9/L. Pre-surgery or if bleeding then a level of 50 × 10^9/L should be aimed for.
Fresh frozen plasma (FFP)	Plasma is the pale yellow liquid part of blood. FFP contains stable components of the coagulation, fibrinolytic and complement systems; the proteins that maintain oncotic pressure and modulate immunity and other proteins. It is used when there are single or multiple clotting factor deficiencies or acute DIC, or for inherited coagulation deficiencies undergoing major	DIC, warfarin reversal, multiple clotting factor deficiencies, e.g. massive transfusion, DIC, TTP, warfarin therapy, liver disease, factor V deficiency.

Product	Details	Indication
Fresh frozen plasma (FFP) – *cont'd*	surgery. Use for immediate reversal of warfarin when prothrombin concentrates are not available. Reactions can include all those seen with a blood transfusion. Usual dose is 10–15 ml/kg body weight.	
Prothrombin complex concentrates (PCC)	Use for immediate reversal of warfarin. It is a combination of blood clotting factors II, VII, IX and X, as well as protein C and S. It is used to reverse the effect of warfarin rapidly reducing INR to 1.0.	Reversal of warfarin with raised INR and bleeding.
Cryo-precipitate	The bag is usually a cloudy yellow colour. Prepared from FFP and contains factor VIII (missing with haemophilia A), fibrinogen, Von Willebrand factor, factor XIII and fibronectin. Used originally for haemophilia. Reactions can include all those seen with a blood transfusion. Target fibrinogen level >1 g/L. Not now used for haemophilia A or Von Willebrand disease as not virally inactivated.	Used to treat low fibrinogen usually seen in the context of liver disease, trauma, DIC and massive fibrinolysis or massive transfusion.

Cross-matching

- Blood transfusion has risks as well as benefits. The report *Serious Hazards of Transfusion* (SHOT) continues to highlight potentially fatal mistakes in the administration of blood.
- Follow your hospital policy on pre-transfusion sample collection, which should detail who can collect samples. Do not use addressograph labels to label blood samples for cross-matching.
- **Vital steps**: identify patient in whom a cross-match sample is indicated. Prepare kit and bring to bedside –do not label bottle yet. Identify patient by asking name and DOB and check with wristband; take blood at bedside and label and date and sign the sample.

Important points on cross-matching blood

- Only cross-match and bleed one patient at a time to minimise the risk of error.
- Label the sample immediately after adding the blood, before leaving the patient. **Never prelabel sample** tubes.
- Label the sample tubes with the following: patient surname and given name in full, NHS number or other unique patient identification number, DOB (not age or year of birth), date and time of collection, signature or initials of the collector.
- As the sample collector you must sign the request form and the sample label to verify patient identification.
- Check identity by asking the patient to state and spell his or her name, and check the wrist band and check that the request form and sample match the patient and wrist band.
- Labelling of request: surname/family name and first name(s) in full, DOB (not age or year of birth), NHS number or address or other unique patient identifier, reason for the request.

References: British Committee for Standards in Haematology (1999) The administration of blood and blood components and the management of transfused patients. *Transfusion Med* 9:227.

Any concerns stop transfusion. Check correct patient and sample. Restart slowly and cautiously if all settles.

Blood transfusion reactions

Initial reactions	Main difficulty is knowing if a simple pyrexia or feeling unwell is a serious transfusion reaction. If unsure, slow blood and observe patient over minutes. If worsening or any haemodynamic compromise then stop and start crystalloid and take senior advice. Minor symptoms are not uncommon. Check the name and the bag and ensure no identification errors.
ABO incompatibility	Acutely unwell, tachycardic and hypotensive and progressively worse. Fever, chills, pain, flushed face, vomiting, diarrhoea all due to complement fragments. If transfusion reaction stop blood. Take full bloods from patient and repeat cross-match. Coomb's test. Coagulation screen. **Start IV NS. Give adrenaline IM if anaphylaxis.** Consider **FUROSEMIDE IV** to initiate diuresis. Discuss with ITU. Discuss with haematologist. *Keep opened unit and any unused units and return to lab for checking*. Can lead to intravascular or extravascular lysis. Intravascular caused by anti-A or anti-B with IgM complement-mediated lysis. Comes on in minutes but may be delayed. Can lead to DIC. Intravascular lysis causes haemoglobinaemia and haemoglobinuria. If hypotension, oliguria and anuria may cause AKI and need FUROSEMIDE IV. ABO incompatibility has a 10% mortality. Extravascular lysis is milder with fever and chills and is usually delayed with anaemia and jaundice and usually due to anti-D. Check all bloods and coagulation screen.
Isolated pyrexia/ rigors	Seen in 1% of transfusions. Check correct patient/transfusion. Restart about 30 min of observations. Slow transfusion, paracetamol, continue if settles. Due to pyrogens and leucocyte antibodies.
Urticaria	Check correct patient/transfusion. Consider IV Chlorphenamine. Continue if settles.
Acute anaphylaxis anaphylactoid reaction	Stop transfusion, treat as for anaphylaxis with **1 L NS IV and HYDROCORTISONE IV**. Consider **ADRENALINE 0.5 ml of 1 in 1000 IM**. May occur in those with IgA deficiency being exposed to IgA. See anaphylaxis in *Section 4.4*.
Bacterial contamination	Fever, hypotension, septic shock, oliguria, DIC. Usually immediate and often lethal. Stop transfusion. Take blood cultures.
Viral contamination	HBV, HTLV, HIV, HCV. Testing is done for these. Use CMV-negative donors for those receiving bone marrow transplants or solid organ transplants on immunosuppression.
Other infections	Include syphilis and malaria and toxoplasmosis.
Transfusion overload	Leads to breathlessness and cardiogenic pulmonary oedema, CXR changes. Treat as cardiogenic pulmonary oedema.
Transfusion-related lung injury (TRALI)	Comes on acutely with breathlessness, non-cardiogenic pulmonary oedema, cough, CXR changes. Due to donor antibodies to white cells. Treat as ARDS.

Transfusion-associated graft versus host disease	Immunocompromised host. Fever, rash on hands, feet and trunk, febrile, liver dysfunction 10 days post-transfusion. Possibly due to viable donor T cells. Supportive treatment. Can destroy recipient's bone marrow. Prevent by giving irradiated blood. See indications below.
Post-transfusion purpura	Later fall in platelets after 10–14 days. Recipient develops antibodies to human platelet antigen 1a. Treat with IVIg or plasma exchange.

Indications for irradiated blood products in adults (*Br J Haematol* 2010;152:35.)

- Immunocompromised, T cell defects (acquired/congenital).
- Blood from close family members, Alemtuzumab (anti-CD52) therapy.
- Irradiated products not needed with IV patients or after solid organ transplantation.
- Stem cell and marrow transplant recipients. HLA matched products, Hodgkin's lymphoma.
- Treatment with purine analogue drugs (fludarabine, cladribine and deoxycoformicin).

26.7 Blood gas interpretation

Normal blood gas

pH 7.35–7.45
PCO_2 35–45 mmHg (4.6–6 kPa)
PO_2 80–100 mmHg (11–13 kPa)
HCO_3 22–26 mmol
O_2 sats 95–100%

Other parameters

- **Base deficit:** >3 normal; −5 to −10 acidosis; <−10 severely ill
- **Anion gap:** Na − [Cl + HCO_3]; normal value is <12 mmol/L

- **Secondary corrections:** an abnormality in pH leads to compensatory changes. Acidosis is detected in brainstem (medulla) and peripheral chemoreceptors and leads to increased ventilation and the excretion of CO_2 from the lungs. There is also bicarbonate retention in the kidneys. This takes hours to days.
- **Measure anion gap** (AG) which is [cations] – [anions] and is normally 12 +/− 2 mmol/L. An anion is a negatively charged ion such as phosphate, sulphate, organic acids, or negatively charged proteins.
- Cations = [Na^+ + K^+]; anions = [Cl^- + HCO_3^-]; some equations omit the small K^+ contribution. Normally, measured [cations (+ve ions)] > [anions (-ve ions)], so there is a normally an 'anion gap'.
- **Calculate alveolar–arterial PO_2 gradient:** P_AO_2–PaO_2. P_AO_2 = (FiO_2 × (76–47) – (PaO_2/0.8). An increase suggests shunting. Normal = 4–10.

Pathophysiology

- The pH = – log [hydrogen ions]. pH varies from 1 which is highly acidic to 14 which is highly alkaline, with neutrality being 7. Blood is alkaline pH of 7.35–7.45. Gastric acid pH = 1.
- We are all net producers of acid, which is excreted both by the kidneys and by removing CO_2 from the lungs. To assess acid–base balance we can measure an arterial blood gas. Once primary respiratory cause excluded then venous gas will give us pH and [HCO_3^-] which may be enough. The pH is the product of renal and respiratory function and metabolic activity and buffering systems.
- Ketone bodies are water-soluble, fat-derived fuels that are used by many tissues for energy generation when there is limited glucose availability. The brain

becomes especially dependent upon ketones for fuel when plasma glucose levels are inadequate.

- *Henderson–Hasselbalch equation*. Note that PCO_2 is dependent on pulmonary function in being able to get rid of CO_2. Hyperventilating will lower $PaCO_2$ and hypoventilation will lead to a rise in $PaCO_2$.

Interpreting an ABG	
Step 1: look at pH	7.35–7.45 : normal or may be compensated pH < 7.35 : acidosis pH > 7.45: alkalosis
Step 2: look at PCO_2	4.6–6.0 kPa: normal > 6.0 kPa: hypercarbia suggests hypoventilation and Type 2 RF < 4.6 kPa: hyperventilation which may be triggered by metabolic acidosis
Step 3: look at HCO_3	22–26 mmol/L: normal <22: suggests metabolic acidosis >26: metabolic alkalosis or renal compensation of a respiratory acidosis
Measure anion gap if metabolic acidosis	AG >12 mmol/L suggests increased acid production or failure to excrete it AG 3–12 mmol/L – usually due to a loss of bicarbonate ions (balanced by increased chloride)

Term	ABG	Causes and management
Metabolic acidosis with **raised** anion gap	*Primary issue is* HCO_3 <22 mmol/L pH <7.35 AG >12 mmol/L	**Clinical:** hyperventilation/Kussmaul breathing. Renal failure, lactic acidosis, diabetic ketoacidosis, alcoholic ketoacidosis, toxins: methanol, carbon monoxide, cyanide, metformin, paraldehyde, iron, ethylene glycol, salicylates.
Metabolic acidosis with **normal** anion gap	*Primary issue is* HCO_3 <22 mmol/L pH <7.35 AG >3–12 mmol/L	**Clinical:** hyperventilation/Kussmaul breathing. Renal tubular acidosis, diarrhoea, small intestinal fistula, pancreatic alkali losses, carbon anhydrase inhibitors, ureterenterostomy, rapid hydration with NaCl, Addison's disease.
Metabolic alkalosis	*Primary issue is* HCO_3 >28 mmol/L pH >7.45 $PaCO_2$ normal	**Clinical:** paraesthesia, tentany. Antacids, dialysis, milk-alkali syndrome, pyloric stenosis/gastric outlet obstruction with vomiting, Bartter's syndrome, adrenogenital syndromes, Cushing's syndrome, Conn's syndrome.
Respiratory acidosis	*Primary issue is* PCO_2 >6 kPa pH <7.35 normal/compensated rise in HCO_3	**Clinical:** hypoventilating, drowsy, hypoxic. Chest disease, e.g. asthma, COPD, airway obstruction, hypoventilation, respiratory nerve or muscle weakness.
Respiratory alkalosis	*Primary issue is* $PaCO_2$ <4.7 kPa pH >7.45 Normal HCO_3	**Clinical:** paraesthesia, tentany. Hyperventilation (anxiety), asthma, CCF, hypoxia, PE, ventilation/perfusion mismatch, aspirin/salicylate overdose.

26.8 Venous access

Venous cannulae

Poiseuille showed that small changes in cannula diameter = large changes in flow.

Colour and size	Flow ml/min	Time to infuse 1000 ml NS	Uses
Yellow 24G			Paediatric
Blue 22G		22 min	Thin fragile veins
Pink 20G	50	15 min	IV drugs and IV fluids routine use
Green 18G	100	10 min	Blood transfusions and IV fluids
Grey 16G	200	6 min	Rapid IV infusion, hypovolaemic shock, ruptured AAA
Brown/orange 14G	360	3.5 min	Rapid blood transfusion, PPH, ectopic pregnancy, AAA

26.9 Choosing a cannula

A pink venflon is unsuitable to resuscitate a patient needing volume replacement. Ideally one or more grey 16G would be used. Flow rates can double if pressure on the bag of up to 300 mmHg is used. Flow is proportional to radius^4 (Poiseuille's law) so a small increase in radius can greatly improve flow and vice versa. Flow is inversely proportional to length and so central lines with long catheters impair flow and are inappropriate for rapid volume replacement. They also carry a higher risk of infection and complications than peripheral lines.

26.10 Nutritional support

Needs	Information	Comment
Water	Usually 2–3 L/day	Increased if other losses, e.g. urinary, gastrointestinal, fistulas
Energy	1750–2400 kcal/day	Titrated to needs
Protein	10–15 g/day of nitrogen in about 90 g of protein	More in severely catabolic states, e.g. burns
Minerals	Na 100 mmol/day, K 60–90 mmol/day, Ca, Mg	Increased K needed with some GI losses
Trace elements	Selenium, iodide, fluoride, iron, zinc, manganese and chromium	Increased for enteral as uptake not 100%
Vitamins	Give all fat and water soluble as per minimal daily requirements (not covered here)	Increased for enteral as uptake not 100%. Vitamin K added to parenteral feeds

26.11 Enteral feeding

- Before commencing nutrition always consider the risks of *refeeding syndrome* and screen the patient. Enteral feeding is used where there is a functioning GI tract but some physical reason (e.g. acute stroke or motor neuron disease, or facial or ENT surgery) that prevents normal swallowing.
- The enteral route is always preferable to the parenteral route if possible. It is important to note that directly feeding the stomach does not necessarily prevent aspiration as gastric contents can reflux and enter the lungs if there are poor protective reflexes.
- **Nasogastric tube:** commonly used but uncomfortable and can cause nasal trauma. Easily dislodged and only used as a temporary feeding measure for up to several weeks. If there is a clearly defined time for which swallowing will not be possible then best to replace with better option. Where outcome is unpredictable and survival unsure it may be used for several weeks, e.g. acute stroke. It is important that these are placed properly and local guidelines followed.
- **Never events**: NG tubes can be accidentally placed in bronchi and feed given – this is regarded as a never event. To show the tip is in gastic lumen an aspirate is obtained and checked for <pH 4 and if any doubt a CXR should show the NG tube in the midline in the thorax and then passing down below the diaphragm. Usual distance from nose to oesophageal junction is about 40 cm.
- **Percutaneous endoscopic gastrostomy (PEG):** medium to long term need for on-going enteral feeding. Performed by gastroenterologists at endoscopy and involves a puncture from abdominal surface through to the gastric lumen. Risks are real and include infection, peritonitis, sepsis, haemorrhage and displacement and the risks of sedation. Other intra-abdominal organs can be punctured. A fibrous fistulous tract forms over about 10–14 days after which replacement of any tube can be undertaken.
- **Percutaneous endoscopic jejunostomy (PEJ):** same as a PEG but tube advanced through pylorus.
- **Radiologically inserted gastrostomy**: ideal where there is a medium to long term need for on-going enteral feeding and the patient, for whatever reason, does not tolerate endoscopy. Performed by radiologists under fluoroscopy and involves a puncture from abdominal surface through to the gastric lumen. Complications and principles similar to PEG.
- **Needle catheter jejunostomy**: fine catheter inserted into jejunum at laparotomy and brought externally through a puncture in the abdominal wall.
- **Enteral feeding regimen**: with a simple polymeric diet consisting of protein and fat and carbohydrate containing essential minerals and vitamins. In those with small bowel disease a more elemental diet may be given such that proteins are given more as amino acids and fats as medium chain triglycerides.

26.12 Parenteral feeding

- **Assess for risk of refeeding syndrome**. Parenteral route really only used where the GI tract is non-functional. Higher risk of complications than enteral feeding particularly sepsis. In terms of feeding it is much less physiological. Not usually considered when needed for less than 1 week. Several routes.
- **Peripheral venous line**: only used with low osmolality feeding as it soon causes thrombophlebitis. The lines are 20 cm in length and can be used for up to 5 days.

- **Peripheral inserted central catheter (PICC):** a 60 cm catheter inserted in the antecubital fossa. The distal end lies within central veins. Hyperosmolar solutions may be used. Thrombophlebitis is less. These can last up to a month and may be inserted before a central venous line is considered.
- **Central venous line:** feeding via jugular/subclavian or femoral line using a silicone catheter. The infraclavicular subclavian route is often preferred and is most practical. A skin tunnel is usually created. The complications are the same as that of inserting any central line here and include infection, haemorrhage, arterial puncture and pneumothorax. Catheter-related sepsis should always be considered if any signs of infection. This will require IV antibiotics and removal of the line.
- **Different preparations** of feed are given depending if central or peripheral access, but all attempt to give about 3 L of feed over 24 h containing between 1700 and 2250 calories with sufficient protein, glucose, lipid, electrolytes, vitamins, water, and fat soluble and trace elements. Steroid and heparin and insulin may also be given. The feeds are usually prepared by pharmacy in liaison with the dietitian and intensivists. These patients are normally on the HDU/ITU or surgical wards.
- **Parenteral feeding** requires frequent monitoring and daily U&Es and glucose, and 2–3 times per week FBC, LFTs, Ca, P, Mg, Zn and glycerides. Monitor nutritional status. Any signs of sepsis requires FBC, CRP, blood cultures and assessment for chest or UTI. Take advice from seniors and microbiology as to management of the catheter. If that is the presumed or proven source then it will need to be removed.

26.13 Managing pain

- Successfully managing pain requires some knowledge of analgesia. Become familiar with a core group of medications. The team looking after a patient should certainly work with the hospital pain team. The perception of pain is multifactorial and often subjective and personal and varies with cause, depression, fears as to causation and control and often cultural and social issues.
- Some patients are stoical and will accept mild to moderate pain if explained without recourse to analgesia. Others will want all discomfort minimised. All effective analgesics carry side effects and these need to be weighed up with their usage. Paracetamol within normal dose range is probably the safest but only appropriate as a single agent for mild pain but can be combined with stronger medications.
- Pain is feared by patients and the experience will vary between those with post-operative pain control and those with pain related to a chronic disease or malignancy.
- Pain control must be appropriate and proportionate. Be aware of the WHO analgesic ladder which you ascend, but manage pain based on severity. Don't forget to consider specific management of fear, anxiety and depression which may well be pain multipliers. Anxiety may be based on mistaken fears which can be addressed. Addiction to opioids when used for pain control is very rare indeed.

WHO pain ladder

Severity	Suggested pain relief
Mild	Paracetamol 1 g 6–8 hourly
Moderate	Paracetamol 1 g 6–8 hourly + codeine 30–60 mg 6–8 hourly or ibuprofen 400 mg 8 hourly. Tramadol 50–100 mg 4 hourly is another possibility
Severe	Strong opioid, e.g. morphine 5 mg 4 hourly PO and then calculate the daily requirement and give as a long acting agent, e.g. morphine sulphate if pain is ongoing or likely to worsen. Others include IV or SC diamorphine +/– non-opioid +/– adjuvant

Managing specific pain

Pain source	Suggested pain relief
Acute MI/ACS	Nitrates, diamorphine 2.5–5 mg IV or morphine 5–10 mg IV, PCI/thrombolysis/CABG
Acute abdomen	IV morphine 5–10 mg + IV cyclizine 50 mg
Bone fracture	IV morphine 5–10 mg + IV cyclizine 50 mg
Bone pain, inflammation pain	NSAIDs, e.g. diclofenac or ibuprofen. Bisphosphonates can help in some forms of bone pain, e.g. myeloma, Paget's disease especially with hypercalcaemia. Try IV pamidronate or zoledronate
Headache of malignancy-related cerebral oedema	Dexamethasone and radiotherapy and codeine
Ischaemic pain	NSAIDs, ketamine, morphine
Liver metastases	Steroids
Local pain	Analgesic infiltration, e.g. lidocaine or nerve root blocks
Metastatic bone disease	Bisphosphonates, e.g. pamidronate 60–90 mg IV, NSAIDs, morphine
Neuropathic pain	Gabapentin, amitriptyline often given at night, pregabalin, steroids and radiotherapy may be useful in malignancy-related neuropathic pain, shingles, trigeminal neuralgia
Non-specific (e.g. back pain)	TENS machine, acupuncture
Renal colic	Consider voltarol 50 mg tds which may also be given PR or diclofenac 75 mg IM. A second dose can be given after a minimum of 30 min if necessary. Alternative is morphine 5–10 mg IV + cyclizine 50 mg IV <u>or</u> voltarol PR

Opiates

- When prescribing opiates the drug, dose and frequency and route of administration should be written clearly. If it is as part of a prescription then the dose must also be spelt out. When pain is expected to be temporary, e.g. post-op or for some other reason it is wise to time limit the drug so that it is reviewed days or weeks later, so that it does not continue indefinitely if not required.

- Weak opiates often are effective both short and long term. However, with dehydration and renal failure they can become toxic, especially in the elderly, and caution must be taken. Always consider codeine as a cause of reduced awareness and delirium and coma and consider a trial of naloxone if unclear. The other main side-effects are constipation and a laxative should be added. They may also cause nausea and vomiting and are often combined with an antiemetic. Diamorphine in reasonable concentrations can be given along with metoclopramide, cyclizine or haloperidol in a syringe driver. Myoclonus may also be seen.
- Strong opiates include **morphine, diamorphine and fentanyl**. They should be commenced at starting doses: morphine 5 mg every 4–6 h which can be given orally or IM or IV or SC. Diamorphine 2.5 mg can be given parenterally only. Both should be increased as needed and titrated to pain.
- Fentanyl is often used transdermally and may be preferred with renal dysfunction and when there are difficulties with oral formulations. However, at times it may accumulate and lead to confusion and coma and the patch should be removed and analgesia needs assessed. With oral medications there is a simple feedback loop. If the medication causes coma then no more medications are taken and the patient recovers until able to swallow the next dose. With parenteral and transdermal routes this pseudo-safety feedback loop does not exist and extra care must be taken.
- Morphine comes as either a faster-acting immediate release formulation which works in minutes and covers about 4 h. Can be started as morphine 5 mg 4–6 hourly. Once morphine need is estimated a longer-acting once daily controlled release formulation can be used. Additional immediate release morphine should be available for breakthrough pain. Patient dose varies with tolerance and renal function and patients may take anywhere from 10 to 5000 mg of morphine per day. Pethidine is sometimes used but has a very short half life.

NSAIDs

Very useful for acute and chronic pain management, but chronic usage can lead to peptic ulcer disease and renal impairment. Best avoided in anyone with CKD or PUD or low platelets or bleeding. If there is dyspepsia then adding a PPI may be useful. Side-effects limit usage in the elderly. Commonly used formulations include ibuprofen PO 400 mg 8 hourly, diclofenac PO 50 mg 8 hourly, diclofenac SR PO 75 mg 12 hourly, diclofenac PR 100 mg OD.

Neuropathic pain

Most anticonvulsants and TCAs have action against neuropathic pain. Gabapentin starts at 100–300 mg at night and is increased slowly to 600 mg 8 hourly or until symptoms control achieved. Amitriptyline starts at 25 mg (10 mg in elderly) and may be increased up to 75 mg; often given at night. Specialists may use pregabalin, ketamine (specialist use only) and carbamazepine 100–200 mg nocte.

26.14 Venous thromboembolism prevention

All patients should be screened for their risk of DVT/PE and managed according to NICE guidance with mechanical or pharmacological agents after a full risk assessment. Avoid pharmacological VTE prophylaxis if the patient has any risk factor for bleeding and the risk of bleeding outweighs the risk of VTE.

Patients who are at increased risk of VTE

Medical patients	Surgical or trauma patients
• If mobility significantly reduced for 3+ days • If expected to have ongoing reduced mobility relative to normal state plus any VTE risk factor (see below)	• If total anaesthetic + surgical time >90 min • If surgery involves pelvis or lower limb and total anaesthetic + surgical time >60 min • If acute surgical admission with inflammatory or intra-abdominal condition • If expected to have significant reduction in mobility or any VTE risk factor present (see below)

VTE risk factors	Patients who are at risk of bleeding
• Active cancer or cancer treatment or obesity (BMI >30 kg/m^2) • Age >60 years, critical care admission, dehydration, known thrombophilias • One or more significant medical co-morbidities (e.g. heart disease; metabolic, endocrine or respiratory pathologies; acute infectious diseases; inflammatory conditions) • Personal history or first-degree relative with a history of VTE • Use of HRT or oestrogen-containing contraceptive therapy • Varicose veins with phlebitis	• Active bleeding, acquired bleeding disorders (such as acute liver failure) • Concurrent use of anticoagulants (such as warfarin with INR >2) • LP/epidural/spinal anaesthesia <4 h ago or expected within the next 12 h • Acute stroke or uncontrolled systolic hypertension (>230/120 mmHg) • Thrombocytopenia (platelets <75 × 10^9/L) • Untreated inherited bleeding disorders (such as haemophilia or von Willebrand's disease)

Choice of method

- **Mechanical VTE prophylaxis**: anti-embolism stockings (thigh or knee length), foot impulse devices, intermittent pneumatic compression devices (thigh or knee length).
- **Pharmacological VTE prophylaxis**: most trusts use LMWH enoxaparin (see *Chapter 29*), however, doses need to be adjusted if there is renal failure. Alternatives include fondaparinux. Dabigatran, rivaroxaban and apixaban have been used in elective hip and knee surgery. Follow local policies.
- **Stroke patients**: there is no fixed standard and practices vary between centres. Compression devices are probably ideal. Some centres use LMWH. In some patients with severe disability and at high risk of VTE even in haemorrhagic strokes LMWH may still be considered after the acute period. Follow local guidance.
- **Pregnancy or up to 6 weeks postpartum**: give VTE prophylaxis if undergoing caesarean section or if any of the following risk factors: expected to have significantly reduced mobility for 3 or more days; active cancer or cancer treatment; age >35 years; critical care admission, dehydration, excess blood loss or blood transfusion; known thrombophilias; obesity (pre-pregnancy or early pregnancy BMI >30 kg/m^2); significant medical co-morbidity (such as heart disease, metabolic, endocrine or respiratory pathologies, acute infectious diseases or inflammatory conditions); personal history or first-degree

relative with history of VTE; pregnancy-related risk factor, including ovarian hyperstimulation, hyperemesis gravidarum, multiple pregnancy, pre-eclampsia; varicose veins with phlebitis.

Reference: NICE (2010) CG92: Venous thromboembolism: reducing the risk.

26.15 Good medical practice

Consent and duties of a doctor

Good advice is given by the GMC. Doctors need to be satisfied that they have consent from a patient, or other valid authority, before undertaking any examination or investigation, providing treatment, or involving patients in teaching and research. The GMC has very useful guidance on the duties of a doctor. Patients must be able to trust doctors with their lives and health. To justify that trust you must show respect for human life and you must:

- Make the care of your patient your first concern and protect and promote the health of patients and the public. Provide a good standard of practice and care. Keep your professional knowledge and skills up to date. Recognise and work within the limits of your competence. Work with colleagues in the ways that best serve patients' interests. Treat patients as individuals and respect their dignity: treat patients politely and considerately. Respect patients' right to confidentiality.
- Work in partnership with patients: listen to patients and respond to their concerns and preferences. Give patients the information they want or need in a way they can understand. Respect patients' right to reach decisions with you about their treatment and care. Support patients in caring for themselves to improve and maintain their health. Be honest and open and act with integrity. Act without delay if you have good reason to believe that you or a colleague may be putting patients at risk. Never discriminate unfairly against patients or colleagues. Never abuse your patients' trust in you or the public's trust in the profession. You are personally accountable for your professional practice and must always be prepared to justify your decisions and actions.

Reference: www.gmc-uk.org/static/documents/content/GMP_0910.pdf

26.16 Medical errors

- 'To err is human' is true. We all make mistakes, the question is how we prevent errors, especially those that can cause patient harm, and what we do when we realise that an error has occurred.
- Errors by definition are unintentional. Multiple issues – health systems are complex, interconnected and multitasking, with lots of competing priorities, and different levels of knowledge and experience.
- One of the commonest sources of error is with medication. Avoid writing up drugs on rounds, sit down and do it later when not distracted. Always examine the drug chart as well as the patient on all hospital rounds.
- It is impossible here to go into the complete list of medical errors, but there are a list of events which should 'never occur'. These are called **'never events' and are listed below**.
- When clinical errors result in clinical harm, alert your consultant immediately. Immediately reduce any possible further harm done. Take advice. Be honest about them with everyone involved – the patient, their family, others in the team, your boss. Document everything, fully.

- Say sorry when things have gone wrong. That one word may make trouble simply disappear. It may hurt to say it, but say it. Sorry does not in itself admit blame or liability.
- Once you start to focus on an error the responsibility rarely lands on one set of shoulders. There may be educational and training issues, work issues, responsibility issues. Most errors occur as several events conspired to happen together and a mistake that would have been caught any day was able to perpetuate itself through until real harm had occurred.
- It has become clear that a simple blame culture does little to perpetuate change and improve things. In many cases, but not all, the error could have happened to most of us and the only differentiating factor has been bad luck.
- Many systems seem set up to allow failure and blaming a scapegoat is, sadly, still a part of healthcare culture which we must try to change.

Never events – the NHS has identified events that should 'never' occur

- Maladministration of potassium-containing solutions
- Wrong route administration of chemotherapy
- Wrong route administration of oral/enteral treatment
- Maladministration of insulin
- Severe scalding of patients
- Overdose of midazolam during conscious sedation
- Opioid overdose of an opioid-naive patient
- Suicide using non-collapsible rails
- Entrapment in bed rails
- Escape of a transferred prisoner
- Falls from unrestricted windows
- Transfusion of ABO-incompatible blood components
- Transplantation of ABO or HLA-incompatible organs
- Misplaced naso- or oro-gastric tubes
- Wrong gas administered
- Failure to monitor and respond to O_2 saturation
- Air embolism
- Misidentification of patients
- Inappropriate administration of daily oral methotrexate

26.17 Discharging patients safely

- Discharging patients safely is a skill developed through knowledge and experience and is really a decision for the registrar or above. Beds are always tight and pressures mean you can only admit the sickest patients if you discharge other patients.
- Before admitting a person ask why: is being onsite going to mitigate some anticipated risk, what is the natural history here, what are the risks? Often there are social and medical reasons. Is admission to a busy, noisy potentially infectious assessment area in the patient's best interest?
- Your hospital should have ambulatory care clinics that can do blood tests, monitor symptoms and continue investigations. Patients should not have to sleep in hospital to have an urgent test done. This is irrational and uneconomic. Patients are admitted only if there is no alternative. Hospitals are sources of new infections, strange environments that will cause significant new cognitive challenges leading to falls, overmedication of elderly patients with insomnia from their agitated neighbours. Admission means packages of care are terminated which can be time consuming to reinstate. Many expect an oasis of peace, quiet and relaxation but this is just not possible on a busy acute assessment unit.

- In terms of hospital admission there is often an 'illusion of safety'. Patients are often placed overnight onto busy wards far from the doctors on take with 2 trained nurses and a healthcare assistant serving 25 or more patients. The patient may be in a side room. If the patient develops a problem it may take time for them to raise help (if the call buzzer is out of reach perhaps) and even longer for the nurse to alert the medical team in another part of the hospital and have them attend.
- The medical team have to prioritise their ill patients in the emergency department with ward patients and this adds to delays. In some instances it is better to let stable and able patients go home, where they will have 1 to 1 care from a sensible spouse or carer who can call 999 and have an emergency ambulance attending within minutes, providing very solid basic medical care if the need arises. This is obviously not appropriate for those with a STEMI or acute severe asthma, but for some patients with less severe conditions it certainly bears consideration.
- The bottom line is that for some patients their own bed at home will be a safer, quieter, more relaxing environment for healing and improvement than a hospital bed. So when sending patients home with their particular illness you need to have a sensible understanding of the natural history of the disease and its expected behaviour. I ask myself – what is the most reasonable worst-case scenario and can I mitigate against it in any way?
- Before you do discharge, the patient has to want to go home. Make sure they know to come back via 999 if there are any problems – make this very clear to the patient and it helps if family support this. Ensure that you have documented a thorough assessment, including what you have told the patient, and make sure all are happy and signed up to the plan. Do not do this if the patient is sick and lives very distant from the hospital or is alone or has cognitive or mental health issues, or there is a lack of family support for the plan.
- An elderly man has new confusion and all the signs and tests point quite clearly to a UTI causing acute delirium. You explain that admission might worsen the confusion and agitation. Patient goes home on oral antibiotics, family member sleeps over at their house to give some support and provides close supervision on the stairs and gives him his medication and meals. They liaise with the GP. He is reassessed by phone call from Intermediate care or the GP to check improvement and has slept well and taken his antibiotics and is improving. In the admission scenario the disorientated patient climbed over cotsides and fell from bed and has a fractured hip and subdural haematoma. Non-admission is good when it can happen but it might be just too difficult and the daughter in this scenario may have other responsibilities, but consider it. The most fundamental question is did I put the welfare and wishes of the patient (not the managers) first.

26.18 Self-discharge

- Hospitals are not prisons and patients (who have capacity until proven otherwise) do have a right to leave at any time. It would be good if they told us why and even told us they were going but some will just go. Most of the time it is frustrating but harmless. Doctors have a duty of care, however, sometimes patients who have on-going needs do decide to leave.
- It is important to define why they need to stay – are they at risk of arrhythmias or do they need urgent tests? Try to find out why – can the patient leave and

do whatever they deem important and come back? The need to leave may be entirely understandable and so try to be reasonable and flexible in your approach, but do negotiate a reasonable level of cooperation. Can they come to ambulatory care next day?

- If the patient decides to leave against advice and there is a risk they will come to serious harm, then explain and document any potential complications that you have explained to the patient. If you feel there is significant risk of harm but the patient has the capacity to appreciate this, then all you can do is document conversations and advice given.
- If concerned then take senior advice. It would be wise to ring the GP then or next morning who may call and visit with the patient. There may be a change of heart. Families can help but you need consent to discuss.
- Most hospitals have a standard form, but even if the patient refuses to cooperate then both you and nursing staff should record contemporaneous notes over what was said and what happened and any advice given. Always make it clear they can and should come back, even though that may mean via A&E if any more problems or a change of mind. Always do a discharge letter to document the events and keep in it any advice and make sure the GP is made aware.
- Problems arise when you suspect that there is impaired capacity. You might consider that the patient is suffering from a temporary capacity issue due to acute delirium (alcohol withdrawal, sepsis, hypoxia, etc.) or has chronic problems, e.g. dementia, and in these cases you should take senior advice. It might be very reasonable to restrain the patient in such a case, either physically or with sedation, but this should be done with senior (preferably consultant) advice and using hospital staff or even the police if needed. At all times you must be able to prove that you acted in the best interests of the patient. If a septic patient leaves and comes to harm you may be blamed for your inaction and have to answer in a coroner's court. If the patient does leave and you have not been able to restrain them then involve hospital security and police. Be seen to be doing all possible to protect the patient. The care of the patient must always be your main focus.

26.19 Suicidal patients

- Suicidal patients who perhaps came in with an overdose should not be allowed to discharge against advice without senior involvement. Involve psychiatry. Take senior advice immediately. If they go you should involve police. Involve the GP. It is rare but it does happen that overdose patients leave the hospital and finish their lives by some other means. You must act.
- All patients admitted with an attempted suicide must be seen by the psychiatry team or equivalent prior to discharge. Senior advice must be taken if there is any attempt to abscond or self-discharge, or if they leave the premises which will usually mean police involvement. These are some of the risk factors for those who go on to commit suicide. Note that most people who commit suicide have seen a doctor in the preceding month.

Factors increasing suicide risk

- A history of depression and substance abuse or borderline personality disorder.
- Age >45 years, living alone.
- Gender: men try more lethal means, women try more often.

- Marital status: never married, divorced, widowed, recently separated.
- Extensive and detailed plans or plans using highly lethal means.
- Family history of suicide, still expressing a wish to die, recent job loss.
- Puerperal, chronic painful illness.
- Recent loss of loved one and the anniversary of the loss.
- Previous attempts – this is one of the best predictors.
- Gay/lesbian youth, Caucasian youth, history of impulsive or reckless behaviour.

Assessment

- **Ask about suicidal ideation:** where concerned, always ask patients about suicide and their intentions. Do they feel life is worth living? Have they thought of ending it? Most patients will discuss. It is very rare, but the person committed to suicide will say whatever gets them out of hospital. Older, single men with financial worries and job loss are one group of concern and you should take experienced advice regardless of what they say.
- **Management:** check your local policy, but anyone with a suicide attempt or suicidal ideation should have a psychiatric evaluation before discharge. Patients may even try to self-discharge. Get immediate help from psychiatry and take senior advice.

26.20 Mental capacity

- An assessment of capacity must be made in relation to a particular decision, at the time the decision needs to be made. Patients are only lacking capacity for the particular question asked.
- The capacity issue must address a specific issue Any assessment assumes that the person has the capacity to make the decision in question until proven otherwise. The Mental Capacity Act Code of Practice describes a test of capacity you can use to decide whether a person is able to make that decision.
- An assessment that a person lacks capacity to make a decision must never be based simply on their age or their appearance, assumptions about their condition or any aspect of their behaviour. The risks and benefits should be discussed in detail to satisfy the questions below.
- In many cases the loss of capacity is partial, it may also be temporary and it may change over time. It can be useful to repeat the assessment on a 'better' day. There are several things to consider when assessing if a person can make a decision:
  - Do they understand the decision they need to make and why they need to make it?
  - Can they understand, use and weigh up the information relevant to this decision?
  - Can they communicate a decision (talking, using sign language or any other means)?
  - Could the services of a professional (speech and language therapist) be helpful? Is a more thorough assessment required, e.g. doctor or other professional expert?
- More detailed information on assessing capacity is available in chapter 4 of the Code of Practice.

26.21 Driving and disease

- The law is quite clear. If a patient has a condition that impairs their ability and makes them unsafe to drive then the doctor has a duty to inform the patient and the patient is legally obliged to inform and follow the advice of the DVLA (Driver and Vehicle Licensing Agency).
- Ultimately it is the DVLA who will determine if the patient can retain their driving licence. All driving advice given (or advice not to drive) should be documented in the notes.
- Licences are normally issued valid until age 70 years unless restricted to a shorter duration for medical reasons as indicated above. There is no upper limit but after age 70 renewal is necessary every 3 years. All licence applications require a medical self-declaration by the applicant.
- This guidance is for a private car or motorcycle. For those with a licence to drive a bus, coach or lorry, all must inform the DVLA because there are more stringent restrictions.
- See www.dvla.org.uk for more information and in particular for the DVLA document entitled 'Fitness to drive', which can be obtained online.
- If you have any concerns you can ring the DVLA medical advisors. When assessing a patient consider if they would be in full control of the car at all times, e.g. can they do an emergency stop? For borderline cases there are driver assessment centres.
- Car modifications can allow a disabled patient to drive to the necessary standard. Advise the patient to also inform their car insurers.

Condition	Advice for private car (usual advice – inform DVLA)	Coach, lorry, bus (usual advice – inform DVLA)
TIA	Can return to driving after 28 days	No driving 1 year
Multiple TIA	No driving 3 months	No driving 1 year
Stroke (fully recovered)	Can return to driving after 28 days if recovery and no impairment to driving ability	No driving 1 year
Stroke (residual neurology affecting ability to drive)	Not to drive – decision to be made by DVLA	Not to drive – decision to be made by DVLA
First seizure or suspected seizure	Can drive after 6 months – should be seen at seizure clinic	Restricted for a minimum of 5 years. Neurological assessment
Epilepsy	No driving 1 year	No driving
Unexplained loss of consciousness	Restricted for 6 months	Restricted for 12 months
Vasovagal syncope	No restriction	No restriction
Visual field defect	No driving until formal assessment – inform DVLA who can advise	No driving until formal assessment – inform DVLA who can advise

Condition	Advice for private car (usual advice – inform DVLA)	Coach, lorry, bus (usual advice – inform DVLA)
Angina	No driving if angina whilst driving	No driving if symptoms
ACS	No driving 1 week if successful angioplasty, or else 1 month and EF >0.4	No driving 6 weeks
Angioplasty	No driving 1 week	No driving 6 weeks
Pacemaker	No driving 1 week	No driving 6 weeks
CABG	No driving 4 weeks – inform DVLA	No driving 3 months; EF >0.4
AICD	No driving 6–12 months (see guidance)	No driving inform DVLA
Hypertension	No restriction	Must maintain resting BP <180/100 mmHg or else inform DVLA
Head injury/ bleed	No driving 6–12 months – inform DVLA	Inform DVLA
Incapacitating arrhythmia	No driving until 4 weeks after controlled	Controlled for 3 months and LVEF >40%
AAA >6 cm	Inform DVLA if >6 cm	Inform DVLA
Brain aneurysm	Inform DVLA	Inform DVLA
Post-surgery	At doctor's discretion about pain and ability. Need to be in complete control of vehicle	At doctor's discretion about pain and ability. Need to be in complete control of vehicle
Diabetes and insulin/ hypoglycaemics	Needs to be aware of hypos. Two or more hypos needing help of another person in past 12 months is a bar to driving – inform DVLA	Full hypo awareness. Regular monitoring. One episode of hypo needing help in past 12 months stop driving and inform DVLA

26.22 End of life care

- End of life care is one of the most challenging aspects of current medicine when the raised expectations of contemporary medical practice comes up against the realities of the limitations of medical science.
- Medicine is fundamentally about adding quality to life and reducing suffering. We must strive to prolong life but not to prolong and draw out an unpleasant death.
- Withdrawal of medical care and supportive management often happens at a time when discussions with the patient are not possible. It is important to involve close family. Keep them informed at all stages.
- Newer strategies such as AMBER (www.ambercarebundle.org) try to pre-empt palliation and involve the patient and close family in discussing end of life care much earlier and need to be promoted to optimise end of life care.
- If the patient has a well-defined terminal illness then the natural history of the disease will be helpful. In some the natural history is less clear, such as stroke or sepsis complicating mild dementia. However, be cautious especially with acute

deteriorations which may have simple remedies, e.g. UTI, hypoglycaemia, opiate toxicity and it can be reasonable to trial therapy for 24-48 h.

- Before an end of life pathway is instituted, make sure you are completely up to date on the patient's letters and notes. If unsure get the GP patient record faxed over. Be well briefed before you talk to family.
- When you do make sure you get the right family – record names of those involved in discussions, it is always best to find out first what they know because they may have additional information for you. Discover what they have been told. What are their expectations?
- If a senior decision has been made to switch to palliation, then the focus is on minimising suffering and symptoms. In most cases IV fluids and feeding are withdrawn and the patient kept comfortable. Continuing fluids will often just prolong death. Good oral care for comfort can continue.
- If there is discomfort then oral or transcutaneous or more often SC diamorphine + antiemetic are given. A local palliative care bundle should be available.
- Patients can survive 7–10 days without fluids. Families should be informed of this timescale. Patients may dry out and temporarily seem to slightly improve but this can be an illusion. It can be reasonable to continue. Take senior experienced advice.

Considerations in the dying patient

- Reduce or stop non-essential usual secondary prevention medications, e.g. statin, aspirin, antihypertensives, etc. Keep only the things that are for symptom control, e.g. a diuretic to avoid pulmonary oedema if fluid intake continues. Judge each case individually.
- Stop inappropriate investigations – remove cardiac monitors and O_2 sats and stop blood tests. Stop observations. Nursing staff should actively monitor for unpleasant symptoms and manage those.
- Stop IV or SC fluids if these are futile treatments because they tend only to prolong death rather than life. Oral fluids and mouth care can be given for care and symptom support.
- Patients at this stage can be given mouth care and analgesia to reduce any discomfort but most have little awareness.
- Make sure DNAR (do not attempt resuscitation) forms are signed and up to date in notes and have been communicated to the nursing staff. Check family are aware and up to date on the status of the patient.
- Are there any religious or spiritual needs? Respect cultural expectations of care of the body after death which will be by the bereavement office. Ensure death certification and any referral to coroner is done as early as possible after death and liaise with the bereavement office.

Diagnosis of death

When on call you will be called to see patients who have died to 'certify them' as dead. These are usually patients who have been resuscitated unsuccessfully or who have died and who are not for resuscitation. In some such as those on palliation the death will have been expected, in others it may not have been. This is rarely an urgent request but one should seek to certify as soon as convenient so that the patient can be moved off the ward to the morgue. Check that family have been informed – they will rarely need to speak to a doctor unless the death is entirely unexpected. If you do have to speak to the family then it is best to set aside some time and find a convenient space to talk to them, preferably with nursing staff to hand. Any contentious issues should be escalated to the responsible consultant to liaise with the family in normal hours.

Certifying death in the UK

- Take your time. See if patient reacts to pain or voice, e.g. a sternal rub. Check central pulse, e.g. femoral or carotid, and test for 1 minute to detect any pulsation to suggest cardiac output. Pupils are usually fixed and dilated and do not respond to light (may not be dilated if previous eye surgery or prosthetic eye).
- At the same time look for any signs of respiration attempts. Listen for the absence of any heart sounds for 1 minute. Note the presence or absence of pacemaker or ICD in case the patient is for cremation. Document your findings and ensure accurately timed and dated and signed.
- Comments such as "rest in peace" and religious comments are not needed. The nurses prepare the body which usually involves closing eyes and mouth. Pumps and syringe drivers are removed but the actual lines are left *in situ*. Orifices are packed with cotton wool. The patient is wrapped in a sheet. The porters will usually come with a special trolley to bring the patient to the mortuary. Often the nurses will close the curtains on adjacent beds whilst this occurs.

Death certification

- Even if you are the person who certified the patient as deceased you cannot do the death certificate unless you personally attended the patient within the past 14 days. Prompt and accurate certification of death is essential.
- The death certificate provides legal evidence of the fact and cause of death, which has legal and statistical importance and enables the death to be formally registered. Only then can the family make arrangements for cremation/burial of the body.
- As a new doctor the 'Bereavement office' will be calling on your services frequently and it is wise to work well with them. They have little flexibility and the death certificate should be done as soon as is reasonably possible – you are required by law to do so.
- Death certification can be done by an F1 or above, but it is important that you take advice from senior members of the team. You are legally responsible for the delivery of the death certificate to the registrar, but the bereavement office staff will often do this and usually it is the family who bring it to the registrar.

Information requested as part of death certification

- **Patient's age at death:** work it out from the notes and check it is correct.
- **Place of death**: record the precise place of death (e.g. typically the name of the hospital and ward or the address of a private house or, for deaths elsewhere, the locality). This may not be the same as the place where you are completing the certificate. It is particularly important that the relative or other person responsible for registering the death is directed to the registrar of births and deaths for the sub-district where the death occurred, unless (from 1st April 1977) they have decided to make a declaration of the details to be registered before another registrar.
- **When last seen alive by me**: record the date when you last saw the deceased alive, irrespective of whether any other medical practitioner saw the person alive subsequently.
- **Information from post-mortem:** you should indicate whether the information you give about the cause of death takes account of a post-mortem. Such information

can be valuable for epidemiological purposes. If a post-mortem has been done, ring option 1. If information may be available later, do not delay the issue of your certificate, ring option 2 and tick statement B on the reverse of the certificate. The registrar will then send you a form for return to the Registrar General giving the results of the post-mortem. If a post-mortem is not being held, ring option 3.

- **Seen after death** (only one option can be ringed): you should indicate, by ringing option a, b or c, whether you or another medical practitioner saw the deceased after death

Ask the bereavement office staff to check your work – it can save you lots of time later on if there are issues.

Referral to the coroner

- You should refer when any of the following occur. In hospital the bereavement office staff will usually assist with this. You may speak to the coroner or their officer who will advise.
- Coroner needs to be informed if: the cause of death is unknown, deceased not seen by the certifying doctor after death or **within 14 days** before death, death was violent or unnatural or was suspicious, death due to an accident (whenever it occurred), death due to self-neglect or neglect by others, death due to an industrial disease or related to the deceased's employment, death due to an abortion, death during an operation or before recovery from the effects of anaesthetic, death due to suicide, death occurred during or shortly after detention in police or prison custody. Any death for which a duly completed medical certificate of cause of death is not obtained.

Cause of death

- This section of the certificate is divided in Parts I and II. Part I is used to show the immediate cause of death and any underlying cause or causes. Part II should be used for any significant condition or disease that contributed to the death but which is not part of the sequence leading directly to death.
- You must state the cause or causes of death accurately and fully to the best of your knowledge and belief and it is wise to take senior advice routinely especially if unsure or any doubts.
- **Underlying cause of death:** consider the main causal sequence of conditions leading to death. State the disease or condition that led directly to death on the first line [I(a)] and work your way back until you reach the Underlying Cause of Death, which initiated the chain of events leading ultimately to death. **The lowermost completed line in Part I should therefore contain the Underlying Cause of Death.**
- Sometimes there are apparently two distinct conditions leading to death. If there is no way of choosing between them, they should be entered on the same line indicating in brackets that they are joint causes of death, e.g. ischaemic heart disease and chronic bronchitis. 'Smoking' may be included if accompanied by a medical cause of death.
- Do not use the following as the single sole cause of death, e.g. asphyxia, debility, respiratory arrest, asthenia, exhaustion, shock, brain failure, heart failure, syncope, cachexia, hepatic failure, uraemia, cardiac arrest, hepatorenal failure, vagal inhibition, cardiac failure, kidney failure, vasovagal attack, coma, renal failure, ventricular failure, liver failure. These are clinical syndromes, which need pathological explanation as to why they occurred. Old age or senility, although

acceptable, should not be used as the only cause of death in Part I unless a more specific cause of death cannot be given and the deceased was aged 70 or over.

- **Part II:** should be used when one or more conditions have contributed to death but are not part of the main causal sequence leading to death. It should not be used to list all conditions present at death. In some cases you can put an interval as to the diagnosis of each in hours, days, months or years before the death occurred. In Part I and II, you should give information about clinical interventions, procedures or drugs that may have led to adverse effects, e.g. warfarin-induced bleeds, etc.

Example of acceptable entries

- 1 a: Cerebral metastases, 1 b: Squamous cell lung cancer, 1c: Smoking.
- 1 a: Respiratory failure, 1 b: Lobar pneumonia, 1 c: Squamous cell lung cancer, 2: Type 2 diabetes mellitus.

Employment-related death

- If you believe that the death may have been due to (or contributed to) by the employment undertaken at any time by the deceased, you should indicate this. Tick the appropriate box on the front of the certificate and then report it to the coroner.

Sign the form

- You must sign the certificate and add your qualifications, address and the date. It would greatly assist the registrar if you could also PRINT YOUR NAME IN BLOCK CAPITALS LETTERS. If the death occurred in hospital, the name of the consultant who was responsible for the care of the patient must also be given.
- Have you remembered your signature, notice to informant, counterfoil? Even now I always get bereavement office staff to check though what I have done. They might spot simple errors, which could cause problems for the family in getting the patient registered. It is so easy to get a date wrong and this can halt a funeral or a cremation ceremony. The bereavement office staff are experts and will help to prevent any problems.

27 Procedures

The content here is to refresh memories and reinforce points to users who have been conventionally trained and are competent in these procedures. Do not perform a procedure in which you have not been trained. Get supervision if you are not competent. Generally get written consent unless dire emergency. Most invasive procedures should not take place out of hours except in an emergency.

In terms of procedures, be aware that the only way to avoid complications is not to do any. Before you undertake a therapeutic procedure which should improve circumstances (e.g. a chest drain) or a diagnostic procedure (e.g. central line placement to measure CVP/pulmonary artery pressures), consider whether the procedure will change management significantly; can you get the information elsewhere? The information you may get might be erroneous due to failure to calibrate or other errors. Complications will happen and you can make a patient even worse, so ensure that the emergency procedure was valid and vital and could someone support or supervise you or be doing it. Procedures are time consuming and this time might be better spent doing other things.

27.1 Questions before any procedure

Five questions you (do not delegate!) must ask before any procedure

- Is it the right patient, is it the right procedure, is it the right (or left) side?
- Have I the right to do it, i.e. has informed consent been obtained?
- Is the patient on anticoagulants or have a coagulopathy?
- Is this the right time: can it wait until working hours?
- Am I the best person to do this (should I get someone more skilled to supervise me)?

27.2 Venepuncture

Equipment

- Sharps bin, cannula, sterile bung and micropore tape (check for known allergies).
- Non-sterile gloves (check for latex allergy), alcoholic wipe 2% chlorhexidine (Clinell), tourniquet, dressing (sterile), cotton wool (sterile), trolley, syringe (10 ml), flushing agent (NS for injection).

Technique

- Explain who you are and explain procedure and get verbal consent. Make sure it is the correct patient. Make sure that the cannula used is appropriate.
- Choose vein and apply tourniquet above vein. Prepare the patient's skin at the selected insertion site with a med swab, wait 30 sec to allow the area to dry. Do not re-palpate the vein or touch the skin.
- Remove the needle guard and inspect the cannula for any faults. Hold the patient's hand/wrist/forearm using the thumb, to keep the skin taut. Care must be taken not to contaminate the site.
- Place the needle tip several millimetres distal to the proposed site for cannulation, with the bevel facing up and elevate the angle of the cannula to

15–25° and insert the cannula into the skin (fragile veins require a lower angle of insertion).

- Once the vein has been located with the needle, lower the angle for insertion. Look for back flow of blood into the cannula chamber, unless the vein is small in which case this may be delayed.
- Hold the cannula steady relative to the vein whilst withdrawing the needle slightly and then slowly advance cannula. If there is any sign of swelling, haematoma, pain or resistance the vein wall may be ruptured. If so, release tourniquet or you will cause a haematoma. Remove cannula. Apply pressure with cotton wool.
- Otherwise, when flashback is seen along the length of the cannula the investigator or delegated person will advance the cannula until it is fully inserted into the vein. Release the skin tension and the tourniquet. Apply gloved digital pressure to the distal end of the cannula to prevent blood spillage.
- Remove the introducer needle and discard into an appropriate yellow sharps container. Now secure a sterile bung to the end of the cannula. Secure the cannula to the patient using a sterile dressing. Flush the cannula with a minimum of 2 ml of NS for injection and capped off.
- Check the patient feels no discomfort, and observe the cannula site for signs of swelling or redness. Ensure that you complete cannula chart and any accompanying documentation.
- If you fail then try again, but if you have tried several times with no success either get some help or come back to the task later. If it is an emergency then get help urgently. You cannot resuscitate a patient successfully without IV access.
- If you have found the cannula is intra-arterial (pulsatile, high pressure, bright red blood) then remove cannula and apply pressure over the site for 10+ minutes until haemostasis. Check distal pulses. Take senior advice if pulseless or distal ischaemia.

27.3 Chest drain insertion

Introduction: ask the five questions (see table above)

- The use of ultrasound-guided insertion is associated with lower complication rates. Useful for effusions and empyema as the diaphragm and effusions can be identified.

Indications

- Pneumothorax: not all pneumothoracies require insertion of a chest drain (see *Section 12.4* on pneumothorax). The differential diagnosis between a pneumothorax and bullous disease requires careful radiological assessment including CT.
- Pleural fluid: malignant pleural effusion, simple pleural effusions in ventilated patients, empyema and complicated parapneumonic pleural effusion, traumatic pneumothorax or haemopneumothorax.
- Peri-operative: e.g. thoracotomy, oesophageal surgery, cardiothoracic surgery. The urgency of insertion will depend on the indication and degree of physiological derangement that is being caused by the substance to be drained.

Procedure to insert a chest drain

- Only to be done by trained or supervised persons.

- Done well there are 3% early complications and 8% late complications. Training reduces complications.

Potential complications

- Incorrect placement with drain outside the pleura, in the fissure, tube kinked.
- Injury to intercostal vessels. Trocar must not be used as risk of spearing heart, liver and other organs.
- Excessive bleeding risk: if known coagulopathy take advice.

Equipment

- Aseptic pack with sterile drapes, iodine or equivalent solution.
- Gauze, scalpel, 2/0 silk and curved needle, 5 and 10 ml syringes.
- Orange and green needles, sterile gloves, chest drain (Seldinger or 'trocar' type).
- Chest drain bottle or bag with flutter valve.

Methods

- **Pre-procedure: informed consent** should be obtained and documented. Check identity of the patient and the site of insertion of the chest drain. Confirm the clinical signs (percuss the chest and listen) and review the latest CXR and clinical indications. As ever, all equipment needed to insert a chest drain should be available before commencing the procedure.
- **Patient positioning:** as comfortably as possible because the procedure may be prolonged. Much will depend on the clinical state of the patient. If possible patient lying back at 45° with the arm on the side used flopped behind head to open up rib spaces. Alternatively, fatigued patient may lean forward resting on some pillows on a table, as long as access to the axilla is preserved. Occasionally the procedure is done with a patient lying on their side with the affected side uppermost. In a trauma situation, or ITU, an emergency drain insertion is more likely to be performed whilst the patient is supine.
- **Premedication:** analgesia should be considered – morphine 5 mg IV with cyclizine if not hypoventilating with appropriate monitoring (pulse oximetry) and resuscitation equipment immediately available. 100% O_2 should be given to all pneumothorax patients if appropriate as it helps resolution.
- **Aseptic technique:** full aseptic precautions (washed hands, gloves, gown, antiseptic preparation for the insertion site and adequate sterile field) in order to avoid wound site infection or secondary empyema.
- **Chest drain:** sizes 10–36 Ch. May be inserted via direct surgical incision (thoracostomy) or using the Seldinger technique incorporating a guide wire and dilator system. Spontaneous pneumothoracies and non-viscous effusions can be drained with relatively small calibre drains via Seldinger method. They are better tolerated and associated with less discomfort, but traumatic pneumothoracies, haemothoracies and empyemas may need larger drains, typically 26F and above.
- **Inserting the drain:** most commonly placed in 4th–5th intercostal space in the mid-axillary line – the lowest axillary hair is useful marker where present. This area is commonly known as the *safe triangle* with anterior border of latissimus dorsi, the lateral border of the pectoralis major, a line superior to the horizontal level of the nipple and an apex below the axilla. Any other placement should be discussed with a chest physician. In an apical pneumothorax, placement of a chest tube in the 2nd intercostal space can be considered but is more difficult to maintain. A specific position may also be required for a loculated effusion.

- **Seldinger chest tube technique:** infiltrate with local anaesthetic using up to 10 ml of 1% lignocaine along the intended track. Remove catheter, dilator, introducer wire and introducer needle from pack and insert introducer needle into the thoracic cavity into the chosen site. Withdraw air with a syringe to confirm placement. Now thread introducer wire through needle lumen into the chest. Whilst holding wire tip and then base, remove needle leaving introducer wire running into chest. Thread dilator over introducer wire, and advance into chest, dilating a track for catheter. Remove dilator. Thread tube over the wire fully into chest ensuring side holes lie within chest cavity. Remove wire. Suture catheter in place. Attach catheter to drainage unit. Obtain post-procedure chest X-ray.
- **Rigid chest tube insertion:** infiltrate with local anaesthetic using up to 10–15 ml of 1% lignocaine along the intended track, make a 3–4 cm incision through skin and subcutaneous tissues between the 4th and 5th ribs, parallel to the rib margins. Continue incision through the intercostal muscles, and right down to the pleura and use dissecting forceps to bluntly dissect down to the pleura and then insert through the pleura and open the jaws widely, again parallel to the direction of the ribs. This will create a pneumothorax if not locally present and allows the lung to fall away from the chest wall somewhat. Insert gloved sterile finger through your incision and into the thoracic cavity. Make sure you are feeling lung (or empty space) and not liver or spleen. Grasp end of chest tube with the forceps (convex angle facing down towards ribs), and insert chest tube through the hole you have made in the pleura. After tube has entered thoracic cavity, remove forceps and manually advance the tube. Clamp distal tube end with forceps and suture and tape tube in place and attach tube to drainage. NEVER USE TROCAR TO INSERT DRAIN. Obtain post-procedure chest X-ray for placement; tube may need to be advanced or withdrawn slightly. Need to be a bit firm but gentle. The chest tube should be placed in the pleural cavity; significant force should never be used as this risks sudden chest penetration and damage to essential intrathoracic structures. The operator should ensure controlled spreading of the intercostal muscles on the superior surface of the ribs to avoid injury to the intercostal vessels and nerves that run below the inferior border of the ribs.
- **The drainage system:** once tube inserted connect to an underwater seal drainage system. This employs positive expiratory pressure and gravity to drain the pleural space. Tube is submerged at least 2 cm below water of the reservoir/collection chamber. The underwater seal acts as a one-way valve through which air is expelled from the pleural space. The collection chamber should be kept below the patient at all times. If the drainage tube comes out of the water then air will re-accumulate in the pleural space.
- **Large pleural effusions:** drained in stages or rapid shifts in pleural pressures and re-expansion of a collapsed lung can cause re-expansion pulmonary oedema, a serious complication. A limit of 1–1.5 L of fluid should be drained before the tube is clamped. If the patient starts to cough or complains of chest pain before this point is reached, drainage should be stopped and may be resumed a few hours later.
- **Portable valve systems** can be used for patients with on-going air leaks or fluid drainage and these use a one-way flutter valve which is generally lower resistance to drainage than with conventional underwater seal units. Ambulatory systems exist.
- **Securing the chest drain:** secure with 1/0 silk suture anchored to the skin and the drain with a suitable non-slip knot technique. This should prevent excessive travel

of the drain in and out of the chest wall. The skin incision can be closed each side of the chest tube usually with one 2/0 silk suture each side. Nylon/Ethilon can be used but is more difficult to tie. Tie sutures securely. Purse string sutures should be avoided because they convert a linear wound into a circular wound which can be painful and leave an unsightly scar.

- **Dressings:** purpose-designed dressings should be used, i.e. *Drainfix* for small bore drains and *Mefix* for large bore drains. Excessive dressings restrict chest wall movement or cause moisture collection. Dressings should allow site inspection. Drain connections should not be covered. A tag of adhesive dressing tape can support the tube and protect it against being pulled out. Patient should be aware to look after the drain and keep the underwater bottle below the chest, avoid compressing the tube by sitting or lying on it and avoid tension on the tube.
- **Analgesia:** ensure regular analgesia is prescribed whilst the chest drain is in place. Dressings should be changed daily for the following reasons: to enable the insertion site to be monitored for signs of infection (swab if any signs of infection), as well as to monitor for surgical emphysema, to ensure the chest drain remains well placed, and the anchor suture is intact.
- **Monitoring/recording:** fluid in tube should swing with respiration due to changes in intra-pleural pressure. Fluid should rise on inspiration and fall on expiration. Bubbling and swinging are both dependent on an intact underwater seal and so can only be picked up if the drain tube extends below the water level in the bottle. Ask patient to take deep breaths and cough and assess. Absence of swinging suggests drain is occluded or is no longer in the pleural space. Try flushing the drain and if no success obtain a chest X-ray to determine the underlying cause. Bubbling in the underwater seal fluid chamber generally indicates an on-going air leak which may be continuous, present on one phase of spontaneous ventilation, or only on coughing. Persistent bubbling throughout the respiratory cycle may indicate a continuing broncho-pleural air leak. Faulty connections and entrained air through the skin incision should also be assessed. If drain inserted for a fluid collection, e.g. effusion or empyema, then record volume and nature of the drain fluid recording. Drains inserted just for fluid should not bubble so the presence of this feature is abnormal and should be recorded. Any abnormal signs or complications should be referred for medical review.
- **Bleeding** from a drain inserted for drainage of a haemothorax (+/− pneumothorax) needs urgent medical review. With fractured ribs most bleeding is from the intercostal vessels, which slows down as the lung reinflates. However, continued bleeding into the drain bottle is indicative of pathology that may need thoracic surgical intervention. After thoracic trauma, more than 1500 ml of blood into the bottle initially or continued bleeding of greater than 200 ml/h requires discussion with the thoracic surgeons. Small bore drains should be flushed regularly with NS; the flush should be prescribed on the Treatment Sheet and carried out by appropriately trained personnel. Full respiratory and cardiovascular observations should be carried out and documented.
- **Clamping chest drains:** as a general rule chest tubes for pneumothorax should not be clamped. Exceptions to this may be when the drainage bottle requires replacement or when testing the system for air leaks. Clamping a pleural drain in the presence of a continuing air leak may result in a tension pneumothorax or possibly worsening surgical emphysema. If a chest tube is clamped it should be under the direct supervision of a respiratory physician or surgeon on a ward with experienced nursing staff. A patient with a clamped tube should not leave the specialist ward

environment. Instructions should be left that if the patient becomes breathless or develops surgical emphysema, the chest tube must be unclamped immediately and the medical team alerted. In cases of pneumothorax there is no evidence that clamping a chest drain at the time of removal is beneficial. Drains for fluid drainage can be clamped or closed to control drainage rate as necessary.

- **Changing the drain bottle:** when changing the drain bottle because it is overfull, temporary clamping of the drainage tube may be necessary to prevent entry of air into the pleural cavity. It is acceptable to clamp the tube between thumb and forefinger. This has the advantage of removing the risk of inadvertently leaving the tube clamped. Local policy should be followed with regard to asepsis and infection control.
- **Suction:** a patient who is free from pain and who can cough will generate a much higher pleural pressure differential than can safely be produced with suction. If a patient cannot re-inflate his own lung or a persistent air leak is preventing re-inflation, high volume, low-pressure thoracic suction in the range of 3–5 kPa (approximately 30–50 cmH_2O) should be used. Prescription of suction is a medical responsibility. Purpose-made low grade suction units (max 30 kPa) should be used when applying to a chest drain. Standard high volume, high-pressure suction units should not be used because of the ease with which it may lead to air stealing and hypoxaemia, the perpetuation of persistent air leaks, and possible damage to lung tissue caused by it becoming trapped in the catheter. Suction that is not working properly or is turned off without disconnecting from the drain bottle is the equivalent of a clamped drain, so when suction is no longer needed it should be disconnected from the drainage bottle. The use of suction may cause continuous bubbling from the tube; movement/swinging of fluid in the tube may not be visible.
- **Mobility:** if appropriate, patients should be encouraged to walk around. If the drain is on suction the patient will be restricted to the bedside. Exercise to prevent complications such as a frozen shoulder or deep venous thrombosis is essential, as are deep breathing exercises to aid re-expansion of the lung.
- **Removal of the chest drain:** removal of the chest drain depends on reason for insertion and clinical progress. Give pain relief before removal of the chest drain. As for insertion, an aseptic technique should be used for removal and the chest drain and drainage kit disposed of appropriately. When the tube is ready to be removed, the patient should be asked to perform a valsalva manoeuvre (to increase the pleural pressure and prevent air entering the pleural cavity) or, if that is not possible, then deep inspiration and the tube withdrawn quickly. The previously placed suture is then tied to close the hole. The operator should be able to tie sutures securely. The wound site should be checked, condition documented and an appropriate dressing applied. An X-ray should be performed following removal of the chest drain to ensure resolution.
- **Surgical emphysema** is the abnormal presence of air within the subcutaneous tissues with the 'Michelin man' type appearance, which may cause upper airways respiratory compromise. Its presence suggests that the drain is inadequate (too small gauge) to deal with size of air leak or occluded or misplaced. Applying suction, inserting a second drain or a larger bore tube, can improve drainage. Worsening surgical emphysema is uncomfortable, interferes with clinical examination of the patient and, at its worst, may track up to the neck and face, potentially causing airway embarrassment and embarrassment to the person who inserted the tube.

27.4 Central venous line insertion

Introduction: ask the five questions (see table above)

Possible sites

- Internal jugular vein, subclavian vein, femoral vein.

Indications

- Measurement of CVP, drug administration, TPN, amiodarone, etc.
- IV fluids when peripheral access poor (poor way to give fluids quickly).
- Insertion of Swan–Ganz catheter to measure pulmonary wedge pressures.
- Insertion of a pacing wire, pre-operative, e.g. CABG in theatre.

Equipment

- Central line pack, sterile drapes, sterile gloves. 5–10 ml lidocaine 1–2%, iodine or equivalent, central line.
- 2 × 10 ml of saline/heparin flush, scalpel, 2–3 × 5–10 ml syringe.
- Green and blue needles and 100 ml bag NS.

Risks

- Skill and luck and experience of the operator can vary as can body habitus and ease of access. Complications higher for emergency vs. elective insertion.
- Risks include infectious, mechanical, and thrombotic complications.
- Obtain chest X-ray (subclavian/internal jugular) to confirm placement and to assess for complications.
- **Infection**. Strict asepsis – hand washing, gown and gloves for all cases. Preferably in appropriate area where a sterile field can be maintained, e.g. anaesthetic room or ITU or CCU procedure room. Avoid attempts in a dimly lit general ward – those days have long gone. Catheter infections due to local site infection or via haematogenous seeding of the catheter.
- Use chlorhexidine skin antisepsis, selection of an optimal catheter site. Ensure daily review of the need of the catheter or removal.

Contraindications to central venous line insertion

- Severe uncorrected coagulopathy: INR >1.6, platelets <50 × 10^9/L (relative contraindication). Femoral or internal jugular site is preferred with a coagulopathy because vessels can be directly compressed in the event of serious haemorrhage which may be arterial.
- **There is NO safe route**. Consider delaying procedure to correct coagulopathy or thrombocytopenia.
- Infected skin over the entry site, thrombosis of target vein, those unlikely to tolerate pneumothorax or lower risk approaches to internal jugular or femoral sites may be preferred.

Potential complications of central venous line insertions

- Arterial puncture when the associated artery lies close (apply pressure and wait 5–10 min), haematoma, pneumothorax, tension pneumothorax, haemothorax.
- Arrhythmia, localised and systemic infection.
- **Thrombotic complications:** risk of venous thrombosis and embolism. Thrombosis can occur first day after cannulation. Lowest risk for thrombosis is the subclavian vein. Early removal of the catheter decreases the risk of catheter-related thrombosis.

General procedure

- Patient must be head down tilt when cannulating neck veins and head up when cannulating femoral vein to prevent air embolism. Raise bed to suitable level for yourself. Head down tilt can compromise breathless patients. Telemetry for any arrhythmias and continue O_2 saturation monitoring.
- Wash hands, asepsis. Cleanse a 15–20 cm or larger area with povidone–iodine solution. Usually the right side is preferred due to more direct line to the atrium, reduces injuring the thoracic duct, is easier in the right handed operator, and dome of lung and pleura are lower than on left.
- Drape the patient with the paper/plastic drape with centre cutout provided. Estimate the length of catheter to be placed to end up with tip above right atrium. Using the blue needle, make a wheal under the skin at the desired spot, and anaesthetise the subcutaneous tissue. Using the green needle, anaesthetise deeper.
- Always withdraw the plunger before injecting to detect if you are in the vein or artery to avoid intravascular injection of 1–2% lidocaine. Open the pack and place the guide wire, dilator, catheter, and scalpel on the sterile drape for easy reach when needed.
- **Ultrasound guidance:** ultrasonography accurately locates the target vein, suggests venous pressure and the presence of intravascular thrombus and is strongly recommended. When using ultrasound guidance, enlist an assistant either to handle the probe or to remove it when it is no longer needed. The vein and artery appear circular and black on the ultrasound image; the vein is much more compressible when gentle pressure is applied to the skin via the probe. The needle appears echogenic and can be followed into the image of the vein. Most useful in internal jugular attempts.
- Using the 18 gauge finder needle (largest needle in the kit) and a small syringe, enter the skin at the top of the jugular triangle. Gradually advance the needle, always gently pulling back on the plunger as you progress. Look for a flashback of dark blood which indicates entrance into the vein. *Bright red or pulsatile flow should suggest carotid artery puncture. Withdraw needle and apply pressure for about 10 minutes before proceeding.* You can pierce the needle through the vein without blood, gradually withdraw; you may still get into the vein as you may have collapsed it on the way in.
- Once in the vessel, hold the needle steady and remove the syringe, holding a thumb over it, to prevent bleeding and reduce risk of embolism, and thread in the **j-tipped guide wire**. It should be a smooth process and if resistance is felt NEVER force it. Guide wire overinsertion can be dangerous. The wire needs to be advanced only far enough to maintain reliable control of the tract from the skin surface to the intravascular space.
- Watch monitor as guide wire is advanced. Ventricular ectopy indicates over-insertion and the guide wire must be withdrawn a few cm. Holding the guide wire, remove needle from skin. Make a small nick with the number 11 blade where wire enters skin with the cutting edge away from the wire. Advance dilator over guide wire with a twisting motion; there will be resistance.
- Remove dilator, holding guide wire and having some gauze 4×4 in your hand to apply pressure to a site that will now bleed after dilation. Place catheter over guide wire; it should advance easily. Hold guide wire at skin entrance and feed it back through distal port of central line (brown cap). When wire comes out, grab it at the end and finish advancing catheter. Remove guide wire and flush line through all 3 ports. Ensure all ports are closed.

- Now suture catheter in place via flange with holes. If more than 1–2 cm of catheter is exposed due to length, either suture the catheter down or use the snap-on flange provided in the kit. Apply a clear dressing.
- Get a chest X-ray to evaluate for line placement and complication. The tip of the catheter should be at the junction of the SVC and right atrium on chest X-ray film. New data would suggest that this is 2 cm below the superior right cardiac silhouette, which is made up by the right atrial appendage.

27.5 Internal jugular vein cannulation

- **Visualise landmarks:** locate the triangle formed by heads of sternocleidomastoid and the clavicle. Entry point is apex. Internal jugular vein runs deep to the sternocleidomastoid muscle. Use of USS is highly recommended. Place patient in head down position to prevent air embolism.
- In obese patients where the landmarks are not discernible, a reasonable rule of thumb is to go three finger breadths lateral from the tracheal midline, and three finger breadths up from the clavicle. Some suggest that patient turn head away from side whilst others suggest keep head in neutral midline position.
- As the head rotates away from neutral, there is an increase in both the overlap and proximity of the internal jugular vein and carotid artery which increases the risk of carotid puncture. Some advocate the use of a small gauge pilot needle to locate the internal jugular vein and an innovative technique to then stabilise it. This small gauge pilot needle may be particularly useful when patients have coagulopathy or when ultrasonography is not available.
- Palpate for the carotid impulse and make sure you are lateral to this. Insert the needle at the apex of the triangle and the needle should point down towards same side nipple with needle at 30° to horizontal. The vein is usually less than 1.5 cm below surface.

27.6 Subclavian vein cannulation

- Complications are higher and so must be carried out by experienced operators only. Benefits are more comfortable for longer term catheterisation than alternative sites and so can be used for dialysis or feeding.
- The adult subclavian vein is approximately 3–4 cm long and 1–2 cm in diameter and is a continuation of the axillary vein at the lateral border of the first rib which it crosses over and passes in front of the anterior scalene muscle. The anterior scalene muscle is approximately 10–15 mm thick and separates the subclavian vein from the subclavian artery, which runs behind.
- The vein continues behind medial third of clavicle where it is immobilised by small attachments to the rib and clavicle. At the medial border of the anterior scalene muscle and behind subscapularis joint, the subclavian unites with the internal jugular to form the innominate/brachiocephalic vein. The large thoracic duct on the left, and smaller lymphatic duct on the right, enter the superior margin of subclavian vein near internal jugular junction.
- **Technique:** head down position, well hydrated if possible. Place towel roll behind scapulae to pull back shoulders which brings clavicles backward. Keep patient's head in neutral position, though some teach to turn head away. Anaesthetise locally with lidocaine down to the periosteum of the clavicle. Locate subclavian vein with a 22 gauge needle and pass introducer needle parallel to retrace path.

- Ensure that the needle is kept very shallow to skin at no more than 10–15° from horizontal. Generally the needle is advanced medially from an entry point 1 cm below junction of middle and medial one-third of clavicle towards the posterior superior angle of the clavicle (the suprasternal notch).
- Advance needle aspirating. The subclavian artery, lung, and brachial plexus are all posterior to subclavian vein; if the vein is not cannulated, at least the other structures will not be hit. Once cannulated use a Seldinger technique as described above.
- The risk of pneumothorax is far greater with this technique. Damage to the subclavian artery may occur; direct pressure cannot be applied to prevent bleeding. Ensure that a chest X-ray is ordered, to identify the position of the line and to exclude pneumothorax.

27.7 Femoral vein

- The femoral vein can be used for central access. The risk of infection is greater at this site. It is a useful site in patients with superior vena caval obstruction. Cardiac monitoring is not needed. The femoral vein is the continuation of the popliteal vein and accompanies the femoral artery in the femoral triangle. The femoral vein ends medial to the artery at the inguinal ligament, where it becomes the external iliac vein. Vein, artery, nerve from medial to lateral.
- **Technique:** extend the leg and abduct slightly at the hip. Adopt full asepsis. Locate the femoral artery, keep a finger on the artery and introduce a needle attached to a 10 ml syringe at 45°, 1.5 cm medial to the femoral artery pulsation, 2 cm below the inguinal ligament. Slowly advance the needle towards the head and posteriorly while gently withdrawing the plunger. When a free flow of blood appears, follow the Seldinger approach, as detailed previously.
- Potential complications include wound sepsis and septicaemia, deep vein thrombosis, femoral nerve or arterial damage, haematoma, arteriovenous fistula. It is certainly an easier site to control in any coagulopathy as pressure can be applied.

27.8 Lumbar puncture

Introduction: ask the five questions (see table above), and also check: is it safe and is there raised ICP with an incipient herniation syndrome?

Contraindications: incipient brain herniation syndrome suggested by seizures, GCS <13, focal neurological signs (including ocular palsies), papilloedema, pupillary dilation, impaired eye movements, coma and low HR and rising BP, older patients, HIV, recent head trauma (CT head required first). Coagulopathy, thrombocytopenia, warfarin, heparin, platelets $<50 \times 10^9$/L. Spina bifida or skin appearances of spina bifida occulta or deformities, local infection or pressure sore, severe cardiorespiratory compromise.

Complications: coning due to brain herniation, epidural haematoma with root or cauda equina compression, subarachnoid haemorrhage, infection (e.g. meningitis), low pressure headache, backache, nerve palsies (e.g. diplopia from CN VI), lumbosacral nerve palsies (extremely rare), dermoid formation.

Patient advice

- Explain procedure and reason for LP to patient. Explain complications including headache and infection. Mention that it is extremely common for a patient to experience a sharp shoot of pain down one leg and if this happens they should let the operator know and that it does not mean something has gone wrong.

- Explain that the needle is placed below the spinal cord and as such the needle cannot enter the spinal cord. It is almost impossible to put a needle through one of the nerve roots and the pain is typically caused by the needle touching the nerve root (e.g. like a cold drink touching an exposed nerve root in a bad tooth). Give the patient a copy of patient information sheet.

Preparation

- Make sure you are clear what samples need to be sent and have relevant tubes ready and inform microbiologist/lab of intended procedure. Do not start without all equipment to hand including manometer.
- Any focal signs or suggestions of coma which could suggest raising ICP, then a CT is needed to exclude space occupying lesion or other signs of increased CSF pressure such as dilated third ventricles, midline shift, etc.

Patient positioning is key to success

- The patient is best positioned lying comfortably on their side, at the edge of the bed with a pillow between knees, back flexed, with the spine horizontal and perpendicular to the couch throughout its entire length.
- The chin should be as close to the patellae as possible in a fetal-like position. Knees and ankles should be symmetrical and together. Careful attention to positioning and explanation to patient before starting significantly increases the chance of success.

Skin preparation

- Give yourself a wide sterile area. For skin preparation use **chlorhexidine or iodine aqueous solution**. It is important to use good technique for sterilising starting in the centre and wiping in circular motion to outside of area.

Position of LP site

- The cord ends at the lower margin of L1. The needle is usually introduced at L3/4 interspace which is indicated by a line drawn joining the tips of the iliac crests. (In adults the spinal cord usually ends at the lower border of L1 so a needle inserted into the subarachnoid space below this level will enter the sac containing the cauda equina floating in CSF.) L3/4 interspace gives a margin of error. If unsuccessful at this level try L2/3.

Procedure

- **Local anaesthetic:** the skin and deeper tissues of the needle track are infiltrated. Use up to 5 ml of 2% lidocaine which should be infiltrated into the skin with a blue needle, waiting for it to take effect and then infiltrating deeper with a green needle. Continually aspirate with the syringe before injecting to ensure not in blood vessel or even CSF (e.g. in thin patient). Allow time for this to be effective.
- **LP needle insertion:** use a sharp disposable fine LP needle (e.g. gauge 22) with a stylet in position; introduce through the skin and advance through the space between the two spinous processes. The top of the bevel should always be parallel to the back (e.g. for a patient horizontal on their side, the bevel will point to the ceiling). The needle point needs to be directed slightly forwards (anteriorly).
- **Insert to a depth** of 4–7 cm; firm resistance which gives way may be encountered as the ligamentum flavum is reached. Beyond this there is a slight give as the needle punctures the dura. The stylet is removed and clear CSF will drip out of the needle if this has been correctly positioned. If no fluid appears or bone is

encountered, it is probable that the needle is not in the correct position. The stylet should be reinserted, the needle partially withdrawn and then advanced with a slightly different angle aiming for the umbilicus.

- **Failure:** the commonest causes of failure are that the needle is not in the midline, the patient's back is not perpendicular to the bed (e.g. twisted at shoulders, or legs not together) or is at too great an angle with the skin. NB. If unsuccessful after 2–3 attempts, take more senior advice before giving up, or ask another more experienced doctor to try. If that is unsuccessful, X-ray screening may be used or contact a friendly anaesthetist. If LP is to evaluate presence of xanthochromia, then further attempts need to be performed at this time and not delayed by more than 2–4 h, otherwise altered blood may be found as a consequence of the 'bloody' traumatic tap and the test becomes unhelpful if xanthochromia is found.
- Once in position and CSF is obtained, the stylet should be placed in the centre of the sterile trolley and kept sterile as it will need to be reinserted prior to taking the LP needle out at the end of the examination.
- **Measure opening pressure:** ensure familiarity with the 3-way tap. Measure and record CSF pressure (normal <20 cmH_2O) using manometry and the patient lying horizontally. **Sample collection:** take 4 tubes and fill each with 3–5 ml (up to 40–50 ml CSF can be safely removed). Label all bottles carefully. Number them 1 to 4 in the order they were filled.
- **Routine samples:** CSF for Gram stain, microscopy and sensitivity, protein, paired sugar (blood + CSF fluoride bottles), cytology sent when indicated at least 10 ml, oligoclonal bands if demyelination suspected and also send serum sample. Xanthochromia – SAH suspected and 3 sequential samples for red cell count. If SAH suspected it is important not to perform the LP within 12 h of the suspected bleed, because time is required to assess presence of xanthochromia. If there are a significant number of red cells from a traumatic tap, as a guide about 10 white cells / 7000 red cells would normally be expected.
- **Other samples**:
  - CSF + serum glucose important – in bacterial/fungal meningitis the CSF sugar is usually <2 mmol/L or <40% blood glucose level.
  - **CSF lactate**: in bacterial and TB meningitis the CSF lactate >3.3 mmol/L. Lactate samples need to go the lab on ice. Inform the lab first.
  - **Microscopy and culture**: CSF may need to be examined for bacteria, fungi, cryptosporidium or tubercules.
  - TB PCR can also be checked but false positives may sometimes be seen.
  - **Latex agglutination** can detect *Haemophilus influenzae* B, *Strep. pneumoniae* and *Neisseria meningitidis* in >75% of affected patients.
  - **Encephalitis**: samples are sent for viral PCR (e.g. HSV, VZV, CMV, etc.).
  - **ACE levels**: neurosarcoid. VDRL – suspected neurosyphilis.
- **Finishing the LP:** once completed **it is essential to replace the sterile stylet before removing the LP needle**. Failure to replace this is one of the main causes of **post-LP headache**. If iodine has been used to clean the skin, it is good practice to swab the LP site with a saline-soaked gauze to remove iodine, if left it may cause skin rashes or burns.

After care

- Lying supine for a short period usually advocated.
- Good hydration is sensible, although not proven to prevent headache.
- Post-LP low pressure headache is severe and always occurs soon after sitting or standing – it should completely disappear on lying flat (or significantly diminish if patient already had headache prior to LP). Whilst this may settle, if it continues

then the longer that treatment is delayed, the less chance of success. Analgesics are to be avoided as they may perpetuate headache.

- Oral caffeine does not prevent post-LP headache. An infusion of IV caffeine is the most appropriate first line management of post-LP headache (e.g. 500 mg in 500 ml NS over 2 h).
- **Persisting low pressure pain:** consider **blood patch** – ask anaesthetists who are experienced at this.

27.9 Abdominal paracentesis

Introduction: ask the five questions (see table above)

Indications

- Therapeutic to relieve excess ascites, diagnostic to take samples for analysis.
- To exclude SBP in anyone unwell with ascites.

Relative contraindications

- Severe coagulopathy, pregnancy, localised cellulitis.

Equipment

- Gauze swabs, sterile dressing pack, sterile gloves, iodine or equivalent.
- Green and blue needles, several 5–10 ml syringes, lignocaine 1–2%.
- Ascitic drain and bag, adhesive dressings.

Procedure

- Obtain consent. Ask patient to micturate first. With ascites when lying supine the fluid is lowest and air-filled bowel floats to the surface. The flanks are dull and fluid filled.
- Safest place to go is right or left inguinal fossa just 2 cm above and medial to anterior superior iliac spine.
- Wash hands and prepare field with iodine. Ensure sterile field and sterile gloves. Identify chosen spot. For a simple diagnostic aspiration, e.g. to detect SBP, a green needle is sufficient with appropriate asepsis.
- Avoid inferior epigastric arteries which run in a pair just a few centimetres lateral of the midline. Apply local anaesthetic down to the point at which you can freely aspirate ascitic fluid. Remove needle and pierce skin with scalpel. Insert drain at 45° aspirating via syringe. Withdraw introducer whilst advancing the drain.

Risks

- Increased risk of post-paracentesis circulatory disturbance with volume removed over 4–5 L. If more removed then consider giving IV albumin.

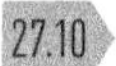

27.10 Arterial blood gas

Introduction: ask the five questions (see table above) and check both radial and ulnar arterial pulses are present.

Arterial blood gas kit

- 1 ml vented, pre-heparinised usually with dry lithium heparin plastic syringe.
- One orange or blue needle (NOTE: longer needles are required for brachial and femoral artery puncture).
- Needle guard to prevent accidental needle stick injuries.
- Vent cap (for evacuation of air bubble), one biohazard-labelled plastic bag.

- Two 1 × 1 sterile gauze, alcohol prep pad, specimen/patient label, iodine pad.
- One adhesive bandage, lab form, ice.

Contraindications

- No absolute contraindications, mostly just extra precautions and hazards.
- Avoid dialysis AV shunt; mastectomy – use opposite side.
- Anticoagulant therapy – hold pressure on puncture site longer than normal.

Preparation

- Introduce yourself and explain what is ordered. Patient cooperation helps.
- Check patient ID, ask patient their name, check patient ID wristband.

Choose artery

- Select site and palpate the right and left radial arterial pulses and visualise the course of the artery. Pick strongest pulse. Radial artery is always the first choice and should be used because it provides collateral circulation.
- If radial pulse weak on right, move to left; if pulse on left weak, then try brachial. Brachial used as alternative site and femoral is the last choice in normal situations. Always have a fallback plan.

Check Allen test

- Applies when using radials. In a conscious and cooperative patient simply compress ulnar and radial arteries at wrist to obliterate pulse and have patient clench and release fist until hand blanches. With radial still compressed, release pressure on ulnar artery and watch for pinkness to return.
- It should pink up within 10–15 sec. If patient unconscious then compress ulnar and radials and elevate hand above head, squeeze hard and release ulnar and lower hand below heart. Palpate left and right radial arteries noting maximal pulse. The one with the stronger pulse will be your site of entry.

Procedure

- Wash hands and put on gloves. Connect needle to syringe ensuring needle kept sterile and eject excess heparin and air bubbles. If using syringe with liquid heparin pull back syringe plunger to at least 1 cm^3 to give room for blood to fill syringe when puncture is made (NEVER recap needle).
- Drape the bed and stabilise the wrist in the position that gives maximal pulse (hyper-extended, using a rolled up towel if necessary) and prepare the site by cleansing the chosen area with an alcohol and/or iodine wipe. Secure needle to syringe and remove cap from needle.
- Pierce the skin at puncture site aiming proximally and keep needle angle constant and bevel of needle up, or into the arterial flow (bevel faces the heart) and slowly advance in one plane. When the artery is punctured, blood will enter the syringe flashback. Slowly allow blood to fill syringe.
- If no blood appears, remove, change needles, and start again. Upon removal of the needle, hold pressure on the puncture site for at least 5 min. Pressure may need to be held longer (>5 min) if the patient is on anticoagulant therapy.

Post puncture procedure

- Remove any air bubbles from sample and cap syringe and dispose of needle in sharps container. Roll syringe to mix heparin with sample and immediately try to lower temperature and metabolism of sample by immersing in ice and ensure rapid delivery to lab. On lab request form indicate: FiO_2, patient temperature and ventilator parameters.

Post procedure

- Check for bleeding, movement of fingers and tingling sensation, pulse distal to puncture. If radial pulse not palpable consider an urgent vascular opinion.

Complications

- **Arterial spasm:** may occur secondary to pain or anxiety. Reassure patient; explain procedure and purpose.
- **Haematoma:** leakage of blood into tissue. You possibly didn't press hard enough and long enough. Ensure using small diameter needle. Ensure proper technique in holding site ×5 min post puncture.
- **Haemorrhage:** patient receiving anticoagulant therapy or patients with known blood coagulation disorders. Two minutes after pressure is released inspect site for bleeding, oozing or seepage of blood; continue pressure until bleeding ceases. A longer compression time is necessary.
- **Other very rare:** laceration of artery, sepsis, infection/inflammation adjacent to puncture site. Avoid sites indicating presence of infection or inflammation. Discuss with vascular surgeons any possible vascular injury.
- **Failure:** consider femoral artery.

27.11 Nasogastric tube insertion

Introduction: ask the five questions (see table above)

Contraindications (or take expert advice)

- Ear, nose and throat abnormalities or infections.
- Suspected oesophageal stricture or pouch.
- Recent oesophagectomy or other surgery.
- Recent fractures of the base of the skull.
- Oesophageal varices, oesophageal perforation or oesophageal surgery.
- Risk of aspiration, suspected atrial–oesophageal fistula.
- Thrombolysed patient – delay NG insertion certainly after stroke thrombolysis.

Procedure

- An NG tube is a long polyurethane or silicone tube passed via the nose and oesophagus into the stomach. Deaths may occur due to feeding tubes displaced into the lungs causing gastric aspiration.
- NG tubes are most commonly inserted by nurses. Sometimes done by doctors, e.g. anaesthetists in theatre. The main indications are: feeding in those, for example, with neurological disease or other cause of impaired swallowing (e.g. stroke); aspirating gastric contents (e.g. obstructed patient) which decompresses the stomach and so prevents vomiting and possible aspiration.
- Nasojejunal tubes are longer versions of NG tubes. They are inserted under endoscopic guidance to lie further in the jejunum and may be useful in feeding patients with pancreatitis.
- Obtain consent – verbal consent is usually sufficient. Practitioners should give patients an appropriate explanation of the insertion procedure, together with the reasons why the tube is necessary. Verbal consent should then be obtained. In some patients actions will need to be done in best interests as consent cannot be communicated.

Preparation

- After washing hands, prepare a trolley including gloves, local anaesthetic jelly or spray, a 60 ml syringe, pH strip, kidney tray, sticky tape and a bag to collect secretions.
- Determine length of NG tube to insert by external measurement from the tip of the nose to a point halfway between the xiphoid and the umbilicus distance. Usually 40–60+ cm. Better to have too long than too short –don't want the tip in the lower oesophagus.
- The patient should sit up. An appropriately sized tube is chosen and the tip is lubricated by smearing aqua gel or local anaesthetic gel. Anaesthetic gel is a drug so if it is used it must be prescribed, and precautions taken such as checking for allergies. The wider nostril is chosen and the tube slid down along the floor of the nasal cavity. The head should not be tilted back. Patients often gag when the tube reaches the pharynx.
- Asking them to swallow their saliva or a small amount of water may help to direct the tube into the oesophagus. Once in the oesophagus, it may be easy to push into the stomach. The correct intragastric position is then verified (see below). The tube is fixed to the nose / forehead using adhesive tapes.
- The stomach is decompressed by attaching the 60 ml syringe and aspirating its contents. Blocked tubes can be flushed open with saline or air.

Verifying correct intragastric positioning: see never events

- There are two recommended ways of confirming the tube position. These are by **pH test and X-ray.** Other methods can be inaccurate and should not be used.
- **Measuring pH**: the NG tube is aspirated and the contents are checked using pH paper, not litmus paper. It is recommended that it is safe to feed adult patients only if the pH is <5.5. Note that taking proton pump inhibitors or H_2 receptor antagonists may alter the pH. Similarly, intake of milk can neutralise the acid.
- **Chest X-ray**: when in doubt, it is best practice to use X-ray to check the tube's location. Patients who have swallowing problems, confused patients and those in ICU should all be given an X-ray to verify the tube's intragastric position. This involves taking a chest X-ray including the upper half of the abdomen. The tip of the tube can be seen as a white radio-opaque line and should be below the diaphragm on the left side.
- **Syringe test**: do not use! This test is mentioned here for historic interest only. Also known as the whoosh test, it has been shown to be an unreliable method of checking tube placement, and the NPSA has said that it *must no longer be used.*
- **Repeated confirmation of position:** correct intragastric positioning should be confirmed at least daily and immediately after initial placement. Before each daily feed – need to wait 1 h before testing pH. Following vomiting/coughing. Decreased O_2 saturation. If the tube is dislodged or the patient complains of discomfort. Never insert the guide wire while the NG tube is in the patient.

Complications

- Misplaced tube and delivery of feed directly into lungs causing pneumonia/ pneumonitis.
- Gastric possibly overfeeding with vomiting also leading to pulmonary aspiration pneumonia.
- Nasal trauma and local mucosal damage when NG inserted roughly or in for a prolonged time. Use lubricants. Gagging or vomiting, therefore suction should always be ready to use.

28 Normal laboratory values

Blood gases (breathing air at sea level)
Blood H^+ 35–45 nmol/L
pH: 7.36–7.44
PaO_2: 11.3–12.6 kPa
$PaCO_2$: 4.7–6.0 kPa
Base excess: +/– 2 mmol/L
Carboxyhaemoglobin: non-smoker <2%
Carboxyhaemoglobin: smoker 3–15%

Serum values
Na: 137–144 mmol/L
K: 3.5–4.9 mmol/L
Cl: 95–107 mmol/L
HCO_3: 20–28 mmol/L
Anion gap: 12–16 mmol/L
Urea: 2.5–7.5 mmol/L
Creatinine: 60–110 µmol/L
Ca: 2.2–2.6 mmol/L
P: 0.8–1.4 mmol/L
Serum total protein: 61–76 g/L

Liver values
Albumin: 37–49 g/L
Total bilirubin: 1–22 µmol/L
Conjugated bilirubin: 0–3.4 µmol/L
ALT: 5–35 units/L
AST: 1–31 units/L
ALP: 45–105 units/L (over 14 years)
GGT: 4–35 units/L (<50 units/L in males)
LDH: 10–250 units/L

Cardiac biomarkers
CK: (males) 24–195 units/L; (females) 24–170 units/L

Others
Cu: 12–26 µmol/L
Caeruloplasmin: 200–350 mg/L
Al: 0–10 mcg/L
Mg: 0.75–1.05 mmol/L
Zn: 6–25 µmol/L
Urate: (males) 0.23–0.46 mmol/L; (females) 0.19–0.36 mmol/L
Plasma lactate: 0.6–1.8 mmol/L
Plasma ammonia: 12–55 µmol/L
Serum ACE: 25–82 units /L
Fasting plasma glucose: 3.0–6.0 mmol/L
HbA1c: 3.8–6.4%
Fructosamine: <285 µmol/L
Serum amylase: 60–180 units/L
Plasma osmolality: 278–305 mOsm/kg

Lipids and lipoproteins: assess overall lifetime risk
Serum cholesterol: <5.2 mmol/L
Serum LDL cholesterol: <3.36 mmol/L
Serum HDL cholesterol: >0.55 mmol/L
Fasting serum TG: 0.45–1.69 mmol/L

Serum tumour markers
α-fetoprotein: <10 kunits/L
Carcinoembryonic antigen: <10 mcg/L
Neuron-specific enolase: <12 mcg/L
Prostate-specific antigen: (males >40) <4 mcg/L; (males <40) <2 mcg/L
hCG: <5 units/L
CA125: <35 units/ml
CA19–9: <33 units/ml

Cerebrospinal fluid
Opening pressure: 50–180 mmH_2O
Total protein: 0.15–0.45 g/L
Albumin: 0.066–0.442 g/L
Chloride: 116–122 mmol/L
Glucose: 3.3–4.4 mmol/L
CSF lactate: 1–2 mmol/L
Cell count: lymphocytes 60–70%; monocytes 30–50%; neutrophils: none
IgG/ALB: <0.26
IgG index: <0.88

Urine
Albumin/creatinine ratio (untimed specimen): (males) <3.5 mg/mmol; (females) <2.5 mg/mmol
GFR: 70–140 ml/min
Total protein: <0.2 g/24 h
Albumin: <30 mg/24 h
Ca: 2.5–7.5 mmol/24 h
Urobilinogen: 1.7–5.9 µmol/24 h
Coproporphyrin: <300 nmol/24 h
Uroporphyrin: 6–24 nmol/24 h
Δ-aminolevulinate: 8–53 µmol/24 h
5-hydroxyindoleacetic acid: 10–47 µmol/24 h
Osmolality: 350–1000 mOsmol/kg

28.1 Haematology values

Full blood count

Haemoglobin: (males) 13.0–18.0 g/dL; (females) 11.5–16.5 g/dL
Haematocrit: (males) 0.40–0.52; (females) 0.36–0.47
MCV: 80–96 fL
MCH: 28–32 pg
MCHC: 32–35 g/dL
White cell count: 4–11 × 10^9/L
White cell differential: (× 10^9/L)
- neutrophils: 1.5–7
- lymphocytes: 1.5–4
- monocytes: 0–0.8
- eosinophils: 0.04–0.4
- basophils: 0–0.1
- platelet count: 150–400
- reticulocyte count 25–85 OR 0.5–2.4%

ESR:
- <50 years: (males) 0–15 mm/1st hour; (females) 0–20 mm/1st hour
- >50 years: (males) 0–20 mm/1st hour; (females) 0–30 mm/1st hour

Plasma viscosity: 1.50–1.72 mPa/s

Coagulation screen

Prothrombin time: 11.5–15.5 sec
INR: <1.4
APTT: 30–40 sec
Fibrinogen: 1.8–5.4 g/L
Bleeding time: 3–8 min

Coagulation factors

Factors II, V, VII, VIII, IX, X, XI, XII: 50–150 IU/dL
Factor V Leiden, Von Willebrand factor: 45–150 IU/dL
Von Willebrand factor antigen: 50–150 IU/dL
Protein C: 0–135 IU/dL
Protein S: 80–120 IU/dL
Antithrombin III: 80–120 IU/dL
Activated protein C resistance: 2.12–4.0
Fibrin degradation products: <100 mg/L
D-dimer screen: <0.5 mg/L

Haematinics

Serum iron: 12–30 μmol/L
Serum iron-binding capacity: 45–75 μmol/L
Serum ferritin: 15–300 mcg/L
Serum transferrin: 2.0–4.0 g/L
Serum B12: 160–760 ng/L
Serum haptoglobin: 0.13–1.63 g/L
Serum folate: 2.0–11.0 mcg/L
Red cell folate: 160–640 mcg/L

Haemoglobin electrophoresis

Haemoglobin A: >95%
Haemoglobin A2: 2–3%
Haemoglobin F: <2%

CSF values

	Normal	Bacterial meningitis	Viral meningitis	TB meningitis	GBS	SAH
CSF	Clear and colourless	Cloudy and turbid	Normal	Normal/ cloudy	Normal	Blood stained
WCC	0–5 × 10^6 per litre Lϕ	Raised Nϕ	Raised Lϕ	Raised Lϕ	Normal	Normal
RCC	0–10 × 10^6 per litre	Normal	Normal	Normal	Normal	Very high 'hundreds'
Protein	0.2–0.4 g/L	High/very high	Normal/high	High, very high	High by week 2	Normal, high
Glucose	3.3–4.4 mmol/L	Low	Normal/low	Very low	Normal	Normal/ low

* Lϕ = lymphocytes, Nϕ = neutrophils.

29 Emergency drugs – quick reference (also see *BNF*)

Prescribing abbreviations

Route
IM = intramuscular
IO = intraosseous
IV = intravenous
PO = oral
SC = subcutaneous

Frequency
OD = once per day (every 24 hours)
OM = once in the morning every 24 hours
ON = once at night
BD = twice per day (every 12 hours)
TDS/TID = three times per day (every 8 hours)
QDS/QID = four times per day (every 6 hours)

Side effects
APX = anaphylaxis
D = diarrhoea
N = nausea
R = rash
V = vomiting

29.1 Antibiotic prescribing advice

In certain cases, for example, a septic patient, you must ensure that the first dose of the appropriate antibiotic(s) is given WITHIN ONE HOUR. It is not enough to write it up. Check availability of that drug on that ward, and check nurses understand urgency of delivering drug to patient. This is especially true for these conditions: suspected bacterial meningitis, septic arthritis, neutropenic sepsis, severe sepsis (of any cause), and also HSV encephalitis.

29.2 Penicillin allergy

Nausea, vomiting or diarrhoea do not, by themselves, constitute an allergic reaction. They are not a contraindication for penicillin use. Anaphylaxis related to histamine release occurs about 30–60 min after administration of a penicillin; symptoms may include erythema or pruritus, angioedema, hypotension or shock, urticaria, wheezing, rhinitis. ERTAPENEM or MEROPENEM is recommended as an alternative to penicillin for some indications. However, if there is a history of an anaphylactic reaction, or an accelerated allergic reaction DO NOT prescribe these drugs. Please discuss alternative antibiotics with a microbiologist. Remember, penicillins (and cephalosporins) can also be nephrotoxic (as they can induce an interstitial nephritis).

WARNING: this is a quick look-up guide for drugs with which you should be familiar and in no way replaces the *BNF*. All drugs should be checked in the *BNF* for safety of use in pregnancy, breastfeeding and renal and liver failure. Allergy is such an obvious contraindication that it is not mentioned. All allergies should be documented.

Drug	Dose	Side effects	C/I and notes
ABCIXIMAB (REOPRO) Monoclonal antibody with antiplatelet activity used in ACS/PCI.	***ACS/PCI:*** 0.25 mg/kg IV bolus administered 10–60 min before the start of PCI, followed by a continuous IV infusion of 0.125 mcg/kg/min (to a maximum of 10 mcg/min) for 12 h.	Bleeding, low platelets, N,V, headache, fever, pulmonary alveolar haemorrhage, ARDS.	High risk of bleeding complications or imminent surgery. Specialist use only – prescribe under senior cardiology direction.
ACETYLCYSTEINE (PARVOLEX) Indicated for suspected paracetamol toxicity. Replenishes glutathione levels.	***First infusion*** (150 mg/kg): add Acetylcysteine concentrate for IV infusion to 200 ml Glucose IV infusion 5%; infuse over 1 h. ***Second infusion*** (50 mg/kg): add Acetylcysteine concentrate for IV infusion to 500 ml Glucose IV infusion 5%; infuse over 4 h. **Third infusion** (100 mg/kg): add Acetylcysteine concentrate for IV infusion to 1 L Glucose IV infusion 5%; infuse over 16 h.	Rash, bronchospasm, anaphylactoid reaction. See paracetamol toxicity section. Reactions more common if infused too quickly.	See paracetamol toxicity section. Use plasma levels and treatment line to judge therapy.
ACICLOVIR Inhibits DNA polymerase in infected cells only. Useful in *Herpes simplex*, varicella zoster (chickenpox and shingles)	***HSV:*** **severe genital HSV***: 5–10 mg/kg IV TDS for 5 days. Non-severe: 200–400 mg PO 5 times daily for 10 days. ***HSV encephalitis****: 10 mg/kg IV TDS for 14–21 days. ***HSV or VZV infections:*** 800 mg PO 5 times daily for 7 days (for HZV in immune-compromised consider IV usage as above).	N,V,R, confusion (IV), phlebitis. Hepatotoxicity, seizures, headache. *Use higher dose or prolonged course if immune-compromised	***Confirm CSF negative for HSV before stopping treatment for HSV encephalitis.***
ADENOSINE Purine nucleoside. Blocks purine A2 receptors. Terminates re-entrant SVTs.	***AVNRT/AVRT:*** start with 6 mg given fast IV into large vein followed by a 20 ml NS bolus (use a three way tap if available). Repeat with 12 mg bolus if indicated. Start with a 3 mg bolus if on dipyridamole, cardiac transplant or central line. Needs cardiac monitoring.	Flushing, angina, headache, palpitations, hypotension, asystole usually temporary, bronchospasm. Warn patient that transient symptoms may occur.	Caution with Dipyridamole: avoid in asthmatics, heart block, pregnancy. In those with asthma/COPD and narrow complex tachycardia then IV Verapamil may be preferred.

Drug	Dose	Side effects	C/I and notes
ACTIVATED CHARCOAL Has surface area of 1000 m^2 per gram. Absorbs certain toxins. Check Toxbase.	50 g PO in 250 ml water or via NG within 1 h of toxin ingestion (2 h with aspirin, opiate, TCA). May be given as multidose 4 hourly.	Pneumonitis if aspirated, constipation (give with laxative), N,V (give with antiemetic)	Other drugs that bind: Methotrexate, Benzodiazepine. Multidose used for carbamazepine, quinine, theophylline ingestion.
ADRENALINE α and β agonist	***Cardiac arrest*:** 1 mg of 1 in 10 000 (10 ml minijet) IV/IO given every 3–5 min in ALS algorithm. ***Anaphylaxis***: 0.5–1.0 mg of 1 in 1000 (0.5–1 ml). Give into anterolateral aspect of muscle bulk of the middle third of the thigh using a green needle in adults. ***Inotrope*:** see below	Arrhythmias. Telemetry and resuscitation equipment needed.	IV usage only for cardiac arrest and in exceptional circumstances in an ITU setting under close observation. Pro-arrhythmic.
ALLOPURINOL Xanthine oxidase inhibitor reduces purine synthesis.	***Gout prevention (2+ attacks)***: 100 mg OD with food. Increase as needed to 300 mg TDS as required. Reduce dose if renal impairment. Use lowest dose to keep uric acid <6 mg/dL. ***Tumour lysis syndrome***: 100–300 mg TDS.	Acute gout, N&V&R, AKI, liver toxicity, gynaecomastia. Increases INR in those on Warfarin **Severe fatal toxicity with AZATHIOPRINE and possibly Ciclosporin.**	An NSAID or low dose of Colchicine 0.5 mg BD can be given for 1–2 months initially along with Allopurinol 100 mg to prevent acute attacks.
ALTEPLASE Tissue plasminogen activator. Breaks down fibrin. Restores vessel patency. Avoid in any tendency to life threatening bleeding especially if non-compressible.	***Ischaemic stroke*:** IV 0.9 mg/kg (max dose is 90 mg) with 10% as IV bolus and 90% over 60 min. ***ACS-STEMI*:** (max dose 100 mg) accelerated infusion (over 90 min) 15 mg IV bolus followed by 0.75 mg/kg (up to 50 mg) IV over 30 min and then 0.5 mg/kg (up to 35 mg) IV over 60 min. If weight >67 kg give 15 mg / 50 mg / 35 mg. ***Compromised PE*:** max dose 100 mg as 15 mg bolus + 85 mg over 2 h.	Haemorrhagic complications, anaphylaxis, angioneurotic oedema, tongue swelling. Heparin should be discontinued during Alteplase infusion.	Recent or current active bleeding or bleeding disorder, trauma, surgery, biopsy. Covered in more detail in *Sections 11.2* (ACS) and *19.8* (stroke).

Drug	Dose	Side effects	C/I and notes
AMINOPHYLLINE Phosphodiesterase inhibitor. Aim for serum levels of 10–20 mg/L. Wait until 4–6 h after infusion started. Stop infusion and wait 15 min and then take level.	***Asthma, COPD and rarely LVF****: Loading dose:* 250 mg IV (5 mg/kg) given over 20 min only if not already taking a theophylline. *Maintenance dose:* 750 mg (0.5 mg/kg/h) over 24 h. Adjust as per levels. Smokers need higher dose; elderly or CCF smaller dose, e.g. 500 mg over 24 h. **Infusion**: make up 500 mg in 500 ml in NS or 5% dextrose as 1 mg/ml.	Headache, anxiety, confusion, restlessness, palpitations, hyperventilation, N&V, life-threatening arrhythmias, hypotension, convulsions.	Anxiety, agitation, arrhythmias. Monitor plasma levels. Omit loading dose if already taking aminophylline/ theophylline.
AMIODARONE Prolonged usage, e.g. infusion, needs a central line.	***Cardiac arrest:*** 300 mg IV/IO after adrenaline to treat VF/pulseless VT in cardiac arrest refractory to defibrillation, then 900 mg over 24 h. ***Tachycardia with pulse and unstable:*** after 3 sync DC shocks give 300 mg IV OVER 20 min then 900 mg over 24 h. ***Wide complex tachycardia with pulse and stable:*** Give 300 mg IV OVER 60 mins then 900 mg over 24 h in 500 ml of 5% dextrose using a syringe and infusion pump through a central vein	Low BP, bradycardia, thrombophlebitis, photosensitivity, thyroid dysfunction, alveolitis, N,V, TdP. *Extravasation causes tissue damage. Follow local treatment policies. Ensure peripheral IV lines are working and flush after usage.*	Amiodarone should not be used in individuals with TdP (polymorphic VT) or a long QT because it prolongs QT interval. Will increase INR and may cause Digoxin toxicity. Watch levels.
AMILORIDE K^+ sparing diuretic.	***CCF, oedema, HTN***: 2.5–10 mg OD PO.	High K^+, low BP, GI upset, low Na.	Watch for Lithium toxicity.
AMITRIPTYLINE Tricyclic antidepressant.	***Migraine prophylaxis***: 10–75 mg PO ON. ***Neuralgia/depression:*** 30–75 mg OD. Higher doses may be used.	Arrhythmias, seizure, sedation, weight gain.	MAOI use in past 2 weeks, epilepsy, phaeochromocytoma.
AMLODIPINE Ca channel blocker.	***HTN***: 5–10 mg OD PO.	Low BP, ankle oedema.	

Drug	Dose	Side effects	C/I and notes
AMOXICILLIN Broad spectrum bactericidal β-lactam antibiotic.	***Infection***: 500 mg – 1 g TDS PO/IM/IV. Severe infection 1 g QDS IV or infusion.	N,V,D, cholestasis, rash with infectious mononucleosis.	Use in mild/mod CAP, UTI, Listeria. Reduce dose in renal failure. Dose and route depend on clinical severity.
AMPICILLIN Broad spectrum bactericidal β-lactam antibiotic.	***Infection***: 500 mg – 1 g PO QDS, 500 mg IM/IV 4–6 hourly, 2 g slow IV 4–6 hourly.	N,V,D, rash with infectious mononucleosis, cholestasis.	Increases INR with warfarin. Infectious mononucleosis. 2–3 week course in listerial meningitis.
AUGMENTIN (CO-AMOXICLAV) Amoxicillin and clavulinic acid.	***Infection***: 375–625 mg TDS PO. ***Severe infection or parenteral:*** 1.2 g IV TDS.	N,V,D, cholestasis, hepatitis, rash with infectious mononucleosis.	Use in mild/ mod CAP, UTI, Listeria. Infectious mononucleosis. Increases INR with warfarin.
ARTESUNATE May inhibit DNA replication and transcription.	***Severe falciparum malaria for adults***: 2.4 mg/kg given IV at 0, 12 and 24 h then once daily thereafter.	Cardiotoxicity (high doses), rash.	
ASPIRIN	***Ischaemic stroke***: 300 mg for 14 days then 75 mg. ***ACS***: 75–300 mg OD. ***IHD***: 75 mg OD.	Gastric irritation, PUD, asthma, tinnitus, toxicity.	Bleeding disorder, PUD, asthma.
ATENOLOL β adrenergic receptor blocker.	***HTN, ACS, SVT/AF/VT***: 2.5–5 mg IV given at 1 mg/min then 50 mg PO 20 min later. PO 25–100 mg OD.	Bronchospasm, fatigue, depression, cold peripheries, bradycardia.	In asthma, bradycardia.
ATORVASTATIN HMG CoA reductase inhibitor.	***IHD, stroke disease, hyperlipidaemia***: 10–80 mg ON.	Myalgia, myositis, pancreatitis, raised LFTs. Myopathy with macrolides or amiodarone.	Liver disease, raised K.
ATROPINE Muscarinic acetylcholine receptor blocker.	***Severe bradycardia***: 0.3–1.0 mg IV/IO repeated as needed. ***Organophosphate toxicity:*** 2–3 mg IV needed. See topic in *Section 20.4*.	Mydriasis, tachycardia, N&V, dry warm skin, urinary retention, bronchodilation.	Caution with myasthenia, ileus. Do not use in asystolic arrest. Large doses may be needed in OP poisoning.

Drug	Dose	Side effects	C/I and notes
BENZYLPENICILLIN β-lactam bactericidal.	***Infection***: 1.2–2.4 g every 4 h only given IV/IM.	N&V&D, rash, convulsions (high dose), renal impairment.	Penicillin allergy. Used in meningococcal meningitis, endocarditis, pnemomococcal infection, cellulitis.
BISOPROLOL β adrenergic receptor blocker.	***HTN, arrhythmias/CCF***: 2.5–10 mg PO daily.	Fatigue, depression, cold peripheries, bronchospasm.	Asthma, bradycardia, heart block.
BUMETANIDE Loop diuretic.	***Acute LVF***: 1–2 mg IV or IM. ***CCF***: 1–2 mg PO OD. Higher doses may be given.	Low K, low Na, low BP, gynaecomastia, urinary retention.	Hypotension, dehydration.
CALCIUM Cardioprotective for high K (>6.5 mmol/L) or ECG changes and high Mg and Ca channel blocker toxicity.	***Cardioprotection / severe hypocalcaemia, tetany***: 10–20 ml of 10% calcium chloride/gluconate slowly over 3–5 min. ***Maintenance***: 100 ml of 10% calcium gluconate in 1 L of glucose 5% or NS. Give 50 ml/h until symptoms resolved or [Ca] > 1.9 mmol/L.	Calcium chloride is often found as min-I-jet on arrest trolley. Give gluconate if prolonged infusion needed.	
CEFTRIAXONE 3rd gen cephalosporin. Penetrates CSF.	***Bacterial meningitis and other severe infections***: 0.5–2 g IM/IV BD.	Rash, anaphylaxis, diarrhoea, pancreatitis.	Cautions in renal failure – reduce dose.
CARBAMAZEPINE Anticonvulsant.	***Epilepsy:*** 400–1200 mg daily in divided doses.	Skin reactions, e.g. SJS, oedema, low Na, N,V, vertigo.	Can worsen myoclonic/absence seizures. Avoid with MAOIs. See *BNF* for interactions.
CEFOTAXIME 3rd gen cephalosporin. Penetrates CSF.	***Bacterial meningitis and other infections***: 1–2 g slow IV/IM QDS (max 12 mg daily).	R, N&V&D, *C. difficile* colitis, arrhythmias.	Reduce dose in renal failure. Use in meningitis, typhoid, UTI, gonorrhoea.
CEFUROXIME 2nd gen cephalosporin	***Infections:*** 750 mg IV TDS or 250–500 mg BD PO.	R, N&V&D, *C. difficile* colitis.	Use for RTI, UTI, severe infections.

Drug	Dose	Side effects	C/I and notes
CHLORPHENAMINE Blocks H1 receptors.	***Anaphylaxis, urticaria, allergic reaction:*** 10 mg slow IV over 1 min or IM. PO at 4 mg QDS if itching persists.	Sedation, urinary retention, dry mouth, blurred vision.	Urinary retention, glaucoma. Sedation – do not drive/ operate machinery. Can increase phenytoin.
CIPROFLOXACIN Fluoroquinolone antibiotic. Gram-negative infections.	***Infections:*** 250–750 mg BD PO or IV 400 mg infusion over 60 min every 8–12 h.	Tendonitis, diarrhoea, QT prolongation, epilepsy.	G6PD, seizures, myasthenia gravis. Caution with theophyllines, NSAIDs, Ciclosporin (see *BNF*).
CLARITHROMYCIN Macrolide antibiotic.	***Infections:*** 250–500 mg BD IV/PO.	As for Erythromycin. Reduce dose AKI/ CKD.	Porphyria, liver failure.
CLOPIDOGREL $P2Y_{12}$ (ADP) receptor blocker. Clopidogrel requires metabolism to its active form.	***STEMI:*** 300–600 mg loading dose in ACS. Otherwise usual dose 300 mg PO and then 75 mg OD. ***Post TIA / ischaemic stroke***: loading dose 300 mg PO and then 75 mg OD.	Bleeding – takes up to 7 days for effect to reduce. Effects reduced by omeprazole.	Active bleeding, trauma, imminent surgery, recent surgery (take advice).
CLINDAMYCIN Lincosamide antibiotic. Binds to 50S ribosomal site. For anaerobic infections, TSS, bone infection.	***Infections:*** 150–450 mg QDS PO. Deep IM/IV: 0.6–4.8 g daily (in 2–4 divided doses); single IV doses >600 mg by IV infusion up to max of 1.2 g.	Stop if any suspicion of antibiotic-associated colitis, diarrhoea, oesophagitis, jaundice, SJS/TEN.	Diarrhoea. Watch U&E and LFTs if treatment >10 days.
CODEINE Weak opiate. Look for use of codeine in any confused or comatose patient. Consider Naloxone.	***Mild–moderate pain***: 30–60 mg PRN or 6 hourly. Consider laxative if dosing >24 h. *Variations in metabolism means some are very sensitive.*	Respiratory depression, coma, constipation, miosis. Low GCS in elderly, renal failure.	Resp failure, asthma, seizures, bowel obstruction – ileus, coma. For acute pain, time limit prescription.
COLCHICINE Inhibits microtubule formation and mitosis.	***Acute gout:*** 1 mg stat PO then 0.5 mg 4 hourly until max dose of 6 mg taken or diarrhoea. A low dose (0.5 mg BD) may be given for weeks before allopurinol started.	N&V, D, GI bleed. Toxicity with Ciclosporin, Erythromycin, statin, others (see *BNF*).	Avoid in pregnancy and AKI/CKD.

Drug	Dose	Side effects	C/I and notes
CO-TRIMOXAZOLE Combined trimethoprim and sulfamethoxazole in 1:5 concentration.	***PCP pneumonia***: 2 × 960 mg (TMP 160 mg, SMX 800 mg) PO TDS. ***Parenteral:*** 20/100 mg/kg/ day IV TDS/QDS. *Check divided dose.	SJS, N&V, agranulocytosis, aplastic anaemia.	Raised INR if taking Warfarin. Phenytoin, Ciclosporin, Azathioprine, Mercaptopurine, Methotrexate toxicity. Check *BNF*.
CYCLIZINE Antimuscarinic. Antihistamine.	***Antiemetic:*** 50 mg slow IV/ IM/PO TDS.	Sedation, dry mouth, urinary retention, N,V.	Metoclopramide preferred in heart failure.
DABIGATRAN Direct thrombin inhibitor.	***VTE prophylaxis post knee and hip replacement:*** see *BNF*. ***Non-rheumatic AF***: 110 or 150 mg BD. Smaller dose in elderly.	Bleeding, indigestion (try taking with food or switch to other NOAC).	Active bleeding, falls, renal failure. Avoid particularly with Verapamil and Ketoconazole and other anti-thrombotics (increased bleeding). See *BNF* or datasheet.
DESFERRIOXAMINE Chelating agent for iron toxicity.	***Iron toxicity***: 1 g (15 mg/ kg/h – 70 kg adult) IM or IV infusion over an hour. Max dose 6 g/24 h or 80 mg/ kg/day.	IM use can be painful, ARDS has been reported.	Chelated iron causes orange/ red urine. IV can release histamine with hypotension.
DEXAMETHASONE Potent glucocorticoid. See *Steroid comparison* table below.	***Dose***: 10 mg IV then 4 mg QDS PO/IM/IV. Dose as per indications. ***Adrenal replacement***: 0.75 mg in a single dose.	See *Steroid comparison* table below.	Sometimes used awaiting synACTHen test as does not interfere with assay.
DIAZEPAM Benzodiazepine. For sedation, anxiety, ongoing seizure or repeated seizure or status epilepticus.	***Ongoing seizure***: 2–10 mg IV over 2–5 min in adult **OR** 5–20 mg PR over 2–5 min in adult if no IV access. May be repeated after 10 min. Can give IV dose PR with a 5 ml syringe connected to a rectal tube introduced only 4–5 cm into the rectum. ***Severe anxiety:*** 1–2 mg TDS PO. Short term.	Drowsiness, amnesia. Be ready to intubate if severe respiratory depression. Continuous monitoring.	**Reversal**: can use Flumazenil (Annexate), however, can precipitate seizures. Caution in elderly or liver/renal failure.

Drug	Dose	Side effects	C/I and notes
DIAMORPHINE Opiate (heroin) which provides analgesia, sedation, dyspnoea, palliation.	***Severe pain***: 2.5–5 mg slow IV over 2–5 min watching for respiratory depression. ***Acute LVF***: 2.5–5 mg slow 1 mg/min. Can repeat after 4 hours. ***End of life care***: given PRN or by syringe driver in doses starting at 10 mg/24 h + anti-emetic.	N&V, respiratory depression, miosis, constipation. Give with Cyclizine or Metoclopramide.	Avoid with respiratory failure or coma. Reversal: Naloxone 0.4–1.2 mg. Dose titrated to response as needed.
DIGOXIN	***AF + CCF, LVF, cardiogenic shock.*** ***Loading dose:*** 500 mcg PO or IV over 30 min. Later dose of 250–500 mcg PO/IV over 30 min 6 h later. ***Maintenance dose***: 125–250 mcg OM. (*Doses are in micrograms*.)	Arrhythmias, heart block (ensure on telemetry), fatigue, confusion.	Risk of toxicity in elderly, renal failure and low muscle mass (see *BNF*). Reduce dose. Serum levels: 1–2 mcg/L at 6 h post dose. Reversal: Digibind.
DOXAPRAM Respiratory stimulant. When NIV not possible.	***Hypoventilatory Type 2 RF***: give 1–3 mg/min IV. Monitor O_2 saturation and ABG.	Agitation, pyrexia, headache, tachycardia, HTN.	Monitor closely on HDU/ITU. Define ceiling of care.
DOXAZOSIN α-1 blocker.	***BPH, HTN***: 1 mg/day increasing to max dose of 16 mg/day in divided doses.	Low BP, headache, dizziness.	
DOXYCYLINE Tetracycline. Long T½	***Bacterial, rickettsial infections, malaria***: 100–200 mg PO for 7–14 days.	N,V, photosensitivity, liver toxicity.	Avoid UV light. Reduced dose in renal failure. Avoid with milk.
ENALAPRIL ACE inhibitor. Increases bradykinin and reduces angiotensin II.	***HTN, heart failure***: 5–40 mg/24 h. Increase dose gradually in heart failure. Watch U&E.	Cough, angioedema, rash, raised K, altered taste, low BP, AKI (esp. with RAS).	Severe aortic stenosis (relative), raised K. Pregnancy as teratogenic.
ENOXAPARIN (CLEXANE) Low molecular weight heparin activates antithrombin III.	***VTE prophylaxis***: 20–40 mg OD (20 mg in renal failure). ***ACS***: 1 mg/kg BD. ***PE/DVT***: 1.5 mg/kg OD but in renal failure max dose is 1 mg/kg/day.	Bleeding, low platelets (HITT), hyperkalaemia, and osteoporosis long term.	Bleeding, HITT. Consider monitoring anti-Xa 4 h post-dose in renal failure, pregnancy, etc.

Drug	Dose	Side effects	C/I and notes
ERYTHROMYCIN Macrolide antibiotic. Penicillin allergy, atypical and other pneumonias.	***Infections:*** 500–1000 mg 6–8 hourly, PO or IV. Increases toxicity of other drugs (see *BNF*).	N,V,D, limits use. Irritant to veins. Inhibits P_{450} enzymes.	Porphyria, liver failure, reduce dose with renal failure. Clarithromycin better tolerated.
FLECAINIDE Antiarrhythmic. Avoid if structural heart disease.	***AF (+/– WPW), SVT and VT:*** 2 mg/kg IV up to 150 mg over 20 min PO 50–100 mg 12 hourly.	Dizziness, oedema, fatigue, GI disturbance.	Exclude structural heart disease (get echo). Specialist use only.
FLUCLOXACILLIN β-lactam penicillin antibiotic.	**Staph. aureus** ***and*** **Strep. pyogenes:** oral dose 250–500 mg QDS. IV dose for severe infections 1–2 g QDS.	N,V,D, cholestasis.	Reduce dose in severe renal failure. Used in cellulitis, impetigo, surgical wounds, adjunct in pneumonia.
FLUMAZENIL Benzodiazepine antagonist. Reverses coma due to benzodiazepines.	***Moderate/severe respiratory depression*:** 200 mcg (0.2 mg) IV over 15 sec and then 100 mcg every minute up to a total dose of 1 mg (1000 mcg).	N,V, flushing. Seizures. Do not use if recent seizure. Consider respiratory support.	Seizure or known epilepsy. Severe liver disease. Avoid use if possible.
FOMEPIZOLE Methanol and ethylene glycol poisoning. Alcohol dehydrogenase inhibitor.	***Poisoning*:** 15 mg/kg IV (up to 1500 mg) then 12 h later 10 mg/kg/IV every 12 h for 4 doses; then 15 mg/kg every 12 h until methanol or ethylene glycol level normal, acidosis cleared, and patient symptom-free; and 10 mg/kg every 4 h while on dialysis.	Headache, N,D, increased drowsiness and bad taste.	
FONDAPARINUX Factor Xa inhibitor.	***VTE prophylaxis:*** 2.5 mg SC OD (give 6 h post-op). ***PE/DVT****:* *<50 kg*: 5 mg SC OD; *50–100 kg*: 7.5 mg OD SC; *>100 kg*: 10 mg SC OD. ***ACS: NSTEMI/USA****:* 2.5 mg SC OD <8 days. ***STEMI:*** 2.5 mg IV then SC OD <8 days.	Reduce dose in renal failure. Causes bleeding, N,V.	Bleeding disorders.

Drug	Dose	Side effects	C/I and notes
FOSPHENYTOIN Prodrug of phenytoin. Fosphenytoin 1.5 mg = Phenytoin 1 mg. FP is less cardiotoxic so can be given quicker.	***Status epilepticus: loading dose:*** 30 mg/kg (20 mg/kg(PE)) IV. Infusion rate of up to 100–150 mg(PE)/min. This works out to be 1500 mg FP (1000 mg PE) in those over 85 kg) given over 20–30 min. ***Maintenance dose***: 4–5 mg(PE)/kg daily in divided doses.	Hypotension, arrhythmias, less than with phenytoin 'purple glove syndrome'. Needs cardiac monitoring.	Reduce dose in liver/renal failure.
FUROSEMIDE Venodilation and diuresis.	**Pulmonary oedema:** 20–80 mg IV. May also be given as an infusion.	Diuresis, low BP, dehydration, low K, low Na.	
GENTAMICIN Aminoglycoside. Nephrotoxic and ototoxic. Stop drug at the earliest sign of toxicity (can develop even in patients with normal Gentamicin levels). Monitoring: the pre-dose level must be ≤1 mg/L before any further dose is given.	***Prophylaxis***: single dose: 3 mg/kg. ***Treatment daily dose***: 5–7 mg/kg (max 450 mg/day). Dose depends on weight, microbiology advice and renal function. Give over 30 min in 50 ml NS. ***Multiple daily dose:*** 3–5 mg/kg/day in 3 doses IM/IV infusion. Those with eGFR <30 ml need to be discussed with microbiology.	Vestibular ototoxicity. Vertigo, ataxia, tinnitus, hearing loss, N,V. Seen with use >3 days. Drug accumulates in the inner ear. Warn those receiving therapy >3 days.	Increased toxicity with loop diuretics, Vancomycin, Ciclosporin, raised INR with Warfarin. CAUTION: aminoglycosides can worsen MG, hypersensitivity, severe renal impairment, loop diuretics. Continuation beyond 3 days must be discussed with microbiology. Dose obese using their 'thin' weight.
GLUCAGON Treat BM <3 mmol/L.	***Hypoglycaemia, cardiac dysfunction due to β-blocker toxicity:*** 1 mg IM/IV/SC.	Low K, low BP, GI disturbance.	Liver disease. Does not work if no liver glycogen reserves.
GLYCERYL TRINITRATE Nitrate.	***Angina/LVF/HTN:*** *S/L:* 1–2 (400 mcg/dose) sprays under tongue. ***Parenteral IV***: 1–10 ml/h (50 mg in 50 ml) for BP/angina/LVF. Onset 1–2 min. **Transdermal:** start with 5–20 mg patches per 24 h.	Headache, syncope, hypotension, tolerance if continued >24 h.	**CAUTION**: avoid if low BP. Close monitoring when given IV or S/L.

Drug	Dose	Side effects	C/I and notes
HALOPERIDOL Antipsychotic.	***Sedation/acute psychosis:*** 2–5 mg IV/IM or even SC daily and may be given in divided doses. ***Elderly***: start at 0.5–2 mg PO/IV/IM/SC.	Tachycardia, low BP, HTN and QT prolonged. Acute dystonias, dyskinesias, NMS.	Parkinson's, epilepsy. In agitated elderly try non-drug strategies. If fails, start with 0.5 mg BD. Liquid formulations useful. Stop when not needed.
HYDROCORTISONE Anti-inflammatory or for steroid replacement.	***Steroid replacement, anti-inflammatory:*** 50–200 mg IV 6 hourly. Use PO/IM for replacement.	See *Steroid comparison* table below.	
IBUPROFEN NSAID.	***Analgesia:*** 200–400 mg TDS. Time limit courses for acute symptoms.	Gastritis, renal impairment, HTN.	AKI, GI bleed, renal disease. Consider PPI.
IMMUNOGLOBULIN IVIg Screen for IgA deficiency. IVIg from the serum of at least 1000 donors screened for HIV, HTLV and hep B and C before pooling.	***Severe infections, GBS, MG, ITP, CIDP***: total dose is 2 g/kg usually given as 0.4 g/kg bodyweight daily for 5 consecutive days. This may be repeated after 4–6 weeks depending on indication.	Nausea, chills, fever, headache, backache in 1% in first 30 min. Aseptic meningitis within 48 h, anaphylaxis, thrombotic stroke, MI and AKI can be seen. Neutropenia.	Selective IgA deficiency. Watch for AKI seen in older, diabetic, dehydrated. Ensure hydrated before starting IVIg.
IPRATROPIUM BROMIDE (ATROVENT) Anticholinergic bronchodilator.	***Asthma, COPD, bronchospasm***: *nebuliser:* 250–500 mcg QDS air-driven in COPD or with oxygen. *Chronic inhaler*: 20–40 mcg QDS.	Antimuscarinic, dilated pupil, uncommon.	BPH, glaucoma.
LABETALOL Mixed α/β adrenergic blocker. **Indications:** acute BP reduction, e.g. for stroke thrombolysis or aortic dissection. Give with cardiac monitoring.	***HTN:*** 20 mg IV dose over 2 min. Additional boluses of 40–80 mg every 10 min as needed up to a total dose of 300 mg. Infusions can be made up as 1 mg/ml. Make up 200 mg in 200 ml NS or 5% dextrose. Give at 5–15 mg (5–15 ml) per hour which can be increased.	Fatigue, depression, cold peripheries, bronchospasm. Do not reduce BP in ischaemic stroke if not for thrombolysis unless SBP >220 mmHg and if so then slowly reduce to <200 mmHg.	Asthma, bradycardia. **Target BP:** aortic dissection: 110 mmHg. Stroke thrombolysis: <185/110 mmHg. HTN encephalopathy: slowly lower SBP to 180 mmHg.

Drug	Dose	Side effects	C/I and notes
LIDOCAINE Class Ib antiarrhythmic Na channel blocker.	***Cardiac arrest*:** 50–100 mg (1–1.5 mg/kg) IV over 2–5 min. Repeat maximum total IV dose of 200 mg.	Slurred speech, bradycardia, twitching, low GCS, seizures suggest toxicity.	May be beneficial in out of hospital VF cardiac arrest.
LISINOPRIL ACE inhibitor.	***HTN, CCF*:** start 5–10 mg OD up to 80 mg per day.	See Enalapril.	See Enalapril.
LORAZEPAM Benzodiazepine.	***Sedation:*** 0.5–2 mg PO/ IM/IV BD. ***Status epilepticus*:** 1–4 mg slow IV (also IM or PO) over 1 min into a large vein.	Respiratory depression, acute narrow-angle glaucoma, sleep apnoea.	Renal failure, respiratory failure, muscle weakness. Be able to manage any respiratory depression.
MANNITOL Osmotic diuretic.	***Cerebral oedema*: 200 ml 20% (40 g) given over 10 min.** This can be repeated. Dose is up to 50–200 g in 24 h.	Diuresis, hypovolaemia, raised osmolarity, high Na.	Mannitol acts within 30–45 min and lasts around 6 h.
MAGNESIUM SULPHATE Indications are multiple.	***VT:*** 8 mmol (2 g) over 15 min then 72 mmol (18 g) over 24 h. ***Asthma:*** 8 mmol (2 g) over 20 min. ***Eclampsia:*** 16 mmol (4 g) over 20 min and then 96–192 mmol (12–24 g) over 24 h.	Hypotension, CNS toxicity, respiratory depression. Toxicity with renal dysfunction. **Reversal: in magnesium toxicity give IV calcium.**	Useful for TdP specifically or VT with hypokalaemia. VT dose can also treat severe hypomagnesaemia.
MEROPENEM Carbapenem broad-spectrum antibiotic. CSF penetration good. Bactericidal.	***Severe infections, meningitis, aerobic Gram +/– anaerobes, neutropenic sepsis*:** 0.5–2 g TDS IV in severe infection.	N,D,V, *C. difficile* colitis, severe low K. Monitor LFTs.	Reduce dose and frequency in renal/ liver failure.
METOCLOPRAMIDE Anti-emetic. D2 blocker.	***Emesis:*** 10 mg IV/IM/PO over 3–5 min.	Acute dystonia. It enhances gastric emptying.	Avoid in bowel obstruction. Avoid age <20 as risk of dystonia.
METOPROLOL β blockade.	***Angina, arrhythmias, HTN, post MI*:** 2–5 mg slow IV over 2 min (max 15 mg). ***Oral dose:*** 50–100 mg BD/ TDS. Daily dose 200 mg.	Can cause fatigue depression, cold peripheries.	Asthma, bradycardia.

Drug	Dose	Side effects	C/I and notes
METRONIDAZOLE Bactericidal.	***Anaerobic infections, abdominal sepsis, C. difficile, Giardia, amoebiasis:*** 400 mg PO TDS or 500 mg IV TDS.	N,V,D, liver toxicity, headache, neuropathy. Raised INR on Warfarin.	Avoid alcohol, lithium and phenytoin toxicity, porphyria.
MIDAZOLAM Benzodiazepine.	***Sedation, epilepsy, palliative care, agitation*:** 1–7.5 mg slow IV over 2–5 min (can also be given buccally, PR or intranasally).	Respiratory depression (consider Flumazenil), amnesia, confusion.	
MORPHINE Opiate.	***Analgesia, sedation, dyspnoea, palliation and pulmonary oedema*:** 5–10 mg slow IV over 2–5 min.	Respiratory depression, seizures, nausea, vomiting, itch, miosis and constipation.	Usually combined with an antiemetic.
NALOXONE (NARCAN) Opiate antagonist.	***Opiate overdose*:** 0.4–2.0 mg IV/IM. Long-acting opiate. Infusion of 10 mg in 500 ml Dextrose over 2–4 h. Higher doses may be needed. ***Opiate reversal in palliative care*:** smaller doses of 20 mcg repeated as needed.	Tachycardia, opiate withdrawal syndrome. Use cardiac telemetry for repeated doses.	IV half-life may be shorter than opiate ingested. Consider infusion. Always consider a test dose in any suspected opiate toxicity.
OCTREOTIDE	***Upper GI variceal bleed*:** 50 mcg bolus with 25–50 mcg/h IV infusion for 3–5 days. ***Carcinoid***: 100–200 mcg TDS.	Hyperglycaemia, abdominal cramps.	Can be used in those with IHD.
OMEPRAZOLE Proton pump inhibitor.	**Upper GI bleed/PUD**: 8 mg/h IV for 72 h. Otherwise 40–80 mg IV bolus. Oral: 10–40 mg OD.	N,V, headache.	Phenytoin toxicity.
PABRINEX Thiamine, riboflavin, pyridoxine, ascorbic acid and nicotinamide.	***Prevention of Wernicke-Korsakoff syndrome:*** give as IV infusion over 30 min or given IM. Prescribe as 1 pair once daily for at least 3–5 days. ***Treatment of WKS:*** of 2 pairs 2–3 times daily for at least 3–5 days	Be prepared for managing anaphylaxis.	

Drug	Dose	Side effects	C/I and notes
PARACETAMOL	***Simple analgesic for mild to moderate pain***: 500–1000 mg 6–8 hourly.	Liver/renal failure with overdose.	
PHENYTOIN High pH so do not give as IM and any IV extravasation will cause tissue damage. The half-life of phenytoin is variable but long enough for most patients to be given a once daily dose.	***Anticonvulsant:*** *loading dose:* 15–20 mg/kg (70 kg = 1400 mg) given over 60 min *with cardiac monitoring* in 50–100 ml NS with infusion pump/ syringe pump into large vein. **Do not exceed** 50 mg/min infusion rate. May cause cardiovascular collapse. *Maintenance dose:* 5 mg/kg daily which works out at approximately **150–200 mg BD.** Dilute with NS (not dextrose).	Low BP, arrhythmias and CNS depression if given quickly. Hypersensitivity, heart. Adjust dose on levels 6 h post dose.	Zero order kinetics so escalating toxicity with small dose increases. These should not exceed 50 mg if daily dose is greater than 300 mg. New steady state may take 5–7 days after dose adjustment.
PREDNISOLONE Steroid.	***COPD/asthma/severe ulcerative colitis***: start 40 mg for 7 days. ***PMR***: 15 mg OD. ***GCA***: 1 mg/kg acutely gradually reduce.	Hypertension, weight gain, delirium, osteoporosis, etc.	GCA get temporal artery biopsy within 7 days of treatment. Prolonged courses consider bone protection.
PRALIDOXIME Reactivates acetylcholinesterase.	***Organophosphate, sarin poisoning***: 1–2 g (30 mg/ kg) IV as 30 min infusion, then 10 mg/h whilst symptomatic. No IV access: 600 mg IM × 3 doses over 30 min.	HTN, tachycardia, diplopia, laryngospasm, headache, N&V.	
PROCAINAMIDE Pharmacological cardioversion.	***Acute AF/atrial flutter/AF and WPW***: 1 g (20–50 mg/ kg) in 250 ml of 5% dextrose over 1 h. Monitor HR, BP and QT. Can cause bradycardia and TdP.	Causes long QT.	Long QT. Can worsen myasthenia gravis.
PROTAMINE Can partially reverse effect of LMWH.	1 mg for every 100 U of anti-factor Xa activity in past 8 h or 1 mg of Enoxaparin or 100 U of UFH in last 4 h.		

Drug	Dose	Side effects	C/I and notes
PROTHROMBIN COMPLEX CONCENTRATES (Octaplex/Beriplex) Replace vitamin K-derived factors.	***Warfarin reversal:*** see local protocols. Used for any bleeding related to Warfarin therapy.		Usually combined with 5 mg IV vitamin K.
QUININE DIHYDRO-CHLORIDE **CAUTION:** Quinine must never be given by rapid IV injection, as lethal hypotension may result.	***Uncomplicated falciparum malaria:*** 600 mg TDS PO for 7 days. ***Complicated falciparum malaria:*** *loading infusion* 20 mg/kg IV (60 kg = 1.2 g) over 4 h (max 1.4 g). *Maintenance* (8 h post loading): IV/PO 10 mg/kg (60 kg = 600 mg) infusion over 4 h TDS. Dilute to 500 ml with NS or glucose 5% and give by controlled IV infusion. If IV not possible then consider IM to the anterior thigh.	Hypoglycaemia, arrhythmias, cinchonism with reversible hearing loss, N,V,D, hypoglycaemia, and visual disturbances.	Send blood films. Take advice from infectious diseases team. Needs ITU management if complicated. Avoid delays. Treat if suspicious.
RAMIPRIL ACEi.	***HTN, CCF:*** start at 1.25–2.5 mg up to 10 mg per day.	As for Enalapril.	As for Enalapril.
RANITIDINE Histamine 2 receptor blocker.	***Peptic ulcer disease, anaphylaxis:*** 50 mg IV TDS or 150 mg BD PO.	N,V,D,R, confusion, hepatitis.	Acute porphyria.
RETEPLASE Activates tissue plasminogen STEMI and PE.	Reconstitute two 10 U vials with sterile water (10 ml per vial) to 1 U/ml. ***STEMI/PE:*** 2 × IV boluses of 10 U. 1st 10 U bolus given over 2 min; 2nd 10 U bolus 30 min later over 2 min. NS flush before and after each bolus. ***PE:*** unlicensed use.	Anaphylaxis, bleeding, haemorrhagic stroke.	
RIBAVIRIN Broad spectrum antiviral.	***Viral haemorrhagic diseases, e.g. Lassa, Hanta, Rift valley:*** 2 g IV infusion and then 1 g QDS, then 500 mg TDS for 6 days. Use after specialist advice.	Significantly reduces mortality in patients with haemorrhagic fever.	Avoid in pregnancy as teratogenic.

Drug	Dose	Side effects	C/I and notes
RIFAMPICIN Broad spectrum antibiotic.	***Augment other antibiotic courses, endocarditis, CAP***: 300–600 mg BD PO/IV.	Red urine.	
RIVAROXABAN Direct Factor Xa inhibitor.	***VTE prophylaxis:*** 10 mg tablets. ***Non-valvular AF:*** 20 mg OD tablets.	Active bleeding, falls. Assess bleeding risk.	
SALBUTAMOL β-2 adrenergic agonist.	***Asthma, COPD, high K***: *nebuliser:* 2.5–5.0 mg QDS or more frequent PRN. Air-driven in COPD or with O_2 in asthmatics. *Inhaler:* 100–200 mcg inhaled QDS or PRN. *Powdered inhaler:* 200–400 mcg inhaled QDS or PRN.	Tachycardia, hypokalaemia, tremor, headache, anxiety.	
SIMVASTATIN HMG CoA reductase inhibitor.	***IHD, stroke disease, hyperlipidaemia***: 10–80 mg ON. Watch LFTs.	Myalgia, myositis, pancreatitis. Myopathy with macrolides or amiodarone.	Liver disease, hyperkalaemia.
SODIUM NITROPRUSSIDE Nitric oxide donor. Overuse can lead to cyanide toxicity.	***Severe HTN, severe CCF***: 0.5 mcg/kg/min, increasing as needed in steps of 0.2 mcg/kg/min to max 8 mcg/kg/min (max 4 mcg/kg/min if used for >24 h). Protect infusion from the light.	Aortic stenosis, HCM, CKD, AKI.	To avoid marked hypotension start at low dose and slowly titrate up.
SOTALOL β-blocker with antiarrhythmic properties. Watch for long QT.	***Fast AF, SVT and monomorphic VT:*** 75 mg IV over 5 h BD. Reduce in renal failure. ***Oral dose***: 40–160 mg BD 24 h.	Fatigue, dizziness, low HR, low BP, polymorphic VT.	Asthma, AV block, bradycardia, long QTc, renal failure. Specialist use.
SPIRONOLACTONE	***CCF:*** 25–50 mg OD. ***Ascites:*** 100–400 mg OD.	Hyperkalaemia, gynaecomastia, N, V, R.	Avoid drugs/ infusions that cause hyperkalaemia.
STREPTOKINASE Activates human plasminogen. Do not use in stroke.	***STEMI, PE and other thrombotic disorders:*** 1.5 MU in 100 ml of 5% dextrose or NS over 60 min IV.	Hypotension, bleeding, haemorrhagic stroke.	Active bleeding, trauma, malignancy. Mild hypotension may need IV fluids.

Drug	Dose	Side effects	C/I and notes
TAMSULOSIN Alpha blocker.	***Poor stream and medical expulsive therapy for stones:*** 0.4 mg (400 mcg) OD.	Hypotension, dizziness, malaise, diarrhoea.	
TAZOCIN Piperacillin (antibiotic) + Tazobactam (inhibits β-lactamases).	***Pseudomonas and neutropenic sepsis:*** PIPERACILLIN 2–4 g + TAZOBACTAM 250–500 mg QDS. Prescribe as: TAZOCIN 2.25–4.5 mg TDS/QDS.	N, V, D, R. As for benzylpenicillin.	As for benzylpenicillin. Reduce dose/ frequency in renal failure.
TENECTEPLASE Assess bleeding risk.	***ACS: STEMI*** (body weight: dose): *<60 kg* 30 mg *60–70 kg* 35 mg *70–80 kg* 40 mg *80–90 kg* 45 mg *>90 kg* 50 mg (give IV bolus dose over 10 sec)	Anaphylaxis, bleeding, haemorrhagic stroke.	Active bleeding, trauma, malignancy. See usual thrombolysis C/I in *Section 11.2* (STEMI).
TEICOPLANIN Bactericidal, glycopeptide antibiotic similar to Vancomycin but longer duration of action.	**C. difficile *infection*:** 200 mg twice daily for 10 days PO. ***MRSA infections, severe burns or endocarditis:*** *weight <70 kg*: 400 mg IV BD for 3 doses then OD; *>70 kg*: 600 mg IV BD for 3 doses then OD.	Nephrotoxic and ototoxic. Plasma – Teicoplanin concentration is not measured routinely.	Avoid other nephrotoxic or ototoxic drugs. Monitor hearing and renal function.
TEMAZEPAM Benzodiazepine.	***Sedation, insomnia*:** 10–20 mg ON.	Drowsiness, respiratory depression.	Use with care in elderly and liver/ renal failure.
TERBUTALINE β2-adrenergic receptor agonist.	***Asthma, COPD*:** *nebuliser:* 5–10 mg air-driven in COPD or with oxygen.	Tremor, tachycardia.	
TERLIPRESSIN Vasopressin analogue.	***Suspected GI variceal bleed:*** 2 mg IV bolus, then 1–2 mg 4–6 hourly for 48 h until bleeding improves.	Cramps, N, V, uterine/bowel contraction, low Na.	Only agent shown to reduce variceal bleed mortality. Avoid if IHD/MI and use Octreotide.
TETRACYCLINE Antimicrobial affects protein synthesis. Doxycycline preferred.	***Acne, tropical infections:*** 500 mg 8–12 hourly PO. Avoid taking with milk or antacids.	N, V, D, headache, oesophagitis.	Avoid pregnancy and age <12, stains teeth, acute porphyria.

Drug	Dose	Side effects	C/I and notes
THIAMINE Vitamin B1.	***Starvation, hyperemesis, alcoholism, Beriberi***: 100–300 mg/day PO in divided doses. IV dose 100 mg/day.	Give Thiamine before giving PO/IV dextrose, glucose.	
TINZAPARIN Low molecular weight heparin activates anti-thrombin III. Often used in pregnancy.	***VTE prophylaxis:*** 3500 U SC 2 h pre-op then OD. ***VTE prophylaxis (ortho):*** 50 U/kg pre-op then OD. ***PE/DVT***: 175 U/kg OD SC and is used in pregnancy with specialist advice.	Bleeding, low platelets (HITT), hyperkalaemia, and osteoporosis long term.	Bleeding, HITT.
TRAMADOL Central acting analgesic. Has mu-opioid agonist activity. Addiction possible if misused.	***Moderate to moderately severe pain***: 25–50 mg QDS. 50–100 mg QDS for moderate to severe pain relief. MAX DOSE 400 mg/day or 300 mg/day in elderly.	Respiratory depression, seizures, anxiety, confusion, incoordination. Only partially reversed with Naloxone.	Avoid if history of seizures. Reduce dosage with renal failure or cirrhosis.
TRANEXAMIC ACID Inhibits plasmin formation and clot lysis.	***Acute severe bleeds, trauma patients, hereditary angioedema, epistaxis***: 20 mg/kg 8–12 hourly PO – for 50 kg adult 1 g tds for 4 days (max daily dose 4 g). ***Traumatic haemorrhage***: 1 g IV over 10 min then infusion of 1 g over 8 h (CRASH-2 trial). ***Oral bleeding***: 1 g orally four times daily.	**CAUTION**: use for gross haematuria as can clot causing obstruction. Reduce dose in renal failure.	Prothrombosis, seizures.
TRIMETHOPRIM	***UTI:*** 200 mg BD PO for 3–7 days. Resistance increasing – consider Nitrofurantoin instead.	Increases INR in those on Warfarin.	Avoid in pregnancy. Caution with azathioprine, methotrexate, mercaptopurine.

Drug	Dose	Side effects	C/I and notes
(Sodium) VALPROATE **Indications:** status and epilepsy prevention, personality disorders.	***Anticonvulsant:*** loading dose 10 mg/kg IV over 3–5 min and then 800–2000 mg/day. ***Long term epilepsy:*** start Sodium valproate 400 mg BD PO and increase dose slowly up to 2 g per day in divided doses.	Ammonia encephalopathy, fluid retention, liver toxicity, N, V, R.	Caution in pregnancy. Therapeutic range 50–100 mcg/ml.
VANCOMYCIN Glycopeptide antibiotic.	**C. difficile *infection*:** 125 mg QDS PO (capsules or give IV form orally) for 10–14 days. ***Infections/MRSA:*** 1–1.5 g IV BD given over 100 min. Administered in a dilute solution slowly to avoid 'Red Man Syndrome'.	Stop if tinnitus develops (ototoxicity). Nephrotoxic. Caution with Gentamicin, Ciclosporin.	Check renal function and trough levels every 48 h. Pre-dose ('trough') concentration should be 10–15 mg/L (15–20 mg/L).
VERAPAMIL CCB. See *BNF* and check all other drugs. Narrow complex tachycardias only.	***SVT when adenosine unsafe***: 5–10 mg slow IV over 2–3 min. Do not combine with β-blockers. ***HTN:*** PO 80–160 mg TDS.	Heart block, bradycardia. *Chronic:* constipation, heart block, hypotension, ankle oedema.	Suspected VT, bradycardia, poor LV function, hypotension, AF or atrial flutter and WPW, acute porphyria.
VITAMIN K Reverse Warfarin or vitamin K-deficient coagulopathy.	***Warfarin reversal/ vitamin K deficiency***: 1–10 mg by slow IV injection over 5–10 min in 100 ml bag of 5% dextrose. Can also give 1–10 mg PO depending on urgency.	INR takes hours to normalise. Consider prothrombin concentrates if immediate effect needed.	

Inotropes/vasodilators

Widely used but efficacy questionable. Never give as IV bolus but as infusion. Work quickly within minutes and half life is very short. Should be given through a dedicated line with a syringe driver with rate carefully controlled. Titrate to effect. Useful to have intra-arterial monitoring of BP. Should be used only on a CCU/HDU or ITU setting.

These drugs do not appear to reduce mortality or improve outcome so use with caution.

ADRENALINE α and β agonist. Low dose mainly beta effects and high dose both. Inotrope and raises SVR.	***IV rate:*** 0.05–0.5 mcg/kg/min. Specialist ITU use only.	Tachycardia, arrhythmias, lactic acidosis.	IV dose should only be used *in extremis*.
DOBUTAMINE Adrenergic agonist augments CO. Used in cardiogenic shock. Predominantly inotropic rather than chronotropic.	***Cardiogenic shock***: 2–20 mcg/kg/min IV infusion. Adhere to local policy for dilution and administration.	Tachycardia, HTN, ectopics, phlebitis as low pH solution and so given through central line. HTN with β-blockers.	Reserved for a critical care/ ITU/CCU setting with continuous monitoring and observation.
DOPAMINE Adrenergic agonist vasodilates renal, mesenteric and coronaries. Medium dose inotropic. High dose raises SVR.	***Low dose in cardiogenic shock/renal failure:*** 2–3 mcg/kg/min IV. ***Inotropic:*** 3–5 mcg/kg/min. ***Inotrope + pressor:*** 5–20 mcg/kg/min. Adhere to local policy for dilution and administration.	N, V, tachycardia, HTN, peripheral vasoconstriction, myocardial ischaemia, arrhythmias.	Severe HTN.
ISOPRENALINE β-1 stimulation increases HR. β-2 stimulation causes peripheral vasodilation and bronchodilation.	***Circulatory compromise due to bradycardia, bradycardia-dependent arrhythmias:*** 0.5–10 mcg/min IV infusion titrated to response. *Severe bradycardia:* 1–4 mcg/min IV infusion. *Shock:* 0.5–10 mcg/min.	Arrhythmias, sweating, tremor, headache and flushing.	**CAUTION:** IHD, diabetes, HTN, hyperthyroidism.
NORADRENALINE Potent α1-agonist which increases SVR. Used in sepsis and low SVR states. Some inotropic effects.	***Used for SBP <70 mmHg with a low SVR state:*** 0.1–1.0 mcg/kg/min. Ensure adequately filled. Adhere to local policy for dilution and administration.	Angina, renal and mesenteric ischaemia. Improves renal and mesenteric flow.	Arrhythmias, ischaemia.
VASOPRESSIN Pure vasoconstrictor.	***Pressor agent used in cardiac arrest***: 40 Units IV. No difference in outcome to adrenaline in cardiac arrest. May be used as an alternative.		

Potentially fatal drug errors

- Excessive opiate dosing – unfamiliar or agents with similar names.
- Getting decimal place wrong, especially weight-adjusted dose, e.g. ×10 digoxin dose in infant.
- Giving drug of which there is a clear history of allergy.
- Giving IV potassium infusion too concentrated or too fast (max is 20 mmol/h).
- Setting pumps wrong, e.g. 100 ml/h rather than 10 ml/h.
- Not detecting hypoglycaemia.
- Giving allopurinol + azathioprine.
- Omitting insulin after failing to recognise diabetes.
- Prescribing methotrexate daily instead of weekly.
- Giving drugs by wrong route in ITU, e.g. intra-arterial or into CSF; always check where the line goes.
- Use of abbreviations (e.g. AZT has led to confusion between zidovudine and azathioprine).
- Not monitoring INR in those on Warfarin.

Steroids compared

Indications: asthma, COPD, cord compression, cerebral oedema, PMR, temporal arteritis, RA, SLE, ulcerative colitis, adrenal replacement.

Side effects: short-term: agitation, insomnia (avoid in evenings if non-urgent), agitation, psychosis, weight gain, hyperglycaemia, fluid retention, HTN, raised WCC, osteoporosis.

Type	Drug	Equivalent doses	Glucocorticoid potency	Mineralocorticoid potency
Short-acting	**Cortisol**	20 mg	1	2
$T_{1/2}$: 0.5 days	**Hydrocortisone**	25 mg	0.8	2
Intermediate-	**Prednisolone**	5 mg	4	1
acting $T_{1/2}$: 1 day	**Methylprednisolone**	4 mg	5	0
Long-acting $T_{1/2}$: 1.5–2 days	**Dexamethasone**	0.75 mg	25–50	0
Mineralocorticoids	**Aldosterone**	0.3 mg	0	300
	Fludrocortisone	2 mg	15	150

Anticoagulation

Warfarin: *Wisconsin Alumni research foundation* – coumarin.

Action: inhibits synthesis of K-dependent coagulation factors II, VII, IX, and X and natural anticoagulants protein C and protein S.

Multiple interactions: varying genetic metabolism, drugs, alcohol, and vitamin K intake affects efficacy.

Monitoring: requires frequent monitoring via INR. Takes at least 72 h to be therapeutic. Give LMWH or UFH cover until therapeutic range achieved. Target INR is 2.0–3.0 for almost all indications though mechanical heart valves can get 2.5–3.5. Bleeding is the most significant problem and significant bleeding is seen in 3–5% per annum. Risk increases markedly after INR of 3.0 and even more so after INR

>4.5. *Skin necrosis* is a rare but significant complication. Warfarin use is avoided in pregnancy especially in first trimester.

WARFARIN INTERACTION	DRUGS: monitor INR after any change in drugs
INCREASE INR, i.e. bleeding. Different mechanisms but all increase INR.	• Broad spectrum antibiotics kill vitamin K-forming bacteria leading to increased bleeding effect. • Others: fibrates, thyroxine, amiodarone, fluconazole, cephalosporins, cimetidine, ethanol, fluvastatin, HMG-CoA reductase inhibitors, lovastatin, isoniazid, macrolides (clarithromycin, erythromycin), metronidazole, quinolones (ciprofloxacin), tricyclic antidepressants.
DECREASE INR	• Barbiturates, carbamazepine, cholestyramine, cigarette smoking, St John's wort , vitamin K corticosteroids, oral contraceptives, phenytoin, primidone, rifampicin, broccoli and green vegetables.

Indications: DVT, PE, cerebral venous thrombosis, cardiac: AF, PAF, metal valves, LV thrombus, axillary vein thrombosis, antiphospholipid syndrome.

Warfarin contraindicated (relative and absolute): pregnancy, any bleeding, GI blood loss, haematuria, anaemia due to possible blood loss, haemorrhagic stroke, frequent falls, imminent need for surgery, safe compliance issues, excess alcohol intake or severe liver disease, high HAS-BLED score. The HAS-BLED score marks increased bleeding risk but also marks those at high risk of thrombosis and often this still exceeds bleeding risk. A difficult area – for specialist assessment.

Side-effects: bleeding anywhere – brain, gut, renal, spine, soft tissue. Bleed risk increases dramatically with INR >3.0. Risk highest in those new on warfarin in the first 3 months of treatment.

Starting warfarin safely: informed consent for patient and clearly document target range and duration. Explain drug/food interactions – need to check INR if new interacting drugs. Avoid the high dose 10 mg: 'start low, go slow' and try a starting dose of 3–6 mg and then after this 3 mg daily. Check INR day 2–3 and adjust warfarin and most will need 3–5 mg per day. Occasionally some need very high doses for same effect. High risk give LMWH (clexane 1.5 mg/kg/day) until therapeutic INR. Ensure follow-up with anticoagulation service.

For most people once the INR is stable, the rate of INR testing can be extended to every 2 weeks and then to every 4–6 weeks. Ensure there is definite follow-up through an anticoagulation clinic to manage the warfarin. Make sure all referrals to anticoagulation clinic have been done. Nowadays if there is a rush to anticoagulate non-rheumatic AF, consider Dabigatran or Rivaroxaban or Apixaban, which can be started immediately and are active within a few hours.

> Always ask your senior if unsure – what is target range and what is duration and make sure documented in notes and discharge/clinic letter.

Duration and INR: in most situations the INR target is 2.5 (target range 2.0–3.0) for treatment of DVT/PE, AF and valvular heart disease. In some situations higher ranges are more appropriate. INR for mechanical prosthetic valves is often 2.5–3.5 with target = 3.0, but dependent on the type of valve replacement used; take specialist advice. Duration of warfarin therapy for a provoked DVT or PE is 13 weeks. For unprovoked DVT or PE the duration again is 13 weeks, but this must be judged case by case – take senior advice. For AF, warfarin is continued indefinitely. **Also see atrial fibrillation** (*Section 11.10*) for CHA_2DS_2VaSc score and HAS-BLED score for AF stroke risk and bleeding risk.

Guidelines for bleeding on warfarin or high INR

Assessment	Action
No or minor bleeding and INR <4.5	Reduce warfarin dose and repeat INR after 1–2 days.
No or minor bleeding and INR 4.5–10.0	Omit warfarin. IV vitamin K at a dose of 0.5 mg sufficient to return the INR to therapeutic range. In those with metal valves may simply omit dose and recheck and avoid vitamin K to avoid overcorrection.
No or minor bleeding and INR >10.0	Omit warfarin and give 2–2.5 mg vitamin K PO or IV to return INR to safe level. In those with metal valves may simply omit dose and recheck and avoid vitamin K to avoid overcorrection. If overcorrection (INR <2) then cover with LMWH.
Life-threatening bleed on warfarin and INR >1.5	Send urgent clotting screen (APTT/PT/INR/fibrinogen). Stop warfarin and give vitamin K 5 mg by slow IV injection over 5 min in 100 ml bag of 5% dextrose (stocked in resuscitation trolley). Try to achieve haemostasis by physical means. PCC (Beriplex or Octaplex) rarely indicated if the INR is less than 2. If bleeding is life-threatening and INR >1.8 then discuss with haematology as may need PCC and 5 mg IV vitamin K. Recombinant factor VIIa is not recommended for emergency anticoagulation reversal. FFP produces suboptimal anticoagulation reversal and should only be used if PCC is not available.

Heparin: low molecular weight

LMWH is administered subcutaneously with near-complete absorption. Monitoring is unnecessary in the vast majority. Where efficacy or safety questioned then measure anti-Xa.

Uses: VTE prevention and treatment, ACS (LMWH in those with a malignancy has been shown to be more effective in preventing VTE recurrence than warfarin, with no increase in bleeding), pregnancy. HIT is significantly less likely with LMWH than UFH. Osteoporosis less with LMWH.

Reversal: Protamine can partly reverse LMWH, e.g. Protamine 1 mg per 1 mg Enoxaparin in previous 8 h; Protamine 1 mg per 100 units Dalteparin in previous 8 h, Protamine 1 mg per 100 units Tinzaparin in previous 8 h.

Heparin: unfractionated heparin

IV heparin is difficult to manage and needs very close monitoring and supervision. It should only be used where this can be carried out diligently without fail and where staff can adjust rates, e.g. CCU or HDU/ITU.

Action: potentiates AT3. Use where immediate anticoagulation needed that can be quickly stopped. Time consuming, labour intensive and fluctuations outside therapeutic range in effect common. Prior to treatment check FBC (platelets), clotting screen and renal function.

Dose: VTE prophylaxis: 5000 U SC BD. Higher doses need monitoring of APTT. Anticoagulation: loading dose 5000 U IV bolus (see below). Check APTT 6–8 h after starting infusion. Aim for therapeutic APTT range of 2.0–3.0. If treatment >5 days then check platelet count daily. Repeat APTT ratio every 6–8 h or after each change in rate, unless APTT ratio is >5.0 when measurement should be made more frequently (1 h after restart).

Side-effects: bleeding, HIT (low platelets – monitor), high K with Protamine. Can be used in pregnancy.

C/I: any raised bleeding risk. Reversal, e.g. Protamine 1 mg per 100 units heparin given in previous 2–3 h.

Dose for 75 kg person (18 U/kg/h): heparin 40 000 units in 40 ml, infuse at 1.4 ml/h (1400 U/h).

APTT ratio	Infusion rate (1000 U/ml)
>5.0	Stop for 2 h; reduce by 0.5 ml/h (500 U) and recheck at 4 h
4.1–5.0	Stop for 1 h; reduce by 0.3 ml/h (300 U) and recheck at 4 h
3.6–4.0	Reduce by 0.2 ml/h (200 U)
3.1–3.5	Reduce by 0.1 ml/h (100 U)
2.0–3.0	NO CHANGE
1.5–1.9	Increase by 0.1 ml/h (100 U)
1.2–1.4	Increase by 0.2 ml/h (200 U)
<1.2	Give 2500 U IV bolus; increase by 0.4 ml/h (400 U)

Drug interactions

Drug A and Drug B	Effect
Allopurinol and Azathioprine	Allopurinol interferes with the metabolism of azathioprine, increasing levels of 6-mercaptopurine resulting in serious blood dyscrasias
Digoxin and Quinidine	Marked increase in plasma concentrations of digoxin
Sildenafil and Isosorbide mononitrate	Dramatic drops in BP and has been associated with some deaths
Potassium chloride and Spironolactone/Amiloride and ACEi	These drugs can in combination lead to severe hyperkalaemia
Theophylline and Ciprofloxacin	Theophylline toxicity
Warfarin and NSAID, Aspirin, Clopidogrel	Increased bleed risk despite no change in INR; expert assessment for combination therapy

Drug A and Drug B	Effect
PPI, e.g. Omeprazole and Clopidogrel	Decreased efficacy of Clopidogrel and the potential for worsened cardiovascular outcomes; consider H2 blocker instead of PPI
Amiodarone and Levofloxacin, Azithromycin, Clarithromycin, Erythromycin	Increased QTc and cause TdP
Carbamazepine or Digoxin AND Clarithromycin, Erythromycin	Increased carbamazepine or digoxin toxicity
Amiodarone and Simvastatin or Lovastatin	Increased statin side-effects, e.g. rhabdomyolysis and myopathy; try Fluvastatin, Rosuvastatin, or Pravastatin
Simvastatin and Amlodipine or Verapamil or Diltiazem (inhibit Simvastatin metabolism)	With these drugs the maximum dose of simvastatin is now 20 mg; higher doses are 'off-label'. Consider Pravastatin, Fluvastatin or Rosuvastatin or Atorvastatin.
IV Verapamil and IV Dantrolene	Potential risk of VF

Index